Contents

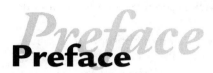

Preface

This book has its origin in a casual comment by Jane Romano, which bemoaned the lack of understanding of health professionals when it comes to educating their patients. The essential need for effectively teaching patients to understand, manage, and live well with their illness is an issue that Romano noted her colleagues struggling with, mostly due to a lack of training and resources. As the issue was further discussed, the conversation became directed toward how to encourage patients to take responsibility for promoting their own best health. Like ripples in water when a pebble is thrown, the discussion expanded toward what was needed to help health professionals gain comfort and skills to effectively establish a teaching relationship with their patients, their families, and communities. And so it came to pass that this book was conceived and born!

There is no getting around the fact that educating patients and families is a necessary aspect of the role of all healthcare providers. Recognizing that guiding patients and families through the complex maze of care and prevention of illness is not a solitary task, this book is intended to benefit a multidisciplinary team of providers. The concepts and theoretical frameworks discussed cross professional roles and are applicable in the many diverse settings where health promotion and prevention of illness are addressed. Many chapters include case studies that demonstrate both successful and unsuccessful applications of information. Both positive and negative cases are used because it is important to understand that not all teaching efforts are successful the first time around. We want not only to provide an analysis of what went wrong in unsuccessful efforts and how the situation could have been handled differently, but also to identify what went right and how those efforts can be preserved and repeated in the future.

Promoting healthy choices and lifestyles comes with many challenges. The individuals we are educating are all different in one way or another. They have varied personalities, levels of education, cultural backgrounds, and resources. The first section of this book describes basic concepts and theories which address these differences as well as provides a common foundation for the education of adults.

The planning, implementation, and evaluation of appropriate and effective learning opportunities require a great deal of time and energy on the part of the healthcare provider. The chapters in the second section of this book provide insights and examples to help you select the tools that will offer the best advantages to your instruction. The key is to capitalize on every interaction with patients, families, and colleagues to assess, deliver, and reinforce education. As you listen to your patients and involve them in determining what information they consider important to know, the information provided in this section will allow you to determine how best to meet the needs of your clients.

As we searched the general patient-teaching literature, we felt it would be helpful to have health professionals discuss of some of the most common disease processes, providing more specifics about illnesses that are of interest to them. The chapters in the third section directly address the unique needs of patients, families, and communities related to education and health promotion for a variety of specific conditions. In addition, health promotion and behavior changes in the community as well as in individuals are explored.

It was our goal to provide a resource of theories and concepts that comprise a foundation for effective education and health promotion, as well as a selection of tools, methodologies, and specific examples that would expand the repertoire and abilities of practicing clinicians responsible for the education of patients, families, and communities. We are honored to bring together clinically based experts from a diverse group of health professions to share their experiences and the evidence that supports their choices and implementation of education and health promotion in their respective fields. We hope that we have been successful and that you will find this to be an accessible, engaging, and useful resource for you and your colleagues in healthcare practice.

Jane Romano
Lynn Foord
Arlene Lowenstein

Acknowledgments

We would like to dedicate this book to our colleagues, both practicing professionals and students, whose boundless dedication to the care and education of our patients and clients inspires us every day.

We would like to acknowledge our contributors not only for their knowledge, expertise, and wisdom, but also for their responsiveness and commitment to this collection of their work. We would be remiss not to also acknowledge the assistance of our editors at Jones and Bartlett who guided and encouraged us in this work. Finally, we owe our gratitude to our families for their invaluable support and fortitude.

CONTRIBUTORS

Judith I. Balboni, RN, BSN
Clinical Educator
Patient and Family Education
Dana-Farber Cancer Institute
Boston, MA

Jo-Ann D. Barrett, RN, BSN, CDE
Diabetes Clinical Improvement and Education Program Manager
Partners HealthCare System, Inc.
Needham, MA

Terry Mahan Buttaro, MS, APRN, BC, FAANP
Assistant Professor of Nursing
School of Health Sciences
Simmons College
Boston, MA

Barbara B. Chase, MSN, APRN, BC, CDE
Adult Nurse Practitioner
Diabetes Management Program Coordinator
Chelsea HealthCare Center
Massachusetts General Hospital
Chelsea, MA

Patricia Christensen, PhD, RN
Distinguished Professor Emerita,
    University of South Carolina Upstate
Adjunct Faculty
Webster University
Greenville, SC

Carol S. Collard, PhD, LMSW
Assistant Professor
WellStar College of Health and Human Services
Kennesaw University
Kennesaw, GA

Susan DeCristofaro, MS, RN, OCN, CLMC
Director, Patient and Family Education
Dana-Farber Cancer Institute
Boston, MA

Anne Marie Dupre, MS, DPT, NCS
Clinical Assistant Professor
Academic Coordinator of Clinical Education
Department of Physical Therapy
University of Rhode Island
Kingston, RI

Flora Carter Flood, DNP, RNC, WHNP
Associate Professor
Oakwood University
Huntsville, AL

Mary E. Foley, MPH, RDH
Dean, Forsyth School of Dental Hygiene
Massachusetts College of Pharmacy and Health Sciences
Boston, MA

Lynn Foord, MEd, PhD, PT
Assistant Professor of Physical Therapy
Director of Online Teaching and Learning
School of Health Sciences
Simmons College
Boston, MA

Kirsten Fowler, MS, CCLS
Child Life Specialist, Surgical Programs
Children's Hospital Boston
Boston, MA

Suzanne Graca, MS, CCLS
Acting Director, Child Life Services
Children's Hospital Boston
Boston, MA

James S. Huddleston, MS, PT
Staff Physical Therapist
Benson-Henry Institute for Mind Body Medicine
Massachusetts General Hospital
Chestnut Hill, MA

Katherine Hurxthal, MPH, APRN, CDE
Nurse Practitioner
Massachusetts General Hospital Diabetes Center
Boston, MA

Karen Janowski, MSEd, OTL
Assistive and Educational Technology Consultant
EdTech Solutions, LLC
Reading, MA

Florence Keane, MBA, DNSc, ARNP
Clinical Assistant Professor of Nursing
Florida International University
Miami, FL

Pamela Kelly, RNC, PNP
Pediatric Nurse Practitioner, Ambulatory Medicine
Children's Hospital Boston
Boston, MA

Gerald P. Koocher, PhD
Professor and Dean
School of Health Sciences
Simmons College
Lecturer on Psychology
Harvard Medical School
Boston, MA

Arlene J. Lowenstein, PhD, RN
Professor and Director, Health Professions Education Doctoral Program
School of Health Sciences
Simmons College
Boston, MA

Nancy Lowenstein, MS, OTR/L, BCPR
Clinical Associate Professor
Boston University
Sargent College of Health and Rehabilitation Sciences
Boston, MA

Mary C. McLellen, BSN, RN, CMT, CPN
Clinical Educator, Inpatient Cardiovascular Programs
Children's Hospital Boston
Boston, MA

Jean Oulund Peteet, PhD, MPH, PT
Clinical Assistant Professor
Boston University
Sargent College of Health and Rehabilitation Sciences
Boston, MA

Shelly Pignataro, RN
Education Coordinator, Surgical Programs
Children's Hospital Boston
Boston, MA

Vivienne B. Piroli, MLS, ALM, HDipEd
Librarian, School of Health Sciences
Simmons College
Boston, MA

Taryn J. Pittman, MSN, RN-BC
Patient Education Specialist
Blum Patient and Family Learning Center
Massachusetts General Hospital
Boston, MA

Madalaine K. Pugliese, MS, MSEd, EdS
Graduate Program Director, Assistive Technology
Simmons College
Boston, MA

Aditi Puri, MS, RDH
Assistant Professor
Massachusetts College of Pharmacy and Health Sciences
PhD Candidate
Simmons College
Boston, MA

John A. Reeder, PhD
Assistant Professor
Department of Psychology
Simmons College
Boston, MA

Jane C. Romano, MS, RN, CAGS (Certificate of Advanced Graduate Study in Health Profession Education)
Education Specialist
Project Manager, Division of Critical Care Medicine
Children's Hospital Boston
Boston, MA

Addie Rosenstock, MS, CCLS
Child Life Specialist, Outpatient Services
Children's Hospital Boston
Boston, MA

Clare E. Safran-Norton, PhD, PT, OCS
Assistant Professor
School of Health Sciences
Simmons College
Boston, MA

Susan C. Scrimshaw, PhD
Interim President, The Sage Colleges
Albany, New York
Past President, Simmons College
Boston, MA

Julie Shurtleff, RN, CPNP
Pediatric Nurse Practitioner, Inpatient Medicine
Children's Hospital Boston
Boston, MA

Susan J. Sommer, MSN, RNG, WHCNP
Nurse Practitioner, Adolescent Medicine
Community Asthma Initiative
Children's Hospital Boston
Boston, MA

Richard L. Sowell, PhD, RN, FAAN
Dean
WellStar College of Health and Human Services
Kennesaw State University
Kennesaw, GA

Danielle Steward-Gelinas, PT, DPT, CAGS
Visiting Nurse Association of Southwestern Connecticut (VNASC)
Waterford, CT
Adjunct Faculty, Physical Therapy
Simmons College
Boston, MA

Debra Wein, MS, RD, LDN
President and Co-founder
Sensible Nutrition, Inc.
Hingham, MA

Martha Young, MS, CCLS
Patient and Family Education Specialist
Jimmy Fund Clinic
Dana-Farber Cancer Institute
Boston, MA

Kathy Zaiken, PharmD
Assistant Professor of Pharmacy Practice
Massachusetts College of Pharmacy and Health Sciences
Boston, MA

Caroline S. Zeind, PharmD, RPh
Chair and Professor, Department of Pharmacy Practice
Massachusetts College of Pharmacy and Health Sciences
Boston, MA

Section *I*

Education Concepts and Foundations

Teaching is both an art and a science. To some it comes naturally, but all who endeavor to be effective teachers need to work at it. We need to understand good teaching, practice it, analyze what we do, and continuously strive to improve our knowledge and skills.

At the foundation of both the art and the science of teaching are core concepts and theories. Knowing theories will not necessarily make anyone a good teacher, but understanding key concepts can help in planning instruction, analyzing what went well and why, and determining what will improve the quality and efficacy of the instruction.

This first section begins with a look at how to get started in teaching by considering theories of adult learning and applying them as we seek ways to promote the qualities of adult learning in all of our patients and clients. Providing education about health issues and health promotion requires recognition of other factors that affect learning, such as stress, illness, and poverty. With this foundation in theories and concepts and an awareness of the influence of these other factors, we can begin to look at the challenges of promoting health literacy and consider how we might use current technologies to address more effectively the health literacy of our patients, their families, and our communities. This section concludes with a look at behavior change—the ultimate goal of health education and health promotion.

Chapter 1

Getting Started

Jane C. Romano

> *People will forget what you said.*
> *People will forget what you did.*
> *But people will never forget how you made them feel.*
> —*Maya Angelou*

INTRODUCTION

A significant aspect of the role of healthcare providers is the education of others. The Federation of State Boards of Physical Therapist Standards of Competence (2000) states this: "The physical therapist educates patient/clients, family, and caregivers, using relevant and effective teaching methods to assure optimal patient outcomes." The American Medical Association's Declaration of Professional Responsibility: Medicine's Social Contract with Humanity (2001) states that physicians commit to "teach and mentor those who follow us for they are the future of our caring profession." *The American Nurses Association Scope & Standards of Practice* (2004): Standard 5B is Health Teaching and Health Promotion. Education is identified as a specific expectation of each of these healthcare provider's role, yet how many have received formal training on how to educate? It is safe to say not many. This issue is one healthcare professions have apparently struggled with for years. In a review of the literature on patient education in 1981, Cohen discusses three principal barriers to patient education, the first being the fact that nurses and other medical personnel are traditionally ill-prepared to teach. As a result of this ongoing problem, the potential for less than ideal outcomes inadvertently exists, and the solutions are not simple. Issues such as the ever-increasing complexity of patients, as well as shortages of both healthcare providers and faculty to teach, are only a few examples of the influences that challenge these professions today.

Thus, are we teachers or are we healthcare providers? Can you be a healthcare provider without being a teacher? We suggest that the answer to the latter question is no. In order to be effective in your role of healthcare providers, you must teach others, including patients, families, colleagues, and students. Jackson and Mannix (2001) examined the influence that the nursing staff had on undergraduate nursing students during their clinical rotation. The study found that nurses were able to empower students by guiding them through patient care. The researchers state that students modeled the behaviors and demeanor of the nurses they encounter in clinical areas. Our ability to influence behaviors and outcomes of those we encounter throughout out practice can be extremely powerful and rewarding provided that we recognize and respect that possibility.

In a perfect world, all programs of healthcare professions would incorporate the fundamentals of what, why, where, when, and how people of all ages learn. Also, healthcare providers would have all of the necessary time and resources that they need to meet the learning needs of their patients and families. Because we recognize that we do not practice in a perfect world, this book is an effort to support these ideals in today's complex, fast-paced world. Throughout the chapters, some basic theories, concepts, and considerations regarding the fundamentals of learning are discussed in an effort to provide a resource to all healthcare providers when educating others. Also, some strategies for planning and implementing patient education in a less than perfect learning environment are explored.

UTILIZING THEORY

Why is theory important when considering patient education? With the current emphasis on evidence-based practice in health care, theory is a logical place to begin. In 2005, the National Institutes of Health (NIH) and the National Cancer Institute published a second edition of an excellent reference titled "Theory at a Glance." This document states that a theory is a "systematic way of understanding events or situations" and "needs to be applicable to a broad variety of situations." It compares theories to empty coffee cups that provide structure and become more useful when filled. The authors also believe that the process of determining which theory or theories are most appropriate to the situation at hand begins with assessment of the situation. The NIH report focuses on health behavior and health promotion theoretical frameworks, which are based on various other disciplines such as psychology, sociology, anthropology, consumer behaviors, and marketing (NIH, 2005).

One of the earliest and most recognized health behavior theories, the Health Belief Model, is discussed by the NIH. Developed in 1950, this theory was used to examine why people were not taking advantage of public health services that were being offered free and in their very own neighborhoods (NIH, 2005). The Health Belief Model is an individual level theory that focuses on the individual's perceptions of the threat the health problem poses. This theory has been expanded on throughout the years and concludes that there are five main constructs that influence people's decisions related to health behaviors. It is believed that people are ready to act if they

- Believe the condition has serious consequences (*perceived severity*)
- Believe taking action will reduce their susceptibility to the condition or its severity (*perceived benefits*)
- Believe costs of taking action are outweighed by the benefits (*perceived barriers*)
- Are exposed to factors that prompt action (e.g., a television ad or a reminder from one's physician to get a mammogram) (*cue to action*)
- Are confident in their ability to successfully perform the action (*self-efficacy*)

Source: NIH (2005)

Thus, what does it take to get an individual to the point of believing they are at risk and need to act in order to bring about a positive outcome? Is this where education fits into the plan? How do you educate someone who does not believe that he or she needs to be educated? This model does provide you with a starting point for what education needs to be planned and delivered. Using this theory will guide your assessment in order to determine where to begin.

Other theories discussed in the NIH report lacked a clear explanation of where education fits into the utilization of these health behavior models. Let us consider a discussion that focuses on Explanatory Theory and Change Theory and their role in planning and implementing activities that support health promotion and behaviors. Explanatory Theory looks at why a problem exists and what can be changed. Change Theory assists with determining the necessary interventions to bring about change. The report points out that no one theory should dominate health promotion and behaviors because every situation is different. **Figure 1-1** is used by the NIH to illustrate how these two theories would be used to plan and evaluate programs. Where does education fit into the scheme of the model? Also, can this model apply to an individual who is being discharged from the hospital or being treated in an outpatient setting, and how does education and learning theory fit in the process?

Wingard (2005) described the ultimate goal of patient education as achieving changes in behavior by providing patients with the knowledge that they need in order to make decisions about their care that will improve their personal outcome. Using this description as a foundation and incorporating the NIH model, consider the case of a 65-year-old man who presents with shortness of breath that has become progressively more problematic to his activities of daily living.

Larry is a former smoker who quit 20 years ago after undergoing an angioplasty. He also spent 21 years in the Coast Guard, several of which were on a ship where he would be housed for sometimes months at a time. It is presumed that Larry was likely repeatedly exposed to asbestos during this time. Based on pulmonary function tests, his past history of smoking, possible exposure to asbestos and his symptoms, Larry was diagnosed with emphysema. With the problem and why the problem exists identified, it is now necessary to assess

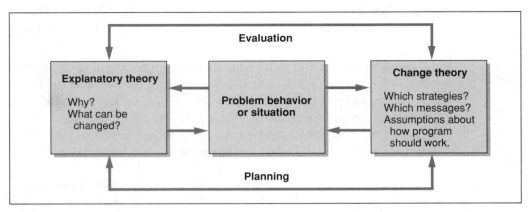

Figure 1-1 Using Explanatory Theory and Change Theory to plan and evaluate programs.

what can be changed. Because Larry has already stopped smoking and is retired, two of the problem behaviors have already been changed. It is determined that Larry is a carpenter and retired locksmith who enjoys spending time in his shop working on various projects, including woodworking. He lives with his wife of 45 years in a single home and has five grown children. His home is approximately 100 years old, has only one bathroom on the second floor, and requires climbing several steps or an uphill driveway to enter. He works part-time as a locksmith, requiring him to carry a heavy box of tools and equipment that he needs onsite. Larry is prescribed metered dose inhalers, nebulizer treatments, and physical therapy to manage his current symptoms.

Your assessment thus far has identified many challenges that Larry and his family will likely face. Using the NIH model, what can be changed? What are the strategies you would use to facilitate this change, and what is the message you wish to convey? Finally, what are your assumptions about how these changes will impact Larry's management of his problematic situation? Based on Wingard's (2005) description, patient education would fit into the category of strategies that you would use in order to bring about a change in behaviors, with the goal being for the patient to be able to manage his symptoms and continue his usual activities. Incorporating patient education into this model requires you to consider the following: What teaching would Larry and his family need to adapt to these changes? What would be the best method of providing the necessary teaching so that the information you provide will be of value to this patient? Who should receive the teaching along with Larry? What is the assumption about how effective the teaching will be and the ultimate outcome is for this individual? Going back to the analogy of theories as a coffee cup providing the structure that becomes more useful when filled, adding educational theories and concepts to the NIH model makes for a much richer brew.

Thus far, we have discussed how theory can be used to determine *why* and *when* patients learn. Let us now consider the critical aspect of *how* patients learn. It is this aspect of improving outcomes and behavior that seems to be focused on the least in the literature related to patient education. We have already discussed how much of health behavior and health promotion theoretical frameworks are based on concepts from areas such as psychology, sociology, anthropology, consumer behaviors, and marketing (NIH, 2005). Examples of the application of these frameworks are easy to find in the literature. Discussions using Maslow's hierarchy of needs (Benson & Dundis, 2003), Schutz's "well-informed" citizen (Henderson, 2006), cognitive aging theory (Knox, 2003), health promotion theory (Davis, 2006), and social cognitive theory (Billek-Sawhney & Reicherter, 2004) are just a few examples of the multiple hits one would get when searching for information on patient education. Absent are the long-standing educational theories that focus on *how* people learn. This is the missing link that is necessary to strengthen patient outcomes and promote health.

In order to discuss assessing the learning needs and abilities of individuals effectively, it makes sense to start with the aspects of growth and development. When planning and implementing learning opportunities for children, it is important to consider the work of the likes of Freud, Erikson, Piaget, Kohlberg, Skinner, and Bandura. These theorists are responsible for laying the foundation for addressing the personal, cognitive, moral, and social development of children. Teaching this patient population requires an understanding of the developmental abilities of the child and to recognize that there is no cookie-cutter method of determining those abilities. It is essential that the assessment of the learner be based on the foundations of growth and development and adapted to address each situation and individual. An important component of this assessment includes input from the family regarding how the child expresses pain and fear, along with how he or she is typically comforted during these times.

The same need for individualization holds true when planning and implementing learning opportunities for adults. In 1970, Malcolm Knowles was the first to theorize about how adults learn (Russell, 2006). The Adult Learning Theory is discussed in more depth in the next chapter. Two other learning theories that are relevant to consider for successful patient education are William Perry's Scheme of Intellectual Development and Benjamin Bloom's Taxonomy of Learning.

Let us first examine Perry's scheme. In his article, "A Nudge Is Best," Robert Kloss (1994) examines how Perry's scheme applies to student's learning as they advance through a series of phases of development: dualism, multiplicity, relativism, and commitment to relativism. Perry believes that students move through these phases as they gain knowledge and a greater understanding of how to use this knowledge. This scheme can also apply to how patients learn. In dualism, Perry describes students as viewing knowledge as truth and believes that teachers have all the answers (Kloss, 1994). This search for truth and answers and this unquestioned belief of an authority figure parallel the relationship a patient often has with healthcare providers. It is important to consider this possible unconditional phase of learning, especially when taking into account generational and cultural influences. The second phase of Perry's scheme is multiplicity where students begin to question their faith in authorities and realize that knowledge is simply a matter of opinion (Kloss, 1994). What is important to consider in this phase of development when examining the parallels is that transitioning into this phase possibly indicates the patient's increasing ability to become an active participant in their care and may be ready to learn how to do so. It is essential to provide information and support and partner with patients as they move into and through this phase of development. Entering the third phase of relativism, students learn to weigh the evidence and figure out what works and does not. Patients in this phase begin to integrate what they are learning from the healthcare providers with what they know about their resources, support systems, and abilities and can begin to contribute to their plan of care. The fourth and final phase of Perry's Phases of Development requires the student to make choices and commitments and to develop a personal world view with the knowledge they have gained (Kloss, 1994). Patients in this phase make a commitment to relativism and become empowered to improving their health outcomes.

When considering the parallels and possible application of Perry's scheme to the education of patients, it is essential to recall the title of Robert Kloss's (1994) article: "A Nudge Is Best." It is important to recognize the significant influence that stress and illness often have on a person's ability to learn and to be supportive during periods of regression or frustration patients may experience. Because of shorter stays and fewer resources, this aspect of "nudging" the patient through the phases of learning can be challenging to some healthcare providers such as those who deliver care in inpatient settings. Ongoing collaboration, communication, and education in both the inpatient and outpatient arenas are critical in today's world to "nudge" or guide patients and families throughout their learning and adapting to managing their health in order improve outcomes.

Another important learning theory is Bloom's taxonomy, which was developed in the 1940s and also focuses on the development of educational objectives and how students learn (Forsyth, 2004). Like Perry's theory, Bloom's approach to learning has many parallels to what influences the education of patients and families. Bloom's theory describes three domains of learning: affective (attitude), which involves growth in feelings and emotions, psychomotor (skills), which includes manual or physical abilities, and cognitive (knowledge), which encompasses mental skills (Clark, 2001). The application of Bloom's taxonomy in education tends to focus predominantly on the cognitive domain in which there is hierarchical learning through six levels (**Table 1-1**). Students progress through the various levels as they become more confident and informed learners.

Table 1-1 Bloom's Taxonomy of the Cognitive Domain

Level	Definition
Knowledge	Remembering information
Comprehension	Understanding information
Application	Using information in concrete situations
Analysis	Breaking down information into component parts
Synthesis	Using information and skills to produce new or original works
Evaluation	Judging value of information based on evidence and personal opinion

Source: Castle (2003).

Consider how this progression might apply to patients and families as they become more confident and informed regarding their health and well-being (**Table 1-2**). Knowledge is gained and accepted as important to the learner and ultimately leads to better outcomes.

Thus far, we have considered only the cognitive domain of Bloom's theory. The majority of literature related to this taxonomy focuses on this domain and its application in educational settings. The affective and psychomotor domains, however, are equally important to include when planning and implementing patient education. **Table 1-3** describes the five categories of affective learning domains as well as the seven categories of psychomotor learning domains.

Table 1-2 The Application of Bloom's Cognitive Domain to Patient Learning

Level	Definition
Knowledge	The patient is able to remember information.
Comprehension	The patient is able to demonstrate that he or she understands this and other information.
Application	The patient is able to use this information in a practical way.
Analysis	The patient gains an understanding of why this information is important to his or her well-being.
Synthesis	The patient is able to use this information to make positive changes in lifestyle in order to achieve and maintain his or her well-being.
Evaluation	The patient is able to make healthy choices based on this information and what he or she has learned.

Source: Castle (2003).

Table 1-3 Bloom's Affective and Psychomotor Learning Domains

Affective Domain

Receiving phenomena	Awareness and willingness to hear, listens to others.
Responding to phenomena	Active participation by the learner, willingness to respond, satisfaction with responding, questions.
Valuing	Worth or value a person attaches to a particular object or behavior. Can range from acceptance to commitment, shows the ability to solve problems.
Organization	Compares, relates, and synthesizes values. Prioritizes, accepts responsibility.
Internalizing values	Shows self-reliance and independence has a value system that controls behaviors.

Psychomotor Domain

Perception	Is able to detect nonverbal cues and adjust/plan appropriately.
Set/Readiness to act	Knows and acts on a sequence of steps. Shows a desire to learn.
Guided response	Able to follow directions/instruction.
Mechanism	Learned response has become habitual and activities can be performed with some confidence and proficiency.
Complex overt response	Performing without hesitation and automatic performing.
Adaptation	Skills are well developed. Able to respond effectively to the unexpected.
Origination	Is able to create new method of dealing with a particular situation or problem. Becomes more creative.

Source: Clark (2001).

We have already determined that the cognitive domain of Bloom's taxonomy is the most heavily relied and focused on in the educational world of planning and implementing learning opportunities. The affective domain could be of more importance to consider for healthcare providers who are planning patient education. After all, how can a person be expected to move through the increasingly more complex stages of cognitive ability if he or she is not ready to listen, actively participate, make a commitment, accept responsibility, and ultimately become self-reliant? For example, the following case:

A mother brings her 6 month old to the doctor for a severe, persistent rash on the child's face. The primary care provider refers the family to a pediatric allergist for evaluation of possible eczema. The child is diagnosed with an allergy to peanuts as the cause of the extreme case of eczema. Because it has been determined during the initial interview that the child is strictly breastfed, the mother is instructed to eliminate all nuts and nut products from her diet and was given a skin care plan to follow daily. Also, an EpiPen® was prescribed for treatment of possible anaphylaxis on accidental exposure. The family leaves with this information and treatment plan and is instructed to return for follow-up in 1 month. The family schedules and keeps the follow-up appointment, and the child's eczema has shown little improvement.

During your assessment, you discover that the mother left the initial visit skeptical that the diagnosis and treatment plan was correct and, although she followed the skin care plan, was not completely compliant with the elimination of nuts and nut products from her diet. She also admits that she rarely carries the EpiPen® with her. Based on Bloom's categories of affective learning, this mother was not willing or able to accept the information she was given and, as a result, could not advance through the stages of learning to reach the ultimate goal of resolving her child's rash. What would you need to do in order to help this family achieve this goal based on this information? What strategies would you use to help the mother to become an active participant in her child's treatment? How can you help this mother become empowered and believe that she has the ability to determine her child's outcome?

Nurses and nutritionists in the allergy program spent additional time with this family to answer their specific questions about how the peanut protein can be passed through the breast milk from mother to child. They also showed them some before and after pictures of children with the same problem as their child that seemed to help the family decide to become more committed to the treatment. At the next follow-up visit 1 month later, the family proudly presented with a beautiful and happy child whose eczema had improved drastically. Their ability to take action and see a marked improvement in their child demonstrated their progress through the various stages of the affective learning domain.

How many of you are thinking back to earlier in our discussion about health behaviors and promotion theories? How does Bloom's affective learning domain differ from the Health Belief Model? Does it differ? Both were developed around the same time and use very similar constructs. One focuses on intellectual levels of learning behaviors (Clark, 2001), and one focuses on individual-level health behavior changes (NIH, 2005). The similarities are striking. Nevertheless, they are different in that one examines why and the other examines how. The development of the Health Belief Model was to help explain why the public was not taking advantage of the services being offered with the ultimate goal of improving health outcomes. Bloom onomy was developed to explain how a student moved through the lear process with the ultimate goal of improving educational outcomes. Both pro vide a foundation for planning and implementing patient education and can be used together to achieve the desired goals and objectives of patient edu- cation, either at an individual, group, or community level.

CONNECTING THEORIES

What does all of this mean to us as healthcare providers? What about as teachers of health? Maybe we need a theory to tie all of the concepts and con- structs together and to make it useful for healthcare providers when educat- ing others. Could we use our own special brew in order to be more effective in our goal of teaching our patients and families? We believe that we can. Using the theory "coffee cup" as our beginning, let's look at creating a model specific to patient education. If we blend Perry's scheme, Bloom's Cognitive, Affective, and Psychomotor Domains, and the Health Belief Model with patient assessment, we might be able to come up with what we need. **Table 1-4** has the multiple concepts and behaviors from all five theoretical frame- works that we wish to combine in order to create an effective strategy for planning and implementing patient education.

As you can see, the information is extensive and appears complicated when presented together. A closer look, however, reveals several redundant characteristics of many aspects of the different constructs. We need to iden- tify and consolidate these redundancies in order to compose a blended frame- work that we can use as our coffee cup. For instance, Perry's dualism, Bloom's receiving phenomena, and the Health Belief Model's perceived sus- ceptibility phases all require the learners to believe that they need help and information in order to deal with a situation and/or condition they are fac- ing. As they move through the various levels and stages of the different frameworks, many of the same behaviors are described by all five constructs. Based on this analysis, consider the proposed blending of the concepts and behaviors in **Table 1-5**.

This proposed model provides a framework that we need as healthcare providers in order to effectively plan and implement patient education based on their abilities and willingness to learn. Think back to the case of the infant with severe eczema as a result of an allergy to nuts. This mother was aware that her child had a problem and sought help. She was able to listen and take in basic information about the care of her child's skin; however, it became neworks

ctive	Bloom's Cognitive	Bloom's Psychomotor	Health Belief Model
	Knowledge The patient is able to remember information.	**Perception** Is able to detect nonverbal cues and adjust/plan appropriately.	**Perceived susceptibility** Believe they are susceptible to the condition.
ind :o hear, listens to others.	**Comprehension** The patient is able to demonstrate that he or she understands this and other information.	**Set/Readiness to Act** Knows and acts on a sequence of steps. Shows a desire to learn.	**Perceived severity** Believe the condition has serious consequences.
Responding to Phenomena Active participation, willingness to respond, satisfaction with responding, questions.	**Application** The patient is able to use this information in a practical way.	**Guided Response** Able to follow directions/instruction.	**Perceived benefits** Believe taking action will reduce their susceptibility to the condition or its severity.
Valuing Worth or value a person attaches to a particular object or behavior. Can range from acceptance to commitment, shows the ability to solve problems.	**Analysis** The patient gains an understanding of why this information is important to their well-being.	**Mechanism** Learned response has become habitual and activities can be performed with some confidence and proficiency.	**Perceived barriers** Believe costs of taking action are outweighed by the benefits.
Organization Compares, relates and synthesizes values. Prioritizes, accepts responsibility.	**Synthesis** The patient is able to use this information to make positive changes in lifestyle in order to achieve and maintain his or her well-being.	**Complex Overt Response** Performing without hesitation and automatic performing.	**Cue to action** Are exposed to factors that prompt action.
Internalizing values Shows self-reliance and independence. Has a value system that controls behaviors.	**Evaluation** The patient is able to make healthy choices based on this information and what he or she has learned.	**Adaptation** Skills are well developed. Able to respond effectively to the unexpected.	**Self efficacy** Are confident in their ability to successfully perform the action.
		Origination Is able to create new method of dealing with a particular situation or problem. Becomes more creative.	

providers.

Multiplicity
Begins to question—indicates patient's increasing ability to become and active participant in their care.

Relativism
Figures out what works and does not.

Commitment to Relativism
Choices and commitments empowered to improving their health outcomes.

Table 1-5 Proposed Blended Framework of Learning in Patient/Client Education

Phase One

- Patient believes that there are consequences to his or her actions/condition/situation.
- He or she seeks medical care and is searching for help with this condition/situation.
- He or she is willing to listen to others.
- You can begin to provide basic information related to the condition/situation.

Phase Two

- The patient begins to ask questions and show a desire to learn.
- He or she begins to become more active participants in their care.
- He or she is able to demonstrate a growing understanding of the information provided and follow a sequence of steps.
- He or she gains satisfaction from being an active participant.

Phase Three

- The patient is able to figure out what works and does not work for him or her.
- He or she is able to identify boundaries and benefits of their actions.
- He or she places value on becoming an active participant.
- He or she is increasingly able to follow directions and apply knowledge to his or her situation/care.

Phase Four

- He or she begins to make choices and prioritize related to his or her health and well-being.
- He or she accepts more responsibilities based on the information and knowledge gained.
- Actions become more automatic and habitual, and he or she responds positively to cues for action.
- He or she shows a better understanding of why the information provided is important to his or her lives.

Phase Five

- He or she is able to use information and knowledge to make changes in order to achieve and maintain health and well-being.
- He or she becomes more confident in his or her abilities.
- He or she demonstrates an increasing self-reliance and independence.
- Increased ability to problem solve and adapt effectively to the unexpected.

Source: Romano (2007)©.

obvious at the follow-up visit that she did not completely believe that her diet was influencing her child's condition. She was not able to advance as a learner through the phases and ultimately improve her child's condition. It was, unfortunately, not until the second visit that the healthcare provider was able to identify this issue and basically, start over with educating Mom. After she was able to see before and after pictures of others with the same allergies, Mom was able to believe that her behaviors could affect her child's outcome.

It was up to her whether that outcome would be positive or negative from this point forward. Using the proposed blended framework, the healthcare provider who worked with this family during their initial visit could have more effectively assessed where the family, in particular the mother, fell on the learning continuum in order to develop the appropriate plan of care.

This progression through more complex phases of learning and ability is reflective of another learning theory that we have not discussed. The Dreyfus Model of Skill Acquisition was developed in 1980 by Stuart Dreyfus, a mathematician and systems analyst, and Hubert Dreyfus, a philosopher (Benner, 1984). This model proposes that there are five levels of proficiency that a student must pass through in the acquisition and development of a skill: novice, advanced beginner, competent, proficient, and expert. Based on this and all of the other models and theories that we have discussed throughout this chapter, the proposed blended framework makes sense as a model that can be used by any healthcare provider as a method of assessing, planning, and implementing patient/client education.

One last behavioral theory that is important to consider at this point is locus of control. Julian Rotter's theory, developed in the 1950s, appears to be the foundation for all of the other theories that we have discussed throughout this chapter. Locus of control refers to an individual's perception about the underlying main causes of events in his/her life (Neill, 2006). An external locus of control is the belief that events are a result of luck, fate, or other external factors that are beyond one's control. An internal locus of control believes that a person's decisions and actions can bring about a positive outcome. Rotter believed that internal and external dimensions exist at opposite ends of a continuum and individuals fluctuate between the two (Neill, 2006). In 1978, Wallston, Wallston, and DeVellis expanded on Rotter's theory by demonstrating that health-related locus of control is multidimensional and identified three independent constructs of: internal—an individual controls their own health; powerful others—the belief that important people such as doctors and nurses can control their health; and chance—belief that fate, luck, or chance controls their health (Malcarne, Drahota, & Hamilton, 2005). This expansion on Rotter's original theory fits nicely into the first phase of the proposed blended framework. Consider the mother who we discussed earlier. She had an external locus of control when she left the first visit. It is up to the healthcare providers to determine this and to assist the mother to move through the dimensions to a place where she developed a stronger internal locus of control. This will enable her to achieve the ultimate goal of education and change her behavior by using the knowledge provided to make decisions about her ability that will improve the outcome (Wingard, 2005).

CONCLUSION

We have determined that a significant aspect of the role of healthcare providers is the education of others and that the majority of current healthcare providers have little to no formal education on how to educate. We are far from the perfect world where the concepts and fundamentals of how, what, why, when, and where people learn are incorporated into academic programs for all healthcare providers. With so many increasing demands on these programs, adapting existing programs is unlikely. Lynch (2007) examines the challenges that face nursing programs related to pediatric content at the undergraduate level. There is concern for competing demands for content that addresses contemporary issues such as an aging population resulting in an increased focus on adult care, bioterrorism, complex ethical–legal dilemmas, genetics, and risk behaviors. Add this to a dwindling supply of faculty to teach health care (many of whom have received little to no formal training on how to educate others) and it is clear that incorporating educational foundation is not a reality in the near future. It is important to continue to advocate for this goal; however, for the time being, we need to rely on available resources and experience to develop a greater understanding and skill when planning and implementing patient education.

Creating change goes beyond the restructuring of undergraduate programs. Providing opportunities for practicing healthcare providers to gain a greater understanding related to the education of patients, families, and colleagues should include professional development opportunities, development of text and online resources, and advanced degree programs. Another way to maximize opportunities to reduce the negative effects of limited health knowledge and skills is to use the curricula of kindergarten through 12th grade classes, as well as adult education and community programs to provide health education and ultimately change behaviors. Ultimately, every interaction with patients, families, students, and the community, whether it is on an individual or group level, can be an opportunity to provide education and information to bring about positive change.

Planning teaching for patients and families requires you to consider many issues. Developmental stage and ability, literacy, including health literacy, primary language, cultural beliefs, stress, and fear are some of the influences that will direct your choices for addressing individual learning needs.

We have added to that an assessment of the patient's locus of control and the use of a theoretical framework as a starting point for the planning and implementation of education.

Theory is typically not a favorite topic of most people. It is, however, essential to consider in the ever-evolving and complex world of health care as we know it. As discussed earlier, evidence-based practice is emphasized and expected to be demonstrated throughout the planning and delivery of all aspects of patient care. Using theory as a systematic way of understanding events or situations (NIH, 2005), we have taken concepts and constructs from different disciplines such as psychology, sociology, health, and education and proposed a framework for patient education. This blended framework can serve as the coffee cup and assist with gaining an understanding of an individual's ability and readiness to become an active participant in their care to ultimately become as independent and as self-reliant as possible.

REFERENCES

American Medical Association. (2001). Declaration of professional responsibility: medicine's social contract with humanity. Retrieved on February 15, 2007, from http://www.ama-assn.org/ama1/pub/upload/mm/475/profresponsibility.pdf.

The American Nurses Association Scope & Standards of Practice. (2004). American Nurses Association, Silver Spring, MD.

Benner, P. (1984). *From novice to expert: excellence and power in clinical nursing practice.* Menlo Park, CA: Addison-Wesley.

Benson, S. G., & Dundis, S. P. (2003). Understanding and motivating health care employees: integrating Maslow's hierarchy of needs, training and technology. *Journal of Nursing Management, 11,* 315–320.

Billek-Sawhney, B., & Reicherter, A. (2004). Social cognitive theory: use by physical therapists in the education of older adults. *Topics in Geriatric Rehabilitation, 20*(4), 319–323.

Castle, A. (2003). Demonstrating critical evaluation skills using Bloom's taxonomy. *International Journal of Therapy and Rehabilitation, 10*(8), 369–373.

Clark, D. (2001). Learning domains or Bloom's taxonomy: the three types of learning. Retrieved January 20, 2007, from http://www.nwlink.com/~donclark/hrd/bloom.html.

Cohen, S. A. (1981). Patient education: a review of the literature. *Journal of Advanced Nursing, 6,* 11–18.

Davis, K. (2006). What is effective intervention? Using theories of health promotion. *British Journal of Nursing, 15*(5), 252–256.

The Federation of State Boards of Physical Therapist Standards of Competence. (2000). Retrieved February 15, 2007, from http://www.fsbpt.org/download/ Standards_of_Competence.pdf.

Forsyth, D. R. (2004). *The professor's guide to teaching psychological principles and practices*. Washington, DC: American Psychological Association.

Henderson, A. (2006). Boundaries around the 'well-informed' patient: the contribution of Schutz to inform nurses' interactions. *Journal of Clinical Nursing, 15*(1), 4–10.

Jackson, D., & Mannix, J. (2001). Clinical nurses as teachers: insight from students of nursing in their first semester of study. *Journal of Clinical Nursing, 10*, 270–277.

Kloss, R. (1994). A nudge is best. *College Teaching, 42*(4), 151–159.

Knox, A. (2003). Building on abilities. *The Journal of Continuing Education in the Health Professions, 23*, 141–145.

Lynch, M. E. (2007). Society of Pediatric Nurses Education Committee: policy Statement "Child health content must remain in the undergraduate curriculum." *Journal of Pediatric Nursing, 22*(1), 87–89.

Malcarne, V. L., Drahota, A., & Hamilton, N. A. (2005). Children's health-related locus of control beliefs: ethnicity, gender, and family income. *Children's Health Care, 34*(1), 47–59.

National Institutes of Health. (2005). Theory at a glance. Retrieved May 28, 2008, from http://www.cancer.gov/theory.pdf.

Neill, J. (2006). What is locus of control? Retrieved February 22, 2007, from http://wilderdom.com/psychology/loc/LocusOfControlWhatIs.html.

Russell, S. S. (2006). An overview of adult learning processes. *Urologic Nursing, 26*(5), 349–352, 372.

Wallston, K. A., Wallston, B. S., DeVellis, R. (1978). Development of the multi-dimensional health locus of control (MHLC) scales. *Health Education Monographs, 6*(2), 160–170.

Wingard, R. (2005). Patient education and the nursing process: meeting the patient's needs. *Nephrology Nursing Journal, 32*(2), 211–215.

Chapter 2

The Search for the Adult Learner

Lynn Foord

INTRODUCTION

A prominent adult educator by the name of J. R. Kidd (1973) once remarked that adult learning is a field of enormous complexity that contains more paradox than consensus, and yet health educators frequently state that we want our students and our colleagues—and often our patients and clients—to be "adult learners." We know that adult learning is not an age-related concept. We know that we want our learners, regardless of their age, to take responsibility for their learning and become empowered to apply or adapt their knowledge and skills to solve problems. All of these qualities are widely considered to be indicative of the adult learner (Brookfield, 1986; Mezirow, 1981).

To gain some understanding of who and what an adult learner is and how one becomes an adult learner, let us consider these four scenarios. Two address teaching and learning in the academic setting, and two describe clinically based instruction. Taken together, they provide a framework for understanding the skills of the instructors of adults and how those skills may be applied in the development of an adult learner.

Scenario 1

Dr. Khalid is an instructor in the School for Health Studies at his university. He knows that his health professions students need to be able to make important decisions about their patients. He cannot possibly teach them everything that they will ever need to know, but he needs to prepare them to be safe and effective clinicians.

Scenario 2

Rosemary is a student in a health professions education program. Her goal is not just to learn the skills her instructors can teach her. She wants to be independent from them, able to make her own decisions about her patients and clients. She never wants to be held back from helping her patients because she does not know something, and she wants to be the kind of practitioner who is always "up on" what is new in her field.

Scenario 3

Jeffrey is preparing an in-service presentation for his colleagues in the hospital where he works. His goal is to share updates on patient assessment techniques and the evidence supporting them. He wants to be sure that he presents information in a way that engages his colleagues and provides them with information they will recall and be able to apply.

Scenario 4

Erica's clinical practice includes teaching patients and families how to manage juvenile rheumatoid arthritis effectively. She needs to be sure that her young patients, their parents, and their siblings all understand how to manage medications, nutrition, and exercise to promote good health and independence.

Adult learning is broadly defined, even by the experts. In our search for the adult learner, we focus on andragogy—the practice of teaching adults. We consider our primary goal to be to develop *self-direction* in our learner as a way to empower them as problem solvers and life-long learners.

The "Charter for Andragogy" proposed by Jack Mezirow (1981), a widely published expert on adult learning, sums up the foundational elements of adult learning that we see reflected in each of these cases. To understand the Charter better, it will be helpful to consider each of Mezirow's points and how they play out in actual practice (**Table 2-1**).

Mezirow's very first point portrays adult education as a process that will decrease the learner's dependency on the instructor. The instructor initiates this process by providing opportunities for the learner to recognize resources relevant to his or her learning that exist *in addition to* his or her instructor, such as

Table 2-1 Mezirow's Charter for Andragogy

Andragogy, as a professional perspective of adult educators, must be defined as an organized and sustained effort to assist adults to learn *in a way that enhances their capability to function as self-directed learners* (original emphasis). To do this it must

1. Progressively decrease the learner's dependency on the educator
2. Help the learner understand how to use learning resources—especially the experience of others, including the educator, and how to engage others in reciprocal learning relationships
3. Assist the learner to define his/her learning needs—both in terms of immediate awareness and of understanding the cultural and psychological assumptions influencing his or her perception of needs
4. Assist learners to assume increasing responsibility for defining their learning objectives, planning their own learning program and evaluating their progress
5. Organize what is to be learned in relationship to his/her current personal problems, concerns, and levels of understanding
6. Foster learner decision making—select learner-relevant learning experiences that require choosing, expand the learner's range of options, facilitate taking the perspectives of others who have alternative ways of understanding
7. Encourage the use of criteria for judging which are increasingly inclusive and differentiating in awareness, serf-reflexive, and integrative of experience
8. Foster a self-corrective reflexive approach to learning—to typifying and labeling, to perspective taking and choosing, and to habits of learning and learning relationships
9. Facilitate problem posing and problem solving, including problems associated with the implementation of individual and collective action; recognition of the relationship between personal problems and public issues
10. Reinforce the self-concept of the learner as a learner and doer by providing for progressive mastery; a supportive climate with feedback to encourage provisional efforts to change and to take risks; avoidance of competitive judgment of performance; appropriate use of mutual support groups
11. Emphasize experiential, participative, and projective instructional methods; appropriate use of modeling and learning contracts; make the moral distinction between helping the learner understand his or her full range of choices and how to improve the quality of choosing versus encouraging the learner to make a specific choice

working with his or her fellow students or consulting professional colleagues. As the learner comes to recognize and learns to trust these other resources, he or she expands his or her knowledge and develops his or her skills by interacting with others in reciprocal, give-and-take learning experiences.

The next step in the development of the learner's independence is for the instructor to lead the learner to recognize and express his or her objectives for learning. The instructor guides the learner in developing a learning contract beginning with a description of what he or she needs to know. After the goals for learning have been established, the learner can plan for how he or she will acquire the knowledge that he or she desires and identify how and where he or she will practice the skills that he or she needs. The instructor will also need to teach his or her learners how to assess their level of skill and their progress toward the goals they had established. To help the students recognize that all of these steps are a part of learning, the instructor intentionally models lifelong learning, self-assessment, and risk taking.

It is a hallmark of adult learners to be motivated by goals for learning that have grown out of concerns in their personal or professional life. In the context of health care, consider the example of a student nurse practitioner and a patient learning about a new medication. The student nurse practitioner who will be responsible for prescribing medications will seek to learn the mechanism of action, appropriate dose, interactions, side effects, and possible complications. Meanwhile, the learning objectives of the patient who will be taking the medication would be focused on how and when to take it and what side effects or complications to be aware of. Although they approach the problem from different points of view, both patient and practitioner need to be able to make decisions about the medication, such as how effective the medication is and under what circumstances to contact the other. As we see later in this chapter, the ability of each party to achieve the understanding necessary to make these decisions can be facilitated by an effective adult educator.

Mezirow describes that a part of taking responsibility for learning and making decisions is owning the concept of oneself as a "doer." Often described as the sense of self-efficacy, this confidence in oneself is learned through believing that you have gained mastery of a set of knowledge and skills. The role of an instructor is to design and maintain a learning climate that provides the opportunity for mastery. For learners to gain a sense of mastery, they must experience encouragement, feedback, and support among all—themselves and their instructors—who participate in the learning process.

To facilitate the learning process, the instructor will provide authentic problems that relate to the learning needs of the student. There will be opportunities for students to learn from one another (reciprocal learning) through participative projects. As students work together to complete their project, they will apply their life experience to understanding the problems and learn from the experience and understanding of their partners.

The importance of learning from others in the development of the adult learner cannot be underestimated. Learning from our colleagues, patients, and clients, rather than from a single authority figure, can be tricky, particularly as healthcare professionals and the patients and clients we work with become more diverse. Mezirow (1981) calls for adult learners to be able to "facilitate taking the perspectives of others who have alternative ways of understanding." More recently, adult learners have been called to develop a sense of intercultural understanding (Ewert, 2007). To illustrate the importance of intercultural understanding, consider this scenario.

> A full airplane is first in line for takeoff when a passenger refuses to place the briefcase in his lap under the seat in front of him. Takeoff is aborted, and the plane is directed to an empty taxiway. After much discussion and negotiation, a bag is removed from the overhead compartment at the man's seat, his briefcase is placed in the compartment, and the bag is placed in another compartment further back in the plane. The delay causes the plane to lose its place in line to take off and significantly delays the flight. Understandably, the other passengers are angry and openly hostile to the passenger, as many are now likely to miss their connecting flights.

The reason for the problem? The man was a devout Muslim, who was carrying the Koran in his briefcase. His religious beliefs prevented him from placing his Holy Book on the floor. The problem was solved as soon as the flight crew realized the passenger's needs. By understanding the point of view of the passenger, they were able to work together to develop a solution.

The lessons of intercultural understanding apply directly to the development of the adult learner in healthcare practice and health promotion who is seeking to learn from and collaborate with colleagues who hold different jobs, have different educational and experiential backgrounds, and increasingly may come from different cultures. Consider the foundational elements to building intercultural understanding (Ewert, 2007):

- Things are often not what they seem.
- We cannot assume that we understand everything that we can see.
- The potential for conflict will increase as people act on what they know and in ways that reflect their own world views.
- Understanding differences demands more than a simple appreciation for other beliefs and practices: It requires specific cultural information as well as the tools of cultural analysis to interpret the meanings that underlie these differences.

- Skills of cultural understanding will not emerge by accident; they must be consciously learned and systematically developed over time.

To use these elements in promoting intercultural understanding in our adult learners, we can provide opportunities for them to practice these skills:

- *Observe.* Look closely at a given situation and seek to separate and eliminate assumptions.
- *Engage in conversation,* as this helps to build relationships. Success in building relationships requires a commitment to ask respectful and appropriate questions and seek to understand the beliefs, interests, and needs of others.
- *Recognize and examine our own assumptions.*
- *Construct logical explanations* for seemingly illogical behaviors by opening our minds to different values and choices.
- *Reconcile differences* by recognizing our own assumptions and understanding the situation.

Mezirow (1981, p. 35 [quoted in Suanmali, 1981, p. 29]) proposes one final challenge to the educator of adults, one that is particularly germane to healthcare professionals: that of making "the moral distinction between helping the learner understand his or her full range of choices and how to improve the quality of choosing versus encouraging the learners to make a specific choice." Surely this is a particular challenge to health educators. We work in a field which includes some absolute "rights" and "wrongs"; our field also includes a great deal of uncertainty and ambiguity. When is it our responsibility to tell our students what is "right," and when do we serve them best by teaching them how to make that decision? This is a question that doubtless has as many answers as there are health educators, and some of us may answer it in different ways at different times.

Mezirow's charter provides a framework for our search for the adult learner. To see how the framework might apply to health educators and a student all seeking the qualities of the adult learner, let us consider our four scenarios.

Dr. Khalid

Dr. Khalid is an instructor in the School for Health Studies at his university. He knows that his entry-level health professions students need to be able to make important decisions about their patients. He cannot possibly teach them everything they will ever need to know, but he needs to prepare them to be safe and effective clinicians.

Dr. Khalid's scenario is one that should be familiar to all healthcare providers from our own experiences of professional education. Students beginning their professional education not only need to learn content and skills, they also need to develop alternatives to their current ways of thinking as they socialize into the profession (Brookfield, 1986). They are seeking to redefine themselves as members of their chosen profession, a transition from the role of student to the role of a health professions student en route to becoming a practicing clinician (Holland, 1999).

In many ways (but not all, as we see later), Mezirow's (1981) Charter for Andragogy is specifically directed toward the needs of students in the academic component of their professional education and describes the challenges of the academic instructor to develop their skills as adult learners. In Dr. Khalid's case, his students seek to become health practitioners who must be able to work independently and must recognize what they need to know to practice safely and effectively. Given the pace of change in healthcare practice, all healthcare practitioners must be able to access resources which inform our practice and assess which of those myriad resources available to us are appropriate to meet our needs.

To promote the development of these qualities of the adult learner, the instructor takes on the role of a facilitator (Brookfield, 1986). In the classroom and laboratory setting, the instructor creates an environment for learning that feels safe and in which participation feels voluntary. Classroom activities are designed to draw connections between the learner's experiences and then to pose challenges to learn more. Whether the goal is the acquisition of cognitive knowledge, psychomotor skill, or affective behaviors (Bloom, 1984), the instructor alternates the learning activities between presentation of content and guided application to authentic problems and periods of review and reflection. The instructor models and leads the review and reflection and then guides students to consider new or different ways to solve the problems. This process continues as the students' knowledge and skills expand and the problems become increasingly complex. Throughout this recursive process, the instructor makes connections between the learners' past experiences and the needs that they will face as practicing clinicians.

Learners develop the ability to make decisions in the face of problems that become gradually less finite and more uncertain. Faced with uncertainty and ambiguity, the learner gradually develops a sense of critical awareness. As exemplified in the case of the religiously devout airline passenger, developing a critical awareness requires students to learn to understand the needs of all parties involved and generate options to develop a response to the case.

As students practice interacting with real problems and taking an active role in their learning, they develop a sense of self-efficacy that provides them with confidence and an experience of success, growth, and development. The sense of confidence empowers lifelong learners who continue to build on their experiences in the academic setting.

Kudos to those readers who are questioning whether this schema is more idealistic than realistic. The development of the adult learner is a progression, but it is a progression that rarely goes smoothly as Mezirow might have us believe. There is still a large piece of information—*how* to make this development progress—that is missing from the discussion so far.

William F. Perry (1999), a well-recognized expert on adult learning, described that learners grow and develop through a predictable pattern which he describes as a series of phases. Professor Robert Kloss builds on Perry's schema, suggesting that phase-specific instructional techniques can "nudge" students into the next phase.

As described by Kloss (1994), the earliest phase of student's learning is Dualism, in which the student perceives that there are right and wrong answers and believes his or her job to be to learn the "right answer." Students in the phase of Dualism are uneasy when asked to think independently of "authority," such as the text or the instructor. Professor Kloss suggests giving students in this phase experience in analyzing situations and learning to recognize different points of view. As instructor, he leads them in understanding and legitimizing alternative points of view.

Following Dualism is the phase of Multiplicity, in which students realize that there is more than one answer and accept the challenge of selecting among recognized authorities to choose the right answer. Students in Multiplicity struggle to learn how to make choices, how to justify them, and how to defend them. During the phase of Multiplicity, Kloss recommends that students have opportunities to debate actions and choices, and learn to discuss and justify alternatives.

By learning to compose well-supported arguments, students enter the phase of Relativism. Learners in the phase of Relativism use the skills that they have developed in analysis and critical reflection to engage in the resolution of complex problems. This may require them to expand their knowledge and skills and learn new ways to apply what they know in order to be successful in resolving multifaceted, ambiguous problems.

We can now add Perry (1999) and Kloss (1994), along with Mezirow (1981) and Brookfield (1986) to the list of those who judge the development of the adult learner to be a progressive development. Perry's schema describes the need for students to learn self-direction to be able to resolve difficult problems, and a primary goal in this chapter is to see how to develop self-direction in our learners. To that end, Professor Gerald Grow (1991) proposes the Staged Self-Directed Learning Model (**Table 2-2**).

Grow's model pairs the development of the learner from dependent to self-directed with the activities of the instructor. The instructor begins as an authority figure, fully controlling the interactions with his students. As they develop as learners, he withdraws somewhat, to take the role of motivator and guide. With increased self-direction from his students, he is able to take the role of facilitator, promoting the students' involvement in their learning and encouraging them to take leadership roles in their learning activities. And for those students who achieve the ability to become self-directed, the instructor makes one final transition to the role of consultant.

If Dr. Khalid is to be successful in developing the qualities of adult learners in his students, he will need to create learning environments that make it safe and easy for his students to learn from each other. He will need to facilitate the development of his students in recognizing what they need to know and acquiring the information they need to understand the kinds of problems they will face in clinical practice. He will provide them with realistic situations in which to practice critical reflection and decision making, and when his students leave his classroom, they will be on their way to developing a sense of confidence and mastery—self-efficacy—that will allow them to practice independently, safely, and effectively.

Table 2-2 Grow's Staged Self-Directed Learning Model

Stage	Student	Teacher	Examples
Stage 1	Dependent	Authority, coach	Coaching with immediate feedback. Drill. Informational lecture. Overcoming deficiencies and resistance.
Stage 2	Interested	Motivator, guide	Inspiring lecture plus guided discussion. Goal setting and learning strategies.
Stage 3	Involved	Facilitator	Discussion facilitated by teacher who participates as equal. Seminar. Group projects.
Stage 4	Self-directed	Consultant, delegator	Internship, dissertation, individual work or self-directed study group.

Source: Grow (1991). Copyright © 1991 by Sage Publications. Reprinted with permission from Sage Publications, Inc.

Rosemary could be one of Dr. Khalid's students. What does her educational development look like from her point of view?

Rosemary

Rosemary is a student in a health professions education program. Her goal is not just to learn the skills her instructors can teach her. She wants to be independent from them, able to make her own decisions about her patients and clients. She never wants to be held back from helping her patients because she does not know something, and she wants to be the kind of practitioner who is always "up on" what is new in her field.

Rosemary clearly already has a vision of herself as a well-informed practitioner who practices lifelong learning. She likely also holds expectations of how she will become that practitioner. Rosemary can use this vision and her expectations of her professional education to prepare herself to meet successfully the challenge of becoming that practitioner and growing as a professional. A set of goals and an idea of how to achieve those goals are two of the characteristics that Mezirow (1981) has identified as distinctive of adult learners.

Early in her professional education, Rosemary should determine, as best as she is able, the values and beliefs that she holds that will guide her in her professional education. She may be led in this reflection by an instructor who requires a journal or learning contract that includes the student's statement of values and beliefs. Some important beliefs for Rosemary to consider would be those regarding her perception of her role as a student, her expectations about the role of her student colleagues and instructors, and her beliefs about the provision of health care. Important values might include her obligations to family and friends, religious commitments, and perhaps commitment to civic organizations. Awareness of the values and beliefs that guide her choices and decisions will help Rosemary to know herself as a learner. Self-awareness shapes the directions that she chooses in her education as a professional and ultimately contributes to her sense of self-efficacy.

Rosemary's sense of self-efficacy will develop from her recognition of what she has learned and how she has grown in facing the challenges she has encountered in her life en route to her professional education. She may be a nontraditional student who has changed careers or returned to school after starting a family. She may be a traditional student who has, since high school, focused her energies on earning the grades and finding the funds to keep going in school just to get to this moment. Students of any age may be dealing with family issues, and essentially all of our students must deal with financial issues. Whatever her challenges, surely her experiences will shape her values, beliefs, and attitudes as a student as well as a practicing clinician.

Knowing that she is capable of growth and change is essential, but Rosemary also needs to know herself as a learner. Self-knowledge will help her find value in the learning activities she encounters and will help her direct her education toward the goals she has set for herself. Mezirow's charter (1981) predicts that early in her educational program Rosemary should consider three questions that will help her know herself as a learner:

1. How do you approach problems?
2. How do you like to learn new information and skills?
3. How do you cope with risk?

By developing responses to these questions, Rosemary will become more aware of her goals and her strengths and abilities as a learner and doer. She may also become aware of the need to extend herself into unknown or uncertain territory and learn ways to cope with the risk of learning new skills under unfamiliar circumstances. Such self-awareness and a sense of self-efficacy are foundational to the success of the adult learner; however, for Rosemary to achieve her goal of being a self-directed, lifelong learner, she will need to collaborate with both her instructors and her fellow students.

Adult learners typically seek a personal connection to the information that is being presented: "How is this information important to me?" To begin to make connections with the information that interests her, Rosemary will build a relationship with her instructors. She might make an appointment at the beginning of the semester just to introduce herself and tell her teachers a little bit about herself. She can also connect with her instructors with thoughtful questions during scheduled office hours throughout the semester. When her instructors know something about Rosemary's prior experiences, her interest in the material, how she expects to use the material, or perhaps some concerns she might have about applying the skills, the instructors can address these issues as they interact with Rosemary and her classmates.

Rosemary can also collaborate with her classmates to enrich her learning experience and develop the learning skills she seeks. Longitudinal studies of student development (Baxter Magolda, 1996) describe that for students to develop fully as independent, self-directed learners, they need a classroom atmosphere characterized by friendliness, generosity, mutual respect, and admiration. The instructor can design a learning environment in which it is possible for these qualities to exist, but it is up to the students to present these qualities and develop the group dynamics which support them. Upbeat, enthusiastic, vocal leaders among the students and a general sense of mutual trust can help to establish a positive attitude about learning and generate collaboration among student colleagues.

Many health professions students must also manage commitments outside of the academic program. The most successful students describe feeling supported by the respect, love, and support of family and friends outside of the classroom (Baxter Magolda, 1996). If she is to successfully meet the demands of health professions education, and ultimately of clinical practice, Rosemary needs to maintain a balance between her work (academic and other), her hobbies, diversions, and "play" activities, and the parts of her life that bring her love—whether through family, friends, pets, or significant relationships. It is never easy to maintain this balance and may be particularly difficult for Rosemary in her role as a student, as she often has so little control over her schedule and the demands on her time.

As Rosemary moves through Perry's phases of learning (1999), she may find that she is fearful of venturing into unknown roles as she progresses from passively receiving information from an authority figure to valuing actively her own thoughts and ideas and using them to make decisions and justify her choices. As she progresses through her educational program, Rosemary must make the transition from college or graduate student, to become a student of her chosen profession, and eventually to become a practitioner in that profession. This requires courage and risk taking, as well as changes in how she learns and how she makes decisions.

A study of the role transition experienced by student nurses conducted by Holland (1999) describes three phases of change from entering student to practicing clinician. The first phase is that of becoming a student nurse, which occurs primarily in the academic setting where the individual chooses nursing and is chosen by the educational program to participate. The next phase, being a student nurse, follows closely in most nursing education programs as the student nurses engage in supervised clinical activities as part of their educational programs. The final stage is completed when the qualified nurse begins to practice without supervision. Educational programs for healthcare providers all vary to some extent, but students of any healthcare profession must work through these same phases.

As she develops her skills as a self-directed learner on the way to becoming an independent practitioner, Rosemary must have the courage to risk taking control of her own learning and trust herself to assume the leadership role that she has previously entrusted to her instructors. She will need courage to overcome anxiety and confidence to be able to survive the risks that lead to her transition to practitioner. She needs a sense that she can overcome barriers and learn new skills—a sense of self-efficacy that begins with her recognition of all she has accomplished to get this far in her education.

Rosemary has many resources for dealing with the challenges she faces and the emotions that accompany her progress, and she will probably need to rely on all of them at some point in her education. Rosemary's instructors are often closest to the academic issues and can help with developing a learning diagnosis and identify the source of her challenges. Rosemary's expectations may be unrealistic, or she may not fully understand the expectations of her instructors. Study habits may need to be improved, or perhaps there is a mismatch between Rosemary's phase of learning and the instruction that her teacher planned. Academic issues are best solved through a collaborative effort between Rosemary and her instructor, and therefore, the more Rosemary knows about herself as a learner, the more she can participate in the collaboration. The more the instructors know about Rosemary, the more accurate they can be in guiding her in resolving her academic problems.

In contrast, Rosemary's friends and family will be an irreplaceable source of support through the challenges of her professional education. They have a distance from her academic life and can help her keep her concerns and emotions in perspective with her personal values and beliefs.

Professional education is, by nature, a challenge. Rosemary's success in meeting her goal of independence as a learner and establishing the skills of a lifelong learner depends on her knowing herself, communicating well with her instructors, and developing strong networks of support both on and off campus.

So far, we have been looking at the development of the adult learner in the academic setting from the point of view of Dr. Khalid and Rosemary; however, continuing education is now a requirement for most healthcare providers. How does the search for the adult learner look when it is conducted in the clinical setting?

Jeffrey

Jeffrey is preparing an in-service presentation for his colleagues in the hospital where he works. His goal is to share updates on patient assessment techniques and the evidence supporting them. He wants to be sure that he presents information in a way that engages his colleagues and provides them with information they will recall and be able to apply.

Jeffrey is also seeking the qualities of adult learners, but his situation is quite different from that of Rosemary and Dr. Khalid. He is teaching a different audience, has a different role as instructor, and has far less time for his instruction; however, the same principles of adult learning can be applied to this situation as well. There is wide variety in how in-service education is offered by different professions in different settings; however, there is a body of literature describing best practices in instructional design. These principles can apply to any instructional unit, and we use them to explore how Jeffrey can design instruction for his colleagues that will be engaging and successful.

One of the best known (and simplest to recall) theories of instructional design is the ADDIE approach put forward by Dick and Carey (1996). ADDIE stands for

- Audience
- Design
- Development
- Implementation
- Evaluation

Following the ADDIE approach, Jeffrey will begin by becoming familiar with his audience. They are practicing clinicians who bring their clinical expertise to the in-service presentation. In addition, each of them has completed some level of training to become a practitioner. Thus, unlike Dr. Khalid, Jeffrey will not need to teach them *how* to learn the content and skills he will be presenting.

Nor will he have the time. The format in which in-service learning is offered varies by profession, as well as by institution. Although, in some cases, there may be regularly scheduled programs of in-service presentations, it is unlikely that Jeffrey will have several months with several hours a week to meet with his learners. Unlike Dr. Khalid, Jeffrey will need to design focused instruction that results in knowledge and skills that can be immediately applied in clinical practice.

Before he begins to prepare his instructional units, Jeffrey will become familiar with the needs and expectations of his audience. If they are colleagues with whom he works closely, he can talk with them to know about their current use of patient evaluation techniques and understand their interest in new or different techniques and the evidence which supports them. It will be helpful for Jeffrey to gather real patient cases that he can use in his instruction; authentic and familiar patient cases will engage his learners and draw them into the teaching/learning experience.

As clinicians, his audience will be looking for "just in time" learning—a presentation focused on information that they can begin to apply immediately in practice. As adult learners, they will want to make connections between what they know and do and the content and skills that Jeffrey will present. They will be most attracted to information that will help them solve recognized problems in their clinical practice, and they will look for valid and reliable evidence that the information that Jeffrey is presenting is supported in the literature.

Based on his understanding of his audience, Jeffrey can now design his presentation. Because he must be so focused and because his audience wants to be able to use what they have learned, Jeffrey will write behavioral objectives that describe his goals for his learners (for more information about how to write behavioral objectives, see Beitz, 1996). Jeffrey will write objectives that reflect the needs and interests of his learners, and he will describe what he wants them to be able to know and do, under what conditions, and how well he expects them to be able to "do" what they have learned. Because behavioral objectives are written to describe measurable outcomes, Jeffrey will also be able to use them to assess the effectiveness of his instruction.

In writing his behavioral objectives, Jeffrey will likely find Bloom's (1984) taxonomy of learning a helpful resource. Jeffrey has learned about his audience, and thus, he will know at what level to direct his instruction. If he were presenting information that is new, he would begin at the level of knowledge or comprehension and move up the hierarchy as his students grasped the material. In this particular case, Jeffrey will know that his learners are already practicing patient assessment; therefore, although he may present some new information at the level of application, he is more likely to direct most of his instruction at the level of analysis or synthesis.

The stages of design and development are often interrelated, as Jeffrey builds from his objectives to develop his content and design a plan for how he will deliver that content. Brookfield (1986) recommends that the adult educator design instruction that promotes critical reflection by carefully selecting among instructional methods such as lecture, discussion, silent reflection, practice with feedback, or activities in pairs or small groups. Jeffrey will deliberately shape the learning environment by assuring learning experiences such as dialogue between instructor and learner and interaction among student's to explore new skills and information that may change one's behaviors and beliefs.

Jeffrey might begin by having participants share their objectives or goals for the in-service—this will help bring the learners together as a group. He might include a discussion during which he and the learners develop a learning contract to clarify what they can expect during the learning experience. Sharing goals and agreeing on a learning contract will help Jeffrey to become familiar with his participants. Based on what he learns from them, he may choose to adapt his presentation and practice activities to build from the knowledge and skills that the participants have brought to the in-service.

In the implementation stage, Jeffrey's presentation will be tightly focused and will incorporate authentic and familiar patient cases. When he is teaching skills, Jeffrey will include a practice component to his instruction. During this time, learners have the opportunity to apply the skills and receive feedback on their performance. His learners will be looking for handouts that will help them transfer the information directly to their clinical practice. Instead of the lists, narrative notes, and PowerPoint slides that might be offered by Dr. Khalid, these learners will be looking for bulleted tip sheets and detailed photos clearly depicting correct performance. After the formal instruction is finished, the learners will be looking for a network of support as they refine their skills in the context of their clinical practice.

Jeffrey's learners will be experienced both as learners and as practitioners and are likely to be capable of self-direction in their learning; thus, as their instructor, Jeffrey can take the role of motivator and guide (Table 2-2). As his learners incorporate the information he shares and begin to practice new skills, his role can transition to more of a facilitator (Grow, 1991).

As facilitator, he can direct the participants to work in pairs or small groups as they interact with new content. This interactive style of learning has participants interacting with the material as well as with their colleagues and allows them to practice new skills with their group members using reciprocal learning. Furthermore, after formal instruction has concluded, these group activities provide the foundation for a network of resources to support learners as they incorporate new information and skills into their practice. As his learners integrate their new knowledge and skills into their practice, Jeffrey's role as facilitator during instruction will transition to the role of consultant. As consultant, he will continue to provide feedback and will be a part of the network of resources available to his learners.

The final phase of the ADDIE model is evaluation. Jeffrey will evaluate the effectiveness of his instruction by comparing observed outcomes to his behavioral objectives. Jeffrey's learners will evaluate his effectiveness as an instructor based on the design, organization, and clarity of his instruction; the quality of the evidence he uses to support the content he has selected; and the value of his feedback as his learners incorporate new information into their practice.

We can see several elements of Mezirow's Charter for Andragogy (Table 2-1) in Jeffrey's instruction of his clinical colleagues. Jeffrey will help his learners define their learning needs through group discussion and perhaps a learning contract. Jeffrey will incorporate experiential learning into his in-service presentations and will provide opportunities for practice in realistic scenarios. Jeffrey will establish and maintain a supportive climate during the learning activities that supports a sense of mastery. He will use interactive group work, creating relationships that will transition into a network for feedback and support in clinical practice.

In contrast to his colleagues in the academic setting, Jeffrey is dealing with learners who already have both academic and clinical expertise in their field. These learners will demand highly focused instruction that must be delivered in a very limited amount of time. They expect to be able to use their information immediately in their practice. Perhaps the most interesting difference is the role of the instructor, who is less likely to be seen as an authority figure than as a colleague and therefore must be especially skilled in the roles of motivator, guide, facilitator, and consultant.

Jeffrey's experience represents one type of clinically based instruction. Erica's challenge is a bit different, and yet it still involves a search for the qualities of the adult learner.

Erica

Erica's clinical practice includes teaching patients and families how to manage juvenile rheumatoid arthritis effectively. She needs to be sure that her young patients, their parents, and their siblings all understand how to manage medications, nutrition, and exercise to promote good health and independence.

Erica's learners need not just to *know*, but to be able to *apply* the information and skills that she is teaching. In this way, they are not very much different from Jeffrey's colleagues or Dr. Khalid's students. Erica's learners are different because they are more likely to be looking for *training* than education. Brookfield (1986) describes the difference between education and training:

> In training, a set of clearly identified skills are transmitted, and adults are required to assimilate these in the manner prescribed by the trainer. . . . In education, by contrast, learners are encouraged to examine the assumptions underlying the acquisition of skills, to consider alternative purposes, and to place skill acquisition in some broader context. (B. 17)

Erica's learners will be looking for an authority figure who can provide them with the basic information and skills that they need to solve their problems. With relatively little instruction, they need to become independent of the instructor, use the information to make decisions and solve problems, and recognize what resources are available to them when they need assistance or guidance. These are the same characteristics that Dr. Khalid and Jeffrey are looking for in their learners, and yet Erica faces some very different challenges in developing these abilities in her learners.

In Erica's clinical area of juvenile rheumatoid arthritis, the entire family is affected by one individual's diagnosis. Thus, Erica's instruction must address the various learning needs of different members of the family as they interact with the patient. Patients and families who may still be struggling with a recent diagnosis are unlikely to have any idea of what their learning needs might be. This is where Erica takes an authoritative role and, as described by Brookfield (1986), prescribes what her learners will need to know; however, her instruction must be fitted to the roles held by each member of the family and to their age-related capacity for learning.

Erica will also need to be attuned to cultural differences between herself and her learners, including the fact that they are lay persons, whereas she is the healthcare expert. She must assess and accommodate the influence of her patient's cultural background and beliefs and be prepared to adjust her teaching in order to provide culturally sensitive care. In preparing and delivering her instruction, she will want to practice the elements of intercultural understanding (Ewert, 2007). It is particularly important that Erica acquires specific information about her patients' culture and practices cultural analysis to gain an understanding of the meanings behind different beliefs and practices. Through conversation with her patients and their families, she can learn about their beliefs and interests and use this information to personalize her instruction.

As she gets to know her patient and the members of his/her family, Erica can use her limited time for instruction to address both the skills she knows they will need, as well as the problems and concerns that they are able to identify. In many cases, Erica may be required to set priorities in her instruction to accommodate limitations in time and each individual's capacity for understanding. She will need to decide who to instruct first and how much instruction to provide each family member. Furthermore, she may need to help the family adjust to their new roles as they cope with the new diagnosis. Each of her learners will need to balance their new responsibilities with their existing roles in the family as well as their commitments and obligations outside of the family, and they may look to Erica for guidance and support in this experience of personal change.

Given that her patients must rapidly become independent in applying the information she has presented, Erica's instruction will be designed to promote her learner's sense of self-efficacy. Erica, like Jeffrey, will build in opportunities for her learners to practice and receive feedback about the skills she has taught them. She can use handouts and informational brochures and perhaps some forms of technology (see Chapter 4) to extend her instruction as her learners become independent from her. She can further promote their independence by informing her learners about community resources, such as the Arthritis Foundation. She will need to be sure that her learners know when to ask for help, who to ask, and where to contact that person. Furthermore, with easy access to the World Wide Web, Erica will need to be sure that her learners know how to determine what information they can trust (see Chapter 4).

All of our instructors will face the challenge Mezirow (1981) proposes in his final element of the Charter for Andragogy:

> To make the moral distinction between helping the learner understand his/her full range of choices and how to improve the quality of choosing vs. encouraging the learner to make a specific choice.

Perhaps, however, it is in the situation of patient/family instruction that this choice becomes most challenging. With limitations in time and resources, are we best meeting our responsibilities by just "telling" the patient what to do, or should we be exploring a variety of options and facilitating his choice? This is perhaps the most intriguing of the challenges faced by adult educators and adult learners. As an in-depth discussion is beyond the scope of this chapter, I leave the question hanging for the reader's further consideration.

CONCLUSION

These are four very different scenarios—four very different ways that health professionals provide instruction. In all cases, nevertheless, we are seeking the qualities of the adult learner. Therefore, what conclusions can we draw?

In spite of the wide variety of teaching conducted by healthcare professionals, there are qualities of the adult learner sought by all of us:

- A sense of his own experiences and motivations related to the learning experience
- The ability to organize new knowledge and skills with what he already knows

- The ability to recognize problems and use all available information to solve those problems
- A sense of self-efficacy: the knowledge that he can solve the problems which face him

Furthermore, in spite of the wide variety of instruction in which we engage, some general tips/rules can make us, as instructors, successful in our search for adult learners:

- Learn about our learners and what expectations, knowledge, and skills they bring to the learning experience.
- Design instruction that fits the needs and level of the learner.
- Provide accurate and helpful feedback to learners.
- Promote independence in our learners.

This chapter began with a recognition that adult learning is a field of enormous complexity that contains more paradox than consensus (Kidd, 1973), and all of our discussion about instruction and adult learners in relationship to these four examples only confirms both the complexity and the paradox. When daunted by the sheer volume of information, we should remind ourselves that becoming better learners and teachers enriches our effectiveness as providers of health care. The breadth and depth of writing about adult learning provide a seemingly limitless resource for us to continue to broaden and develop our skills as both learners and instructors.

REFERENCES

Baxter Magolda, M. B. (1996). Epistemological development in graduate and professional education. *Review of Higher Education, 19*(3), 283–304.

Beitz, J. M. (1996). Developing behavioral objectives for perioperative staff development. *AORN Journal, 64*, 87. Retrieved August 5, 2007, from Expanded Academic ASAP database.

Bloom, B. S. (1984). *Taxonomy of educational objectives*. Boston: Allyn and Bacon.

Brookfield, S. D. (1986). *Understanding and facilitating adult learning*. San Francisco: Jossey-Bass.

Dick, W., & Carey, L. (1996). *The systematic design of instruction* (4th ed.). New York: Harper Collins College Publishers.

Ewert, D. M. Building intercultural understanding: the passenger in row 22. *Adult Learning, 11*(2), 2007–2030.

Grow, G. O. (1991). Teaching learners to be self-directed. *Adult Education Quarterly, 41*(3), 125–149.

Holland, K. (1999). A journey to becoming: the student nurse in transition. *Journal of Advanced Nursing, 29*(1), 229–236.

Kidd, J. R. (1973). *How adults learn* (Rev., updated, completely rewritten ed.). New York: Association Press.

Kloss, R. J. (1994). A nudge is best. *College Teaching, 42*(4), 151.

Mezirow, J. D. (1981). A critical theory of adult learning and education. *Adult Education Quarterly, 32,* 3–24.

Perry, W. G. (1999). *Forms of ethical and intellectual development in the college years: a scheme.* San Francisco: Jossey Bass.

Suanmali, C. (1981). *The core concepts of andragogy.* Unpublished Doctor of Education, Teachers College, Columbia University.

Chapter 3

Impact of Poverty on Learning

Carol S. Collard & Richard L. Sowell

INTRODUCTION

One of our primary roles as health educators is to pursue new and better ways to facilitate the learning process. Toward that goal, we often study ways to respond better to individual learning styles as a way to uncover each individual's full potential for acquiring knowledge. Of equal importance, however, is our need to develop an enhanced understanding of the impact that context has on an individual's learning (Caffarella & Merriam, 2000). In no other teaching–learning situation is achieving desired learning outcomes more important than in health-related education.

An understanding of how poverty impacts adult learning is useful in that it further illustrates the role of context in the learning process. Jarvis (1987) argues that "learning is not a psychological process that happens in splendid isolation from the world in which the learner lives but that it is intimately related to the world and affected by it" (p. 11). For educators, context is critical to knowing that learning is also a social process that must take into account the environment in which the student functions; therefore, to achieve fully the desired goals of promoting health or assisting individuals to regain their health, health educators will need to understand the influence of poverty (context) on an individual's ability to comprehend and implement health messages or treatment instructions. The impact of poverty on health can be multifocal and long lasting, affecting an individual's learning and motivation to undertake healthy behaviors starting in early childhood and establishing health behavior patterns for life.

UNDERSTANDING POVERTY

According to the 2006 report of the U.S. Census Bureau, the poverty line for a family of three is an annual household income of no more than $16,242. This is determined largely by a 40-year-old formula developed by the USDA that measured the costs of meeting a minimal diet. The use of this measure is controversial in that it is largely believed that it fails to take into account the larger share of today's dollars that a family must spend on housing, health care, and transportation (Brooks, 2004; Rank, 2005). Many experts agree that if the measure was ever adjusted to reflect today's real standard of living that the poverty rate would be significantly higher.

During the 1960s, a "War on Poverty" was declared to reduce the ranks of the poor. As a result of that effort, there was notable success in reducing the ranks of those living in poverty through the late 1970s; however, the economic slowdown in the early 1980s, combined with reductions in spending on social welfare and the growth of single-parent families, led to a stagnation of and a subsequent rise in poverty rates. Most recent estimates are that in 2006 approximately 12% of Americans live at or below the poverty line (U.S. Census Bureau, 2008). In truth, many more households know the vulnerability of being "one paycheck away" from financial devastation and/or homelessness. It is important to understand that many of the poor do work. In fact, many individuals that we encounter in our everyday lives represent the "working poor."

Poverty can be either chronic or transient. Employment and family structural changes are frequently influential in ending spells of poverty (Rank, 2005). Two thirds of the households living in poverty are able to rise out of it when the wages of a family member increased or when the family structure changed, typically by marriage or the departure of a child from the household (Rank, 2005). Given this context, many households apparently have experienced spells of poverty, whereas others have endured a chronic state of impoverishment. Life-changing events such as divorce or job loss could push a household into a temporary spell of poverty. A smaller number of households do experience prolonged states of poverty that last for years or transcend generations. These families are often characterized by significant barriers such as limited literacy and vocational skills or physical or mental illness; however, any spell of poverty experienced by an individual or family has the potential of having a dramatic impact on health and health behaviors. The need to provide food and shelter for the individual or family unit often takes priority over or leaves limited resources for accessing health care or implementing health-related messages or treatments.

Poverty persists as a social problem largely because of the complexity of our evolving economic, political, and social structures. According to Brooks (2004), "In wealthy nations such as the United States where there is no absolute scarcity of food, shelter, health care, or opportunity, poverty results from the politics of distribution" (p. 9). Furthermore, political ideology and religion help shape the values that dictate how the poor are perceived. It is therefore difficult to find enduring solutions for poverty because of society's judgmental regard that poverty is primarily as a result of individual moral failing (Danziger et al., 1994) rather than economic circumstance. Symbolic language continues to be used to perpetuate negative stereotypes (Corcoran, 1995; Gans, 1995) and the perception of an "undeserving" poor. Gans (1995) asserts that such terms as "welfare queens," "underclass," and "culture of poverty" serve to segregate and imply behavioral and moral deficiencies on the part of the poor. In the United States, poverty is also politicized by race. "Urban" has become the code word for "black." Although disproportionately represented among the poor, poverty is not the exclusive domain of persons of color or single mothers. Poverty impacts all racial and ethnic groups and family configurations, whether they live in the city or in rural areas. With this understanding, health education practitioners need to assess all clients comprehensively to determine accurately whether poverty or the residual influences of having lived in poverty are significant variables that require attention in any health education plan or health intervention strategy.

Human Costs of Poverty

Rank (2005) describes three experiences associated with poverty in American life that negatively impact the human experience: (1) doing without daily necessities, (2) enduring elevated levels of stress, and (3) experiencing diminished potential.

Doing Without

Everyday those who live in poverty have to do without or compromise on access to basic necessities that nonpoor households take for granted. Essential needs such as food, clothing, shelter, health care, and transportation are often not met. This situation means that meeting the basic essentials of life becomes the focus of daily life.

Elevated Stress

The inability to meet basic needs compounds the stressors of everyday life. This added weight strains marriages, impacts parenting, and contributes to physical and mental illnesses.

Diminished Potential

The combination of prolonged deprivation and excess stress can inhibit an individual's personal development. That stunting of growth can lead to poor physical and mental health, academic, and vocational underachievement and to a higher degree of likelihood that the experience of poverty will persist.

Poverty and Academic Achievement

Much has been written about the disparities of academic achievement among economically disadvantaged youth. Research has shown that children growing up in chronic poverty run a heightened risk of repeating a grade, being placed in special education classes, and dropping out of high school (Huston, 1991) than their nonpoor counterparts. It is generally believed that those disparities can be attributed in part to the differences in the quality of the education provided to low-income youth but also to the comparative differences in life stressors that many low-income children must endure (Brooks, 2004; Corcoran, 1995; Huston, 1991). As the most vulnerable member of the family unit, children of economically disadvantaged households also have higher rates of exposure to hunger and malnutrition, substandard or cost-burdened housing, a parent's joblessness or limited employment opportunities, and neighborhood crime and violence (Corcoran, 1995; Gans, 1995; Wilson, 1987) than their nonpoor counterparts. These life stressors create a difficult environment that is not conducive for learning and affect what the child determines is important to learn. Such an environment can also provide the context in which distrust of social systems and outside information sources can develop.

Low-income adults who choose to pursue higher education often must cope with the same stressors and may also have the additional stress of being a parent. Parental stress may be further magnified if the adult seeking higher education is heading a single-parent household. These kinds of stressors may be among a number of obstacles that could inhibit academic success.

Additionally, these stressors can function as barriers to understanding and accepting health information and/or adherence to treatment regimes.

INTEGRATING THE CONTEXTUAL APPROACH TO LEARNING

Examining how poverty impacts learning helps to demonstrate the need to integrate the two perspectives of adult learning: the individual and the contextual perspectives (Caffarella & Merriam, 2000). The *individual perspective*, which is the predominate approach of most educators, calls for a need to understand the varying learning styles of the individual. The *contextual perspective* acknowledges the influences of external or environmental factors such as race, class, or gender on individual learning. To be effective, health educators need a clear understanding of these perspectives, but more important, they need to work to integrate appropriately these two perspectives in developing plans of health education for individuals and groups.

The Individual Perspective

The individual perspective is the foundation of many adult learning theories, including andragogy (Knowles, 1970), self-directed learning (Tough, 1971), and transformational learning (Mezirow, 2006). According to Caffarella and Merriam (2000), these perspectives are grounded in the premise that "learning is something that happens primarily internally" and that "all adults can be effective learners no matter their background or situation" (p. 56).

The Contextual Perspective

The contextual perspective has two different dimensions: the *interactive* and the *structural* (Caffarella & Merriam, 2000). The interactive dimension considers the context in which learning occurs. The situation or environment that the learner is in is just as important to the learning process as what the individual learner and/or educator contributes. The structural dimension incorporates an understanding of how race, class, gender impact the learning process, affecting not only the way we learn but even what we learn. Caffarella and Merriam (2000) cite scholars such as Freire (1970), Goldberger (1996), and Tisdell (1998), who have embraced the structural perspective.

Rather than having to choose one over the other, increasingly, educators are discovering that the integration of both individual and structural perspectives is vital in achieving a complete and holistic approach to working with the adult learner (Caffarella & Merriam, 2000). In the context of students living in poverty or near-poverty situations, there will be those whose individual intellectual competence and capacity for coping with stressors will help transcend environmental barriers. For others, strategies may have to be devised to facilitate coping with the external obstacles in order to help them achieve academic success. As educators of adult learners, each learning situation must be assessed from both perspectives, which considers how individual learners learn, as well as how the "context shapes learners, instructors, and the learning transaction itself" (Caffarella & Merriam, 2000, p. 62).

Applying the Contextual Perspective

Although any learners may be susceptible to challenges and crises while undertaking academic pursuits, economically disadvantaged learners must often cope with more limited resources for problem solving. The following represents potential obstacles, both interpersonal and environmental, that may impede academic success.

Interpersonal Obstacles

- Impaired cognitive development
- Physical health issues
- Low self-esteem
- Higher external locus of control
- Mental health concerns

Individuals who have experienced chronic poverty may have to cope with interpersonal obstacles such as cognitive impairment and physical illness due to a history of prolonged malnourishment or inadequate medical attention. The constant exposure to negative reinforcements and the experiences resulting from prolonged deprivation may contribute to lower self-esteem and sense of powerlessness over one's destiny. Over time, negative life experiences may also contribute to mental health concerns such as depression or posttraumatic stress disorder. Often these conditions are not attended to either for financial reasons or because they have not been diagnosed (Brown, 2003).

Environmental Obstacles

- Limited economic resources
- Unstable housing or homelessness
- Limited social support
- Family crises
- Discrimination

Unstable income or unemployment can adversely affect a student's ability to become or remain successful. Rarely does a low-income adult have the economic resources to be a full-time student without also having to work. The hours devoted to work may compromise a student's time for study or completion of assignments. Unemployment may cause student to be excessively absent from class while looking for work or drop out of school. An insecure, overcrowded, or substandard housing situation can impose stress that impairs concentration or ability to attend. Limited social support to assist with child care or other care giving duties, housekeeping chores, or other family demands may cause frequent absences and affect completion of tasks or study time. Family crises such as a death in the family, domestic violence, or divorce could more significantly derail a low-income student who has fewer resources to cope. A student may be affected by discrimination when academic expectations are set too high or too low based on biased or incomplete assessments of a student's ability. In either instance, the student's academic experience may be negatively affected.

OPPORTUNITIES FOR THE EDUCATOR

Merriam and Caffarella (1999) acknowledge that as we learn more about the adult learner and how their life experiences and circumstances impact their motivation for and ability to learn we will be better able to construct relevant learning experiences and opportunities. "Teaching strategies that allow participants to connect the material to their own life experiences, allow for reflective time, confront differences, and bring together theory and practice seem to provide useful starting points" (p. 127) to engage and motivate students. Representing the interactive domain of the contextual approach to learning, these strategies acknowledge the student as partner and contributor in the learning process: Case studies, role plays, and small group work provide opportunities for different experiences and alternate points of view to be shared.

Parenthetically, educators must understand that a low-income student's life experiences may be more stressful than their nonpoor counterparts and may also impact their ability to learn, not their desire. Frequent absences, tardiness in completing assignments may be the result of inadequate support at home, not lack of interest. Open communication with the student to understand better the context of his or her life situation and, when feasible, a small measure of flexibility may mean the difference between retaining or losing the student.

Health Education and Poverty

There is a critical need for health educators to understand the impact poverty and the stressors that result from poverty have on their clients' ability to understand and implement health teaching successfully. Most individuals that encounter situations requiring health teaching do so because of a health crisis or potential health issue. Such situations naturally invoke concern and can lead to heightened stress in any client; however, in the client whose life situation is already economically and socially tenuous, the situation that has resulted in the need for health teaching only serves to compound the stress of their daily lives. Adherence to medical treatments or changes in health behavior is a major focus on health education. To achieve such desired outcomes, clients have to both understand information and be able to implement the behaviors. Cognitive impairment, low self-efficacy, mental health issues, and a higher propensity to be influenced by external others represent potential interpersonal obstacles to implementing desired health behaviors successfully. Likewise, limited economic resources, unstable housing situation, and limited social support can be significant environmental obstacles that prevent clients from focusing on health information and/or having the ability to carry out health directives. For example, economically disadvantaged individuals may be faced with the choice of purchasing medications or health-related services or buying food for their family. In such cases, not following through with health directives does not represent nonadherence, but rather a reasonable decision in context of the individual's life situation.

Nevertheless, understanding the influence of poverty on the success of health education is only the first step for the health educator. Equally as important is the implementation of strategies to identify and respond to clients who are coping with stressors related to poverty or whose ability to learn has been negatively influenced by their life situation. Health educators need to assess the economic status of all clients using assessment techniques that do not disrespect or embarrass clients who have limited resources. It may be even more important to develop a supportive teaching environment that helps to build trust with clients living in poverty than with their non-poor counterparts. Health educators need to seek out resources and services that can be used to assist poor individuals in achieving health and treatment goals. It may be important to not only identify available resources for the client, but rather assist the client in accessing needed resources and services.

Additionally, health educators should be able to adapt their health messages to place information in the context of the realities of the client's life situation. Adult education theory (Knowles, 1970) supports that learning is more successful when it can be related to the individual's life experiences. For many economically disadvantaged clients, their life experiences are influenced by a lack of resources, doing without, and making survival choices daily. This situation is the context in which they have to assess the significance and reasonability of health education messages. Health educators' assessments and teaching strategies require careful attention to this reality if they are to be successful in assisting clients in implementing health information and treatment protocols.

Healthcare Resources for Low-Income Households

According to the AFL-CIO (2008), 47 million (15%) Americans do not have health insurance. Low-income households often require additional supports to assist them with coping with healthcare needs. A variety of public and private resources are available to assist low-income individuals with obtaining information and/or financial assistance with their healthcare issues. Table 3-1 provides a list of potential healthcare resources that can be used by health educators in assisting their clients.

Table 3-1 List of Health Care Resources to Assist Disadvantaged Clients

Health Care Resource	Contact Info
Prescription Assistance	
Patient Assistance Program Center	www.rxassist.org
Rx Outreach	www.rxoutreach.org
Partnership for Prescription Assistance	www.pparx.org
Health Care Information	
AFL-CIO	www.aflcio.org/issues/healthcare/resources/ justforyou.cfm
National Diabetes Information Clearinghouse	http://diabetes.niddk.nih.gov/dm/pubs/financialhelp/
Health Care Services	
Bureau of Primary Health Care	1-800-400-2742 or www.bphc.hrsa.gov
Department of Veteran's Affairs	1-800-827-1000 or www.va.gov.
Health Coverage	
Medicaid	Contact local Department of Human Resources
Medicare	www.medicare.gov/
Hospital Care	
Hill-Burton Federal Program for free or reduced-charge medical services	1-800-638-0742 or visit www.hrsa.gov/hillburton/default.htm

SUMMARY

The prevalence of poverty in our society increasingly impacts not only those we serve but also those with whom we work. Most recent statistics indicate that nearly 37 million (U.S. Census Bureau, 2008) Americans live in poverty. Economic, political, and social forces have more influence on who is poor than personal character imperfections. Three common experiences that are associated with poverty in American life negatively impact the human experience: (1) doing without daily necessities, (2) enduring elevated levels of stress, and (3) experiencing diminished potential.

In addition to identifying ways to meet the needs of the adult learner, educators, generally, and health educators, particularly, must also recognize the importance of understanding the role context plays in the learning process. The conditions and stressors that often accompany life in poverty can impair an adult learner's ability to achieve academic success or implement behaviors that are desired. Economically disadvantaged adult learners must often cope with a wide range of interpersonal and environmental obstacles. Within the healthcare context, obstacles to understanding health messages or directives may be even greater. A lack of adherence to medical regimes can often be, in part, attributed to the healthcare professional and the client having very different goals, beliefs, and priorities. Additionally, clients in the healthcare system may be faced with explanations and directives stated in medial jargon that is often incomprehensible and meaningless. Health educators are obligated to learn more about the adult learner and how their life experiences and circumstances impact their motivation for and ability to learn. Furthermore, they are challenged to develop an awareness of the impact of poverty on learning and then consciously incorporate strategies to adequately respond to poverty-related obstacles to learning (health education) in client plans of care.

Case Study 3–1

Jodi is a health educator in the outpatient diabetic clinic of a large urban hospital system. Jodi was assigned to do follow-up education with Sonya, a 38-year-old woman who had been treated for hyperglycemia for the past 6 months. She had been placed on oral medication to help control her elevated blood glucose levels. Sonya had also been provided with information about her condition and what measures were needed to help lower her elevated glucose level. On previous visits to the clinic, two other health educators conducted one-on-one education briefings with Sonya about steps that she could take to control her blood glucose without having to start taking insulin injections. Sonya had been told that she should increase her level of exercise by having a set program of exercise each day. She was advised on the role of good nutrition in controlling her glucose and given booklets to take home that outlined recommended dietary practices for persons with elevated blood glucose levels. The health educator also reminded Sonya that her physician had indicated that it would be necessary for her to lose 20 pounds as part of her exercise and dietary control program if she was going to control her blood sugar level. Nevertheless, on this visit to the clinic, Sonya had not lost any weight, and her A1C value showed that her hyperglycemia was getting worse. The clinic physician determined that it was time to place Sonya on insulin injections.

Sonya pleaded with the medical staff not to put her on insulin and let her have one more chance to control her blood sugar without having to take injections. Based on her high level of anxiety and stress at the thought of taking insulin injections, the physician agreed to give her 3 more months to make progress in controlling her blood glucose; however, if she had not make significant progress by her next clinic visit she would have to begin blood glucose monitoring daily and control her sugar levels with insulin.

Jodi met with Sonya. She reviewed Sonya's chart with the progress notes describing her condition, treatment, and health education at each of her previous clinic visits. In her assessment of Sonya, Jodi determined that Sonya understood the seriousness of her situation and that she really wanted to take the necessary measure to control her blood glucose without shots. Jodi noted in her initial interaction with Sonya that she had expressed concern that she could not afford to go on insulin. Sonya had said several times, "I have to do something. I can't afford to take insulin for many reasons." Although Sonya was neatly dressed, Jodi looked back at her chart and noted that Sonya was a single mother who had two adolescent children. Her occupation was listed as waitress/cook. Based on this information, Jodi undertook a social assessment of Sonya understanding that Sonya's failure to reach previously identified goals to control her blood glucose level may be more related to her life situation than to her lack of understanding of what was required or willingness to undertake needed behavior changes.

Jodi acknowledged Sonya's concern and spent some time talking to her about her family, work, and living situation. Jodi found that Sonya was working two jobs as a waitress/cook in a fast-food restaurant. She was divorced with two preteen

(Continues)

Case Study 3–1 (*Continued*)

children and was not receiving child support or any other assistance from her ex-husband. Now free of what was a relationship prone to domestic violence, Sonya stated that she was happy not to have any communication with him. Sonya did not have family in the local area and thus was having difficulty keeping up with the household expenses, as well as trying to be a supportive mother to her children. Sonya confided in Jodi that she had not consistently taken her oral medication because she could not afford to buy the medication and pay her bills. She tried to make sure her children got meals, but she often found it necessary to eat at work. She knew that fast food was not good for her but felt she had no choice. Certainly, there was limited time for a formal exercise program or shopping and preparing foods that would help keep her blood glucose under control as recommended by the previous health educators. Jodi realized that like many other clients who struggled with limited financial resources and little social support Sonya would require more than just knowledge to be able to take the steps necessary to address her health issues.

To that end, Jodi assured Sonya that she understood her situation and was going to help her develop a plan that offered the potential for her to reach her goal of controlling her blood glucose without insulin. She validated Sonya's ability to take the necessary steps with some help. Here rather than just providing information and direction to Sonya, Jodi assessed the entire person and identified the role Sonya's life situation played in her inability to control her blood glucose. Jodi set out to develop in partnership with Sonya a plan that was realistic in the context of Sonya's life situation.

First, Jodi worked with Sonya to identify potential programs that would help her get her oral medications for free or at a lower cost as part of a prescription-assistance program. She made an appointment for Sonya with the local Diabetes Association to insure that she got linked to resources for both peer support and assistance with dietary issues. Jodi made sure that Sonya not only received information on how she might improve her diet but also helped develop strategies on how this could be done while limiting the cost. Additionally, Jodi helped Sonya identify potential sources that would help her obtain assistance with the cost of her housing or help her identify, safe low-cost housing. Jodi was very aware that the daily stress Sonya experienced had an adverse effect on her health. Such stress was also an obstacle to her weight loss goals and was having an adverse affect on her glucose levels. Jodi knew that for Sonya to be successful in controlling her blood glucose, she would need to gain some sense of stability in her life situation. Additionally, Jodi gave Sonya her telephone number in the clinic and offered to be there when needed to talk through problems in implementing the steps they had agreed on to address her inability to control her blood glucose.

Sonya came back to the clinic 3 months later. Her blood glucose continued to be higher than desired; however, she had moved into a new apartment, had lost 10 pounds, and was excited about the progress that she had made. Sonya had gotten assistance with purchasing her medications, and she reported taking them as prescribed. She limited the amount of food she ate at her work and had learned how to cook for her family foods that helped her control her blood glucose levels and that were healthy for her children. Based on Sonya's progress, her physician agreed to let her continue work to control her glucose levels without being placed on insulin. Jodi had succeeded in helping Sonya positively address her health situation by understanding how an individual's life situation can influence their ability to adhere to health education messages and directives. Jodi realized that the environmental obstacles to reaching desired health outcomes are often greatest in disadvantaged individuals who struggle to provide the basic necessities of life for themselves and their family. Jodi astutely implemented this understanding by probing deeper into Sonya's life situation to determine what contextual obstacles she faced that prevented her from successfully responding to information provided by her physician and the health educators in the clinic.

REFERENCES

AFL-CIO. (2008). *Hot facts: America's broken health care system.* Retrieved April 22, 2008 from http://www.aflcio.org/issues/healthcare/facts_hot.cfm.

Brooks, S. (2004). *Poverty and schooling in the U.S.: contexts and consequences.* Mahwah, NJ: Lawrence Erlbaum Associates.

Brown, D. (2003). A concentrated model of mental well-being for African American women. In D. Brown & V. Keith (Eds.). *In and out of our right minds: the mental health of African American women.* New York: Columbia University Press.

Caffarella, R., & Merriam, S. (2000). Linking the individual learner to the context of adult learning (pp. 55–70). In A. Wilson & E. Hayes (Eds.). *Handbook of adults and continuing education.* San Francisco: Jossey-Bass.

Corcoran, M. (1995). Rags to rags: poverty and mobility in the United States. *Annual Sociology Review, 21,* 237–267.

Danziger, S., Sandefur, G., & Weinburg, D. (Eds.). (1994). *Confronting poverty: prescriptions for change.* Cambridge, MA: Harvard University Press.

Freire, P. (1970). *Pedagogy of the oppressed.* Translated by Myra Bergman Ramos. New York: Herder and Herder.

Gans, H. (1995). *The war against the poor: the underclass and antipoverty policy.* New York: Basic Books.

Goldberger, N. (1996). *Knowledge, difference, and power: essays inspired by women's ways of knowing.* New York: Basic Books.

Huston, A. (1991). *Children in poverty: child development and public policy.* New York: Cambridge University Press.

Jarvis, P. (1987). *Adult learning in the social context.* London: Croon Helm.

Knowles, M. (1970). *The modern practice of adult education: andragogy versus pedagogy.* New York: Association.

Merriam, S., & Caffarella, R. (1999). *Learning in adulthood: a comprehensive guide* (2nd ed.). San Francisco: Jossey-Bass.

Mezirow, J. (2006). An overview of transformative learning. In P. Sutherland & J. Crowther (Eds.). *Lifelong learning.* New York: Routledge.

Rank, M. (2005). *One nation, underprivileged.* New York: Oxford University Press.

Tisdell, E. (1998). Poststructural feminist pedagogies: the possibilities and limitations of feminist. *Adult Education Quarterly, 48,* 139–156.

Tough, A. (1971). The adult's learning projects: a fresh approach to theory and practice in adult learning. Toronto: Ontario Institute for Studies in Education.

U.S. Census Bureau. (2008). *Poverty highlights.* Retrieved April 22, 2008, from http://www.census.gov/prod/2007pubs/p60-233.pdf.

Wilson, W. (1987). *The truly disadvantaged: the inner city, the underclass, and public policy.* Chicago: The University of Chicago Press.

Chapter 4

Methods for Working with Cultural Diversity

Susan C. Scrimshaw

INTRODUCTION

Culture permeates everything about how each of us views and approaches health, illness, prevention, and healthcare systems. Everyone—healthcare providers, patients, families and, community members—brings cultural understanding and experience to their responses to health maintenance and illness. Because of this, healthcare providers must be aware of their own health beliefs and behaviors in order to listen to and understand their patients (Paul, 1955).

This chapter begins with some key definitions of concepts such as culture, culture change, ethnicity, and cultural processes. It then goes on to illustrate the importance of cultural influences in health care. It concludes with approaches healthcare providers can use to understand users of health care and to negotiate treatment options.

CULTURE

There are probably as many definitions of culture as there are cultures. A review of these definitions reveals a number of common elements, which are described later.

In the most basic sense, culture is everything that is socially learned and not genetically transmitted. Culture includes shared meanings, values, and ideas. People who share a common culture exhibit patterns of behavior that are guided by these shared ideas, meanings, and values. Culture includes language, norms guiding social interactions, and material culture such as how housing is organized and objects we use. In every culture, there is pressure to learn the culture and to conform to cultural norms. There is also pressure to believe that one's culture includes the "right" way to do things. Thus, most cultures are innately conservative.

Cultural norms, beliefs, and behaviors often exist at an unconscious level, which means that people are not always aware of why they do things and why some things are so important to them. To complicate matters, culture is far from static. Cultures are constantly changing through exposure to other cultures, new discoveries, and changes in norms and behaviors over time. For individuals, their own sense of culture is constantly being modified through lived experiences (Garro, 2003).

The concept of lived experiences revolves around the fact that we may be born into one or more cultures and live in several others (think about a contemporary young woman who was born and raised in Boston, whose mother was born and raised in India, and whose father is of East Indian extraction but was born and raised in Kenya). As we move from culture to culture, we often find ourselves surrounded by multiple cultures. We are influenced to some degree by all of these. As we move into professions, we also come under the influence of shared values, beliefs, skills, and other cultural elements within a profession. All of these shape how we think, what we know, how we interact, and how we feel. Both clinical practice and health promotion and prevention activities involving culture, ethnicity, and behavior need to take into account the dynamic nature of these and to see them as processes rather than as static categories.

Ethnicity implies some sharing of lived experience and learned traditions, including meanings and values. There is a great deal of overlap between ethnicity and culture, but ethnicity may also include some common factors such as country or region of origin, shared language, shared phenotype (outward physical characteristics). In the United States, ethnicity may be a self identification or may be defined by others.

In all of this, race is not a very accurate or useful concept. Steven Jay Gould summarizes it this way (Koch, 1995):

> Races aren't definable, and even if definable, not very well defined. Racial variation is the original geographic variation of

the species that spread, presumably from an African center, all over the world. . . . When you measure the actual genetic differences among people, they're astonishingly small.

From the perspectives of providing health care, a family or genetic history is far more important than any attempt to put someone in a meaningless category like race. For example, take a young woman who has an American Black mother and a father whose family is predominantly Ashkenazi Jews. Genetically, she should be tested for the Tay Sachs gene to determine risk to her future children. Nevertheless, she self-identifies as "black." At first glance, a healthcare provider would not see her as being a potential Tay Sachs carrier. She is one of many, many examples of people whose family or genetic history is far more important than their "racial" or ethnic self-identification.

This brings us to the fact that diversity in the United States is culturally and socially constructed. People are "placed" into ethnic and "racial" groups because we have cultural and social ideas about who belongs in those groupings, not because there is scientific evidence to create such groupings. Even the federal Office of Management and the Budget, which mandates these groupings, admits that there is no scientific basis for racial categories (1997 OMB Directive). Anthropologist Alan Goodman (2001) refers to these groupings as "sociopolitical realities." Unfortunately, the fact that race is not a valid concept for scientific measurement does not negate the fact that racism exists and shapes how people are seen, defined, and treated.

CULTURAL COMPETENCE

All of us bring our cultural experiences to our work in health care. Just as patients have beliefs and behaviors surround health and illness, so do we. Just as patients have social norms around respect, age and gender norms for communication, what is "late" and what is "pain," so do we. Our own cultural backgrounds, which may already be a complex blend, then are influenced by professional training, which brings an overlay of Western biomedical culture. It is critical to be aware of all of this as we attempt to maximize our cultural competence in health care and health maintenance.

Cultural competence in health care describes "the ability of systems to provide care to patients with diverse values, beliefs and behaviors, including tailoring delivery to meet patients' social, cultural, and linguistic needs" (Betancourt et al., 2002); therefore, cultural competency must include understanding and appreciation of health beliefs and behaviors in their cultural contexts and respectful strategies to negotiate optimum health in the context of these beliefs and behaviors. In order to do this, we must understand our own biases.

For example, many years ago, work by Zborowski (1952) demonstrated that different cultures have different perceptions of pain and different attitudes toward the meaning of pain. In general, the group they called New Englanders or "Old Americans" tended to deny the symptoms of pain and were generally opposed to taking medication. A healthcare provider from a culture where pain is more easily acknowledged might miss critical symptoms when interviewing someone from a culture where pain is denied.

Cultural competency means not only listening for symptoms, but also involves treating people in ways that are respectful with in their culture. In the U.S. biomedical culture, we tend to be very focused on solving the problem. In many other cultures, such as Latin America, Asia, and Africa, solving a clinical problem is important, but so is respectful treatment. This may include greeting a patient by name (with appropriate titles of respect, not always just the first name) and asking a few general questions about his or her well-being before beginning to discuss the clinical issue at hand. In many cultures, it is difficult for people to understand how a health practitioner can diagnose and treat a patient without ever touching him or her. As technology gets increasingly more sophisticated, medical encounters in which there is little or no physical examination are more frequent. Anthropologists often advise healthcare providers to conduct some sort of brief physical exam, even if it is something as simple as taking a pulse.

Perhaps the easiest way to approach this aspect of cultural competency is to bring common courtesy and respect to every medical encounter. It helps to think about what you would want for yourself or for a close relative. There is no question that current time pressures on the medical encounter make this more difficult, but also in the smallest word or gesture can make a big difference to an anxious patient. Practitioners also worry when they do not speak the language of their patient. Obviously, a good interpreter is very important, but many times patients report that the smile and the tone of voice and the general manner in which a practitioner treats them count far more than linguistic competence.

Healthcare providers in the United States today also have another strong resource: each other. People from many cultures mingle in today's healthcare settings. It is important to respect each other's deep cultural knowledge, to ask questions, and to create opportunities for learning and dialogue.

CULTURAL BELIEFS AND BEHAVIORS AROUND HEALTH AND ILLNESS

Vast literature in medical anthropology exists on the topic of cultural beliefs and behaviors around health and illness in cultures both in the United States and around the world. A recent summary of these can be found in Scrimshaw (2006).

In brief, definitions of health and illness vary not only by culture and ethnicity, but also by gender, age, and sometimes other factors such as socioeconomic status. They also vary by common illnesses in a given culture. For example, in parts of Africa, where malaria is endemic, mild cases of malaria are not necessarily defined as illness. If everyone has it, it becomes the norm. Unfortunately, we are beginning to see this pattern with diabetes in some communities in the United States. It is so common that people talk about "high sugar" as something you expect to get.

There are several tools to help us understand our perspectives on health and illness, as well as our patients. The first of these is the anthropological concept of *insider* and *outsider* views (Scrimshaw & Hurtado, 1987). *Insider* (*emic* in anthropological terminology) applies to the culture as viewed from within. It refers to the meaning that people attach to things from their cultural perspective. The *outsider* perspective (*etic* in anthropology) refers to the same thing as seen from the outside. Rather than meaning, it conveys a structural approach, or something as seen without understanding its meaning for a culture.

For example, I was conducting an in-service training on cultural competence to the staff at a hospital in Chicago where many patients are from Latin America. Before the training began, a stop in the restroom found a spotlessly clean facility. During the lunch break, another stop revealed small piles of toilet paper in the corner of each stall. I asked the staff why they thought this occurred, and they talked about "dirty" habits from other countries, their outsider view. Then I explained that in many public facilities in Latin America, toilets will stop up if paper is thrown into them. Instead, every bathroom has a wastebasket in each stall for toilet paper. From the insider perspective, the hospital's patients were being considerate, not deliberately "dirty." What was required was good signage and health education explaining that these Chicago toilets could, indeed, handle the paper. Aha!

The *insider–outsider* concept leads to another set of definitions. *Disease* is the outsider, usually the Western biomedical definition. It refers to an undesirable deviation from a measurable norm. Deviations in temperature, white cell count, red cell count, bone density, and many others are seen as indicators of disease. *Illness* on the other hand, means "not feeling well." Thus, it is a subjective, insider view. This sets the stage for conflicts between the two views. Someone can have an undesirable deviation from a Western biomedical norm and feel well. Hypertension, early stages of cancer, HIV infection, and early stages of diabetes are all instances in which people may feel well but have a disease. This means that healthcare providers must convince patients to treat a problem that is not causing symptoms.

It is also possible for someone to feel ill and for tests to fail to identify a disease. Western trained healthcare providers have a hard time dealing with this. Is it a "psychosomatic" problem? Is nothing wrong, but the patient wants attention? Sometimes another possibility is that Western biomedical science has not yet developed the correct test or measurement. Diseases such as AIDS, anxiety attacks, and chronic fatigue syndrome were all labeled psychosomatic at one time and now have measurable deviations from a biological norm. Similarly, painful menstruation used to be labeled "subconscious rejection of femininity" but is now associated with elevated prostaglandin levels and can be helped by a prostaglandin inhibitor.

In some instances, also, there are clusters of symptoms that are cultural learned responses to stress. They may get expressed in words like "*susto*" (literally in Spanish, "fright" refers to symptoms resulting from fright) or "spirit possession." These, too, may cause symptoms that cannot be analyzed through traditional medical means but that may indicate distress that needs treatment.

There are many insider ways to describe even symptoms that have clear diagnoses and names in the Western Biomedical system. Part of the work of a healthcare provider is to listen for these and to translate or decode them. Scrimshaw (2006) contains a listing of all of the categories of these from the medical anthropological literature, along with brief descriptions of each.

People bring their beliefs to bear on health through decisions that they make to maintain health and through decisions made when they, or someone close to them, becomes ill. In the past, sociologists referred to this decision-making process as "hierarchy of resort," but in reality, people engage in *patterns* of seeking solutions to illness (Scrimshaw & Hurtado, 1987). They may try an herbal tea at home, get something over the counter, see a doctor, and then ask someone to pray for them. There is no hierarchy here, just persistence in trying to solve the problem.

If patients come to you and feel that you do not understand them, cannot help them, or disrespect them, they will try something else. Also, if they do not understand what is expected of them, they may not take medication properly or at all. As the next section of this chapter describes, clear and culturally competent communication is essential.

COMMUNICATION

Health literacy is defined as "the degree to which individuals have the capacity to obtain, process, and understand basic health information and services needed to make appropriate health decisions" (U.S. Department of Health and Human Services, 2010). It is estimated that 90 million American adults may lack the needed literacy skills to effectively use the U.S. health system (Committee on Health Literacy, Board on Neuroscience and Behavioral Health, 2004).

It might be easy to think that the "problem" is then the patient, that people need to learn to read and understand health information better. In reality, health literacy is about more than literacy levels for individuals—it is about how healthcare providers communicate and about people's understanding of health concepts, regardless of literacy or educational levels. In many ways, it is about languages (medical and lay, English and over 200 others) and cultures that become barriers to understanding. We have multiple problems:

1. *There is a difference between medical versus lay terminology.* Someone with a PhD in physics may not understand what "diastolic" or "bronchodilator" or "iatrogenic" mean, to name just a few terms. What are HDL and LDL? How do they get that way? What is total cholesterol, and how do you add up the numbers? Why do the "ideal" numbers keep changing? Clear communication begins with plain speaking.
2. *We have individual and cultural differences around concepts.* What does maintain a "moderate" weight mean? To an anxious teen who wants to model, moderate weight may mean something clinically dangerously low (from the outsider, health practitioner perspective). To some women from Latin America or the Middle East, moderate weight will be heavier than U.S. norms, whereas a U.S. woman who fears she weighs too much might be viewed as dangerously thin in those cultures.
3. *There are meanings.* While working with prenatal care programs in Mexico, my team struggled with communicating the concept of risk in pregnancy as we developed materials to help women identify symptoms that meant that they should seek care. It turned out that the direct translation of "risk" into Spanish, or "*riesgo*," did not carry the same meaning.

When we explained the concept to women, they said: "Oh, you mean "*peligro.*" Peligro translates directly as "danger."

4. *There are language issues.* While doing research on seizure disorders in adolescents from three cultures, it became clear that the word "trauma" has two different meanings. It can mean psychological shock, or trauma, or it can mean physical trauma, such as a blow to the head. The exact same word "trauma" is used in Spanish, with the same two potential meanings. When talking with epileptic patients and their parents from Latino cultures, the neurologists used the word "trauma" as a cause of seizures, meaning "a blow to the head." The Latino parents, however, heard the psychological meaning and thought their children had been traumatized psychologically by some fright or shock.

All of these differences in how we express and hear each other affect our understanding of patient concerns and complaints, accurate diagnoses, patients' understanding of treatment, and follow-up to care. Not only is quality of care affected, but so is patient safety and patient and provider satisfaction.

Cultural and other factors that can lead to communication errors include the following:

- Language
- Gender
- Age (younger, older)
- Economic status
- Social class
- Ethnicity/culture (not just language)
- Blind
- Deaf, hard of hearing

Communication errors can have serious consequences. One asthma medication has a label indicating "take two puffs twice a day." Does this mean one puff two times or two puffs each time for a total of four? The meaning is ambiguous, but the consequences of overdosing or underdosing can be serious. In another example, many people have expressed confusion over how and when to eat grapefruit if someone is on Lipitor or a similar medication.

One study in California found an average of 31 errors per pediatric clinic visit. Two thirds of these had clinical consequences. They included the dose and duration of prescribed drugs and missed information on patient allergies.

Errors were most common with untrained interpreters. For example, an oral dose of amoxicillin for an ear infection was translated as 1 teaspoon three times a day in the ears. Twice a day for 3 or 4 days was translated as "in 4 days" (Flores et al., 2003).

BECOME A CULTURALLY COMPETENT HEALTHCARE PROVIDER

An anthropologist and physician team wrote a seminal article in 1981 arguing for a meaning centered approach to clinical practice (Good & Good, 1981). Their advice is summarized in the discussion that follows.

Good and Good (1981) note that

Groups vary in the specificity of their medical complaints.

Groups vary in their style of medical complaining.

Groups vary in the nature of their anxiety about the meaning of symptoms.

Groups vary in their focus on organ systems.

Groups vary in their response to therapeutic strategies.

For example, the "old Americans" described by Zborowski will describe pain in functional terms. For an eye infection, they will say, "It's hard to thread a needle," whereas members of one of the more expressive cultures studied said this: "My eye hurts." Both the specificity and the style are different. Their anxiety also varied. Old Americans dismissed the pain and refused medication. Members of another of the cultures studied interpreted the symptoms with fear of the worst possible outcome. "My eye hurts. I have a brain tumor. I'm going to die." They refused medication because of fear of the side effects. Thus, these groups showed different responses to therapeutic strategies.

There are also cultural differences in focus on organ systems. Good and Good talk about a Chinese woman on cardiac medication who kept complaining of pain to her heart. Her healthcare providers kept changing her medication to no avail. Finally, the anthropologist discovered that her son had died, and she was describing emotional pain, not physical, using the heart as a focus. In Latin America, women will often locate discomfort in the uterus. They may have indigestion, a bladder infection, or something else, but the uterus is the focus.

Given the propositions discussed previously, the conclusion is that human illness is fundamentally semantic or meaningful. It may have a biological base but is a human experience. As a result, clinical practice is inherently interpretive (Good & Good, 1981). Healthcare providers must understand the difference between language and culture and address both.

They must work with individuals and families to define problems and develop solutions. This results in a "to do" list for health practitioners.

1. Elicit patients' requests.
2. Elicit and decode patients' semantic networks.
3. Distinguish disease and illness and develop plans for managing problems.
4. Elicit explanatory modes of patients and families, analyze conflict with biomedical model and negotiate alternatives.

For example, a teenager is brought in by her parents because she "fell out" at school and the school said she had to be checked before she could come back. Her parents think she is fine. Falling out is normal when people are stressed. When you ask about falling out, you learn the insider view that it means fainting for a brief time, that it happens when people feel stressed, and that it just means that they need some attention. You agree that such things indeed can happen (show respect for the insider view, and people can faint under stress as a culturally learned response). You also explain that sometimes losing consciousness can mean that something is wrong with your body or your brain, and you want to check it out and be sure. They agree to let you run some tests, and you rule out a seizure but discover that she is diabetic. You then proceed to explain diabetes, emphasize the need for treatment, and refer the young woman to a specialist. All of this may be more difficult than it sounds!

This example describes a success. For an excellent account of a communication failure, read *A Spirit Catches You and You Fall Down: A Hmong Child, Her American Doctors, and the Collision of Two Cultures* (Fadiman, 1997).

In general, dialogue with patients has been found most effective to verify understanding. Having patients explain/demonstrate prevention and treatment options is essential. Finally, multiple sources of reinforcement work best for health behavior change. The diabetic young woman described previously will need to hear from her doctor, a dietician, a health educator, peers, written literature, and other sources to reinforce her understanding and acceptance of her treatment. There are even computer games for children with diabetes and asthma to help them understand their diseases.

SUMMARY AND CONCLUSIONS

Providing culturally competent care improves the overall quality of care through a better understanding of patient concerns, knowledge, understanding, and complaints. Patient understanding of treatment, diagnosis, and patient follow-up to care needs is far more effective when clear and respectful communication has taken place. Both patient and provider satisfaction also improve.

Cultural competency must include understanding and appreciation of health beliefs and behaviors in their cultural contexts and respectful strategies to negotiate optimum health in the context of these beliefs and behaviors. All health professionals must learn cultural competency, including understanding health behavior, and the ability to communicate clearly. In the long run, both those seeking health care and those providing it benefit.

REFERENCES

Betancourt, J. R., Green, A. R., & Carrillo, J. E. (2002). *Cultural competence in health care: emerging frameworks and practical approaches.* The Commonwealth Fund, New York, NY.

Board on Neuroscience and Behavioral Health. Institute of Medicine. Institute of Medicine of the National Academies. Committee on Communication for Behavior Change in the 21st Century: Improving the Health of Diverse Populations. (2002). *Speaking of health: assessing health communication strategies for diverse populations.* Washington, DC: The National Academies Press.

Committee on Health Literacy, Board on Neuroscience and Behavioral Health. (2004). *Health literacy: a prescription to end confusion.* In L. Nielsen-Bohlman, A. M. Panzer, & D. Kindig (Eds.). Washington, DC: Institute of Medicine of the National Academies, The National Academies Press.

Fadiman, A. (1997). *A spirit catches you and you fall down: a Hmong child, her American doctors, and the collision of two cultures.* New York, NY: Farrar, Straus, and Giroux.

Flores, G., Laws, M. B., Mayo, S. J., Zuckerman, B., Abreu, M., Medina, L., & Hardt, E. J. (2003). Errors in medical interpretation and their potential clinical consequences in pediatric encounters. *Pediatrics, 111,* 6–14.

Garro, L. (2003). Narrating troubling experiences. *Transcultural Psychiatry, 40*(1), 5–43.

Good, B. J., & Good, M. J. D. (1981). The meaning of symptoms: a cultural hermeneutic model for clinical practice. In L. Eisenberg & A. Kleinman (Eds.). *The relevance of social science for medicine* (pp. 165–196). Dordrecht, Holland: Reidel.

Goodman, A. (2001). Biological diversity and cultural diversity: from race to radical bioculturalism. In I. Susser & T. C. Patterson (Eds.). *Cultural Diversity in the United States* (pp. 29–49). Malden, MA: Blackwell.

Koch, J. (1995). Stephen Jay Gould: the interview. *The Boston Globe Magazine.* December 31, 14.

Paul, B. (Ed.). (1955). *Health, culture, and community* (pp. 71–103). New York: Russell Sage Foundation.

Scrimshaw, S. C. (2006). Culture, behavior, and health. In M. Merson, R. Black, & A. Mills (Eds.). *International public health: diseases, programs, systems and policies* (2nd ed., pp. 43–64). Sudbury, MA: Jones and Bartlett Publishers.

Scrimshaw, S. C. M., & Hurtado, E. (1987). *Rapid assessment procedures for nutrition and primary health: anthropological approaches to programme improvement.* Tokyo: UCLA Latin American Center, the United Nations University, and UNICEF.

U.S. Department of Health and Human Services. (2000). *Healthy people 2010: understanding and improving health.* Washington, DC: U.S. Department of Health and Human Services. Available from: www.healthypeople.gov/

U.S. Office of Management and Budget. (1997). Revisions to the standards for the classification on federal data on race and ethnicity. *Federal Register, 62*(131), 36847–36946. Washington, DC: Author.

Zborowski, M. (1952). Cultural components in responses to pain. *Journal of Social Issues, 8,* 16–30.

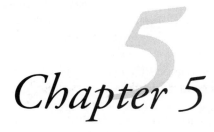

Chapter 5

Supporting Patient Literacy Using Technology

Madalaine Pugliese & Karen Janowski

INTRODUCTION

It is commonly recognized that the use of printed health education materials or information pamphlets can result in readability or usability challenges (Sand-Jecklin, 2007; Pignone et al., 2006; Shohet & Renaud, 2006; Powers & Bosworth, 2006). Nevertheless, healthcare organizations continue to provide patients with less than effective health education materials. Today's more global and mobile society creates the need for more innovative approaches to health education.

Our increasingly diverse population also brings a range of issues to consider. For example, English is not the primary language for many patients. Nevertheless, these patients still need to describe symptoms and understand medical care instructions. Every patient depends on the healthcare provider to communicate understandable information. It is critical that the communication between patient and healthcare provider be effective in order to work toward positive outcomes. Assessing the patient's ability to exchange information about health literacy is the primary consideration to this type of effective communication (Cassey, 2007).

Oftentimes, economic or political factors at an institution may interfere with the development of effective educational materials. In some cases, there is a lack of resources or a lack of support for the development of the modified materials. The time and expense of testing the efficacy of draft materials may be believed to be prohibitive due to the competitive necessity to endure financially over other organizations. In other cases, leaders may assume that another organization will create the more detailed or perhaps more expensive materials in support of less literate patients. If this translated material is not created when the need is determined because perhaps budget does not permit, this might isolate patients that require a modification to educational literature (Gal & Prigat, 2005). The process for development of support materials that contain factual, expert, credible, and accurate information seems to be causing the usability challenges. It may be that the creator of the materials needs to know more about using the certain features available in existing tools in which these materials are created. Knowing certain features in design tools, such as the ability to use a thesaurus to find a word that might be clearer in creating instructions, could make an enormous difference. Creating effective health education materials ought to be considered not merely as a specialized process or mechanical procedure, but also as an ethical obligation between health organizations and patients. The effectiveness of health education resources must be evaluated based on their ability to influence a patient's understanding of his or her health condition (Gal & Prigat, 2005).

Why are health education pamphlets and other print materials needed? In "Health Literacy: A Prescription to End Confusion," the Institute of Medicine reports that "people with low health literacy are hospitalized more often and for longer periods of time, use emergency departments more frequently, and, for those with asthma or diabetes, manage their diseases less proficiently." Quite obviously, the absence of accommodations for low patient literacy can have direct financial impact on any organization.

Health education materials are essentially intended to facilitate a health organization's ability to convey accurate medical information to patients. The Joint Commission has emphasized, within its accreditation standards, the importance of fulfilling the fundamental right and need for patients to receive oral and written information that they can understand. Furthermore, accredited organizations are explicitly encouraged to ensure patient understanding (The Joint Commission, 2007); however, effective health education materials also serve to maintain the integrity and efficiency of the organization. Strong and effective health education materials provide credibility, leading to the business opportunity to market or promote the organization with potential stakeholders. Administrative ambitions could include the goals of making the public more conscious of available services, attracting new patients, or pointing patients in appropriate directions. Traditionally, a flier or pamphlet is a concrete or substantial artifact that can highlight an organization in such a manner to increase stature and have influence on internal policy and even potential distribution of resources. Used as a means of communicating an image to other professional institutions, often such materials are seen as potentially providing for both patient education as well as a marketing tool (Gal & Prigat, 2005).

Significant numbers of patients, however, may not be able to understand critical information because of vocabulary, writing approach, or presentation. Guidelines for the creating, writing, and testing of readable and user-friendly resources are available (Duffy, 1985), and studies have demonstrated the successful outcomes when implementing these guidelines from the perspective of more effective learning (Thompson et al., 2004). Although most organizations were uncertain how many years of education would be needed to ensure understanding of the printed materials, several estimated a range of 8th- through 12th-grade levels. No specific rationale was offered for these estimates (Gal & Prigat, 2005).

Why do organizations continue to produce health education materials with ineffective results that appear inappropriate for their intended function? How might technology play a role in changing these dynamics in such a way that patients better understand their own health care? If there are ways that technology can better facilitate patient literacy, it is important that we identify not only some possibly useful tools but also some potential strategies for implementation. This chapter is dedicated to defining or perhaps redefining patient literacy in the 21st century, identifying potentially useful technologies in support of patient literacy, discussing the impact of legislation that supports the implementation of these strategies, and making recommendations for pragmatic next steps that organizations might consider toward improving patient understanding.

WHAT IS PATIENT LITERACY?

A definition of health literacy has been offered by the Institute of Medicine (2004) in its report "Health Literacy: A Prescription to End Confusion":

> Health literacy is defined as the degree to which individuals have the capacity to obtain, process, and understand basic health information and services needed to make appropriate health decisions.

People need to be able to understand the information that is provided to them. Because traditional print materials assume some measure of literacy, the challenge to the consumer lies in the ability to recognize and understand the health information that is presented. When our purpose is to create materials that promote understanding of their own health and the health of their families, we need to focus on creating materials that match the patient's ability in reading to learn. The alternative—inappropriate design that requires a patient to learn to read—is not effective and not acceptable. We must make sure that health education materials focus on effective communication of critical information and avoid forcing the reader to struggle through decoding meaningless information that has been presented in challenging ways.

At the heart of any reading or literacy activity is the understanding or meaning taken from the print and graphic information contained in the document. In order for learning to occur, a patient must be aware that the purpose of the activity is to obtain meaning. The reader must learn how to read specifically as it relates to the task of learning from the pamphlet. This is commonly called reading to learn as opposed to the mechanical task of learning to read (Collins, 1994). A significant consideration in reading to learn is the patient's previous experience or motivation. Research suggests that successful readers tend to relate information in print to previous knowledge; less successful readers showed little tendency to use their knowledge to clarify the printed materials when presented with new information (Collins, 1994).

As we can see in **Table 5-1,** literacy issues affect a significant portion of American society. These patients must be supported in reading to learn about their own medical conditions.

Table 5-1 Assessment of Adult Literacy

- A large segment of the American population has basic (29%) to below basic (14%) prose literacy skills.
- An additional five percent are nonliterate in English.
- About half of the U.S. adult population has difficulty using text to accomplish everyday tasks.
- The ability of the average American to use numbers is even lower—33% have basic, and 22% have below basic quantitative skills. These skills include the ability to solve one-step arithmetic problems (basic) and simple addition (below basic).
- Most Americans (44%) fall into the "intermediate" level of prose literacy. That is, they can apply information from moderately dense text and make simple inferences.
- Even those who are most proficient at using text and numbers may be compromised in the understanding of healthcare information when they are challenged by sickness and feelings of vulnerability.

Source: National Assessment of Adult Literacy (2003). National Center for Education Statistics, U.S. Department of Education.

Low literacy and low health literacy are two distinct issues. For example, a patient may demonstrate adequate literacy skills but be challenged by health-related concepts and instructions, resulting in errors in healthcare decisions (Schwartzberg et al., 2007).

Low health literacy occurs when individuals have difficulty understanding health-related information, resulting in inappropriate health decisions. It is not enough for the patient to be aware of the lack of understanding or inability to comprehend. In fact, a patient must be able to advocate for materials that match his or her ability to understand the information that is being communicated. This fact can not be overemphasized as we know that low literacy is associated with lower levels of health (Hemmings & Langille, 2006).

In making important healthcare decisions, patients are often faced with a variety of text-based materials, including patient education brochures, medication labels, consent forms, and discharge information. A number of informal assessment strategies might provide insight as to a patient's literacy abilities:

- Does the patient attend appointments or education meetings as they are scheduled? In other words, does the patient understand how to read the scheduled date and time and then follow up appropriately?
- When literature is presented, does the patient read key information? Does the patient instead tuck the flier inside a pocket and mention that it will be read later? This might be a clue that the patient requires support outside of that provided during the appointment. Patients may be reluctant to disclose their difficulties with reading; to avoid embarrassment, they may immediately pocket the information and avert disclosure of literacy challenges.
- Can the patient articulate his or her medication protocols or schedule? Does the patient seem to understand the timing for taking prescription medications or follow-up recommendations? If the patient has difficulty repeating or paraphrasing instructions, this may be an indication that there is a lack of understanding. For example, an informal health literacy evaluation through observation and presentation of print materials might be a sign that a specific language is needed as well as limited ability to read in any language (Cassey, 2007).

Empowering patients to become informed participants in their own health care is essential but must go beyond merely simplifying the language used in instructional materials. Literacy can be improved when patients are assisted in making connections between previous experience and new information being presented to them.

Hoffman and Worrall (2004) admit that it is common practice to provide patient education only in the verbal format despite recommendations to include supplemental written materials. Written materials offer an economical solution to patient instruction as well as other advantages, including the following:

- Message consistency
- Reusability, portability
- Flexibility of delivery
- Permanence of information that may be more easily remembered

Hoffman and Worrall (2004) further identify several factors that should be included in well-designed, effective health education materials, including the following:

- Clearly stated prose
- Accurate content
- Readability at the 5th- to 6th-grade level
- Use of bulleted lists where possible
- Summaries of the main points
- Clear layout and typography
- Quality illustrations that enhance the reader's understanding
- Features that require a response from the reader such as a blank area to write questions, answer a short quiz, or list three things that the reader should do next

Features that optimize patient understanding have been identified and described; however, what happens in the presence of difficulty using orally presented information due to memory, comprehension, sensory, or cognitive deficits? What happens in the presence of difficulty accessing printed materials due to low literacy, vision, learning or cognitive deficits, or physical limitations? Before we can address these questions, we must reexamine what it means to be literate in the 21st century.

REDEFINING LITERACY IN THE 21ST CENTURY

Educational Testing Service's Center for Global Assessment defines literacy as the ability to use "digital technology, communications tools, and/or networks to access, manage, integrate, evaluate, and create information in order to function in a knowledge society" (International Information and Communication Technologies Literacy Panel, 2002, p. 2). Even though the classic definition of literacy still resonates, people today must be able to make sense of information and communicate thoughts using an array of media.

Classically, literacy involves a person's capacity to read, write, listen, and speak. This definition has evolved over time. In the early 20th century, simple literacy indicated a person's ability to write his or her own name. By the mid 20th century, this evolved to mean the decoding of print and the ability to articulate ideas in writing (21st Century Literacy Summit, 2002).

The impact of technology is reflected in current use of the Internet as a health information resource. Information found on the Internet has doubled in volume every year since 1990. Its content is unquantifiable and requires new literacy skills in order to make good use in harvesting appropriate information. In light of the power that comes with access to such rich and extremely useful information, it is critical that people acquire sufficient skills to take advantage of this medium to support learning new information. The knowledge and skills that are fundamental for meaningful use of this medium have typically been considered as a new form of information literacy for the 21st century. A person must be able to acknowledge or understand when information is needed and have the ability to search for and then access that information. The American Library Association's Presidential Committee on Information Literacy adds that a person must be able to effectively use or apply information once it is found (California School Library Association, 2004). With the increased focus on understanding in today's more global society, it is important to understand that everyone can benefit from learning 21st century literacy skills in order that they effectively apply or take advantage of information access in support of their daily needs.

As we have already established, however, a patient's ability to take advantage of any information might present a variety of challenges. How might we use technology to facilitate better patient understanding in today's media-rich world? How might we use the technology to create better access to information and mitigate patient understanding? Why use technology for literacy?

Patient education incorporates the teaching of health-related knowledge from a variety of sources to the patients, as well as incorporating the necessary skills for applying this information into their lives. Nurses and therapists often play a significant part in the creation of imaginative strategies that facilitate patient learning. Multimedia technologies are powerful tools for designing meaningful materials that can be incredibly influential and effective in educating patients.

For example, the use of technology as a patient education tool provides many advantages over traditional health education methods in the presence of low literacy or other special needs. The most common methods of instruction are language-based and consist of verbal directions, printed text, or a combination of both. Many patients struggle with comprehending and retaining verbally presented information, and those with low literacy may experience limited comprehension of written instruction. Houts et al. (2006) evaluated the effects of picture use on health education and found that when compared with text alone, a combination of pictures with text or oral directions significantly increased the recall of health education content.

In a metastudy of 32 research articles published in peer-reviewed journals that evaluated computer-based patient education, Lewis (2003) found significant changes in knowledge acquisition and in clinical outcomes, as well as improvement in self-care behaviors when patients used computer-based health education programs. Furthermore, there were documented improvements in social support of participants who engaged in online computer support groups. One study described the benefit of an interactive graphic and audio program to overcome low literacy. Computer-based patient education was found to be effective for all ages, including older patients with limited computer familiarity. The author concluded that "computer-based patient education is an effective strategy for presenting information and improving knowledge outcomes" (Lewis, p. 95).

One caution expressed by Lewis concerned the readability level of web-based material. Her concern is supported by a study conducted by Graber et al. (1999) evaluating 50 samples of patient information on the Internet. The investigators found that on average the readability level of information on the Internet was at the 10.2 grade level, well above the comprehension level of many patients.

When patients are in a clinical setting, we cannot assume that they have processed verbally presented information. The use of text alone offers a limited two-dimensional environment that may be challenging for some patients who will be expected to follow prescribed exercise regimens, postoperative precautions, or rehabilitation programs.

The use of multimedia resources to reinforce what they have learned in the clinical setting can address a variety of learning styles. Patient understanding is greatly enhanced by combining verbal directions with video representation of the expected patient activity. Presenting information in this manner taps into the benefit of offering multiple methods of representation and promotes patient engagement to augment patient understanding.

For example, there are computer-based video software programs (iMovie on the Macintosh and Movie Maker or PhotoStory in Windows) that are simple to use and offer the potential of building a patient care video library that can offer such accommodations as multiple language tracks, closed caption, and described video. It is also possible to use digital cameras, digital video recorders, or cell phones to record information visually as it is presented. One inexpensive option is the Flip Video (http://www.theflip.com/). This is easily connected to any computer via a USB connection. The software is instantly installed and easily downloaded to create a review video in a CD format or post it online. This offers an additional method to support patient adherence to instruction and correct performance of exercise or self-care skills on discharge or when the clinician is no longer readily available. This concept is further discussed in Chapter 14. A study conducted by Maasland et al. (2007) suggests that the amount of exposure to multimedia health instruction may also influence the effectiveness of the instruction. Maasland et al. (2007) evaluated the effectiveness of a multimedia computer based program on the health education of patients who sustained a transient ischemic attack or a minor stroke in a randomized, controlled study. They found no significant differences in acquired health knowledge between the experimental group that completed a 20-minute multimedia program and received health education from a physician and the control group that only received health education from a physician. This study suggests that a one-time exposure to a brief multimedia program that included slide shows and oral information is insufficient for improving health literacy.

There may also be value in using video instruction to teach patients physical exercises that may be part of a home exercise program. Lysack et al. (2005) compared the use of computer-aided video instruction using a television and videotape recorder with routine rehabilitation practice to follow a home exercise program prescribed after a total hip or total knee replacement. The control group received daily inpatient care consisting of 30 minutes of physical therapy, 30 minutes of occupational therapy, and two 1-hour group exercise classes daily until discharge. At discharge, they received a printed handout of home exercises. The experimental group received identical rehabilitation, as well as a customized videotape of the exercises to be performed on discharge. No statistical differences in compliance and satisfaction were found between the two groups 4 weeks after discharge. The mean age of participants was 64.8 years. Despite the lack of clear benefit of video exercise instruction in this population, it will be helpful to continue to explore and seek to identify populations that will benefit from digital video modeling.

Many times patients seek information from online resources or are referred to the Internet by healthcare providers. According to Agarwal and Day (1998), "hands-on" experience gained while using the Internet "provides a better understanding of the subject matter and makes the learning process more active."

The importance of evaluating the readability of online materials can not be overlooked. Graber et al. assessed the readability level of 50 randomly selected web-based medical information sites and found that they were written, on average, at a 10th-grade, 2nd-month reading level using the Flesch reading score and the Flesch-Kinkaid reading level. Evaluating online readability levels and adapting material appropriately remain priorities.

The fact remains that the healthcare provider is responsible for directing patients to valid and reliable sources, including those accessed through the Internet. The Internet includes current, reliable information as well as misleading or unreliable information. Cassey (2007) exhorts healthcare professionals to become knowledgeable about high-quality, accurate, peer-reviewed online health resources. How does one determine the reliability of a particular website? The ability to conduct an effective online search that leads to up-to-date, accurate information is an essential skill for health educators today; therefore, when evaluating Internet Health Information that may be shared with patients, it is vital to consider the following questions (adapted from http://www.fda.gov/oc/opacom/evalhealthinfo.html):

1. Who runs the website? Is this information prominently displayed? Review the "About Us" link to find out who authors the site.
2. What is the purpose of the site? Determine whether the site is trying to disseminate information, sell a product, or raise money. The most reliable sites are those that disseminate information with clear language devoid of promises or sales pitches.
3. What is the URL of the website? Sites that end in .gov are sponsored by the federal government. Sites that end in .edu are associated with universities or medical schools. Sites that end with .org are run by nonprofit groups and often include a focus on research and health education. Be cautious about .com sites, as these are usually commercial sites and may try to sell particular products.
4. How is the information on the website documented? Look for references from medical journals, and review the medical credentials of those who contribute to the site.
5. How current is the information on the website? Is the review date posted? This date is often found at the bottom of the web page. Check to ensure

that the hyperlinks are not broken. Many broken links suggest that the site is not maintained or up-to-date.

6. How does the website choose links to other sites? Does the site include advertising or paid links? Review the linking policy in the "About This Web Site" section.

7. Does the website collect information about visitors and, if so, for what purpose? Websites that require subscriptions or memberships collect personal information about their visitors. Review the "Privacy Statement" on each website.

8. Is it possible to contact the website owners? Review the "Contact Us" link to ensure the ability to contact the site owners.

WHAT ARE SOME USEFUL TECHNOLOGIES AND STRATEGIES FOR IMPLEMENTATION?

Healthcare professionals have the responsibility to be proactive in presenting information in ways that increase patient understanding, despite the presence of limited literacy, low health literacy, and sensory, cognitive, physical, or other learning disabilities. Technology offers the power to provide improved educational understanding for those patients that might need it the most.

Developments in assistive special education technology first began in the early 1970s. In 1988, assistive technologies were defined under the Technology-Related Assistance for Individuals with Disabilities Act of 1988 (see the legislation section of this chapter). Ever since, the field of assistive technology has experienced significant growth as important new tools have been developed. The use of assistive technology tools has become widespread. Assistive technology specialists, skilled in assessing unique needs and finding tools that mitigate challenges, are working in schools and public agencies to support individuals with learning or literacy challenges, including people with diverse cultural situations, who have experienced unfulfilled needs. Professionals must find ways to consider multiple approaches during the teaching process in order to make important information as accessible for patients as possible. Using technology tools may assist patients and families to understand and perhaps use existing resources better in order to become well informed with regard to their health or related healthcare issues (Parette et al., 2005). (Every state and US territory has an Assistive Technology Act Program [AT Program] funded under the provisions of the Technology-Related Assistance Act of 1988 and reauthorized under the AT Act of 2004. Refer to the AT Program in your state for additional assistive technology resources and services that are available.)

Along with these specialized assistive technologies, we have numerous options to consider in support of patient literacy and education, including but not limited to computers, hand-held language support aids, and mp3 players. Access to information and communication can be facilitated in a multitude of ways. Using learning technologies is successful when patients can use or apply information effectively in their own lives (see Chapter 15).

Consider, for example, sensory challenges. If vision presents a challenge to a patient's ability to use printed text, this information might be offered in a digital form so that computer-based screen reading software can offer the content in an auditory form. The screen reader provides synthesized speech translation of any content found on the screen.

Alternatively, if hearing presents a barrier for communicating with a patient, the text-to-speech features that are built into computer operating systems might support literacy. Patients who are hearing impaired as well as those diagnosed with a learning disability can take advantage of built-in text-to-speech support tools that are available in all computers thanks to the Americans with Disabilities Act (see the legislation section of this chapter). Text-to-speech technologies convert visual digital text into auditory synthesized speech using a range of features that can assist a patient with researching and ease of reading information. If print information is not in a digital form, the use of a scanner and optical character recognition (OCR) software can literally convert a needed flier into a digital file. OCR software converts printed, paper-based text into editable digital text and comes installed on some scanners. It is essential to use good-quality OCR software when converting a printed brochure that may include tables or other graphics. Two examples of excellent OCR software include ABBYY FineReader Professional Version and Omnipage Pro (the most recent versions of each). After the file is digital, it becomes flexible. Text can be enlarged; a voice can be attached for multisensory feedback. Furthermore, text can be copied and pasted into a word-processing document where additional manipulation is possible. Fonts, font colors, and color backgrounds can be selected that promote text access.

Cognitive challenges present a completely different set of barriers in the patient education process. Although patients with cognitive challenges also experience barriers with access to print information, there are a range of solutions afforded by technology. Special software such as Writing with Symbols by Mayer-Johnson, Inc. (http://www.mayer-johnson.com/) can be used to support or enhance text with pictures or universal symbols in order to provide graphic interpretation of the information. For example, tasks that a patient might need to follow during home care might be simplified or broken down into manageable chunks of information by providing a picture-supported schedule. If the information has been converted to a digital format, two features built into Microsoft Word can be of benefit. It is possible to use the autosummarize feature found under the Tools toolbar in Word, which changes the volume of information, depending on the length of the summary selected, to a more readable level that is easier to understand. The Readability Statistic feature allows one to easily determine the readability level of the text and make adjustments as necessary to ease conversion to a more simplified language presentation.

Patients with physical challenges can activate such computer operating system features as Sticky Keys, which is designed to turn a simultaneous set of keystrokes into a sequence instead. This permits the patient to use only one pointing device to activate one key at a time to give a command rather than of having to hold down more than one key at a time. Suppose a patient has significant motor challenges in using his hands for typing, yet he or she wishes to search the Internet for medical information related to his or her health. Perhaps this patient uses a pointing device in order to access each key, one at a time. How then could this single pointing device be used in circumstances when the patient is required to type one key while holding down another? These simultaneous key strokes, for example, typing the shifted character @ symbol, are impossible for this patient to type. Activating Sticky Keys permits this patient to use his or her pointer to first press the shift key, which is then electronically held down for him or her. While that first key is being electronically held down, then he or she can press the next key as a sequence, but because of Sticky Keys, the computer thinks that the patient typed the two keys simultaneously together. This example is one of several features that are freely designed and included in computer operating systems so that anyone can use the equipment with equal facility. Chapter 15 discusses additional information with regard to built-in accessibility features.

Beyond these free, built-in modifications offered within computer operating systems, an enormous variety of commercially manufactured access devices are available in support of any physical barrier to using computers. Light-tech devices such as key guards can lie across the keyboard, helping to prevent unwanted keystrokes. A key guard lets a patient rest his hand across the guard while poking through a hole just over the key in order to press it. More high-tech devices such as alternate keyboards, mouse replacements, screen modifications, and other adaptive devices are typically prescribed for individual users by assistive technology specialists following an intricate assessment process. Although some patients will require this assessment simply to access a computer, certain access devices such as a track ball, joystick, or a touch screen to replace the mouse or enlarged key labels for the keyboard might prove useful in any teaching and learning environment.

Communication devices offer tools for facilitating two-way information exchange between healthcare providers and patients with speech challenges. These devices combine a visual target with synthesized speech so that a non-speaking patient might be able to initiate and participate in critical conversation. Communication devices are equipment designed to help patients with speech or writing difficulties to exchange concepts. At its very simplest, augmentative communication can be a page with picture choices or alphabet letters that a person points to. It can also involve highly sophisticated speaking computers with on-screen symbols for communication. An impressive range of devices offers options from light-tech tools that are simple to operate through to high-tech dynamic display devices that are significantly more intricate. A light-tech tool might be a battery-operated button and only speak one simple, but very important message. For example, a single emergency message recorded under single button might permit the patient to quickly let you know when he feels sick. One popular single message device is called the BIGmack communicator by AbleNet (http://www.ablenetinc.com/). A high-tech tool, typically prescribed by an augmentative communication specialist, might be a portable computer running an intricate communication symbol-based software program that speaks any message designed by the user. Boardmaker with Speaking Dynamically Pro software by Mayer-Johnson, Inc. (http://www.mayer-johnson.com) offers thousands of symbols and hundreds of templates for making electronic communication boards in a choice of over 40 languages. Symbols may be placed with no text, one language above the symbol, or any two languages above the symbol. A variety of universal symbol sets or photographs can be used either in print or mounted on a device for basic language exchange during health related interviews. For example, a patient with speech limitations might point to a picture that shows a person with a sore body part, whereas the communication device artificially speaks the message "my head hurts." Specific symbol sets are available for varying conditions in order that patients can communicate detailed specific information with regard to their medical condition. Another way that communication devices might play a role is in providing an opportunity for two-way question and answer exchanges. Questions from patients about their diagnosis and specific recommendations can be clarified because tools facilitate the exchange. Impressive amounts of research exist that examine successful partner-assisted communication techniques. Prompting hierarchy indicates that sometimes a single symbol is enough to evoke understanding of a concept. Depending on the patient, at other times, more deliberate partner-focused questions are needed. Efficient communication outcomes can enhance the quality of life for individuals who have significant speech and language challenges.

Hoffman and Worrall (2004) have shown the importance of incorporating features that require patient's response to printed materials, such as completing a quiz or identifying three things that they will do as a result of learning the information; however, some patients may experience barriers to providing their response. To resolve this challenge, several technologies might be employed to assist computer-based writing, such as word prediction or picture-based software. Word prediction software programs (such as WordQ [http://wordq.com] or Co:Writer [http://donjohnston.com]) supply a ready vocabulary bank that a patient might use to assist with producing written text. Picture-based writing software, such as Writing with Symbols (http://www.mayer-johnson.com) or Pix Writer (http://www.slatersoftware.com/), that provides representation of key vocabulary in symbols or pictures might support a patient in communicating his or her thoughts using pictures. Activating built-in text-to-speech features and hearing written words "read" back will allow a patient to correct errors more easily.

As we researched information for this chapter, the authors were surprised to learn how little information is available describing methods for adapting written materials to maximize accessibility for all patients. Much has been written about effective communication strategies such as simplifying language, speaking slowly, reading material out loud, using a teach back model, underlying key points (Schwartzberg et al., 2007), or designing effective printed materials using best practice principles (Hoffman & Worrall, 2004), but there was no research that addressed the critical need to adapt instructional materials using readily available technology to overcome barriers to material access. Hopefully, these suggestions will highlight an area that is frequently overlooked in the field of health education.

WHAT RESEARCH AND LEGISLATION SUPPORTS TECHNOLOGY IMPLEMENTATION?

Setting the Stage: Legislative Mandates

There are several legislative mandates that have increased awareness about accessibility and individuals with disabilities. Section 504 of the Rehabilitation Act of 1973, which required all federal agencies to make information technology accessible for individuals with disabilities, is widely regarded as the first civil rights legislation that addressed disability issues in the workplace. In 1998, Section 508 was added to the Rehabilitation Act to define electronic and information technology, in part, as "any equipment or interconnected system or subsystem of equipment, that is used in the creation, conversion, or duplication of data or information." In addition, "(ii) individuals with disabilities who are members of the public seeking information or services from a Federal department or agency (must) have access to and use of information and data that is comparable to the access to and use of the information and data by such members of the public who are not individuals with disabilities" (http://www.section508.gov, retrieved December 5, 2007). The addition of this standard triggered the development of new technologies that continue to promote access to data and information for all individuals.

The Technology-Related Assistance for Individuals with Disabilities Act of 1988 (Tech Act) (P.L. 100-407) provided the first formal definition of assistive technology devices and services. Assistive technology devices were defined as "any item, piece of equipment, or product system, whether acquired commercially off the shelf, modified, or customized, that is used to increase, maintain, or improve functional capabilities of individuals with disabilities." Assistive technology services meant "any service that directly assists an individual with a disability in the selection, acquisition, or use of an assistive technology device."

One of the purposes emphasized in this act was to "increase awareness and knowledge of the efficacy of assistive technology devices and assistive technology services among:

I. Individuals with disabilities and their family members, guardians, advocates, and authorized representatives;
II. Individuals who work for public agencies, or for private entities (including insurers), that have contact with individuals with disabilities;
III. Educators and related services personnel;
IV. Technology experts (including engineers);
V. Employers; and
VI. Other appropriate individuals."

For the first time, federal funds were released to states to develop training and delivery systems for these devices and services. The Tech Act required states to develop consumer-oriented programs providing technology services for all individuals with disabilities. The Assistive Technology Act of 1998 reinforced the merits of this act by extending the commitment of the federal government through continued funding of permanent, comprehensive, statewide programs of technology-related assistance.

In 1990 the Americans with Disabilities Act, which prohibits discrimination based on disability was passed. Disability is defined as "a physical or mental impairment that substantially limits a major life activity." The ADA is divided into five titles addressing issues of employment, public services and transportation, public accommodations, telecommunications, and miscellaneous provisions. Once again, the concept of equal access for all was reinforced through this legislation.

Additional federal laws mandated assistive technology for students with disabilities. The Individuals with Disabilities Education Act (IDEA) of 1990 first delineated the role of the school to provide assistive technology for students with disabilities. These protections were expanded and strengthened with the reauthorization of IDEA in 1997, at which time a provision was added to the law that required Individualized Education Program teams to consider assistive technology for *all* students with disabilities. The provision remains in the most recent reauthorization of IDEA 2004.

SUMMARY AND NEXT STEPS FOR IMPROVING PATIENT LITERACY

Research various community resources for your patients who are unfamiliar with how to use computers and the Internet. Make a list of places that they might go to learn more about becoming comfortable computer users. Consider checking with adult education centers, local libraries, and after-school adult education programs.

Print materials for patient education must be accessible to all and therefore available in multiple formats. What are some alternate formats to consider? First, consider using the built-in Auto-Summarize and Readability Statistics features in Microsoft Word in order to convert difficult passages into a more comfortable and understandable use of words and language. Even the built-in thesaurus/synonyms found when right clicking within a word might provide support in simplifying complicated text. Also, consider using a text-to-symbol writing tool in order to embed symbolic or picture translated concepts within the print. Whether or not a patient has a reading challenge, picture-supported text helps any patient to understand key concepts quickly.

If patient support materials involve a series of steps to be taken or procedures to follow, consider multimedia formats to convey these important procedures. Record how to implement these steps with an inexpensive video camera such as the Flip Video using the appropriate materials and vocabulary. After the video is captured and downloaded to the computer, it is possible to manipulate the video to promote patient understanding depending on the needs of the patient. For example, create a CD for the patient to watch, or upload the video to the Internet (see Chapter 15) or your organization's website for the patient to watch at home for exercise or program review. If a patient is unable to comprehend the complex terminology, have him or her narrate the video during filming. This will provide the patient ease of review in his or her native language on his or her return home. Patients can then pause, rewind, and review instructions repeatedly until he or she is comfortable with these detailed instructions.

You might collect and post a set of web resources in order to help a patient focus his or her search for follow-up information. Because these materials are digital, they can be updated easily and then archived and collected over time in order to create a growing media library of patient informational resources. Posting resources on your organization's website can help make them available for patients who may wish to access this information anytime from anywhere. Imagine a set of videos, audio recordings, text instructions, or even photographs that brings patient education information alive in order to facilitate accurate and effective follow-up care.

REFERENCES

21st Century Literacy Summit. (2002). 21st century literacy in a convergent media world [white paper]. Berlin, Germany: Author. Retrieved April 14, 2003, from http://www.21stcenturyliteracy.org/white/WhitePaperEnglish.pdf.

Agarwal, R., & Day, A. E. (1998). The impact of the Internet on economic education. (Research in Economic Education). *Journal of Economic Education, 29*(2), 99–111.

California School Library Association. (2004). *From library skills to information literacy: a handbook for the 21st century* (2nd ed., pp. xi–xvi). Spring, TX: Hi Willow Research and Publishing.

Cassey, M. Z. (2007). Building a case for using technology: health literacy and patient education. *Nursing Economics, 25*(3), 186–188.

Collins, N. D. (1994). Metacognition and reading to learn. *ERIC Clearinghouse on Reading, English, and Communication Digest #96,* EDO-CS-94-09 June 1994.

Duffy, T. M. (1985). Readability formulas: what's the use? In T. M. Duffy & R. Waller (Eds.). *Designing usable texts* (pp.113–143). Orlando, FL: Academic Press.

Gal, I., & Prigat, A. (2005). Why organizations continue to create patient information leaflets with readability and usability problems: an exploratory study. *Health Education Research, 20*(4), 485–493.

Graber, M. A., Roller, C. M., & Kaeble, B. (1999). Readability levels of patient education material on the world wide web. *The Journal of Family Practice, 48*(1), 58–61.

Hemming, H. E., & Langille, L. (2006). Building knowledge in literacy and health. *Canadian Journal of Public Health. Revue Canadienne De Santé Publique, 97*(Suppl 2), S31–S36.

Hoffman, T., & Worrall, L. (2004). Designing effective written health education materials: considerations for health professionals. *Disability and Rehabilitation, 26*(19), 1166–1173.

Houts, P. S., Doak, C. C., Doak, L. G., & Loscalzo, M. J. (2006). The role of pictures in improving health communication: a review of research on attention, comprehension, recall, and adherence. *Patient Education and Counseling, 61*(2), 173–190.

Individuals with Disabilities Education Act of 1990. Retrieved December 5, 2007, from http://atto.buffalo.edu/registered/ATBasics/Foundation/Laws/atlegislation.php#IDEA.

Institute of Medicine. (2004). Health literacy: a prescription to end confusion. National Academies Press. Retrieved November 23, 2007, from http://www.jointcommission.org/NewsRoom/PressKits/Health_Literacy/facts_figures.htm.

International Information and Communication Technologies Literacy Panel. (2002). Digital transformation: a framework for ICT literacy. Princeton, NJ: Educational Testing Services (ETS). Retrieved April 11, 2003, from http://www.ets.org/research/ictliteracy/ictreport.pdf.

Lewis, Deborah. (2003). Computers in patient education. *Computers, Informatics, Nursing. 21*(2), 88–96.

Lysack, C., Dama, M., Neufeld, S., & Andreassi, E. (2005). Compliance and satisfaction with home exercise: a comparison of computer-assisted video instruction and routine rehabilitation practice. *Journal of Allied Health, 34*(2), 76–82.

Maasland, E., Koudstaal, P. J., Habbema, J. D. F., & Dippel, D. W. J. (2007). Effects of an individualized multimedia computer program for health education in patients with a recent minor stroke or transient ischemic attack: a randomized controlled trial. *Acta Neurologica Scandinavica, 115*(1), 41–48.

Parette, H., Huer, M., & VanBiervliet, A. (2005). Cultural research in special education technology. In D. Edyburn, K. Higgins, R. Boone (Eds.). *Handbook of special education technology research and practice* (pp. 81, 98). Whitefish Bay, WI: Knowledge by Design.

Pignone, M. P., & DeWalt, D. A. (2006). Literacy and health outcomes: is adherence the missing link? *Journal of General Internal Medicine, 21*(8), 896–897.

Powers, B. J., & Bosworth, H. B. (2006). Revisiting literacy and adherence: future clinical and research directions. *Journal of General Internal Medicine, 21*(12), 1341–1342.

Sand-Jecklin, K. (2007). The impact of medical terminology on readability of patient education materials. *Journal of Community Health Nursing, 24*(2), 119–129.

Schwartzberg, J., Cowett, A., Vangeest, J., & Wolf, M. (2007). Communication techniques for patients with low health literacy: a survey of physicians, nurses, and pharmacists. *American Journal of Health Behavior, 31*(9), S96–S104.

Section 504 of the Rehabilitation Act of 1973. Retrieved December 5, 2007, from http://en.wikipedia.org/wiki/Rehabilitation_Act.

Section 508 of the Rehabilitation Act. Retrieved December 5, 2007, from http://www.section508.gov.

Shohet, L., & Renaud, L. (2006). Critical analysis on best practices in health literacy. *Canadian Journal of Public Health Revue Canadienne De Santé Publique, 97*(Suppl 2), S10–S13.

The Americans with Disabilities Act. Retrieved December 5, 2007, from http://www.ada.gov/pubs/ada.htm.

The Joint Commission. (2007). What did the doctor say? Improving health literacy to protect patient safety. Retrieved December 7, 2007, from http://www.jointcommission .org/NR/rdonlyres/D5248B2E-E7E6-4121-8874-99C7B4888301/0/improving_ health_literacy.pdf.

The Technology-Related Assistance for Individuals with Disabilities Act of 1988. Retrieved December 5, 2007, from http://www.section508.gov/docs/AT1998.html.

Thompson, H. S., Wahl, E., Fatone, A., Brown, K., Kwate, N. O., Valdimarsdottir, H. (2004). Enhancing the readability of materials describing genetic risk for breast cancer. *Cancer Control, 11*, 245–253.

Chapter 6

Stress and Illness

Jane C. Romano

In a hospital which welcomes to its care people of all nations, all creeds, all ages—infants, children, adults—men and women, rich and poor, there will be many types of patients. Each will demand our greatest sympathy, tact, and understanding. They will vary widely in previous experience and education, in disposition and characteristics, in prejudices and fears, in health habits and needs, and in the diseases or accidents from which they are suffering. While all must consider equal consideration, these factors of racial or personal differences all call for special consideration in their treatment. The patient may be alone or accompanied by one or more anxious friends. They also should receive special consideration.

From *The Principles and Practice of Nursing*, (1935)

INTRODUCTION

The idea that stress is an integral aspect of health care is not new to our day and age. In the opening quote, which was taken from a nursing text that was published over 70 years ago, Harmer (1935) wrote of the need to consider the patient's as well as the families' past experiences, prejudices, and fears when providing care. Wilson-Barnett (1984) presented three central components of stress: the first being the element of threat, which includes the realization that one is sick enough to require hospitalization and fear of the unknown. The second is focused around the concept of loss—of health, liberty, independence, the company of loved ones, pleasure, comfort, and privacy. The third is the challenge of assuming the role of patient which requires adjusting and/or coping with the demands of the situation. Wilson-Barnett (1984) concluded that in order to minimize the stress of the experience patients need information on what is and will be happening during their healthcare encounter.

The needs of individuals and families related to the stress that goes hand and hand with being a patient have clearly not changed much over the generations, and many of the strategies to help alleviate stress have not changed. What has changed, however, are the increasingly complex needs of the people who we care for, as well as their access to information beyond the healthcare environment. The key is to be aware of the influence that stress can have on a person's ability and willingness to take in and process the information that is necessary to maintain their best possible state of well-being. It is essential to factor in this as well as other potential barriers to learning when planning and implementing patient education.

COPING AND STRESS

It is nearly impossible for human beings to enter into the healthcare system and not have some level of stress. Whether it is for a routine physical exam or an emergency room visit for an acute illness or injury, some stress is always associated with the experience. The level of stress often determines the path that healthcare providers need to take when planning and implementing patient education. Assessing this potential obstacle of the patient's capacity to learn is an important initial step in the process of empowering a patient to make informed decisions. It is essential for healthcare providers to recognize this and respond appropriately in order to minimize stress and ultimately maximize patient learning.

Case Study 6-1

Theresa is a 75-year-old woman with a history of asthma as a child that has exacerbated in her adult years. She has been prescribed both an albuterol inhaler with a spacer for fast-acting relief as well as Advair for maintenance of her symptoms. At her annual checkup, Theresa is obviously wheezing and has difficulty completing sentences. During your discussion, Theresa mentions that she has not been compliant with her maintenance medication but does occasionally use the albuterol for relief. She also shares that she does not use the spacer with her inhaler for no particular reason. Eventually, it comes out that Theresa is resistant to using the "steroid" because of the "side effects" it can cause. It is determined that Theresa's husband had passed away a few years ago after a long battle with emphysema and had been on oral steroids many times during the course of his illness. He also used inhalers and nebulizer treatments often for relief of his symptoms. Theresa was afraid of "ending up like him." With this new understanding of her knowledge related to asthma as well as her previous experience with the medications her husband took, a plan of education and support can be developed for Theresa that takes all of these influences into consideration. Knowing her source of anxiety and stress related to her ability to manage her symptoms is critical to improving her outcomes.

We exist in what Woolf et al. (2005) describes as a culture of consumerism in the United States, where people are encouraged to take control over their choices. Health care is being redirected from a patient–clinician relationship toward a patient-centered model. There is more opportunity for patients to access information about issues related to their health through the wonders of computers and the Internet. Today's generation is looking for more information from other sources besides their primary care physician. This new expectation of patients coming to the healthcare experience with more knowledge can influence patient education in either a positive or negative way. Sometimes, what is learned from these sources is not always accurate and can also be significantly skewed to one method of treating or managing a specific issue. Your initial assessment of the patient and family should include what information they have and clarify any misconceptions that can create increasing stress and barriers to learning.

Another important aspect of assessing your patient's ability to learn includes his or her past experiences with the healthcare system. In 1989, Johnson and Lauver examined how patients cope with the stress of dealing with physical illness using self-regulation theory. This theory relies on the processing of information to explain human behavior. The central concept involves a schema, a cognitive structure of complex knowledge that is a result of experience—in other words, a plan based on what the person has learned and/or experienced. The focus of attention, organization of incoming information, the retrieval of stored information, and goal setting behaviors are guided by schemata (Johnson & Lauver, 1989). Remaining focused on objective aspects versus subjective emotional aspects of a situation contributes to more effective coping strategies. Restructuring attitudes, clarifying misconceptions, and emphasizing what can be done versus what cannot be done increases the patients' understanding of information to support their schema (Saarmann, Daugherty, & Riegel, 2002).

The knowledge and experience patients brings with them can influence their current situation. In 2006, Nash, Williams, Nicholson, and Trask examined the impact that pain-related anxiety had on a patient's ability to cope with chronic severe headaches. The authors found that this multidimensional construct includes physiological, cognitive, behavioral, and affective manifestations related to a person's past experience with pain. The patients in the study reported fear, avoidance of activities and limited functioning as a result of anticipating high levels of pain that had previously occurred with their headaches. On a somewhat positive note, some patients reported hypervigilance with early indication of pain. It would make sense that this concept of pain-related anxiety would influence all persons who have experienced pain either chronic or acute and should be considered and assessed by healthcare providers when planning and implementing patient education.

This concept of pain-related anxiety can also realistically be taken to another level that is experience-related anxiety. Ultimately, pain is an experience that is not pleasant and welcomed, as are many other events in life. The information and impressions that an individual acquires from all health-related experiences can influence their ability to cope.

In 1990, Gonzalez, Goeppinger, and Lorig discussed psychological theories and their application to patient education. Eight different coping strategies were identified: confronting, distancing, self-control, seeking social support, accepting responsibility, escape-avoidance, problem solving, and positive reappraisal. Self-control, accepting responsibility, problem solving, and positive reappraisal were considered the more effective and efficient methods of coping and required the patient to take charge of his or her situation, to determine what he or she can and cannot control, along with setting and working toward personal goals. Gonzalez et al. (1990) felt that the ability to solve problems is one of the most useful coping strategies when dealing with illness. They believed that, at the time, most patient education taught specific solutions rather that the process of problem solving.

More recently, Feely (1997) and Marchese (2006) examined Peplau's Theory of Interpersonal Relations and its application related to patient stress. According to Feely (1997), Peplau recognized that stress and needs create both tension and energy that can be used either positively or negatively. The role of the healthcare provider is to help the patient identify what the source of the tension is and to develop positive strategies to deal with the cause. This is where the interpersonal relationship between the patient and healthcare provider is central to Peplau's theory (Feely, 1997). Building and maintaining a therapeutic relationship can improve communication and enhance the patient's ability to learn how to develop and adopt new patterns of behavior that will reduce their stress levels and ultimately improve their outcomes.

The concept of the interpersonal process proposed by Peplau requires the progression through four phases: orientation, identification, exploitation, and resolution (Marchese, 2006). During the initial orientation phase, the nurse and patient are essentially strangers. The healthcare providers begin to get to know the patients and establish themselves as a resource. This phase is where the patient and family begin to recognize their need for help with a specific health-related problem and require assessment of prior experiences and knowledge and readiness to learn. The patient and family are involved in the process of determining what they need to learn as well as how and when they would like to be given specific information. The phase of identification is where the patient is increasingly able to focus on the problem and therefore becomes a more active participant in his or her care as well as begins to trust the healthcare provider. During the exploitation phase, comfort and trust between the patient and healthcare provider have been established. This creates the opportunity to empower the patient and family by promoting more independence. The final phase of resolution brings the patient to an increased self-reliance and a decreased need for the healthcare provider. Goals that were made have been met, and there is an opportunity for setting new goals.

It is clear that healthcare providers play an important role when working with patients and families to identify and maximize their coping strategies when dealing with illness. Early as well as ongoing assessment is a critical aspect of determining behaviors that work or impede effective coping.

CAREGIVERS AND STRESS

It is not only the stress of the patient that needs to be considered when planning and delivering patient education. Extended lifespan, decreased lengths of stay in the hospital, and an increased focus on outpatient management of health-related issues have a significant impact on the experience of a patient's family. Caregiver questions, concerns, and fears are just as important as the patients when providing education. In a study related to parental stress in a pediatric intensive care unit, Aldridge (2005) examined key stressors that these parents experienced. Issues such as the often unplanned admission, the severity of the illness that warranted intensive care, and the limitless number of tests and procedures that are done appear to be significant contributors to parental stress levels. A summary composed by Aldridge (2005) of parental needs and stressors in the pediatric intensive care unit included the following:

Information/uncertainty over outcome

- Not being present when a physician examines the child
- Receiving inconsistent information

- Not knowing how long the child will be in the hospital
- Not knowing what to expect (Will the child die? Will the child have a disability?)
- Not knowing how life-threatening the child's illness is

Alteration in parental role

- Seeing the child in pain
- Being unable to care for the child
- Being unable to communicate with the child
- Not knowing how to help the child

Access to the child

- Being separated from the child during examinations or procedures
- Being unable to visit at will
- Hearing the child cry when the parents leave

Appearance of the child

- Noticing the changes in the child's behavior or appearance

It is safe to say that most, if not all, of these statements listed by Aldridge (2005) can apply to pretty much any patient population and caregiver, not just parents. Taylor, Nolan, and Dudley-Brown (2006) examined the influence of a spouse's response to an illness on patient outcome. It was reported that an individual's adjustment to illness as well as recovery was significantly impacted by the spouse's response to the situation. The ability to influence recovery may be hindered by the spouses's own level of stress, challenges, and coping demands. Also important to consider is the nature of the illness: Is it acute or chronic? The Institute of Medicine report "Crossing the Quality Chasm: A New Health System for the 21st Century (2001) states that chronic conditions are now the leading cause of illness, disability, and death in the United States. Although all caregivers will experience some level of stress related to the illness, those dealing with chronic illness typically suffer from higher levels of stress (Chan, 2000) and require ongoing support.

The importance of considering the stress levels of caregivers and addressing the needs of these critical individuals is essential for healthcare providers to recognize when planning and implementing patient education. As stated earlier, the needs of parents in response to the stressors identified by Aldridge

(2005) can apply to any person who is ultimately responsible for the care and well-being of the patient. Parents and caregivers need access to accurate and ongoing information related to what the patient's prognosis is, to procedures and tests being done, as well as to what equipment is being used and why. They need their questions answered honestly and timely. They also need to know what to expect over the long run, when the patient goes home. Or are they going home? Parents and caregivers need to know that their family member is getting the best care and that staff cares about the patient. They should be provided access to the patient and can also be encouraged to participate in the patient's care whenever and wherever this is appropriate. Finally, Aldridge (2005) points out that parents and caregivers need their own physical needs met. They need to have access to food and drink as well as a place to rest if appropriate.

Considering the stressors and needs of caregivers is essential to providing effective family-centered care. It is important to recognize that these people, especially parents, are the quintessential experts on what works best for their family members. Miceli and Clark (2005) describe parents as having knowledge important for understanding how best to care for the child that *only they can provide*. It is safe to say that this would be true for many family members who are the primary caretaker of the patient. It is essential to not only recognize this but to capitalize on it when planning and implementing patient education.

Another important aspect to mention when discussing how stress can impact one's ability to learn is how stress affects a healthcare provider's ability to teach. Studies examining this issue are plentiful throughout the literature and seem to agree that stress in the workplace has a negative influence in many ways. It can impact the employee's health and well-being as well as create the perfect opportunity to make mistakes (Elfering, Semmer, & Grebner, 2006). Increasingly, complex patient populations, a shortage of healthcare providers, as well as an aging existing workforce, are all factors that contribute to stress and burnout (Milliken, Clements, & Tillman, 2007). This undoubtedly negatively impacts the patient's experience and outcome.

When assessing a patient's readiness and ability to learn, it is also important to be aware of your own stress level and to determine whether there is a more appropriate time or person to provide the education the patient and family needs. Wicks (2006) believes that the question is not if but when stress will appear and take a toll on those working in healthcare. It is essential to appreciate, minimize, and learn from this stress in order to support providers in developing personal self-care strategies to enable them to effectively continue their role as helpers and healers. Along with taking care of yourself, it is essential to know and use your resources in order to provide the best possible opportunity for you and your patient to have a positive experience in the long run.

The needs of all caregivers are important to include in the assessment, planning, and implementation of patient education. The ability of this group to influence outcomes is clear and can often make or break a patient's ability to weather the storm of illness successfully. Providing family-centered care can increase the caregivers' capacity to become empowered in order to support their child, spouse, sibling, parent or whomever.

HEALTH LITERACY AND STRESS

Nearly half of all American adults—90 million people—have difficulty understanding and using health information, and there is a higher rate of hospitalization and use of emergency services among patients with limited health literacy, says a report from the Institute of Medicine (Nielsen-Bohlman, Panzer, & Kindig, 2004). Limited health literacy may lead to billions of dollars in avoidable healthcare costs.

More than a measurement of reading skills, health literacy also includes writing, listening, speaking, arithmetic, and conceptual knowledge. Health literacy is defined as the degree to which individuals have the capacity to obtain, process, and understand basic information and services needed to make appropriate decisions regarding their health (Office of Disease Prevention and Health Promotion, 2001). At some point, most individuals will encounter health information that they cannot understand because of the complexity of the content. Traditionally, the focus on the issue of literacy has been older adults, patients with limited formal education, and individuals for whom English is not their primary language (Murphy-Knoll, 2007). Even well-educated people with strong reading and writing skills may have trouble comprehending a medical form or doctor's instructions regarding a drug or procedure (Cutilli, 2005). It is essential that healthcare providers consider their patients' beliefs, values, and cultural influences in order to determine the most appropriate and effective way to deliver information and education related to their health and well-being.

Effective communication is essential in delivering quality health care. Low health literacy makes this challenging for providers as well as patients. How can patients and families make informed decisions about their care if they cannot understand what their options are? How can healthcare providers ensure the safety and well-being of their patients after they have left the healthcare environment? The Joint Commission considers it a fundamental right and need of patients to receive both written and oral information about their care in a format that they can understand (Murphy-Knoll, 2007).

Rothman et al. (2007) developed a tool kit for addressing low literacy issues in diabetic patients. The strategies identified to improve communication and ultimately comprehension of education provided include the following:

- Focusing on selected critical behaviors
- Decreasing the complexity of information
- Avoiding the use of jargon
- Limiting the number of items taught in each setting
- Using real examples
- Using the "teach back" technique where the patient needs to correctly teach back what has been taught to them so that it can be assured that they understand the instructions or information they were given

It is essential for providers to consider how the information is delivered as well as received when planning and implementing education for patients and families. Be cognizant of the impact that stress and anxiety can have on learning in addition to the complexity of the information and instruction you are planning. Assessment of the level of literacy as well as health literacy is the first step in determining how to proceed. Using strategies such as pictures, diagrams, handouts, and return demonstration can be effective methods of assessing the patient and family's understanding of what they are expected to do. Using interpreters is essential when English is not the first language of the individual being taught. Using family members as interpreters can often lead to misinformation being translated; therefore, it is essential to use trained interpreters. In an effort to keep patient education centered and effective, it is important to *ask* the patient and family what they feel they need to learn and what the best way is to help them achieve this, and then essentially connect the dots. There is significant value in this strategy if you can be certain that the person understands what you are asking. This can help to build trust and strengthen your ability to be a resource in the process of moving the patient and family along to gain increasing self-reliance.

CONSIDERING ALTERNATIVE THERAPIES

It is important to consider other approaches to assisting individuals in healthcare setting to manage stress and anxiety related to illness. There are many various alternative methods of dealing with stress and illness. Often, these therapies and practices can assist patients and families to navigate through the healthcare world effectively. Reiki, therapeutic touch, therapeutic massage, acupuncture, meditation, and guided imagery are a few examples of the types of alternative therapies that are currently practiced. In a study examining the reduction of anxiety in women who have heart disease using mindfulness meditation, Tacon et al. (2003) reported that anxiety was determined to have a significant role in the onset of this morbidity. The participants showed decreased anxiety as well as increased coping skills and ability to control negative emotions.

These methods of relaxation and stress reduction are noninvasive and harmless to the individual. They are also believed to promote healing. In a time of dealing with illness that is very often associated with a loss of control, these therapies can provide patients and families with strategies that can help them gain some control over at least part of their healthcare experience. Many hospitals and healthcare environments are increasingly recognizing the value of alternative therapies and developing resources for patients and staff in order to provide this method of coping with stress effectively. With that being said, these therapies should support traditional treatment regimens and not replace them. Also, the effective application of alternative therapies requires specialized training that needs to be respected when considering their use. Healthcare providers should be aware of what is available to patients and families within their institution in order to safely offer these methods of reducing and managing stress.

Case Study 6-2

Placing intravenous lines in infants and children can be particularly challenging. Rose, RN, is able to insert the IV quickly and with minimal distress to the patient. Parents and patients request Rose on subsequent admissions to place their IVs. "What's your trick?" a new grad asked her. "Massage" she answered. The new grad was astonished, "How do you have time to give a massage? It's busy enough! No one has time for such a thing!" Rose smiled and explained, "When I massage the patient's arm, hands, or feet it vasodilates the area. It also calms the patient and helps distract them from the procedure."

By using a massage technique, from start to finish, the IV placement may take 10 minutes versus 30 minutes on a distraught patient. Using this technique reduces stress and anxiety for both patients and families.

Another possible method of assisting individuals deal with stress and anxiety is the use of expressive writing techniques. Smyth and Helm (2003) examined focused expressive writing (FEW) as a way to help process emotions related to stressful events. FEW involves having a person write about his or her thoughts and feeling regarding something that he or she perceives as a stressful and/or traumatic event that he or she is dealing with. Research has shown that using expressive writing techniques with chronically ill patients had a positive influence on their physical and psychological being. For example, women with breast cancer who practiced FEW were found to have fewer medical appointments and somatic symptoms related to their diagnosis (Smyth & Helm, 2003). This method of reflection and expression has also been found to be helpful for healthcare providers as a means of coping with difficult clinical situations. The keys to using FEW to support coping are to

- Encourage the person to reflect on both their thoughts and feelings about the stressful experience or event.
- Explain that the writing is for them only and does not have to be shared with anyone else.
- Forget structure, spelling, grammar, and so forth. Just write what they are thinking and feeling however they would like.

Expressive writing is a simple and inexpensive activity that anyone can do. It crosses educational, cultural, and socioeconomic barriers and has been shown to have a positive effect on coping and problem solving as well as physical and psychological well-being.

LOCUS OF CONTROL

In the 1950s, John Rotter developed the behavioral theory of locus of control. It is important to consider the concept of a patient's control beliefs when planning and implementing education for patients and families. Locus of control refers to an individual's perception about the underlying main causes of events in his or her life (Neill, 2006). An external locus of control is the belief that events are a result of luck, fate, or other external factors that are beyond one's control. An internal locus of control believes that a person's decisions and actions can bring about a positive outcome. Rotter believed that internal and external dimensions exist at opposite ends of a continuum and individuals fluctuate between the two (Neill, 2006). In 1978, Wallston, Wallston, and DeVellis expanded on Rotter's theory by demonstrating that health-related locus of control is multidimensional and identified three independent constructs: (1) internal, an individual controls his or her own health; (2) powerful others, the belief that important people such as doctors and nurses can control their health; and (3) chance, belief that fate, luck, or chance controls their health (Malcarne, Drahota, & Hamilton, 2005). It is believed that individuals can exist in one or more of the dimensions simultaneously. Determining a patient's locus of control should be done early on in the assessment process. This will help to guide healthcare providers when planning and providing education and information. If a person does not believe that he or she has any or little control over his or her outcome, the approach would be much different than for that of a person who demonstrates an internal locus of control and can effectively partner in their care.

Health-related locus of control is considered an important variable in the adjustment to health problems as well as compliance with treatments (Malcarne, Drahota, & Hamilton, 2005). It is another tool that healthcare providers can use to support individuals to manage effectively in their role as a patient or as caregiver to a patient. It is important to assess and address the control beliefs of everyone who is influenced by the challenges of being a patient can bring.

CONCLUSION

Ironically, education can influence anxiety and can also be influenced by anxiety. Sometimes too much information and decision-making responsibilities precipitate increased stress and anxiety. On the other hand, new unexpected information can cause stress and anxiety to creep up. The fact remains that patients and families need information and education in order to eventually gain control of the influences that stress can have on their healthcare experience.

Marchese (2006) states that key aspects of providing information and education to patients and families who are experiencing stress include the following:

- Recognize, validate, and accept the stress, fear, tension, and anxiety that the patient is experiencing.
- Foster a collaborative relationship with patients and families by being supportive and encouraging active participation in establishing and evaluating their plan of care, questioning and problem solving, and using trial and error.
- Use the principles of adult learning that focus on readiness, repetition, and reinforcement to determine when, what, how, and why to provide information and instruction.

In addition, it is essential to consider the aspects of health literacy and locus of control that can be sources of stress and can significantly influence the task of planning educational opportunities for patients and families.

Stress related to illness is not a new concept but a more complex concept in today's society. Aspects such as the realization that one is sick enough to require hospitalization, fear of the unknown, and the concept of loss along with the challenge of assuming the role of patient present multiple stressors for individuals. The need to provide necessary information on what is and will be happening during their healthcare encounter is clear.

Healthcare providers are faced with continuous challenges when identifying and managing the various influences stress can have on a patient and family's ability to gain the necessary skills and knowledge to navigate successfully the often stormy healthcare experience. We are in the position to offer support and guidance that can assist with this journey; therefore, it is essential that healthcare providers recognize and respond to the needs of those weathering the storm in order to assure the best possible outcome. Initial and ongoing assessment and evaluation of the patient and family's barriers to learning as well as the knowledge and understanding that they have gained is key to focusing education on what is important to the individuals.

The goal of empowering patients and families to become less reliant on healthcare providers and more independent related to their situation needs to be shared by everyone. The stress and anxiety that comes with this responsibility is critical to address if the journey is to have a safe and acceptable outcome. Remaining focused on what can be done alone with restructuring attitudes and clarifying misconceptions will serve to increase the patient's understanding of information while minimizing the stress associated with the experience.

REFERENCES

Aldridge, M. D. (2005). Decreasing parental stress in the pediatric intensive care unit: one unit's experience. *Critical Care Nurse, 25*(6), 40–50.

Chan, R. C. K. (2000). Stress and coping in spouses of persons with spinal cord injuries. *Clinical Rehabilitation, 14,* 137–144.

Cutilli, C. C. (2005). Do your patients understand? Determining your patient's health literacy skills. *Orthopaedic Nursing, 24*(5), 372–377.

Elfering, A., Semmer, N. K., & Grebner, S. (2006). Work stress and patient safety: observer-rated work stressors as predictors of characteristics of safety-related events reported by young nurses. *Ergonomics, 49*(5–6), 457–469.

Feely, M. (1997). Using Peplau's theory in nurse-patient relations. *International Nursing Review, 44*(4), 115–119.

Gonzalez, V. M., Goeppinger, J., & Lorig, K. (1990). Four psychological theories and their application to patient education and clinical practice. *Arthritis Care and Research, 3*(3), 132–143.

Harmer, B. (1935). *Text-book of the principles and practice of nursing* (3rd ed. Revised). New York: MacMillan.

Institute of Medicine. (2001). *Crossing the quality chasm: a new health system for the 21st century*. Washington, DC: National Academies Press.

Johnson, J. E., & Lauver, D. R. (1989). Alternative explanations of coping with stressful experiences associated with physical illness. *Advances in Nursing Science, 11*(2), 39–52.

Malcarne, V. L., Drahota, A., & Hamilton, N. A. (2005). Children's health-related locus of control beliefs: ethnicity, gender and family income. *Children's Health Care, 34*(1), 47–59.

Marchese, K. (2006). Using Peplau's theory of interpersonal relations to guide the education of patients undergoing urinary diversion. *Urologic Nursing, 26*(5), 363–371.

Miceli, P. J., & Clark, P. A. (2005). Your patient—my child. *Journal of Nursing Care Quality, 20*(1), 43–53.

Milliken, T. F., Clements, P. T., Tillman, H. J. (2007). The impact of stress management on nurse productivity and retention. *Nursing Economics, 25*(4), 203–210.

Murphy-Knoll, L. (2007). Low health literacy puts patients at risk: The Joint Commission proposes solution to national problem. *Journal of Nursing Care Quality, 22*(3), 205–209.

Nash, J. M., Williams, D. M., Nicholson, R., & Trask, P. C. (2006). The contributions of pain-related anxiety to disability from headache. *Journal of Behavioral Medicine, 29*(1), 61–76.

Neill, J. (2006). What is locus of control? Retrieved February 22, 2007, from http://wilderdom.com/psychology/loc/LocusOfControlWhatIs.html.

Nielsen-Bohlman, L., Panzer, A. M., Kindig, D. A. (2004). Health literacy: a prescription to end confusion. Washington, DC: National Academies Press.

Office of Disease Prevention and Health Promotion. (2001). Healthy People 2010: Understanding and Improving Health (2nd ed.). U.S. Health and Human Services Department.

Rothman, R. L., Huizanga, M. M., Elasy, T. A., et al. (2007). *Literacy and numeracy toolkit for diabetes: provider's manual*. Retrieved September 24, 2007, from http://www.mc.vanderbilt.edu/diabetes/drtc/preventionandcontrol/files/dlnet-instructions.pdf.

Saarmann, L., Daugherty, J., & Riegel, B. (2002). Teaching staff a brief cognitive-behavioral intervention. *MedSurg Nursing, 11*(3), 144–151.

Smyth, J., & Helm, R. (2003). In session: psychotherapy in practice. Focused expressive writing as self-help for stress and trauma. *Journal of Clinical Psychology, 59*(2), 227–235.

Tacon, A. M., McComb, J., Caldera, Y., & Randolph, P. (2003). Mindfulness meditation, anxiety reduction and heart disease: a pilot study. *Family & Community Health, 26*(1), 25–33.

Taylor, L., Nolan, M., & Dudley-Brown, S. (2006). Evidence on spouse responses to illness as a guide to understanding and studying spouse responses to living organ donation. *Progress in Transplantation, 16*(2), 117–126.

Wallston, K. A., Wallston, B. S., DeVellis, R. (1978). Development of the multidimensional health locus of control (MHLC) scales. *Health Education Monographs, 6*(2), 160–170.

Wicks, R. J. (2006). *Overcoming secondary stress in medical and nursing practice: a guide to professional resilience and personal well-being.* New York: Oxford University Press.

Wilson-Barnett, J. (1984). Alleviating stress for hospitalized patients. *International Review of Applied Psychology, 33,* 493–503.

Woolf, S., Chan, E. C. Y., Harris, R., Sheridan, S. L., Braddock, C. H., Kaplin, R. M., O'Connor, A. M., & Tunis, S. (2005). Promoting informed choice: transforming health care to dispense knowledge for decision making. *Annals of Internal Medicine, 143*(4), 293–300.

Chapter 7

Creating Change for Positive Health Behaviors, Including Ethical Practice

Gerald P. Koocher

INTRODUCTION

Creating change in human behavior involves a complex interplay of information and motivation. People's beliefs, habits, and preferences all play important roles that influence the choices they make. The roots of these choices may involve biological, cultural, economic, environmental, and social forces, as well as education and understanding of scientific facts. Simply giving people scientific data about their health or telling them what to do will rarely lead to sustained changes in behavior and does not take account of their values and needs as unique individuals. Similarly, we know some strategies that grab people's attention can also provoke anxiety that will not sustain change while inducing personal discomfort (e.g., "you're going to die if you don't"). Changing people's behavior toward improving health behavior also has significant economic importance. Poor adherence to medical regimens accounts for substantial worsening of disease, increased mortality, and increased healthcare costs.

Looking only at medication-related hospital admissions in the United States, one estimate holds that from 33% to 69% result from poor medication adherence, leading to an additional cost of approximately $100 billion a year (Osterberg & Blaschke, 2005). This chapter highlights the factors that make a difference and discusses ethically sensitive strategies for promoting effective healthy change.

HOW CAN WE EFFECTIVELY PROMOTE HEALTH BEHAVIOR?

One of the most successful transtheoretical models for conceptualizing health behavior change originated with the work of Prochaska and his colleagues (Prochaska, DiClemente, & Norcross, 1992; Prochaska et al., 1994; Prochaska, Prochaska, & Johnson, 2006). The first stage, precontemplation, characterizes individuals who have not given significant thought to altering their behavior or who may even deny the significance of the relevant health problem or a need to alter their behavior. The second stage, contemplation, suggests a beginning level of recognition or acknowledgment of a problem without a clear personal commitment to take action. After the person decides that he or she "does something" about the health problem, he or she moves into the preparation stage that involves planning or strategizing about taking action. The next stage involves active efforts to alter prior habits or behavior problems. Once begun, the focus of intervention becomes sustaining the new behaviors. Ultimately, as the new behaviors become routine and solidify as new habits, we reach the termination stage.

Table 7-1 illustrates the model of six stages of change, along with suggestions for promoting progress at each stage. For example, in attempting to engage someone who seems resistant to considering changing behavior (i.e., precontemplation), one might consider engaging the patient in a discussion about the consequences of doing nothing. Similarly, patients who have begun to take action will benefit significantly from external recognition of their efforts and progress.

From an ethical perspective, such discussions must recognize and respect each patient's personal, social, and environmental context. What may seem an obvious need for change from the perspective of a healthcare provider can easily ignore the realities of patients with compromised ability to take the next step given some critical realities in their lives. The next section of this chapter focuses on stepping into patients' frames of reference and recognizing the potential attributions that may contribute to their not following the change-oriented advice of healthcare practitioners.

Table 7-1 Stages of Change Model

Stage of Change	Characteristic Internal Questioning	Suggestions for Promoting Progress
Precontemplation	Who cares? Ignorance is bliss; keep the status quo.	Encourage re-evaluation and self-exploration; recognize risks of doing nothing.
Contemplation	Do I really want to do this? What are the benefits and risks?	Consider the pros and cons of change as potential positive outcomes.
Preparation	Okay, I want to try to do things differently. Now what?	Identify any obstacles, acquire necessary skills, and begin taking small steps.
Action	I want to do it, but can I? Let's try and see how this goes.	Modifying previous behavior, practice the core change skills, improve feelings of self-efficacy, and focus on long-term benefits.
Maintenance	Can I sustain this change? How did I ever do without it?	Sustaining new behavior with social support and coping strategies. Follow-up and document patients' successes, prevent relapse, self-reinforcement assured.
Termination	I have done it?	The new behavior becomes a self-reinforcing habit.

CONCEPTUALIZING THE CASE

Getting a new medical diagnosis or experiencing a progression or exacerbation of symptoms in a chronic health condition often demands adaptation to the change in health circumstances (one's own or a family member's). Such news often involves new or revised treatment plans that require adherence with medical advice to restore or maintain health. One sometimes hears healthcare providers use the term "noncompliant" to refer to patients who fail to follow fully a prescribed course of treatment or recommendation; however, substituting the term "adherence" for "compliance" suggests better collaborative engagement with patients. Compliance suggests going along with or acquiescing to a request or demand with a degree of passivity. Adherence, on the other hand, implies an active process of faithful attachment or devotion with an implicit therapeutic alliance forged between patients and care providers.

Osterberg and Blaschke (2005) note that research reports of adherence rates for individual patients generally cite percentages of prescribed medication doses or treatment actually taken over a specified period. The same measurement approach applies to other therapeutic interventions (e.g., physical therapy or psychotherapy sessions attended), although mere attendance at an appointment does not necessarily betoken full, active engagement in treatment. Some attempt to refine measurement of adherence by focusing on accuracy of dose taking (i.e., prescribed number of pills each day) and sequencing or timing (i.e., taking medication within a specified interval or sequence). Because most reports of adherence rates come from clinical trials, the data can prove misleading. For example, not every patient qualifies for trials, and the nature of the trial itself can lead to recruitment and response biases. One would expect that the adherence rates in research studies may run misleadingly high because of attention focused on participants, but even so, the average adherence rates reported in clinical trials run only 43% to 78% among patients receiving treatment for medical chronic conditions (Osterberg & Blaschke, 2005).

It is not surprising that no uniform consensual standard exists for what constitutes adequate adherence to medical treatment. Some research reports of clinical trials consider rates above 80% acceptable, whereas others require 95% adherence critical (e.g., in treatment studies of HIV infection). In clinical practice, some degree of adherence may prove better than nothing (e.g., I would like my sedentary patient to exercise daily, but getting on the treadmill for 20 minutes twice a week is better than not at all.).

CONSIDERING THE PERSONAL DIMENSIONS OF AN ILLNESS

In order to best motivate our patients, we must understand their perspectives and how they attach meaning to their medical condition. We can begin to frame our grasp of these issues by considering the implications along a set of continua. **Table 7-2** lists a number of the most salient dimensions. The nature of onset, duration, natural course, predictability, prognosis, route of transmission, burdens of care, obviousness, and social tolerance for the condition can all play important roles in how patients define themselves and respond to their condition. In addition to the actual implications of an illness in terms of treatment realities, the special meaning of the condition to the patient has critical importance that may not be readily apparent.

Consider middle-aged people who are newly diagnosed with diabetes. Apart from the acute medical care associated with events leading to the

Table 7-2 Dimensions of Illness

Attribute	Continuum	Implications
Onset	Acute to gradual	Adherence rates typically run higher among patients with acute conditions.
Duration	Brief—intermittent—lifelong	Persistence among patients with chronic conditions often declines dramatically after the first 6 months of therapy.
Course (or natural history of the illness)	Static—progressive—relapsing/remitting	Will anything the patient does (or does not do) stabilize or slow the progress of an illness or sustain remissions?
Predictability	Known and predictable or unknown and unpredictable	Can treatment reduce disruption in the lives of patients or families by unpredictable medical events?
Prognosis	Normal life span to terminal	Can following a prescribed treatment plan extend my life or improve my quality of life?
Transmission	Genetic—traumatic—contagious	Does the manner of transmission or origin of the condition create emotional issues or barriers such as guilt or fear.
Burdens of care	None to extensive	How significant are the burdens placed on the patient or family members by the medical regimen, need for monitoring, required appliances, need for personal assistance, and so forth?
Obviousness	Blatant to invisible	Can others notice the condition or can I keep my privacy?
Societal tolerance	Stigmatizing to acceptable	Does having this condition add a burden of social stigma?

diagnosis, avoiding complications demands lifestyle changes and chronic attention to medical status. Nevertheless, the disease is invisible, the consequences of nonadherence may not become quickly evident, and a family history of the disease may trigger particular meaning, anxiety, or resignation to the patient.

A patient who contracts an HIV infection as the result of unsafe sexual contacts must adhere promptly to an effective medical regimen or face a downward-spiraling course. At the same time, he or she may have strong emotional reactions associated with the person who infected him or her and his or her own relationships to others that he or she may have put at risk. Disclosure of HIV infection status to others will also likely convey a social stigma that would not accompany disclosure of a diabetes diagnosis.

TYPOLOGIES OF NONADHERENCE

The healthcare provider will need to consider how the various attributes of any given medical condition affect a patient's adjustment in terms of the meanings he or she attaches to the illness and the way society (including the healthcare system) responds to them. A critical incident survey focused on teenagers and young adults with cystic fibrosis and suggested three types of medical nonadherence that may generalize across patients and medical conditions (Koocher, McGrath, & Gudas, 1990). The key translational assumption is that identifying the basis for deviating from the prescribed course of treatment is the first step in improving the patient's adherence.

The first type of nonadherence flows out of ignorance or inadequate knowledge about the proper implementation of treatment or the rationale for the components. For example, do the patient and family have access to information about the condition and treatments in comprehensible form? Did they receive both oral and written instructions in the language and at a reading level that they could readily use? Did the information include a rationale for the treatment or simply a list of actions without rationales? Did the information provider(s) encourage the patient or family members to ask questions and make an effort to tailor the presentation to individual needs, or did the information arrive as a one-size-fits-all message?

The second type of nonadherence generally resulted as a form of psychosocial resistance related to patient or family members' attributions, motivations, defense mechanisms, or even (although rarely) frank psychopathology. Are people in denial, hopeless, angry, frightened, or affected by other emotional issues that make a solid working alliance with their caregiver challenging. Such nonadherence can arise as the result of practitioner behaviors, patient issues, or family tensions.

The third and final type of failure to follow medical advice involves educated nonadherence. This refers to situations in which the patient understands the recommended treatment but makes a competent, well-reasoned decision in favor of quality of life, as opposed to the prescribed regimen. In such situations, one must consider whether the patient (or family in the case of minor children) has adequate reasoning capacity to consent, can articulate personal values or preferences, has explored reasonable alternatives, and has made a decision congruent with moral and legally standards.

If the patient does not understand rationales for the treatment regimen, no amount of psychological counseling will improve adherence. Similarly, when a patient feels depressed and hopeless, giving educative information about all the bad result that will flow from nonadherence will only make things worse. When a competent patient chooses quality of life over aggressive medical intervention, those wishes demand respectful attention of medical care providers.

ETHICAL PRIORITIES

Table 7-3 provides a list of seven fundamental ethical principles often cited from the work of Beauchamp and Childress (2001), along with an expanded set of eleven framed by Koocher and Keith-Spiegel (2008). Although the lists have much in common, Koocher and Keith-Spiegel focus less on the Western value of autonomy drawn from self-government and democratic ideals and more of providing patients with personal choice. They also add the dimensions of compassionate care, pursuit of excellence, and acceptance of accountability as central values.

One illustration drawn from the writings of Arthur Kleinman (1988) helps to make the point of ethical sensitivity across cultures in medical care. He describes the cultural gaps in addressing a patient's illness between the

Table 7-3 Ethical Fundamentals

Traditional Ethical Fundamentals per Beauchamp and Childress	Adaptation and Reframing per Koocher and Keith-Spiegel
Autonomy	Allow people choice
Beneficence	Do good
Nonmaleficence	Do not do bad
Justice	Be fair (equality) in practice
Fidelity and responsibility	Show loyalty
Integrity	Behave in a trustworthy manner
Respect for the rights and dignity of others	Show respect for others
	Accord dignity
	Treat others with caring and compassion
	Pursue excellence
	Accept accountability

Western world and acceptable practice in China and Japan, where traditional values mandate avoiding direct discussion of illness with the patient in many contexts. In the United States, we would traditionally place paramount importance on patients' autonomy. In Japan, for example, great importance would be placed to informing key family members, rather than directly discussing such matters with the patient, particularly in end-of-life matters. In such circumstances, compassionate care would dictate following the cultural values of the patient.

The pursuit of excellence means not only doing good and seeking to avoid harm but going the proverbial extra mile to assist in healing the patient. Similarly, acknowledging personal responsibility and even apologizing when appropriate constitute clear indicators of ethical striving. These principles should cause us to use sensitivity, wisdom, and the forging of thoughtful alliances with our patients, rather than attempting to rely on authoritative pronouncements, threats, or appeals to their worst fears and uncertainties.

INQUIRING ABOUT NONADHERENCE

Sadly, medical care providers generally have little ability to recognize non-adherence, and research interventions aimed at improving their recognition rates have had mixed results. Studies have used pill counts, ascertaining rates of refilling prescriptions, patient questionnaires, electronic medication monitors, and asking patients to keep medication diaries. One can sometimes directly observe treatment in institutional settings, but more often than not we rely of delayed indirect methods of measuring adherence (e.g., hemoglobin A1c measurement in diabetes). Simply asking the patient will often prove inadequate by virtue of memory errors or simply fearing a critical response or loss of approval from the caregiver.

A more productive course of action might involve asking the patient directly in a way that recognizes perfect adherence is not expected. Consider asking this: What has your doctor asked you to do in order to best manage your illness (or to stay healthy)? What are the hardest pieces of medical advice to follow? Which parts do you skip or miss most often? With the answers to such question in hand one can craft an intervention optimally suited to the patient's situation. The solution may involve improved patient education, altered dosing schedules, improved communication between physicians and patients or similar steps that respond the basis for nonadherence. Most strategic plans to improve adherence will likely involve combinations of behavioral interventions, efforts to increase the convenience of care, or providing educational information about the patient's condition and the treatment.

Prochaska, Norcross, and DiClemente (1994) list nine specific behavioral strategies to employ as needed:

1. *Consciousness raising*—helping to increase the information patients have about themselves and their problem.
2. *Social liberation*—increasing social alternatives for behaviors that are not problematic.
3. *Emotional arousal*—recognizing, experiencing, and expressing feelings about one's problems and potential solutions.
4. *Self–re-evaluation*—assessing feelings and thoughts about oneself with respect to the problem at hand.
5. *Commitment*—choosing and committing to act with a belief in ability to change.
6. *Countering*—substituting alternatives for problem behaviors.
7. *Environment control*—avoiding triggers or situations that elicit problem behaviors.
8. *Reward*—rewarding self or earning recognition and reward from others for making changes.
9. *Helping relationships*—enlisting the help of supportive others (including both professionals and components of the patient's social networks).

REFERENCES

Beauchamp, T. L., & Childress, J. F. (2001). *Principles of biomedical ethics* (5th ed.). New York: Oxford University Press.

Kleinman, A. (1988). *The illness narratives: suffering, healing, and the human condition.* New York: Basic Books.

Koocher, G. P., McGrath, M. L., & Gudas, L. J. (1990). Typologies of non-adherence in cystic fibrosis. *Journal of Developmental and Behavioral Pediatrics, 11,* 353–358.

Koocher, G. P., & Keith-Spiegel, P. (2008). Ethics in psychology and the mental health professions: standards and cases (3rd ed.). New York: Oxford University Press.

Osterberg, L., & Blaschke, T. (2005). Adherence to medication. *New England Journal of Medicine, 353,* 487–497.

Prochaska, J. O., DiClemente, C. C., & Norcross, J. C. (1992). In search of how people change: applications to addictive behaviors. *American Psychologist, 47,* 1102–1114.

Prochaska, J. O., Norcross, J. C., & DiClemente, C. C. (1994). *Changing for good.* New York: Avon.

Prochaska, J. O., Velicer, W. F., Rossi, J. S., et al. (1994). Stages of change and decisional balance for 12 problem behaviors. *Health Psychology, 13,* 39–46.

Prochaska, J. M., Prochaska, J. O., Johnson, S. S. (2006). In W. T. O'Donohue & E. R. (Eds.), Assessing readiness for adherence to treatment. In Levensky (Eds.), *Promoting treatment adherence: a practical handbook for healthcare providers* (pp. 35–46). Thousand Oaks, CA: Sage.

Section *II*

Teaching Methodologies

T he planning, implementation, and evaluation of appropriate and effective learning opportunities require a great deal of time and energy on the part of the healthcare provider. To meet the educational needs of our patients and clients while balancing our multiple commitments, it is helpful to draw upon the success of others.

The chapters in this section present and discuss examples of teaching methodologies used in a variety of settings, and build upon the fundamental concepts presented in Section I. They provide specific information, examples, and resources for you to adapt to your own teaching needs, settings, and the populations with whom you work. In our increasingly multicultural society, all of our teaching must be sensitive to cultural differences among our learners. As we seek to make the best use of time and resources, we can prepare our instruction to address a single individual or to accommodate a group or community. As we seek to best connect with our learners, there is a wide variety of instructional tools we can select from; we might use any of a variety of instructional technologies, or even incorporate play.

The vast amount of health information available to providers and patients is both a blessing and a curse—if we are to be effective in teaching patients about accessing health information, we must know about resources available to us, how best to access them, and how to judge the reliability of the source. Regardless of who we teach and where we conduct our instruction, we can all benefit from recognizing the "teachable moment," being able to teach "on the fly," and knowing how to "make learning stick."

Chapter 8

Individualized Instruction

Danielle Steward-Gelinas & Jane C. Romano

INTRODUCTION

Health professionals have a distinct responsibility and opportunity to educate patients about many issues. Effective presentation of information is critical to an individual's ability to carry out treatment protocols and to develop positive lifestyle changes related to his or her health. In order to educate patients, it is important to be aware of the uniqueness of individuals and to use appropriate strategies and resources. Much of the onus falls on the healthcare provider to determine the best methods to deliver the necessary information and education to patients.

Historically, teaching was often very individualized and included a multitude of different methods, including words, sounds, actions, and pictures. Often in the form of apprenticeships, skills and information were presented, absorbed, and passed on through many generations. In very early years, the acquisition of these skills was a matter of survival. Times have changed, and although our learning is not always necessarily about survival, it plays a significant role in how we choose to live our lives.

Teaching patients occurs on many different levels and in many different environments. You teach patients about surgeries, procedures, diagnoses, exercises, and the importance of health and wellness in clinics, hospitals, schools, communities, and workshops. As a healthcare professional, it is important that you address all of the necessary components of individual learning. Some of the many issues that can influence the efficacy of our teachings include primary language, available resources, literacy skills, physical abilities, cultural and socioeconomic factors, emotional issues, and locus of control. This chapter is designed to address effective teaching of individuals in all settings. Issues such as assessing your learner, various strategies to consider, teaching tools and evaluative techniques are examined.

ASSESSING INDIVIDUAL'S LEARNING PREFERENCES

Before you begin teaching, it is critical to know your audience. Teaching individuals provides you with an opportunity to truly understand your patient's interests and concerns. Take every interaction as a chance to learn more about your patient and to provide valuable information. Even during the busiest clinic visit or on a full inpatient floor, it is essential to take time to talk with your patient. Effective teaching does not always require large amounts of time and can be delivered in shorter, very focused interactions. Gaining information about an individual initially will help you to determine and design your teaching strategy (Vella, 2002).

A thorough and holistic assessment is the first step in planning and implementing all patient care, including education. Cognitive, physiological, psychological, environmental, and cultural influences need to be considered when performing initial as well as ongoing assessment (Whittemore, Bak, Melkus, & Grey, 2003). Information such as knowledge base, skills, beliefs, lifestyle patterns, as well as readiness to change, is essential to determine during early interactions with patients.

People use many different methods to learn information and can often require some combination of techniques to experience an effective learning event. Think about how you learn best. Do you prefer to listen to a lecture, watch a video or slide presentation, interact in a discussion, or some combination of these methods? Most people benefit from a combination of teaching strategies; however, it is important to determine whether an individual prefers to learn by listening (auditory), watching (visual) or doing (kinesthetic) in order for teaching to be most effective.

Literacy skills are essential to assess in order to determine an effective approach to delivering education. Low literary skills are associated with poor health and lead to decrease compliance with treatment (Pawlak, 2005). Simply asking individuals about their literacy skills is not the answer because most will try to hide their inabilities. People with limited reading skills typically take words literally, skip uncommon words, attempt to sound out words, and tire easily with written instructions (Schultz, 2002). They will often try to guess their way through oral instructions and do not ask questions in fear that their low literacy skills will be discovered. When planning education for individuals with low literacy skills, use a variety of methods of delivering and reinforcing the information. Videos, demonstrations, verbal explanations such as step-by-step audio tapes, and pictures can help to improve understanding and retention. It is best to choose a quiet time when there is less chance of interruptions because individuals with low literacy skills are often more difficult to engage and are easily distracted (Schultz, 2002). It is important to personalize the message, give direction in small steps, and encourage frequent feedback in order to assure that limited readers understands what is expected of them.

In order to best determine your approach, listen to your patient. Listening is an active process and can help you determine your priorities when planning patient education. It is essential to recognize that patients have their own ideas of what they believe is important for them to know (Pender, Murdaugh, & Parsons, 2006). This is particularly crucial when faced with the dilemma of educating a patient with multiple health issues. This requires the healthcare provider to deliver information that focuses on what the *patient* is most concerned about versus what they believe most important. Research has shown that individuals have better health outcomes when they are included in decision making and planning (Whittemore et al., 2003). Keeping teaching patient centered will increase the likelihood of successful behavior changes, which in turn will motivate the individual to learn more about his or her health. Taking the time to get to know your patient is critical to create the most beneficial learning experience effectively.

ASSESSING READINESS: THE PRECEED ASSESSMENT MODEL

Multiple theories are related to a person's ability to change his or her health behaviors. Bellamy (2004) discusses a practice model that can be used to improve compliance on a one-to-one basis. The individual's readiness for behavioral change is assessed in three phases.

- *Phase 1: predisposing factors*—the following three questions are asked: (1) Does the person believe that he or she is susceptible to disease or illness if the behavior change is not adopted? Does he or she believe that problems associated with noncompliance are severe? Does the person believe the benefits of the change outweigh the risk? Education is planned based on the answer to all three questions.

- *Phase 2: enabling factors*—the person's skills and resources as well as any barriers to change are assessed. If the skills and resources are determined to be inadequate, the person will need additional support before moving on to phase 3.
- *Phase 3: reinforcing factors*—the person's understanding and expectations of the intervention are assessed to assure that they are realistic. If they are not, the patient requires additional education in order to bring about effective behavior change (Bellamy, 2004).

This model provides a solid foundation for determining an individual's readiness to learn about his or her health in order to plan and implement an appropriate, effective educational plan.

THE ABILITY TO PROBLEM SOLVE

In addition to determining a readiness to learn, it is essential to assess an individual's ability to identify and solve problems that he or she may encounter during his or her patient experience. The ability to solve problems effectively is considered one of the most useful strategies for coping with illness (Gonzalez, Goeppinger, & Lorig, 1990). It is important to teach problem-solving skills and not just specific solutions to problems. This is where a person's locus of control can have a positive or negative influence on his or her ability to solve problems. A belief that there is no ability to control an outcome will create obstacles the healthcare provider will need to consider when planning and implementing patient education. Whittemore et al. (2003) identifies the following key points to focus on when supporting a patient's ability to solve problems:

- Set specific, relevant, and realistic goals with an incremental approach to achieving them.
- Promote self-monitoring using strategies such as having the patient keep a journal or diary in order to help identify factors that can assist or interfere with lifestyle change.
- Encourage an individual to identify situation or events that may promote unhealthy behaviors.
- Identify environmental and personal cues that increase the likelihood of compliance with healthy behaviors.
- Determine rationalizations for unhealthy behaviors and replace them with positive self-statements.
- Encourage the involvement of supportive family and friends in the healthy behavior.

Even the best made plans will be of no value if the potential problems to its implementation are not explored. Create opportunities to partner with the patient and collaboratively identify strategies that will enable him or her to maximize his or her ability to overcome barriers and optimize his or her health outcomes through effective problem solving.

STRATEGIES TO CONSIDER

The environment in which health education is conducted is vitally important to successful outcomes (Pender et al., 2006). Ideally, individualized instruction occurs in a quiet, uninterrupted setting where the healthcare provider can truly listen to the patient in order to prioritize and maximize teaching. When you are lucky enough to have the opportunity to educate patients in this type of setting, it is critical to avoid information overload. It is best to limit instruction to maximize learning, which reinforces the need to prioritize learning and remaining patient centered.

Less than ideal settings are what we are more familiar with as healthcare providers practicing in an increasing complex environment. Busy clinics and inpatient units where noise and interruptions are normal are the more common setting for the delivery of patient education. The challenges of effectively delivering education in these settings are not insurmountable. The key again is to keep instruction patient centered. It is also essential to maximized learning by using visual, auditory, and kinesthetic methods of delivering information. Written materials, computers, videos, and return demonstrations should be used to supplement verbal instruction in order to make learning more individualized.

When considering the use of methods such as computers and videos, it is essential to assess the individual's access to these technologies. Willis (2006) states that 56% of people ages 50 to 64 have access to the Internet and computers. In addition, in the year 2000, the majority of people over the age of 65 did not have access to these sources of information. In order for these teaching strategies to be most effective, assessment should include the person's level of education, employment status, occupation, and type of household they live in (Willis, 2006). Individuals with higher levels of education who are currently working in a job where computer skills are required and who have computers in their household are more likely to benefit from these teaching methods.

Your ability to think quickly on your feet can often either make or break the desired outcome of any instruction. Even the best made plan can go astray; thus, it is wise to have a plan B, C, and D. When explaining a

diagnosis, technique, or exercise, it is essential to assess the patient's understanding of the subject through observation. Nodding accompanied by a
blank stare can indicate a lack of understanding. Asking the patient to
restate or demonstrate the information allows the provider to clarify misconceptions or confusion. Your patients will not always respond to the same
teaching technique, and thus, it is necessary to be prepared to use many different methods of getting your message across.

Research has offered some varied learning theories that may provide
insight into how to prepare for teaching your patients. Planning education
for adults is significantly different than planning learning opportunities for
children in which it is necessary to consider stages of growth and development in order for teaching to be effective. Knowles (1980) describes the key
to adult learning as learning based on personal experience. When adults are
engaged in the learning planning and design, they are more apt to develop an
interest and better understanding of the information presented. By personalizing the learning experience and presenting each component in a manner
that is relevant to your patient's interests and abilities, you can improve your
effectiveness as an educator.

TEACHING METHODS

As stated earlier, effective teaching requires taking into account various ways
of delivering information. Consider the following four methods of presenting
education: verbal, written, pictures, and actions. First and foremost, it is
important to deliver the information in a manner that is easy for the individual to understand. Verbal instructions are perhaps the most common means
of providing information. As healthcare professionals, we are able to discuss
issues such as diagnoses, medications, therapies, and prognoses with our
patients. To provide verbal instructions effectively, you first must consider the
patient's primary language, education level, and comprehension. Research
shows that Americans typically read and understand information that is 3 to
5 years below their last year of formal of education (Cutilli, 2005). Too often,
healthcare professionals use medical terminology that is difficult for even the
most literate patient to grasp. Many well-educated and high-level literate individuals have trouble understanding medical jargon (Cutilli, 2005). When
explaining a component of their treatment plan to an individual, take note of
the terms that they use to describe things when they ask questions and use
their words to clarify or reinforce teaching. Use the support of an interpreter
when English is not the individual's primary language. The onus is on the
healthcare provider to be aware of how he or she delivers the desired message

as well as their patient's ability to process and understand the message in order to bring about a positive change in behavior.

Written instructions can be a nice supplement to verbal instruction and help to reinforce key points that are covered during verbal instruction. This can include booklets, leaflets, and information handouts. Written instruction is a cost-effective and time-efficient method of communicating health information (Griffin, McKenna, & Tooth, 2003). They also provide flexibility for the individual allowing them to refer to the information when they need to and to learn at their own pace. The key to effective written materials is to keep it simple and clear. It is recommended that in order to benefit the majority of users written material should be written at a fifth- or sixth-grade level (Griffin et al., 2003). This will also make it easier to translate written materials into languages that meet the needs of your patient population. Other considerations are the layout and design of the content. Effective written instruction is not jam packed with content and focuses on the key points.

Pictures can provide a resource that can transcend age, language barriers, and educational differences. Illustrations address the areas of attention (did the patient read the instructions), recall (can the patient repeat the instructions), and adherence (did the patient perform the activity correctly) (Houts, Doak, Doak, & Loscalzo, 2006). They can assist a patient in understanding specific directions and schedules more effectively. The pictures may not guarantee adherence to a program but may help to provide a better understanding of instructions.

Action in conjunction with the previously mentioned methods may be the most effective means of accurately relaying and measuring the impact of appropriate information. When instructing a patient in a medication schedule, have the patient organize medications in a method that best makes sense to them while accurately reflecting the correct regimen. An exercise program can be best demonstrated by the actions of the therapist and a return demonstration by the patient. When these actions have been performed, reinforce your instruction with verbal and written instructions as well as including pictures. This comprehensive combination of instruction will increase the likelihood of attention, recall, and adherence to the education. It is important to ask your patient to recall and demonstrate, when appropriate, the information that has been presented. You may think that you have been effective in teaching your patient, but if he or she is unable to recall the information or adhere to instructions, learning has not taken place. Repeat the information in as many different methods and as often as possible. In addition, education needs to be reevaluated and reinforced with every opportunity.

Case Study 8-1

Dr. Smith is an 80-year-old woman who was recently involved in a motor vehicle accident. She was teaching at a local community college before her admission. Her primary care nurse has learned that she did not suffer a head injury, and while in the hospital, she was diagnosed with diabetes and hypertension. Upon discharge, she will need to manage her pain medication as well as new medications for her diabetes and hypertension. Because this patient is a well-educated individual, the nurse assumes that she will easily understand directions and begins providing her with instruction. Dr. Smith nods and smiles during the interaction. The nurse leaves feeling as though she will be fine with her new medications and the detailed schedule discussed. Within 1 week of discharge, Dr. Smith is readmitted to the hospital because of complications with her medications.

In this case, Dr. Smith indicated an understanding through her nonverbal communication, but no follow-up or support was provided. She was not given written instruction, nor was she asked to repeat the instructions back to the nurse. During her repeat admission, various strategies were used to deliver education where Dr. Smith was provided verbal as well as written instruction and was required to demonstrate an understanding of her medication regimen.

Involving your patient in the education process will help to ensure a more successful outcome. Making sure the information you provide is relevant to that particular patient and is delivered in a manner that is tailored to his or her specific needs is critical to bringing about positive health behavior change.

USING GROUPS TO STRENGTHEN INDIVIDUALIZED INSTRUCTION

Research has shown that group education has both pros and cons. Instruction delivered in group forums is more cost-effective than individualized instruction (Moseley, 2003). It can also serve to motivate patients with the same diagnosis by providing the opportunity to share experiences, problem solve, and form friendships that will help to make patients realize that they are not alone in their experience (Peltier, 2006).

Group education enables the facilitator to focus their instruction on a specific topic or treatment that is common to the participants and can include various teaching strategies. It does, however, limit their ability to tailor the education to the specific needs of individuals. Moseley (2003) found that, despite the positive aspects of group instruction, it is not as effective in bringing about lifestyle changes as one-on-one teaching. The combination of individual and group instruction was found to enhance a patient's ability to bring about changes in their health behaviors.

One of the keys to effective group instruction is a skilled and knowledgeable facilitator. The role of the facilitator is to help the group to communicate, examine, and solve problems and to make decisions (Spangler, 2003). The role also involves helping group members get to know each other, stay on task, and be more creative, efficient, and productive. It is essential to know when to deliver instruction and when to allow the group to share and process the information as well as their experiences in order for this type of education to be effective.

SIMULATION AS A LEARNING TOOL

Simulated experiences have been used as a training tool in several different occupations throughout the years. The military, nuclear power plants, and the aviation field continue to use mock scenarios of critical incidents to better prepare for unexpected yet potential events. Academic programs for healthcare providers also employed this teaching method to simulate everything from critical incidents to basic clinical skills.

The possibility for using the simulated experience as a learning tool is limitless and does not always require high-fidelity equipment to be effective. Many rehabilitation programs have Easy Street Environments that provide a lifelike, everyday world within a safe rehabilitation setting (Northwest Hospital and Medical Center, n.d.). Actual city streets exist in a controlled environment and include daily activities such as a restaurant, grocery store, hair salon, bank, car, gas pump, and bus. Obstacles such as heavy doors, high curbs, high and low shelves, varied flooring, and turnstiles provide the patient with a chance to manage real-life situations.

Even without access to environments like Easy Street, simulation can still be an effective teaching tool. For example, using various restaurant menus can help an individual practice making appropriate choices related to their health issues when eating out. It requires the healthcare provider to be creative when planning and implementing individualized education.

Simulating actual situations as a teaching method is patient centered and addresses multiple learning styles. It provides a safe environment where trial and error reinforces learning. This method of delivering education enables the information to be tailored to the specific needs of the individual and can be easily adapted and evaluated for its effectiveness.

PROVIDING EDUCATION AND SUPPORT FOR CARETAKERS

An aspect of the patient experience that we have not yet considered is that of the caretakers. The stress of illness affects more than just the patient.

Education and interventions should be planned to address not only the needs of the individual but also the needs of his or her caregivers (Neef & Walling, 2006). The primary caretaker has the ability to influence recovery and may be less able to do so because of his or her own challenges related to the stress placed on them (Taylor, Nolan, & Dudley-Brown, 2006). Patient education needs to extend beyond the individual to include the people who have the potential to sway health behaviors in order to have the most impact. Addressing the needs of those who are responsible for care will foster resiliency, provide valuable resources, and promote positive outcomes for everyone concerned (Pender et al., 2006).

EVALUATING INDIVIDUALIZED LEARNING

Education is only effective if it brings about a change in health behaviors. It is essential to evaluate the impact of individual learning in order for it to be achievable and sustainable when they are not under your care. It can be difficult to overcoming the urge to give in to at-risk behaviors and temptations of the real world. It is particularly challenging for low-income and disadvantaged individuals because of limited resources in the social and physical environment (Pender et al., 2006).

In a study that examined the self-efficacy of patients with chronic obstructive pulmonary disease, Wong, Wong, and Chan (2005) found that an individual's compliance with treatment regimens increased with a nurse initiated telephone follow-up. Something as simple as a phone call from a healthcare provider can serve a dual purpose. It can provide an important link to the support, reinforcement, and validation that individuals may need to be successful in adapting their health behaviors. In addition, it can provide an opportunity for the provider to evaluate the effectiveness of their teaching.

A method for evaluating change that can be easily applied to education is a quality-improvement strategy that was originally developed by Walter Shewhart in the 1930s called the Plan, Do, Study, Act (PDSA) Cycle (The Improvement Network, 2004). The four stages of this model involve the following: (1) plan—decide what you wish to accomplish after determining the nature and size of the problem as well as what will need to be done to accomplish the desired change; (2) do—put the plan into action; (3) study—did the plan work; and (4) act—adapt, adopt, or abandon the plan. Keep in mind that even the best made plans do not always bring about the desired effect on the first try. The fourth stage of the cycle is where it can be determined whether change has taken place and this change has brought about the desired outcome of the original plan. If it is determined that the original accomplishments were not achieved or turned out to be unattainable, you begin the cycle again using this new information to develop, try out, and evaluate a new plan.

The PDSA cycle is just one method of evaluating desired learning outcomes. It does not matter which method you choose to evaluate your teaching. What does matter is that you take the time to determine whether the goal of the education is attainable and sustainable for the individual.

CONCLUSION

As healthcare professionals, we have a wealth of information that is necessary to share with our patients in order to bring about positive lifestyle changes related to their well-being. It is important that we are able to share that information in the most effective manner possible. There is no cookie-cutter approach to teaching that will present this information effectively to every member of society, but a combination of techniques make teaching far more effective for most individuals. It is the responsibility of those planning and implementing patient education to be aware of the uniqueness of individuals as well as the various ways in which people learn. Effectively presenting information that an individual needs to adopt positive lifestyle changes requires the healthcare provider to determine the most appropriate and effective methods to deliver the necessary information.

One of the keys to successful education is to remember that every interaction is an opportunity to teach. Taking the time to get to know an individual's thoughts and ideas about being a patient is the cornerstone of gaining critical insight into the best way to plan and implement education. Each time you interact with a person, whether it is during a scheduled clinic visit, an inpatient stay, or a follow-up phone call, it is essential to capitalize on this time to reinforce and/or evaluate the impact of your teaching. Doing so delivers continual support to individuals in their efforts to change behaviors. It also provides the healthcare provider opportunities to strengthen their ability to educate effectively the individuals under their care.

REFERENCES

Bellamy, R. (2004). An introduction to patient education: theory and practice. *Medical Teacher, 26*(4), 359–365.

Cutilli, C. C. (2005). Do your patients understand? Determining your patients' health literacy skills. *Orthopaedic Nursing, 24*(5), 372–377.

Gonzalez, V. M., Goeppinger, J., & Lorig, K. (1990). Four psychological theories and their application to patient education and clinical practice. *Arthritis Care and Research, 3*(3), 132–143.

Griffin, J., McKenna, K., & Tooth, L. (2003). Written health education materials: making them more effective. *Australian Occupational Therapy Journal, 50,* 170–177.

Houts, P. S., Doak, C. C., Doak, L. G., & Loscalzo, M. J. (2005, May 8). The role of pictures in improving health communication: a review of research on attention, comprehension, recall, and adherence. *Patient Education and Counseling, 61,* 173–190.

Knowles, M. S. (1980). *The modern practice of adult education: from pedagogy to andragogy* (2nd ed.). New York: Cambridge Books.

Moseley, G. L. (2003). Joining forces: combining cognition-targeted motor control training with group or individual pain physiology education: a successful treatment for chronic low back pain. *The Journal of Manual & Manipulative Therapy, 11*(2), 88–94.

Neef, D., & Walling, A. D. (2006). Dementia with Lewy bodies: an emerging disease. *American Family Physician, 73*(7), 1223–1229.

Northwest Hospital and Medical Center (n.d.). Easy Street Environment brochure. Accessed February 9, 2008, from http://www.nwhospital.org/news/brochure/final%20EasyStreet%20brochure.pdf.

Pawlak, R. (2005). Economic considerations of health literacy. *Nursing Economics, 23*(4), 173–180.

Peltier, M. (2006). More than weight loss: a steady diet of support and achievement. Accessed January 23, 2008, from www.nursinghomesmagazine.com.

Pender, N. J., Murdaugh, C. L., & Parsons, M. (2006). *Health promotion in nursing practice.* Upper Saddle River, NJ: Pearson Prentice Hall.

Schultz, M. (2002). Low literacy skills needn't hinder care. *RN, 65*(4), 45–48.

Spangler, B. (2003). What is facilitation? Beyond intractability. Accessed February 2, 2008, from www.beyondintractability.org/essay/facilitation.

Taylor, L., Nolan, M., & Dudley-Brown, S. (2006). Evidence of spouse responses to illness as a guide to understanding and studying spouse responses to living organ donation. *Progress in Transplantation, 16*(2), 117–125.

The Improvement Network. (2004). The plan, do, study, act cycle. Accessed February 10, 2008, from http://www.tin.nhs.uk/index.asp?pgid=1130.

Vella, J. (2002). *Learning to listen, learning to teach.* San Francisco: Jossey-Bass.

Whittemore, R., Bak, P. S., Melkus, G. D., & Grey, M. (2003). Promoting lifestyle change in the prevention and management of type 2 diabetes. *Journal of the American Academy of Nurse Practitioners, 15*(8), 341–349.

Willis, S. L. (2006). Technology and learning in current and future generations of elders. *Generations* (Summer), 44–48.

Wong, K. W., Wong, F. K. Y., & Chan, M. F. (2005). Effects of nurse-initiated telephone follow-up on self-efficacy among patients with chronic obstructive pulmonary disease. *Journal of Advanced Nursing, 49*(2), 210–222.

Chapter 9

Teaching with Groups

Nancy Lowenstein

INTRODUCTION

Groups offer an effective method of teaching a variety of topics in health promotion and health education. With the increased focus on self-management of chronic disease, groups are often an effective way to deliver this education. Group counseling and group processes were introduced early in the 1900s in the medical realm, with much of the work on using groups for counseling stemming from the 1950s and later (Gazda, Ginter, & Horne, 2001). Groups offer an opportunity for enhanced learning because of sharing of information between group members, brainstorming of ideas and solutions for health-related issues, shared thinking, and challenging of assumptions and myths held by individual members. There are disadvantages to groups as well, but they are far outweighed by the advantages. Some of the disadvantages include time and energy, group conflict, poor leadership, and unclear goals. This chapter addresses some of these issues.

Running successful groups requires skill and knowledge of group interaction and group process and group dynamics. Groups can be any size (from two on up), and the teaching techniques will vary with the topic, type of group, and size. Engleberg and Wynn (2007) describe several different types of groups, some of which are addressed in this chapter (**Table 9-1**).

Table 9-1 Group Types

Group	Membership/Purpose/Examples
Primary group	Family and friends: provide "affection, support, and a sense of belonging" (p. 9)
Social groups	Share common interests; do common activity (e.g., sorority, team, and garden club)
Self-help groups	All members share the same problem/issue (e.g., Alcoholics Anonymous, multiple sclerosis support group).
Learning groups	Members acquire information on a topic (e.g., parenting class and college class).
Service groups	Help others, often associated with a cause (e.g., Habitat for Humanity, PTA, Rotary clubs).
Work groups	Groups that form at work to achieve tasks (e.g., committees, task force).
Public groups	Groups work done before the public (e.g., school committee, regulatory board).

RUNNING GROUPS: ISSUES AND ANSWERS

The most common types of groups that are used for teaching health promotion are family/friends, self-help/support, and learning groups. These types of groups fit best with teaching health promotion strategies as they include important characteristics, such as sharing of information, common goals, shared motivation, and participants that have the same conditions.

For groups to function well, however, a skilled leader with knowledge of group dynamics and group process is key to a successful group. In this section, we explore the following aspects of group dynamics: group norms, leadership, and teaching techniques.

Group Norms

Members of a group all arrive with their own past experiences of being a group member. These groups had their own unique set of norms, those implicit and explicit rules that groups abide by in order to run most effectively. Some norms are universal, such as the expectation that a group starts at the stated time, not an hour later. Other norms may have been particular to a specific group, such as a team, where winning is the implicit group norm. An implicit norm is a way of behaving within the group that is not formally or verbally stated but that is known by group members anyway (Posthuma, 2002). An example of an implicit group norm would be raising your hand in a classroom in order to be recognized or everyone taking the same seats each time. It is not usually stated but is either universally known or evolved without being stated.

Table 9-2 Effective Group Norms

Norm	Reasons
Start and end time	Stating the norm for start time allows group members to feel comfortable if they are running late, that they are not holding up the start of the group. Stating the exact end time will allow members to arrange transportation or other activities and allows the leader to stay on schedule.
Talking time	Clearly stating a time limit for each member to talk allows time for all members to participate in the group and prevents one member from dominating a discussion. This can be done by stating a "time rule" such as a 1.5, 2, or 5 minute rule (each member can talk for that specific amount of time), and then they need to let someone else talk. They can talk again if there is time.
Rules for being recognized to speak	Establishing the norm for speaking such as raising hands, going in a circle, being recognized by the leader will allow all members to feel comfortable with being recognized to speak.
Use of names	Sets the tone for formality. First or last names, use of name tags, how to address leader.
Break times	Clearly stating if there will be breaks, how they are determined, or when they will occur.
Learning contracts	This may be useful if there is homework or other aspects of the learning that benefits the participants in their learning.
Confidentiality	Stating a confidentiality policy establishes a safe environment for members to share honestly.

An explicit norm is a clearly stated rule or procedure, and all members are aware of it (Posthuma, 2002). An example of an explicit norm would be the group agreeing to start and end the group exactly on time. In this case, a discussion would have taken place and this "rule" agreed on by all members.

Therefore, for a group to run effectively as quickly as possible, it is best for the group to state the norms that it wishes to abide by. Norms that help a group run well are noted in **Table 9-2**.

Group Leadership

There are many different theories of group leadership (Gershenfeld, 2004) and work defining the qualities of a good leader; however, there is no clear consensus as to the "ideal" qualifications for successfully leading a group.

Successful leadership of a group depends on the purpose of the group, the type of group, and group members. Learning to be an effective group leader is a skill that takes experience and practice. This section outlines some of the qualities and skills for effective group leadership.

Leader and leadership are terms with different meanings. One refers to an individual being followed by others, and the second refers to the "process of influencing the task and social dimensions of a group to help it reach its goal" (Fujishin, 2001, p. 122). When beginning the task of leading a group, it is important to look at the goals of the group and the presentation style. For a group that involves member participation and active participation as its learning focus, then a more facilitative or democratic leadership style is best. For a group that is more teaching than interactive, a more directive or "teaching" style is useful.

Research on leader and leadership has focused over the years on three main areas: that of the leader personality traits, the group situation (task group at work, support group, team, etc.), and style of leadership. The trait theory states that leaders have particular personality traits, such as intelligence, warmth, or assertiveness; however, there are many examples of leaders who do not demonstrate these traits. The situational theory postulated by Hersey and Blanchard looks at the circumstances or situations in which leadership is needed, such as a team and business. In this theory, it is held that different group members become leaders in different situations or for different tasks. The leadership style attributes three different styles of leadership: autocratic, democratic, and laissez-faire. Each of these styles puts the leadership of the group in different hands. In the autocratic style, there is a definitive leader who makes the decisions and tells the group what to do. In the democratic style, the leader shares leadership with the group, and decisions are made on a consensus basis. In the laissez-faire style, the leader lets the group take charge (Engleberg & Wynn, 2007; Schwartzberg, Howe, & Barnes, 2008). A fourth way of looking at leadership and groups is to look at the leader–member continuum described by Tannenbaum and Schmidt (1958) and modified by Schwartzberg et al. (2008) to suit non–business-oriented groups. This model looks at the continuum of leader–member participation. The more "leader centered" a group is, the less involved the group members are in the decision-making process. As the group becomes more "group" or member centered, the less influence the designated leader has on group decision making and the more this person acts as a guide and mentor to the group (**Figure 9-1**).

There is no "best" or "worst" leadership style, but the most effective one depends on the type of group and the goals of the group. When the leader

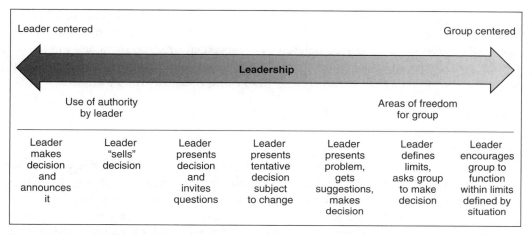

Figure 9-1 Leadership–member continuum.
From: Schwartzberg et al. (2008) (with permission) and Tannenbaum and Schmidt (1958).

determines the group goals and tasks then the group requires a more directive type of leadership. A typical example of this type of group would be a
team or a group comprised of individuals who need structure and guidance
(young children, adults, and children with cognitive disabilities, etc.). As the
group becomes more member centered, the role of the leader becomes less
authoritative and more facilitative. An example of this type of group would
be students working on a project, a task group given a goal and no more, or
a family or peer group that needs guidance or education. The skills of leadership require knowledge of self and group dynamics and the interplay of
these complex factors.

Teaching Techniques

It is most important to teach to the group at an appropriate level. Teaching
groups comprised of adults, adolescents, or children will all require different
techniques. Some groups may be a mix of these age groups, such as families,
support groups, or groups geared toward children and their parents, and it
will be necessary to use techniques that appeal to all group members. People
learn better by doing than they learn by listening. When teaching health
behaviors, it is helpful to have members practice the skills you want them to
develop and to practice them in the context in which they are to be used.
Changing behaviors requires considerable practice, support, and time.

It is important to realize that each group and group session should have a beginning, middle, and end. The behaviors of members in newly formed groups versus groups that have been meeting for several sessions will be different. Additionally, group sessions that have a set routine are more efficient and predictable and therefore more comfortable to group members.

GROUPS

Beginning

In newly formed groups, members do not know each other; they may be awkward, not very talkative, or forthcoming with honest sharing. In talking about their health condition, they may minimize their own functioning in an effort to seem better. When starting a group whose members do not know each other, it is good to start the group with an introductory activity that allows members an opportunity to get to know each other. These are often called icebreakers, and there are many books and websites that offer these types of activities. **Table 9-3** has a few of these icebreaker ideas.

Middle

As the group has more meetings, members begin to know each other and feel comfortable, becoming more open. Group members are more trusting of

Table 9-3 Icebreakers

Icebreaker Name	Procedure
Member scavenger hunt	Develop a list that starts with the statement "find someone who . . . ." Then provide a list of attributes such as "likes pepperoni pizza," "has blue eyes," "has 2 siblings," and so forth.
	Then have members move around and find group members who match the different descriptions; they should write the names when they find someone who matches the descriptions.
Getting to know you	Have group sit or stand in a circle. Take a ball, bean bag, or some easy object to catch. The first person says their name and throws the object to anyone in the circle. The object is caught and that person says "thank you X, my name is Y, and I am throwing the ball to YOU."
	The object is thrown to another person in the circle, and this continues until all members of the group have had a chance to say their name.
Two truths and a lie	Each group member is given an index card and writes down two true statements and one lie. One person shares their card, and the group guesses which is the lie. Have all members share their card.

each other and are therefore more likely to share personal information and support each other and make suggestions to solve health-related problems. There is joking and sharing and an open atmosphere.

Ending

As the group's meetings are coming to a close, it is important for members to acknowledge the support that they have received from each other and to have time to bring closure to the experience. Often members will share names and contact information or even continue to meet on their own. Having some sort of closing "ceremony" often helps to bring closure to the group and allows members to have a sense of completeness. This can be accomplished with a certificate of completion, a party, a group hug, or some other activity that brings closure.

GROUP SESSIONS

Each group session also has a beginning, middle, and an end. Routine is helpful in establishing norms and expectations for group members and for relieving individual anxiety. Group members know that the group will have a set format and do not have to be concerned with what is going to happen each session.

Beginning

Each session should be started with some sort of introduction to the day's topic and format, as well as time for members to ask questions on previous session's learning or activities.

Middle

After the introduction and questions, the group embarks on the learning/activity for the current session. There are different techniques that the leader/facilitator may use, including flip charts, worksheets, games, discussion, and more.

Ending

Each session should end with a wrap-up or summary of that day's material, time for questions, an explanation of any homework, and a reminder of when the next session will meet.

Table 9-4 Group Problems and Possible Solutions

Problem	Possible Solution
Leader is unskilled.	If leader is just developing his or her skills, it is best to have a skilled co-leader.
Leader is not familiar with teaching materials.	Leader should know and be confident in the information to be taught before the group starts. If this is not possible, then involving a co-leader who does know the material is a possible solution.
Individual group members do not get along.	If this involves two members who do not get along, try addressing each individual member separately outside of the group. If this involves the group itself, have a discussion during one of the group meetings to resolve the issues.
One or two group members monopolize group interactions.	Limit all group members to a specific time limit for talking and/or number of times in each group session.
Group member has cognitive problem or is in some other way not appropriate for group.	Group member may need to be asked to leave the group, but it is best if there is another group or learning opportunity for them to go to.
Group norms are not adhered to.	Discuss and identify implicit and explicit norms. Clarify all norms, both implicit and explicit.

PROBLEMS THAT CAN ARISE WITH GROUPS

Many problems or obstacles can arise when working with groups that may affect the effectiveness of the group learning. These issues can revolve around problems around leadership or the leader's effectiveness, difficulties that arise from individual members, or issues around group dynamics that impact the group. **Table 9-4** has examples of problems and possible solutions. This is in no way a comprehensive list, and ways to resolve problems will depend on a variety of factors that cannot be completely anticipated. Additionally, these solutions are based on the author's experiences with leading groups.

SUMMARY

Successfully teaching groups is a skill that takes knowledge of many aspects of group process and group dynamics. These skills can be learned by mentoring with someone who is a skilled group leader. Additionally, through reading one of many different books on the topic (see resources) or by taking a class at a college or university or continuing education workshop, an individual can learn in more detail the skills needed for effective group teaching. Establishing trust and an open, honest atmosphere and routine is important for effective group function.

WEBSITES

A great website for more icebreakers is http://wilderdom.com/games/Icebreakers.html.

A website for a PDF booklet on leading groups with topics on communication, facilitation, problems, and more is http://www.selfhelpconnection.ca/leadingagroup.htm.

ADDITIONAL RESOURCES

Engleberg, I. N., & Wynn, D. R. (2007). *Working in groups* (4th ed). Boston: Houghton Mifflin.

Fujishin, R. (2001). *Creating effective groups: the art of small group communication.* San Francisco: Acada Books.

REFERENCES

Engleberg, I. N., & Wynn, D. R. (2007). *Working in groups.* Boston: Houghton Mifflin.

Fujishin, R. (2001). *Creating effective groups.* San Francisco: Acada Books.

Gazda, G. M., Ginter, E. J., & Horne, A. M. (2001). *Group counseling and group psychotherapy: theory & application.* Boston: Allyn & Bacon.

Gershenfeld, N. (2004). *Groups: theory and experience* (7th ed.). Boston: Houghton Mifflin.

Posthuma, B. W. (2002). *Small groups in counseling and therapy: process and leadership* (4th ed.). Boston: Allyn & Bacon.

Schwartzberg, S. L., Howe, M. C., & Barnes, M. A. (2008). *Groups: applying the functional group model.* Philadelphia: FA Davis.

Tannenbaum, R., & Schmidt, W. H. (1958). How to choose a leadership pattern. *Harvard Business Review, 36,* 96.

Chapter 10

Teaching on the Fly

Jane C. Romano

INTRODUCTION

A good teacher looks at every interaction as an opportunity to enlighten, instruct, and empower their students. As healthcare providers, we need to be equally aware of this philosophy and develop the ability to capitalize on the often limited and stressful time we have with the patients and their families that we care for.

The many influences on the delivery of health care in this complex world are, for the most part, negative. The growing older population may seem like a positive outcome; however, it has put an enormous strain on the provision of health care. The introduction of managed care was intended to improve the delivery of services and reduce costs. From a healthcare provider's perspective, the limitations and restrictions have created many new challenges while delivering those services (Harrison, 1999). This has also created an increasingly important need for us "teachers" of patients and families to capitalize on teachable moments.

Case 10-1

School nurses have extremely challenging roles taking care of the children, staff, and families in their school communities. They wear many different hats and have the potential to have a powerful influence on health behaviors and outcomes. On a typical day, an elementary school nurse responds to an emergency on the playground. While hurrying to the situation, the nurse could see a crowd of fifth-grade children surrounding one of their classmates lying on the ground next to the climbing structure. From a distance, she could see that the young boy had a severe injury to his arm. After managing the situation and sending the student off in an ambulance to the emergency room, many of his classmates began to ask the nurse questions about what bone was broken and what kind of fracture it was. She was surprised at the specificity of the questions, only to find out that the class was in the middle of a science unit about the human skeleton. The nurse consulted with the teacher about scheduling time to come and talk to the class about bones and fractures. She contacted the family of the student who was injured to let them know that she would be spending some time with the class and asked how they felt about including the student's experience, which included an open reduction. The student and his family were excited about the opportunity to help the class learn more about the experience. They even asked the doctor for copies of the x-rays to show to the class. The lesson was fun, interactive, and informative for all.

London (1999) defines the teachable moment as "a moment when the learner's readiness is at a peak. When teaching synchronizes with readiness, the most effective education occurs" (p. 78). It is an invitation to teach what is personally, socially, and culturally meaningful to the learner at that moment. The key to capitalizing on a teachable moment is to recognize and capture the opportunity. These moments usually occur during a conversation and are all around you whether you know it or not (London, 1999). They are most often not planned and are very informal. It is important to learn to recognize and take advantage of these very ripe chances to provide patient education. Teachable moments can and should be a time of mutual empowerment for the patient/family and the healthcare provider. When a person asks a question, makes a comment, or demonstrates a particular behavior, these are all opportunities to clarify or reinforce behaviors or information related to their care. For instance, if a patient asks a question about a specific food, this is a perfect time to discuss nutrition. When giving medications or treatments and when performing a procedure, explain what you are doing or giving and why.

Benner (1984) describes the role of the nurse as a teacher–coach. In this aspect of their role, nurses are able to minimize anxiety and fear by taking what is foreign to the patient and making it familiar. She believes that much of the value of teaching–coaching is found embedded in good nursing care versus formal teaching activities. Benner identifies several competencies that are essential aspects of the teacher–coach role—the first being timing, which involves capturing a patient's readiness to learn (in other words, recognizing and capitalizing on teachable moments). This role of the teacher–coach applies to all healthcare providers and creates the opportunity to educate patients on what to expect, clarify misconceptions, and offer explanations related to their illness. It also presents chances to introduce and enforce lifestyle changes that may be necessary for this patient to become empowered and gain control over his or her illness.

An important aspect of providing for patients is to be astutely aware of the fact that they, like you, are human beings. They come into the healthcare situation with challenges that, although they are different than the challenges we face when providing care, are much more important to them as individuals. It is equally important for those providing care to consider that the routine care we provide is far from routine for most of the patients we care for. Nursing theorist Hildegard Peplau concentrated on the human aspect of patients and nurses and shifted the focus of providing care from what nurses do *to* patients to what nurses do *with* patients (Timmins, 2004). Consider how you would feel if you were in a patient's shoes or a family member of this patient. What would you expect from the healthcare team? How would you like to be treated? It is important not to let the human aspects of your relationship with patients and families get lost in what we so routinely do in our roles.

The reality of the complex environment we practice in requires us to do much of our teaching on the fly, which can be effective if done right and done often. In many ways, it is much more interpersonal and responsive to the patient's individual needs and a moment when the learner's readiness is at a peak. There are several key concepts that are important to consider in order for teaching on the fly to be effective and worthwhile. These include the following in no specific order:

- Start at the beginning: discharge teaching begins on admission.
- Keep education patient centered.
- Listen to your patients and families.
- Every interaction is an opportunity to teach.
- Communicate, communicate, communicate.

These concepts seem to align well with Knowles Principles of Adult Learning that includes a perceived need to learn, progressing from the known to the unknown and simpler to the more complex along with participation, opportunities to practice, reinforcement, and immediate feedback (Freda, 2004). Using these aspects of teaching and learning when developing and delivering patient education can provide you with a solid foundation to accomplish a positive outcome.

START AT THE BEGINNING: DISCHARGE TEACHING BEGINS ON ADMISSION

An important aspect of starting at the beginning is the opportunity to establish a therapeutic relationship with the patient. This requires you to consider the patient's perspective and strengths, as well as his or her readiness to learn. Rogan Foy & Timmins (2004) describe this as using a holistic approach to care that is achieved by engaging the patient as an individual in an effort to understand his or her unique needs and goals.

The idea that discharge teaching begins on admission allows you to maximize the time that you have with patients and families. This applies whether it is on admission to an inpatient setting or an initial visit with a physical therapist. In 2001, the Institute of Medicine reported that hospital discharge often meant an abrupt transition without information on how patients should care for themselves. This disturbing information truly reinforces the need for education assessment, planning, and implementation to begin at the first meeting between providers and patients and families. This requires education to be viewed not as a separate task but as an integrated component of delivering care. From the first interaction through the last, healthcare providers should be assessing, addressing, and documenting not only patient care needs but also their educational needs. Providing patient education is an ongoing process that evolves and adapts throughout the patient's healthcare experience.

KEEP EDUCATION PATIENT-CENTERED

Patient-centered care requires respect for a patient's values, preferences, and expressed needs. It is defined as valuing people as individuals, and it is regarded as the optimum way of delivering health care (Kelleher, 2006). The Institute of Medicine (2001) identified patient-centered care as one of six specific aims for improving the healthcare system in the 21st century. The report describes this as care that is respectful of and responsive to individual patient preferences, needs, and values to ensure this information guides all clinical decisions. This requires healthcare providers to go beyond the concept of administering care to actually partnering with a patient and family to determine what works best for them. This includes determining how this can be best accomplished in order to arrive at what the *patient and family* considers the best outcome. Some patients may not want or need to learn all we think need to be taught. They may have already had experience with this particular illness either personally or with a family member (Freda, 2004). There may be other barriers such as literacy, cultural issues, or primary language to consider. When providing education, it is essential to consider what is important from the patient's perspective. All of this involves a synergistic dance between patient, family, and provider in order to recognize and respond to the needs, preferences, and values of patients without sacrificing quality care.

Ellers (1993) wrote that the key to patient-centered education is always keeping the patient's perspective in mind. She asked what patients need and care most about. She identified the following as critical components:

- The need for information and an understanding about how to incorporate that information into their lives
- To know what to expect
- The need of different amounts and kinds of information
- Patient-centered education that focuses on the needs, goals, and motivation of the patient versus those of the program or provider
- Education that is evaluated from the perspective of the patient
- Educational planning and commitment throughout the organization

LISTEN TO YOUR PATIENTS AND FAMILIES

The art of listening is a critical aspect of effectively communicating with others. It involves listening with not only your ears but also your eyes as nonverbal cues can be just as powerful and important as verbal cues. Writer and educator Dr. Peter Drucker (American Public Health Association, 2005) believes that the most important thing in communication is to hear what is *not* being said. The art of listening involves all of the senses. It is also important to be aware of your own feelings and thoughts, body posture, and eye contact (Stickley & Freshwater, 2006). Active listening focuses on what is being said along with how it is being said and received. It is not automatic or passive and involves a range of behaviors such as using prompts or phases to encourage more explanation, nonverbal behaviors such as nodding, reflections, and understanding a different perspective. Rogan Foy and Timmins (2004) describes the need to be truly present in order to effectively listen. This can often be a challenge in a healthcare setting for many reasons. Professional and personal competing demands often influence one's ability to be truly present and actively listen to a patient or family member. We are, after all, human beings. The art of listening requires balancing the human relationship with a patient and/or family while maintaining professional boundaries.

London (1999) believes that the key to knowing what and when to teach and to save time teaching is listening to your learners. She explains that they will tell you what they think is important and what they need to know. Listening will tell you what and how to teach them most effectively and also serves to strengthen therapeutic bonds and build partnering relationships.

An important aspect of effectively listening to others is allowing for silence. This is not an easy thing to do in any situation, especially a busy healthcare setting. Silence can be a resting place for patients and can provide an opportunity for reflection. It can provide time to think about what has been said and what will be said next. It is important that healthcare providers recognize the value, although sometime discomfort, of silence and not feel as though they need to interject.

EVERY INTERACTION IS AN OPPORTUNITY TO TEACH

When healthcare providers view every interaction as an opportunity to teach, they become much more influential to patient outcomes. Much of patient education occurs in the process of conversations and informal interactions, any of which can turn into a teachable moment. London (2004) believes that all learners should be informed that most of their instruction will occur informally in the context of the care they are provided. The secret to integrating teaching into your interactions with patients and families is active involvement in learning. To accomplish this, the information and/or activity need to be of interest to the learner. It is important to keep it brief, to make connections and make information fit (this helps the patient and family to make an informed decision), and to encourage the learner to practice and apply to new knowledge or skill.

Factors that can improve the effectiveness of patient education include keeping the information simple, using repetition to reinforce the activity or message, and being specific (Rogan Foy & Timmins, 2004). It is also important to speak in terms that the patient can easily understand. We tend to get caught up in the use of medical jargon, and this can often be a barrier to effective patient education.

Gregor (2001) identified six different types of exchanges that can result in informal education occurring:

- Asking questions
- Offering explanations

- Giving information
- Providing instruction
- Setting expectations
- Demonstrating the correct performance

Often, several of these activities occur in one conversation. An example of this is demonstrated in Case 10-2.

Case 10-2

A mother brings her 10-year-old son Joe to the allergy and asthma clinic for a routine visit. The following is a conversation that occurred between the nurse and mom regarding Joe's medication regimen:

Nurse: Is Joe using his spacer with his inhaler?

Mom: He uses it at home but does not take it with him outside the house. It is too big to carry back and forth to school. I am afraid he will lose it, so we keep it home.

Nurse: The importance of the spacer is to make sure that Joe is receiving the correct dose of his medication. It is difficult for anyone to use an inhaler correctly, and we recommend spacers for all our patients, even adults. The medication in an inhaler is under pressure, so it is not easy to coordinate puffing and inhaling the correct way to get the best results of the dose. The spacer device helps keep the puff of medication contained until Joe can inhale it slowly, which makes sure that he is receiving the right dose.

Mom: I get it. I am still concerned that he will lose it if he takes it out of the house, and then we will really be stuck.

Nurse: Is there a nurse at Joe's school who could keep an extra spacer and maybe even an inhaler in the health office so that he does not have to take it back and forth to school?

Mom: There is a school nurse, and I suppose I could ask if this could be done. I am not sure my insurance will cover getting a second inhaler and spacer.

Nurse: We can check on your coverage and see. In the meantime, I am going to review with you and Joe the correct method for using the inhaler with the spacer.

In a brief amount of time, the nurse was able to solicit important information about Joe's treatments, explain why it was important, provide information and instruction, set expectations, and have Joe and his mom demonstrate correct use of a spacer with an inhaler. Ultimately, the outcome for the patient and family as well as the healthcare provider is positive. As a final step, the nurse should document this interaction so that the information can be reinforced at future visits by every member of the healthcare team.

COMMUNICATE, COMMUNICATE, COMMUNICATE

All of the time and energy that you put in to understanding what is important to your patient and providing the necessary education is almost moot if this information is not communicated to the entire healthcare team. It is essential that you are able to build on one another's teaching. Ongoing communication is the cornerstone of effective and efficient patient education. It allows teaching to be reinforced, clarified, and enhanced by various members of the multidisciplinary team.

Case 10-3

Kate goes to a patient's room to administer medications, and when she enters the room, she sees that the patient is sitting in his chair using his incentive spirometer. Although she is happy to see that the patient is following his postoperative therapy routine, Kate notices that he is not using the equipment properly. To make sure, she asks the patient to demonstrate and sees that the patient is blowing as hard as he can rather than slow and steady like he should. Kate explains using the spirometer serves to get the patient's lungs back into their best shape and that a long, steady breath is more effective than a hard quick breath to accomplish this. After a few more attempts, the patient is able to demonstrate the use of the spirometer correctly. Kate documents in the chart that she reviewed with the patient the correct use of the spirometer so that this teaching can be reinforced by other members of the healthcare team.

Lee (2004) discusses the importance of a patient's impression of their hospital experience. He believes that it is what people say or do not say that creates an impression. Lee describes one hospital's persistent disappointing results on a post discharge survey of patients related to the staff's concern for patient's privacy. They determined that people do not notice concern unless we say something. The hospital focused on teaching staff to communicate with patients more effectively in order to change their perception of their concern for privacy. An example would be when a nurse closes a patient's door out of concern for the patient's privacy when there is a lot of commotion at the nurse's station during report. Because the patient was not told that the door was shut out of concern for his or her comfort, there is the opportunity for them to image negative reasons for the nurse's actions. Simply telling the patient why the door is being closed or even asking the patient if he or she would like the door closed would alleviate any misconceptions the patient may have. By concentrating on improving communication with patients and families, this hospital was able to improve patient's perception of the staff's concern for their privacy.

It is not only the patient's impressions and perceptions that are effected with improved communication, but also the other members of the healthcare team. It is important not to assume that your patient who is a newly diagnosed diabetic has met with the diabetes nurse specialist and has had all of their questions answered. It is essential to close the loop on all communication in order to minimize gaps in care as well as to support your patient and family in dealing with this new information. Building on each other's assessments and teaching requires ongoing communication among the multidisciplinary team. London (2004) believes that this is most effectively accomplished through continually documenting what you do. In order to teach with every encounter, team members need to be aware of their own teaching and communicate their progress to the rest of the team through documentation.

COVERING ALL OF THE BASES

Thus far, this chapter has focused mainly on recognizing and capitalizing on teachable moments; however, it is important not to rely on this teaching method alone. Although they are wonderful and ripe opportunities to educate, they can create the risk of incomplete teaching (London, 1999). It is essential that a formalized education plan be developed early on in the patient's healthcare encounter and be used to guide teaching throughout the experience. The plan should be considered a living document that needs to be continually updated and adapted to the ongoing needs of the patient in order to be effective. An effective education plan involves the utilization and application of research and evidenced-based practice specific to the patient's healthcare needs as well as their learning needs. It should identify key family members and supports that should be included in patient education. Often, these people are determined during your interactions with patients and families and can be a result of a teachable moment.

Along with patient-centered care, we also need to be aware of family-centered care when planning and providing education. Parents are the foremost experts on their child's well-being and have an important understanding of how best to care for their child (Miceli & Clark, 2005). When planning for education of an older person, it is often just as important to include their spouse or children in the activities. A family-centered approach supports the role of the primary caregiver by partnering with him or her to plan and deliver care based on what works best for everyone concerned.

TEACHABLE MOMENT CAUTIONS

It is also important to recognize when not to teach. This can be considered a teachable moment for you instead of the patient. Issues such as fatigue, stress, pain, visitors, and meals can be inopportune times to provide information. Being tuned into cues from the patient can reduce frustration for everyone and sometimes requires the healthcare provider to forgo the teachable moment. This is one of many opportunities for communication with the healthcare team in an effort to inform other members of what you have discovered about some barriers to the patient's learning as well as remaining educational needs of the patient.

Another caution about teachable moments is to be sure that you are teaching the correct information. If a patient or family member asks a question about something you are unsure of, it is appropriate to say that you are not sure and that you will find out and get back to them after you have more information. The key in this situation is to follow through and bring the correct information back to them in some form, even if it means having another member of the healthcare team provide the information. If you are unsure or uncomfortable about an aspect of their care, remember that you are a member of a team and have many resources available to you to assure that the patient gets what he or she needs.

Case 10-4

A nurse who had been working on a pediatric surgical unit for less than 6 months needed to do teaching with a family on caring for their child who had an appendicostomy, a rare procedure that involves creating a stoma opening in the appendix in patients with chronic bowel disorders. The nurse had never cared for a patient after this surgery, and she anticipated being asked questions by the family that she felt unprepared to answer. She sought out the unit-based educator to help her figure out the best approach to providing the teaching. The nurse and the educator went into the patient's room to discuss what had already been covered. From there they told the family that they would gather supplies and be back in a little while to do the teaching. The nurse and the educator developed a lesson plan that was appropriate for the patient. They determined what they would highlight during the teaching with the family and then gathered the necessary supplies. After a review of the plan, they went into the room where the nurse reviewed the materials with the family, participated in demonstration with return demonstration from the family, and offered opportunities for questions. The family did have a couple of questions in which the nurse was unsure of the answer, and the educator was able to support the nurse and the family. After they left the patient's room, they talked about how the teaching went, and the nurse expressed how relieved she was to have it completed. She also felt that she had a much better understanding of the surgical procedure and postoperative care required for patients with an appendicostomy.

Another challenge to the healthcare provider when trying to maximize your teaching time with patients and families is recognizing when to proceed with teaching at the least opportune times. Benner (1984) believes that an important aspect of effective patient teaching is deciding when to go ahead even when the patient does not appear ready. Too often, the message we need to convey is not what the patient and family had hoped for or expected; however, the information that is relevant to their lives related to the health issue still needs to be delivered. Being aware of and using available resources are critical. This is when it is also especially important to recognize that most patients do not live in isolation and that their social support system is vital to the delivery and effectiveness of patient education (Rogan Foy & Timmins, 2004).

CONCLUSION

All of these concepts are intertwined and equally important and yet equally difficult to accomplish. Individualizing care begins with a good assessment and requires you to consider multiple issues that are important to the patient and family. It also often requires the healthcare provider to set aside their predetermined or typical method and approach to patient education in order to meet the needs of individual patients and families. In order to be effective, patient education needs to be more that just providing information; it needs to be interactive and patient centered. It involves developing a relationship with and partnering with patients in order to determine what their needs, wants, and desires are related to their health and well-being. This requires ongoing communication between the patient, their families, and the multi-disciplinary healthcare team. This also requires a great deal of time, energy, and planning on the part of the individuals involved in the process.

We need to embrace the idea of moving from what we do *to* patients to what we do *with* patients. By considering every interaction an opportunity to enlighten, instruct, and empower patients and families, we can effectively navigate through the limitations, restrictions, and challenges we face in the healthcare environment today. Although it may seem impossible and complex, it really requires us to be human and to recognize those that we care for as human, too. Ask yourself questions: How would you feel if you were in the patient's shoes or a family member of this patient? What would you expect from the healthcare team? How would you like to be treated?

REFERENCES

American Public Health Association. (2005). Quotes to think about and use: leadership quotations on communication. *Health Administration Newsletter*. Retrieved on August 28, 2007, from http://www.apha.org.

Benner, P. (1984). *From novice to expert: excellence and power in clinical nursing practice*. Menlo Park, CA: Addison-Wesley.

Ellers, B. (1993). Innovations in patient-centered education. In M. Gerteis, M. S. Edgman-Levitan, J. Daley, & T. L. Delbanco (Eds.). *Through the patient's eyes: understanding and promoting patient-centered care* (pp. 96–118). San Francisco: Jossey-Bass.

Freda, M. C. (2004). Issues in patient education. *Journal of Midwifery and Women's Health, 49*(3), 203–209.

Gregor, F. M. (2001). Nurses' informal teaching practices: their nature and impact on the production of patient care. *International Journal of Nursing Studies, 38*(4), 461–470.

Harrison, J. K. (1999). Health policy. Influence of managed care on professional nursing practice. Image in *Journal of Nursing Scholarship, 31*(2), 161–166.

Institute of Medicine. (2001). *Crossing the quality chasm: a new health system for the 21st century*. Washington, DC: National Academies Press.

Kelleher, S. (2006). Providing patient-centered care in an intensive care unit. *Nursing Standard, 21*(13), 35–40.

Lee, F. (2004). *If Disney ran your hospital: 9½ things you would do differently*. Bozeman, MT: Second River Healthcare.

London, F. (1999). *No time to teach: a nurse's guide to patient and family education*. Philadelphia: Lippincott.

London, F. (2004). How to prepare families for discharge in the limited time available. *Pediatric Nursing, 30*(3), 212–214, 227.

Miceli, P. J., & Clark, P. A. (2005). Your patient—my child: seven priorities for improving pediatric care from the parent's perspective. *Journal of Nursing Care Quality, 20*(1), 43–53.

Rogan Foy, C., & Timmins, R. (2004). Improving communication in day surgery settings. *Nursing Standard, 19*(7), 37–42.

Stickley, T., & Freshwater, D. (2006). The art of listening in the therapeutic relationship. *Mental Health Practice, 9*(5), 12–18.

Chapter 11

Making Learning Stick

Arlene Lowenstein & John A. Reeder

INTRODUCTION

Today's world moves faster than ever and healthcare providers are in a race with time. In order to increase the profit margin, providers are encouraged to treat patients more and more efficiently, delivering the same services in briefer meetings and over shorter periods of time. Meanwhile, new treatments join or replace the old ones as research and technology race along, with new discoveries coming at an accelerated pace. What does efficiency mean, however, and how can we, as healthcare providers, keep up with the changes and bring our new knowledge to our patients and their families? Most importantly, how can we help our patients to achieve the long-lasting changes in behavior that reflect their new knowledge?

Patients may leave the office or hospital with a prescription for medication; however, how much time and attention was given to teaching them about their illness and medications, and how they and their families can cope? Has attention been given to prevention of illness and support for lifestyle changes? When and where can we address health promotion to our communities, and how do we fit all this in?

Unfortunately, the answer is this: We cannot fit this all in, but the emphasis on efficiency in health care does not necessarily preclude effective patient education. We can maintain and even enhance it by developing a better understanding of strategies that can help patients, families, and communities learn and retain knowledge about their health needs, healthy lifestyles, and a healthy society. We can learn about resources that can be used or developed to work with our patients when they will not return to us for months or longer. We can follow up with patients and encourage positive behavior change or assess barriers that are interfering with that change, and we can work to increase motivation for change. The purpose of this chapter is to provide information and strategies to help individuals, their families, and communities retain and better use the important healthcare information that they have been offered. **Table 11-1** outlines important areas to address in this process.

Table 11-1 Guidelines to Enhance Learning

The healthcare provider as teacher

- Have awareness of the need for learning and teaching in their practice.
- Identify the specific patient, family, or community need for education.
- Understand the content needed to be taught.
- Understand the time frame needed and available.
- Identify appropriate printed or web explanatory materials to be referred to after contact.
- Identify resources that can be used by patients, families, or communities to continue and reinforce learning.

Educating patients, families, and communities

- Understand differences in patient's objective versus educator's objective.
- Assess motivation for the learning process and encouraging participation.
- Identify obstacles to learning including the effect of memory, age, literacy, cultural and language issues, poverty, and stress.
- Encourage behavioral change.
- Use teaching strategies to enhance retention of learning, which may include the use of reflection, recall and personalization, making the educational materials specific to the patient's background and experiences. Pictures and entertaining materials, used with discretion, may create a more upbeat atmosphere for positive learning, reduce the amount of necessary reading, and increase interest and motivation for change.
- Evaluate learning in the time available, what was said, what was left out, how learning was accepted by the recipient and what needs to be done and how.

Using collaboration and resources to extend learning opportunities

- Understanding how much contact with healthcare providers is available, identify additional material to be learned and who can do it.
- Can technology be used?
- Follow up over time, establish communication and feedback methods, including effectiveness of referrals.

THE HEALTHCARE PROVIDER AS TEACHER

Be Alert to the Need for Learning and Teaching in Your Practice

A new diagnosis is a cry for education. The language of health care and the science of illness are unfamiliar to most patients, and they and their families need to learn what is happening to them, how it can be controlled, and how to minimize the effects of the illness on their lives. We have seen a positive growth in resources, such as the Internet, television, and articles available to the general public that have raised health educational awareness of the consumer; however, patients' greater access to educational resources can also contribute to a climate of confusion. Available information may need interpretation and explanation of how it actually relates to the affected individual.

Is a drug advertised on television really appropriate for a patient's condition, and will its side effects be safe and tolerable for that individual? Does a dramatic newspaper or Internet article about a medical study really provide correct information for all? Are the results appropriate for a wide or limited population, or is it too soon to know whether the treatment will really be effective over time? If patients misattribute information learned in one context, such as a magazine article, to another context, such as a consultation with their doctor, they might unwittingly change their behaviors in ways that negatively impact their health and treatment. How do we, as healthcare providers, explain that to our patients?

Identify the Specific Patient, Family, or Community Need for Education

For individuals as clients or patients, it is important to assess what they know about their illness and positive lifestyle behaviors or lifestyle behavior changes that may be needed to improve their health and manage chronic or severe illness. A teacher needs to assess constantly the learner's knowledge, keeping an updated model of how the learner mentally organizes new information and identifies misconceptions. Good teaching requires a type of meta-cognitive empathy, being aware of what the learner does and does not understand.

A good way to begin is by asking them to tell you what they think they know about their health, how they feel about it, and what they want or think they need to know more about. Absolutely do not start by telling them what you think they need to know—that will come later. Listen carefully to identify appropriate thoughts that may need strengthening or reinforcing, misunderstandings that may need correction, and lack of knowledge that may need education or referral to appropriate resources. It is very important to ask about family and support systems. Explore what individuals believe their families know or do not know about what is happening and what the clients/patients want or do not want them to know. With the client's approval, family or members of the support system who are easily available can be queried directly, or other appropriate measures to contact them may be needed if feasible.

Providers need to be alert to patterns of illnesses or needed lifestyle changes within their practice and be alert to patterns of patient reactions. Patterns can be discovered by recognizing similarities among the provider's clients or patients and looking to see how often those similarities occur with others. Another important pattern to be aware of is the patient's response to referrals and other healthcare agencies or services with which they may be involved. Consumers are generally not exposed to evaluations of community healthcare services, but they know their own experiences. It is the healthcare provider who may be able to identify similar success stories or complaints among clients that may need to be addressed with those agencies or services. By observing patterns and assessing responses, themes can be identified that point out the need for additional information, study, or referrals. Identification of patterns can also lead to determining the need for group or community education or research and feedback to agencies if appropriate.

Understand the Content Needed to Be Taught

Healthcare providers are responsible for keeping up-to-date with new medications, treatments, and health promotion issues, and evaluating what will work best for their practice. Along with traditional healthcare content for specific diseases and health promotion, some of the new knowledge also needs to be made available to clients and patients. Patients come from different age groups and cultural, socioeconomic, and educational backgrounds. They may require different approaches to the amount and presentation of material. For example, a copy of an article from a professional journal may be helpful and interesting reading for one patient but an intimidating source of confusion and frustration to another. The amount of healthcare information available can be overwhelming, and it is up to the healthcare provider to decide what is most important for patients to know and what would be good to know but is not critical. In other words, the provider's role as educator involves thoughtfully filtering information for patients on an individual basis.

Understand the Time Frame Needed and Available

After the important content is decided, providers need to be aware of how much time it will take to deliver the information and how much repetition will be necessary. How often do your patients come to see you? Who else do they see regarding their health care, and how often? Can educational sessions be scheduled? What additional information would be helpful? Where can they get it if not from you, and how can that be fitted in? Fitting the information needed to the time frame available is not easy, and alternate methods and referral sources may be needed to work with patients to provide needed information. Too often, educational material is delivered offline in the form of pamphlets, newsletters, or one-time consultations. It is crucial to appreciate that learning is a gradual process, and the consideration of appropriate time frames must be incorporated into individual treatment plans.

Identify Resources That Can Be Used by Patients, Families, or Communities to Reinforce Learning

Resources can be found by way of individuals, organizations, government agencies, print materials, and Internet sources among others. Patients can be referred to healthcare providers in different disciplines who may be able to provide a broader approach to the problems, have access to information that can add to or reinforce learning and behavior change, and can also work with families to help patients build support systems. Physical or occupational therapists, nutritionists, and social workers may be able to provide practical assistance and therapy for patients in dealing with their environment and making adjustments for the effects of their illness. Nurses, clinical specialists, counselors, and psychologists may also provide information, therapeutic interventions, and encouragement, which can help reduce anxiety levels so that patients and families can be more receptive to learning and behavior change.

Many nonprofit organizations have been developed around specific disease entities. These organizations often have printed educational materials available and Internet sites that patients can use to reinforce learning about and living with that disease. Even more importantly, they may also offer services that patients and their families can take advantage of for care and/or for financial help with needed supplies.

The U.S. Government Printing Office offers information on health and safety, including educational materials for some specific diseases. Healthcare providers need to become familiar with and screen a number of Internet sites in their specialty. Provider screening is important to be sure the information is appropriate for use by those patients and families who need additional information. Internet sites are not regulated and misinformation as well as appropriate, valuable information can be found. Healthcare providers referring patients to Internet sites need to be sure those sites are reliable, up-to-date, and accurate.

It is very important for providers to know where patients are getting information about their condition, including lay literature and sources outside of traditional health care. Follow-up is important when patients have been referred to resources or have been given or found resource materials. In this respect, patient education is a collaborative effort, a series of conversations that demand good listening skills. Follow-up should explore the likelihood of misunderstandings, reinforce appropriate learning, but also evaluate the resources and patients' reactions, including positive and negative experiences of the referrals or materials.

EDUCATING PATIENTS, FAMILIES, AND COMMUNITIES

Understand Differences in Patient's Objective Versus Educator's Objective

Providers have a responsibility to explore the potential for learning, and recognize readiness to learn in their patients. An important component is assessing what the patient wants to learn (Barnstable, 2003). Patients may not share their provider's view of what is important for them to know. Life experiences, family, friends, and the print, television, and Internet media can influence what they want to know and think they know.

Lichtenfeld's PEEK is an acronym for a readiness to learn model that is easily used and can be adapted for health education. Readiness to learn can be identified by being aware of and assessing the following areas (adapted from Lichtenfeld, as cited in Barnstable, 2003) (**Table 11-2**):

- The *P* stands for *physical readiness* and includes a person's health status, physical ability to learn, and the complexity of what needs to be learned.
- The first *E* stands for *emotional readiness*, including anxiety, motivation for learning, and available support system.
- The second *E* is for *experiential readiness*, including past experiences, cultural influences, and coping and control mechanisms.
- The *K* stands for *knowledge readiness*, including the level of the individual's current knowledge, cognitive ability, preferred learning styles, and learning disabilities.

Assess Motivation for the Learning Process and Encourage Participation

Along with readiness to learn, patient assessments can begin to uncover patient motivation to know more about their specific condition or a healthy

Table 11-2 Learning Assessment Model

1. Start by asking the patients what they know about their health status and condition.
2. Confirm with them what you think they said—use PVCs: perception, validation, and clarification.
    a. Check your *perception* by stating what you think you heard them say.
    b. Have them *validate* that is what they said.
    c. If they do not agree, *clarify* your perception to meet theirs.
3. Assess patient's response to illness and clarify misconceptions.
4. Determine what you feel they need to know and what adaptations to their lifestyle may be needed.
5. Consider use of the Harm Reduction Model—what is the most critical education and behavior change need, and is there something related that can be accomplished quickly and successfully in a short period of time?
6. Assess ability for understanding printed or web explanatory materials to be referred to after contact (i.e., literacy, language, and education level).
7. Assess ability to use technology, such as e-mail, the Internet, videos, and podcasts that could be used to reinforce learning.
8. Assess patient's ability to access potential resources for further education and follow-up. Includes time, transportation, and financial availability.

lifestyle. Some patients are anxious to learn everything they can about what is happening to them, whereas others may want to avoid the entire issue. Some will want a pill to solve everything and want to avoid the work needed for learning and behavior change. Some will want family involvement, and others may prefer to keep the information to themselves in order not to worry others. Scaring patients into behavior change by emphasizing the complications or death that can occur if the condition is not taken care of can be frightening to patients and may actually de-motivate rather than encourage them to learn more. This may send them further into anxiety and denial. It is important for patients to understand that behavior change is very difficult and does not happen overnight; instead, change occurs with perseverance and support—it can happen and make a positive difference in their lives.

In order to motivate patients to adhere to needed changes to reduce the likelihood of onset or complications of disease processes, Prochaska's stages of motivation for change can provide a structure to understand and apply (Prochaska, Norcross, & Diclemente, 1994). The beginning point for patients is precontemplation. Patients at this stage do not have enough information to recognize the need for a better lifestyle, or they deny that need. With their provider's help, they may be able to move to the contemplation stage where they begin thinking about what is happening and what needs to be done. If the health promotion message gets through, they can then move to the next stage, beginning to plan what needs to be done and what they can reasonably do, develop support systems, and eventually take action to manage their health issues (Prochaska et al., 1994). It does not end there. This is an ongoing process that in subsequent physician and provider visits will require assessment and reinforcement of positive changes.

Identify Obstacles to Learning, Including the Effect of Memory, Age, Cultural and Language Issues, Literacy, Poverty, and Stress

In the role of teacher, a healthcare provider also needs to assess the *cognitive* factors that determine how successfully a patient will learn new information. Even healthy people with normal cognitive functioning are susceptible to certain limitations of memory, along with changes associated with age. These factors influence how patients understand their health conditions and perhaps more importantly how they comply with treatment plans. By taking memory and age into account, providers can adopt appropriate teaching styles that enhance learning and provide greater motivation for behavioral change.

Social and emotional factors, such as cultural background, literacy, poverty, and stress, can also affect learning potential. Effectively and actively communicating needed information when working with patients who do not have a good command of the English language can be challenging. Cultural home remedies and beliefs may be in opposition to traditional western medicine, and accommodation may be necessary. A low level of literacy will impede a patient's ability to gain information from printed materials, and poverty issues may mean making a choice between medicine or food, making positive health changes inaccessible. These barriers to learning are discussed in more detail in the following passages.

Memory

All learning depends fundamentally on memory processes, but these vary dramatically from one person to another and are prone to common types of errors. Healthcare providers who understand memory processes can transfer critical knowledge to patients more effectively, even in a single consultation. As a result, their patients retain what they have learned longer and more accurately. There is a more direct health benefit, however. A patient's memory processes provide the all-important internal cues that initiate behaviors such as taking medication, performing therapeutic activities, and following preventive regimens. The success of treatment hinges on the way providers apply what they know about memory, with all its strengths and weaknesses, to patient education.

Memory is not just an information storage system. Ongoing thought requires multiple pieces of information to be held in readiness while the thinker shifts attention from one to another. Even the simple act of listening requires the ability to remember the beginning of a sentence when the speaker reaches the end of it. The term *working memory* refers to the temporary storage of information so that it can be organized, elaborated on, and stored for future reference. From a teacher's perspective, working memory is the gateway to knowledge. The way new information is organized in working memory reflects the way learners are thinking about it for the first time, which influences whether they will subsequently remember it, forget it, or (perhaps worst of all) *mis*-remember it.

One important function of working memory is to *refresh* a piece of information by momentarily thinking back to it after attention has shifted to something else. Refreshing a piece of information keeps it available for further processing in working memory, where it can be integrated with related ideas. There is experimental evidence that refreshing also provides a long-term memory benefit. In one study (Johnson, Reeder, Raye, et al., 2002), researchers asked participants to read aloud as a long sequence of words was presented on a screen, one at a time. Some words only occurred once. Some occurred twice in a row, and others were followed by a dot. The dot was a signal to refresh the preceding word by thinking back to it. Participants took slightly longer to say words in response to the dot compared with reading them for a second time, reflecting the additional mental work of refreshing the word in working memory. Later, in a memory test, the words from the sequence were mixed with new words, and participants decided whether they recognized each one. Not surprisingly, they recognized words that they had read twice more accurately than words that they had only read once. More interestingly, they recognized words that they had refreshed most accurately of all. These results demonstrate that long-term memory depends on the way people process new information when they first encounter it. Being given repeated presentations of information helps, but refreshing new information themselves provides additional learning benefits.

Working memory has an important limitation, but one that can be overcome if the teacher takes it into account. There is a maximum number of information chunks that working memory can hold. The so-called magic number is 7 ± 2, meaning that a person can only keep track of 5 to 9 chunks at a time (Miller, 1956). After those chunks are filled, any new information will cause interference and confusion. Fortunately, the capacity of each chunk can be increased to hold more information, but existing knowledge is required. For example, a list of letters like H, I, M, and N would take up four chunks for a person who treated them as individual details. In contrast, a healthcare provider might mentally reorganize them as N.I.M.H., the acronym for the National Institute of Mental Health. Then the letters would only take up one chunk, freeing three others to accommodate additional information. Because healthcare providers have considerable medical expertise compared with patients, they can chunk related information more efficiently and keep track of more complex ideas about health, illness, and treatment. As teachers, they should be aware that this advantage also presents a challenge. It can lead them to overestimate the clarity of their explanations and advice to patients, who are not organizing the information in working memory as efficiently. Keeping this difference in mind is crucial to effective teaching.

To overcome the limitations of working memory, providers should present new information at the patient's pace and avoid irrelevant details or lists of items. It helps to repeat information, but especially if the right kind of repetition is used. In *massed repetition*, the same information is rehearsed again and again during the same learning experience. *Spaced repetition* is spread out over a longer time frame so that the same information is rehearsed during different learning experiences. Experimental research has shown spaced repetition to be better for memory than massed repetition (Seabrook, Brown, & Solity, 2005). Providers can apply this finding to patient education whenever multiple consultations are possible. It does little good to repeat some fact or instruction again and again during a single visit. Reminding a patient about it during each visit, however, is more likely to support learning over the course of time. Encouraging patients to refresh new information themselves can be even more effective than repetition. Providers should refer back to earlier ideas after discussing something else, prompting patients to think about those ideas again before moving on. In addition to facilitating the comprehension of those ideas, the act of refreshing will improve their long-term retention.

Finally, providers can use their expertise to help patients organize new information in working memory more efficiently and meaningfully. Spare them unnecessary detail in the interest of maximizing their attention to the most important points and encourage them to think about how various details are related or combine to form new ideas. For example, a list of symptoms should be presented so that similar ones are mentioned together, with the most critical ones occurring at the beginning or end of the list. If two symptoms reflect the same underlying condition, that connection should be made explicit so that they can be chunked together. If two medications are intended to address the same symptom, that connection should likewise be emphasized. Not only will the association provide a richer context for appreciating their purposes, but it will increase the likelihood that each medication will cue a patient to remember the other. Most importantly, providers should encourage patients to relate new information to their own knowledge and experience, which can provide the richest organizational framework for chunking and provide the greatest long-term memory benefit.

A related cognitive phenomenon that informs effective teaching styles is the *generation effect*, a tendency for people to remember information better if they previously thought of it themselves instead of passively receiving it. The generation effect has been consistently observed across a number of experimental situations. In one early demonstration (Slamecka & Graf, 1978), participants were presented with pairs of words (like HOT/COLD). Some pairs were incomplete (like SAD/HA___), requiring participants to think of the missing letters themselves. In a subsequent memory test, they recognized more words that they had completed themselves (like HAPPY) than words that they had merely read (like COLD). The generation effect illustrates a truism in education: Active learning is superior to passive learning, and students should be treated as participants in the learning process rather than as sponges for information. The application in patient education is clear. Patients should be asked to paraphrase what they are learning, rather than "parroting" it. They will learn more about their health condition if they go through the experience of explaining it in their own words. Of course, they may lack the expertise to explain it with the same jargon or detail that a professional would, but good instruction will guide them to an understanding that makes sense in the context of their own knowledge and experience. As much as possible, providers should involve patients in the process of planning their own treatment, giving them options to weigh and select rather than simply prescribing a predetermined plan. Patients will remember their medication and therapy regimens better if they collaborate on developing a schedule, rather than being assigned one.

The generation effect generally aids learning by making information easier to remember. Another memory process, *source monitoring*, involves the ability to identify the origin of remembered information. Accurate source monitoring can be critical in patient education because the value of remembering some detail about a condition or treatment depends entirely on whether it was learned from a reliable source (like a doctor) or an unreliable one (like a television commercial). Researchers have observed that people often remember information without knowing how they originally learned it, or worse yet, misattributing that information to the wrong source. These so-called *source errors* might lead patients to unwittingly jeopardize their own health. The challenge is compounded by the wide range of educational (and not-so-educational) resources available today and the varied reliability of popular media claims about health and the social sciences. Providers should be aware of this potential for confusion and take steps to minimize it. Some studies have suggested that source errors are less likely when people explicitly consider the possible origins of remembered information, rather than simply evaluating whether it came from a specific source (Hashtroudi, Johnson, & Chrosniak, 1990). Patients should be encouraged to focus not only on *what* they have learned, but on *where* they learned it.

One last characteristic of memory is worth mentioning because it suggests a simple strategy for enhancing patient education, particularly for helping patients to remember important behaviors like taking medications and following treatment plans. People are more likely to remember something when in the same setting that they previously thought about it or when some aspect of a previous experience is reinstated. This phenomenon, called *encoding specificity*, was demonstrated in an unusual experiment involving a swimming pool (Godden & Baddeley, 1975). Participants were divided into two groups: One was sitting comfortably by the side of the pool, whereas the other went underwater (with the aid of scuba gear). Both groups were presented with a list of words to study. In a subsequent test, participants from each group tried to recall the words in either the same setting (poolside or underwater) or the opposing one. Those who originally studied the words poolside recalled more of them there than in the pool. In contrast, those who originally studied the words underwater recalled more of them there than poolside. Encoding specificity turns out to be a robust effect, with environmental cues serving as reminders for all kinds of information. Taking advantage of the effect is a useful way to remember things. For example, if patients need to make a habit of taking medications or performing treatment activities on a regular basis, suggest that they always do so in the same situation—the same room, under the same circumstances, at the same time of day—and to pay attention to those consistencies. As a result, they will be more likely to remember responsibilities spontaneously as a matter of habit.

Age

It is commonly believed that aging is accompanied by a global decline in cognitive function, especially in memory. In part, this impression is influenced by the public's awareness of the dramatic ravages associated with *dementia*, but normal, healthy aging is another matter. Although it is true that cognitive processes change across the lifespan, it is simplistic to assume that an older person's memory inevitably declines into unreliability. It is more accurate to say that memory changes in specific ways, and although those changes can produce certain impairments, other memory processes continue to operate normally. Taking these changes into account in patient education is especially critical now, with the ranks of older patients swelling in proportion to other age groups.

As it was described earlier, memory is not just stored information; it is a record of how that information was originally processed. In other words, memory is shaped by the way a person thinks about an experience while it is happening. Younger adults tend to focus on the *perceptual* and *semantic* aspects of events, and as a consequence, they perform well on conventional memory tests that emphasize perceptual and semantic details. In contrast, older adults are more concerned with the *personal* and *interpersonal* aspects of events: their mood, their thoughts, how they feel about what is happening, how they think other people feel about it, and so on. When they are subjected to conventional memory tests or when they face everyday demands that require memory for perceptual or semantic information, they may perform relatively poorly. In addition, focusing on thoughts and feelings can have a negative effect on certain kinds of source monitoring, such as when people try to distinguish between memories for real and imagined events (Hashtroudi et al., 1990). In fact, a variety of age-related deficits in source monitoring have been observed among older adults (Spencer & Raz, 1995).

Older adults may attribute such functional changes to "senior moments," but the truth about memory and normal aging is not quite so dire. There is evidence that older adults' source-monitoring performance improves when they are prompted to consider the various characteristics of their memories besides thoughts and feelings. Perhaps perceptual and semantic details are not actually forgotten, but are merely given less attention when older adults remember information about the past (Hashtroudi et al., 1990). The point is that age-related changes in source monitoring may be associated with shifts in focus, not global impairments. By guiding an older adult's attention to the different aspects of past events, it might be possible to minimize age-related difficulties in remembering (Craik, 1984). Healthcare providers should be aware that older patients tend to focus on thoughts and feelings and encourage them to use those responses as cues for remembering new information. At the same time, it is a good idea to emphasize specific details and concepts, drawing attention to them with the understanding that they might not be central to the older patient's subjective experience. Above all, keep in mind that some memory changes are specific in nature, even though they produce effects that could be interpreted as forgetfulness or cognitive slowing. Normal aging is not associated with a decline in general intelligence.

There is a kind of memory that does, unfortunately, decline with age, but understanding this change can help educators minimize its impact. When older adults are presented with a lot of information to think about at once, they may have difficulty keeping it all available in working memory by refreshing it. The impairment is subtle and quite specific. In one of the studies described earlier (Johnson et al., 2002), participants read a long list of words that included some repetitions of the same word and some dots signaling them to think of the preceding word. In addition, some words were presented in a visually degraded form so that they were difficult to read. In many ways, younger adults (aged 18–21) and older adults (aged 67–84) performed similarly on this task. Both groups read a word more quickly the second time, for example, and both groups were able to read degraded words more easily if they had recently seen the same word. Both groups took longer to refresh words than to read them a second time, reflecting the additional processing involved. Apparently, the older adults' memory functions were largely preserved compared with younger adults. The specific difference, however, involved the extra processing time associated with refreshing the preceding word. The delay was significantly longer for older adults and by a greater margin than the overall age difference in reading new and repeated words. Moreover, older adults did not enjoy the long-term memory benefit from refreshing that younger adults did. Apparently, there is some age-related impairment of the refresh process that has negative consequences for learning. It is interesting to note that an area in the prefrontal cortex has been identified with refreshing (Raye, Johnson, Mitchell, et al., 2002), and there is evidence that the same general region is subject to increasing neuropathology over the course of normal aging (Raz, 2000).

In another study (Raye, Mitchell, Reeder, et al., 2008), participants were sometimes presented with three words at once, followed by a dot signaling them to think of the word that previously occupied the same position on the screen. Because the signal came after all three words had disappeared, refreshing required an extra step. The relevant information in working memory needed to be selected from among the irrelevant information. Not surprisingly, all participants responded more slowly when selection and refreshing were combined this way compared with refreshing a word that had been presented alone. An interesting age difference was observed, however. Unlike younger adults, older adults exhibited the same selection delay when a presentation of three words was followed by a repetition of one of them, or by a new word, instead of a dot. This result is surprising because, in those situations, their task was only to read the word on the screen, not to select a preceding one in working memory. It is consistent with other evidence, however, that older adults have difficulty ignoring or inhibiting irrelevant details (Hasher & Zacks, 1988). Educating patients well depends on understanding the specific changes that occur in memory function as part of the normal aging process but also on appreciating that other memory processes and cognitive functions are generally preserved.

Literacy, Language, and Culture

In this country, literacy is usually thought of as the ability to read, write, and speak English, but it can also be difficulty with understanding the reading material, an inability to process complex items, and difficulty in problem solving a large segment. A study by the Institute of Medicine (2004) found that 29% of Americans have basic literacy skills, and 14% are below basic, with 5% who do not speak or read English, which adds up to almost 50% of the population that has low literacy skills. Low literacy impacts more than learning from printed health materials. Unfortunately, healthcare providers often take reading ability for granted; however, because of shame and embarrassment, persons often hide the fact that they cannot read or have trouble reading. Davis et al. (2006) related literacy issues to patient safety by describing how misunderstandings of drug labels on prescription bottles led to patients taking the wrong medication or dose. The Joint Commission has recently begun to pay attention to this issue and place emphasis on providers needing to become aware of literacy issues as a way to reach the commission's goal of reducing medical errors. *What Did the Doctor Say? Improving Health Literacy to Protect Patient Safety*, a booklet developed by the commission, is available for free download at http://www.jointcommission.org/PublicPolicy/health_literacy.htm (The Joint Commission, 2007).

Is translation by a reliable source and printed resource materials available when needed for persons whose native language is not English? Providers need to recognize that patients with English as a second language may appear to understand because they will smile back and sometimes nod, even though they did not understand the conversation, but are trying to be polite. It is very important for the educator to *speak slowly, not loudly*. To assess if the message came through, ask the patient to repeat what he or she thought he or she heard. Use PVCs (perception, validation, and clarification) to be sure that the message is understood. Is the patient's *perception* the same as the provider's? *Validate* that with the patient. If the perception is not the same, *clarification* is needed. This process may be repeated to be sure understanding has taken place.

Providers need to be aware of certain cultural beliefs and home remedies that could interfere with positive healthcare practices, but it is helpful to listen to the patient's viewpoint. Cognitive dissonance can occur when patient beliefs do not match provider beliefs, and compromise may be needed to keep the required behavior change to a manageable level for the patient and family. Family beliefs and influences may also need to be assessed. Providers should resist the temptation to dissuade patients from harmless behaviors just because they are not recognized by the medical community as effective treatments. If a behavior does no harm but is reassuring to a patient, then it is consistent with good health care.

Poverty, Literacy, and Stress

A recent U.S. Census Bureau press release reported that blacks have the lowest income and that 25% of blacks and 26.6% of Native Americans live in poverty. Although the poverty rate stabilized for some groups, the number living in poverty increased for seniors 65 and older—3.6 million in 2005, up from 3.5 million in 2004 (U.S. Census Bureau, 2006). In addition, immigrants, legal and illegal, living in poverty may not have access to programs developed to provide health services for low-income persons. Poverty may interfere with achieving satisfactory levels of positive health behaviors. Doctor's visits may be skipped because of cost, and medications may not be available unless funds can be secured for purchase. Social services may need to become involved to assist in ensuring appropriate healthcare services for low income persons.

The homeless population has special needs to be addressed. What is the client's source for running water and sanitary facilities? Can medications be purchased, and how often do they need to be taken? Is this feasible, given the lack of housing? For example, how can insulin be stored with no refrigerator, and how can needles and syringes be managed? Insulin pens have multiple doses of insulin for easy use, but how will loose needles be stored? How can nutritional needs be met? Plans to address these issues need to be developed and resources made available to deal with some of the root causes and to begin to promote a better and safer lifestyle.

Stress and anxiety often accompany a new diagnosis and/or treatment, and it is important to assess the level. High stress and anxiety may be debilitating and may interfere with listening and memory, but moderate stress and anxiety may actually provide the impetus for seeking adherence to the therapeutic regimen and movement toward healthy lifestyles and behavior changes. Illness often causes turmoil in families as well as within the mind of the individual. Observe reactions to information given in stressful situations to patients and their families. Too much information can increase anxiety. Providing information over a longer time frame may be better absorbed for increased understanding and allows for repetition and evaluation to increase learning retention.

Encourage Behavioral Change

Habits are very hard to break, and adding medications, therapeutic regimens, and lifestyle changes can be daunting for patients. The Harm Reduction Model was developed for work with substance abuse and with HIV/AIDS patients, who are expected to change sexual behavior and take large amounts of medication with unpleasant side effects (Des Jarlais, 1995; Mallinson & Hawthorne, 1996; Newcombe & Parry, 1988; Sowell, Spicer, & Lowenstein, 2004).

The first principle behind the model is that total change of unhealthy behaviors should not be the only objective of health education for this population, as many persons are committed to their lifestyle and will ignore information and education requiring change. Although behavior change may be the final objective, the second principle holds that small changes are better tolerated and may be accomplished; in other words, better some change than none. Clients may be asked to choose behaviors they feel they can accomplish, knowing that they will ignore those they have no attention of changing. To encourage harm reduction further, providers can present alternative ways of behaving that may satisfy the need for the behaviors. For instance, if HIV/AIDS clients are unwilling to give up unprotected sexual activity, they can be told of activities that can provide pleasure and gratification other than direct, unprotected intercourse and be able to reduce the amount of unprotected activity without loss of pleasure (Sowell et al., 2004).

Both substance abuse and HIV/AIDS are conditions subject to stigmatization in the community and unfortunately with health providers as well. Working with these populations can be frustrating because change is exceedingly difficult and relapses occur frequently. Moral issues with HIV/AIDS and manipulative behaviors of substance abusers may cause providers to have negative views of this population. The provider or staff frustration and dislike may become visible to patients by way of angry, annoyed, irritated, or deprecating comments. Patient experiences with providers' discomfort led to the final principle of the Harm Reduction Model, the provision of user-friendly services, supportive rather than judgmental and the establishment of trust so that contact with the healthcare provider will be continued (Sowell et al., 2004).

The Harm Reduction Model can be used for patients with other conditions or unhealthy lifestyles. The principles are applicable to obesity treatment and smoking cessation. The model can also be used with patients who have difficulty adhering to their suggested therapeutic regimes and prescribed medications. The use of the term compliance has been criticized because it implies power and yielding or obedience to authority, and patients can react negatively to this concept (Falvio, 2004). Patients can be asked what healthy behaviors they think they can adhere to, rather than comply with. This puts the power ratio in the patient's hands. Small victories, without having to do everything at once, may allow patients to feel more comfortable with their ability to change behavior and reduce the discouragement of not being able to do what is expected, leading to giving up. Over time, patients can be encouraged to try more positive health behaviors, but even if this does not happen, the harm caused by unhealthy behaviors may be reduced to some degree.

TEACHING STRATEGIES TO ENHANCE RETENTION OF LEARNING

Teaching strategies to enhance retention of learning may include the use of reflection, recall, and personalization. Reflection is a technique used when patients are asked to think about, or reflect on, what is going on in their lives because of their illness or unhealthy lifestyle. They can then be encouraged to try problem solving to work with the disease condition and need for behavior change. Reflection and recall can work well with older patients and used to refresh memories of what was taught and learned. In subsequent visits, providers can ask patients to recall what was told to them, bringing the material back to conscious thought. This can also work in a family group, where they can help each other refresh their memories.

Personalization makes the educational materials specific to the patient's background and experiences. Personalizing can make a condition seem more real to patients because it clearly relates to the fact that their disease or lifestyle is directly affecting them and their families (Kammerer et al., 2007). Individual diet planning is a technique that uses personalization. The plan is developed around the patient's likes and dislikes. Medication administration needs to be worked around the patient's schedule and what is happening in their lives. How can insulin be taken at dinner when a person goes directly from work to a restaurant for dinner? Persons with English as a second language may need written health education materials in their native language. The experience can be made more at ease if someone who speaks their language assists them in working through the material and is able to answer questions. Native English speakers also benefit from having the healthcare provider go through the pamphlets and other materials with them, clarifying concepts and involving the patients in planning ways to improve their health.

Pictures and entertaining materials, used with tact and good judgment, may create a more upbeat atmosphere for positive learning, reduce the amount of necessary reading, and increase interest and motivation for change. Many persons are visual learners, and reading text can be difficult. Pictures can illustrate and reinforce points that need to be made and can enhance recall.

Humor can reduce anxiety and stress, increase interest, make learning a pleasant experience, and when used constructively, help build a positive self image (D'Amico & Jaffe, 2007; Hillman, 2001). Cartoons are frequently found in education materials and can bring a smile or laugh. Humor in conversation can help relaxation and make the learning environment a shared pleasant experience that can be remembered. Although joke punch lines may fade away, the context of the learning may be remembered; however, there can be another side to be aware of when using humor. Gender, culture, ethnicity, and context can affect how humor is received (Ziegler, 1998). Words and meanings may be completely different even in closely related language such as British English and American English. A boot is a type of footwear in American English and an automobile trunk in British English. Additionally, words often have more than one meaning. If the meaning of words is important to the integrity of a joke, it may not make sense or be understood to those who speak a different language or even a different dialect. The chapters and case studies in this book address many different teaching and learning strategies and techniques that can be used with individuals and groups and in many different learning situations.

Evaluate Learning in the Time Available, What Was Said and What Was Left Out

How Learning Was Accepted by the Recipient and What Needs to Be Done and How

Evaluation of learning is crucial to making learning effective. Having patients recite some, not all, of the important concepts that they learned, and their plans for working with it can reinforce the learning, which can then remain with the patient after leaving the office. Time does not allow for an extensive recitation, but patients can be asked to mention the *most important thing* they feel they learned in the conversation and what was the *most confusing*, which can then be clarified.

Creating ways to keep in contact allows for reinforcement of learning and correction of misunderstandings or misinformation. Patients need to know how they can have their questions answered after they leave the site. Can they call or use other sources or technology? The person on the other end, the one answering questions, needs to be user friendly and encouraging and *must avoid* "talking down to" the individual or allow patients to feel they are being criticized or scorned for asking "silly questions."

Becoming aware of how patients and families perceive their interaction with providers is not easy, but necessary. An uninviting environment, often because of unpleasant or rushed staff, may make patients uncomfortable and discouraged. The power equation is in favor of the provider over the patient because of knowledge and potential control of life threatening issues. Patients will not openly express their discomfort or dislike because of that power ratio for fear of retaliation; however, negative perceptions of the inter-action can show up with a pattern of missed appointments, lack of progress of change, or other subtle cues. Anonymous patient satisfaction surveys may help expose the atmosphere, either positive or negative. Surveys are not fool-proof because many patients may not or cannot answer and may not trust the survey to be truly anonymous, but they can be helpful.

Evaluation can provide an understanding of teaching goals and behavior changes achieved or not and provide a direction for planning future learning opportunities and selection of teaching strategies. It also identifies the need for referrals and resources to enhance the learning experience and provide additional information and assistance with continuing behavior change.

Using Collaboration and Resources to Extend Learning Opportunities

Understand How Much Contact with Healthcare Providers Is Available and Identify Additional Material to Be Learned and Who Can Do It

A patient may see many healthcare providers in the course of an illness. Patient care is often fragmented among primary care, specialists, nurses, and allied health providers. Consistency in the teaching and learning message among providers who work with patients is important; otherwise, confusing or contradictory information may occur. Care guidelines circulated among providers and documentation of use may encourage consistency in therapeutic regimen and message. In this era of patient privacy, permission may be needed from the patient to share records and reports of interaction. The need for sharing information may need to be explained to patients to gain their approval and set limits on what can or should be shared.

The presentation of a large amount of healthcare information can be overwhelming and confusing to a patient. This may be especially true for older persons, but anxiety and stress in all patients interferes with learning and impacts the amount that patients can absorb and work with. Learning sessions may be scheduled with other health professionals within the practice or through outside referrals.

The *ABCs of Cardiovascular Risk Reduction Care Bundle* was developed as a risk-reduction guideline for use with postcoronary artery bypass graft patients (Poe et al., 2007). These guidelines included consistent medication prescription and lifestyle counseling. The use of this packaged approach required adherence to guidelines and documentation of use by all professions in the care of these patients. Improvement occurred when the guideline medications were prescribed and lifestyle counseling was implemented. Patients appreciated and used the information booklet given to them when leaving the hospital. Patient adherence to medications and lifestyle change showed significant improvement, except for smoking cessation, where only minimal improvement occurred (Poe et al., 2007).

Can Technology Be Used?

The world we live in today is very different from the past, especially in the area of technology. The younger generation has grown up with the Internet, e-mails, text messages, blogs, and podcasts. They are often considered digital natives, whereas some of the older generation have begun to use more technology as digital immigrants, but some do not use much, if any, technology. Explore whether the use of technology for health education is feasible in your practice, and learn which patients can use it, even at a low level; e-mail may afford a communication method for patients to ask questions and for providers to communicate and follow up.

Selected web pages and video URLs, DVDs, and podcasts may be given to patients to view for additional information or to reinforce what was taught. The provider can develop a web page newsletter, updated at intervals and a notice e-mailed to patients, with a link to the newsletter. More and more podcasts are being developed, with both video and sound, making obsolete the older audio tape cassettes many of us were used to. Podcasts are a growing business, and the numbers and variety will increase in many areas in the future. Websites are available that provide instruction on creating the podcasts so that providers can personalize a podcast specifically for their practice and patient use. Commercial podcasts with health education programs may be available for purchase. Nonprofit agencies may also develop podcasts or DVDs that can be given out free of charge. Regardless of the type of technology used, providers need to evaluate if, what, and how patients are using it and if misconceptions are occurring.

Follow Up Over Time, Establish Communication and Feedback Methods, Including Effectiveness of Referrals

A key component in collaboration between healthcare professions for healthcare education is the development of a method to share what has been taught and what needs further teaching. Lowenstein and Hoff (1994) found poor communication between hospital and community health nurses regarding discharge planning and patient teaching carried out in the hospital. Seventy-two percent ($n = 161$) of hospital nurses answered that they effectively participated in discharge planning, which included health teaching with their patients; however, 85% ($n = 89$) of the community nurses in the same geographic area did not think that teaching had been done, because their post-discharge patient assessments could find little or no evidence of such teaching. There was no patient follow-up from the hospital nurses, and there was no feedback from the community nurses to hospital nurses about the lack of effectiveness of teaching while the patient was in the hospital (Lowenstein & Hoff, 1994; Lowenstein, Hoff, & Jackson, 1995). When healthcare providers do not receive feedback about their teaching, they will be unaware of problems and inefficiencies and may continue to provide ineffective teaching without realizing it.

Pharmacists who provide medication education to patients, in combination with the traditional healthcare teaching by nurses and physicians, have been able to show improvement in adherence. In one study, pharmacists were involved in providing medication education before hospital discharge. After discharge, patients received a follow-up phone call from a pharmacist asking about medications patients were taking, including adverse effects and difficulties in adherence. They also checked for discrepancies between the medicines the patient was taking at home and the discharge medication list. Problems with medications were discussed with the patients, and the pharmacist was able to schedule follow-up appointments or laboratory tests when needed. Emergency visits for medication-related issues diminished in the study group (Peterson, 2007).

Another study showed that adherence to tuberculosis treatment significantly improved when a pharmacist was involved together with the traditional method of physicians and nurses providing patient education on medication use. Pharmacists provided medication information on discharge from the hospital, but also followed up at out patient clinic visits where patients' pharmaceutical care issues could be further addressed (Clark, Karagoz, Apikoglu-Rabus, et al., 2007).

Establishing a regular routine for at least one follow-up with patients discharged from the hospital can provide hospital personnel important information about the effectiveness of the education process, the course of the patient's recovery, and the effectiveness of referrals. Information can be gathered by phone or in person when follow-up visits are scheduled at short intervals; however, it is important to make that information available to the providers who worked with the patient on the hospital unit.

It can be helpful to use a short, survey style guideline with specific open-ended questions that can be carried out in person or by phone. When a problem is noted, questioning can probe deeper into the situations. A standard format will also allow for the development of patterns needing to be further explored when similarities among patient answers appear.

Mailed surveys can be used; however, the response rate is often low, and the communication is usually one way and not effective in helping patients work through any problems or issues they mention in the survey. For computer literate patients, e-mail surveys may be used. That provides the opportunity to establish two-way conversations on specific issues and a way to keep the door open to further contact and communication.

CONCLUSION

Educating patients is important not only for increasing their knowledge, but for shaping their behavior. Informed patients have a better understanding of their conditions and treatment plans, but perhaps more importantly, they are more likely to remember what they need to do in fulfillment of those plans. Unfortunately, the drive for increased efficiency in health care presents a genuine challenge to providers who take their role as educators seriously. Nevertheless, it is possible to "do more with less" in that role by understanding what makes patients ready and willing to learn and how to present new information in a manner that interests and motivates them, leading to long-term retention, accurate remembering, and reliable self-care. Patient education may have the most immediate benefits of any kind of learning in society. Without a doubt, the pedagogical responsibilities and opportunities of healthcare providers are among their most crucial functions. They are not just expert practitioners; they are teachers.

Each diagnosis or prescription brings with it a need for explanation and demystification. A patient's education begins with an assessment of current knowledge and, before any new information is imparted, some careful debunking of misconceptions that may have been learned from a myriad of unreliable sources. This work must be careful; insensitively discrediting their beliefs or unnecessarily alarming them about the severity of their conditions can be counterproductive and even dangerous to their health. Patient education is necessarily a two-way conversation, not a lecture, and part of the healthcare provider's job is to listen carefully. In addition to building a model of their patients' understanding, providers who are good listeners can be alert for patterns in their patients' feedback that could inform institutional improvement and innovation.

The next job, of course, is to provide new information that has been appropriately filtered for the individual patient. The available time frame must be considered, along with the patient's readiness to learn, motivation, language and memory, age, cultural and socioeconomic background, and stress level. Learning depends on memory, and memory depends on how well the learner organizes new information when it is first encountered. The provider, having more expertise, is in the perfect position to help the patient see how different pieces of new information can be "chunked" together. Given that time for one-on-one discussions is likely to be limited, the availability of additional resources beyond the provider's direct attention must also be taken into account, including new technologies.

Finally, as an educator, healthcare providers require knowledge and skill to encourage long-term retention through reflection, recall, and personalization and to encourage behavior change by focusing on harm reduction. If at all possible, developing a collaborative approach will be most effective, especially when repeated assessments can be made during regular follow-up consultations.

Many aspects of health care are compromised, unfortunately, in a climate of time pressure and cost efficiency. Effective patient education does not need to be a casualty, however. By following some of these guidelines, healthcare providers can add a little pedagogy to their realm of expertise, and their patients will only benefit. From this perspective, learning is part of recovering, and teaching is an act of healing.

REFERENCES

Barnstable, S. B. (2003). *Nurse as educator: principles of teaching and learning for nursing practice* (2nd ed). Boston: Jones & Bartlett.

Clark, P. M., Karagoz, T., Apikoglu-Rabus, S., & Izzettin, R. V. (2007, March 1). Effect of pharmacist-led patient education on adherence to tuberculosis treatment. *American Journal of Health Systems Pharmacy, 64,* 497–506.

Craik, F. I. M. (1984). Age differences in remembering. In L. R. Squire & N. Butters (Eds.), *Neuropsychology of memory* (pp. 3–12). New York: Guilford Press.

D'Amico, M., & Jaffe, L. (2007). Lighten up your classroom. In M. J. Bradshaw & A. J. Lowenstein (Eds.), *Innovative teaching strategies in nursing and related health professions* (pp. 79–91). Boston: Jones & Bartlett.

Davis, T. C., Wolf, M. S., Bass III, P. F., Thompson, J. A., Tilson, H. H., Neuberger, M., et al. (2006). Literacy and misunderstanding prescription drug labels. *Annals of Internal Medicine, 145,* 887–894.

Des Jarlais, D. (1995). Harm reduction: a framework for incorporating science into drug policy. *American Journal of Public Health, 85,* 10–12.

Falvio, D. R. (2004). *Effective patient education: a guide to increased compliance* (3rd ed.). Boston: Jones & Bartlett.

Godden, D. R., & Baddeley, A. D. (1975). Context-dependent memory in two natural environments: on land and underwater. *British Journal of Psychology, 66,* 325–331.

Hasher, L., & Zacks, R. (1988). Working memory, comprehension, and aging: a review and a new view. In G. H. Bower (Ed.), *The psychology of learning and motivation* (pp. 193–225). New York: Academic Press.

Hashtroudi, S., Johnson, M. K., & Chrosniak, L. D. (1990). Aging and qualitative characteristics of memories for perceived and imagined complex events. *Psychology and Aging, 5,* 119–126.

Hillman, S. M. (2001). Humor in the classroom: facilitating the learning process. In A. J. Lowenstein & M. J. Bradshaw (Eds.), *Fuszard's innovative teaching strategies in nursing* (3rd ed., pp. 54–62). Sudbury, MA: Jones & Bartlett.

Institute of Medicine. (2004). *Health literacy: a prescription to end confusion.* Washington, DC: National Academies Press.

Johnson, M. K., Reeder, J. A., Raye, C. L., & Mitchell, K. J. (2002). Second thoughts versus second looks: an age-related deficit in reflectively refreshing just-activated information. *Psychological Science, 13,* 64–67.

Kammerer, J., Garry, G., Hartigan, M., Carter, B., & Erlich, L. (2007). Adherence in patients on dialysis: strategies for success. *Nephrology Nursing Journal, 34*(5), 479–486.

Lowenstein, A., & Hoff, P. (1994). Discharge planning: a study of nursing staff involvement. *Journal of Nursing Administration, 24*(4), 1–6.

Lowenstein, A., Hoff, P., & Jackson, W. (1995, March). *From hospital to home: a study of hospital and community nurses' perception of discharge planning.* Paper presented at the Fourth Annual Conference of the Quality of Worklife Research Unit: Worklife in the 1990s. Toronto, Canada.

Mallinson, K., & Hawthorne, J. (1996). A realistic approach toward injection drug users. *Canadian Nurse, 92*(2), 22–26.

Miller, G. A. (1956). The magical number seven, plus or minus two: some limits on our capacity for processing information. *Psychological Review, 63,* 81–97.

Newcombe, R., & Parry, A. (1988). *The Mersey harm-reduction model: a strategy for dealing with drug users.* Paper presented at the International Conference on Drug Policy Reform. Bethesda, MD.

Peterson, A. M. (2007, March 1). Improving adherence in patients with alcohol dependence: a new role for pharmacists. *American Journal of Health Systems Pharmacy, 64*(Suppl. 3), 523–529.

Poe, S. S., Dawson, P. R., Cafeo, C., Sealander, D., Curtis, C., Meyer, P., et al. (2007). Use of the ABC Care Bundle to standardize guideline implementation in a cardiac surgical population: a pilot study. *Nursing Care Quality, 22*(3), 247–254.

Prochaska, J. O., Norcross, J. C., & Diclemente, C. C. (1994). *Changing for good: a revolutionary six-stage program for overcoming bad habits and moving your life positively forward.* New York: Harper Collins.

Raye, C. L., Johnson, M. K., Mitchell, K. J., Reeder, J. A., Greene, E. J. (2002). Neuroimaging a single thought: dorsolateral PFC activity associated with refreshing just-activated information. *NeuroImage, 15,* 447–453.

Raye, C. L., Mitchell, K. J., Reeder, J. A., Greene, E. J., & Johnson, M. K. (2008). Refreshing one of several active representations: behavioral and fMRI differences between young and older adults. *Journal of Cognitive Neuroscience, 20*(5). 852–862

Raz, N. (2000). Aging of the brain and its impact on cognitive performance: integration of structural and functional findings. In F. L. M. Craik & T. A. Salthouse (Eds.), *The handbook of aging and cognition* (2nd ed., pp. 1–90). Mahwah, NJ: Lawrence Erlbaum Associates Publishers.

Seabrook, R., Brown, G. D. A., & Solity, J. E. (2005). Distributed and massed practice: from laboratory to classroom. *Applied Cognitive Psychology, 19,* 107–122.

Slamecka, N. J., & Graf, P. (1978). The generation effect: delineation of a phenomenon. *Journal of Experimental Psychology: Human Learning and Memory, 4,* 592–604.

Sowell, R. L., Spicer, T., & Lowenstein, A. J. (2004). Nursing perspectives in the care of persons with HIV infection. In G. Wormser (Ed.), *AIDS and other manifestations of HIV infection* (4th ed., pp. 1029–1044). Boston: Elsevier.

Spencer, W. D., & Raz, N. (1995). Differential effects of aging on memory for content and context: a meta-analysis. *Psychology of Aging, 10,* 527–539.

The Joint Commission. (2007). What did the doctor say? Improving health literacy to protect patient safety. Retrieved February 10, 2008, from http://www .jointcommission.org/PublicPolicy/health_literacy.htm.

U.S. Census Bureau. (2006). *Income climbs, poverty stabilizes, uninsured rate increases.* Retrieved February 2, 2008, from http://www.census.gov/Press-Release/ www/releases/archives/income_wealth/007419.html.

Ziegler, J. (1998). Use of humor in medical teaching. *Medical Teacher, 20*(4), 341–348.

Chapter 12

Play—An Educational Tool in Health Care

Suzanne Graca, Kirsten Fowler, & Addie Rosenstock

INTRODUCTION

Play—a powerful word in the world of the child—has been considered "critical for children's expression, mastery, and learning about their experiences" (Rollins, Bolig, & Mahan, 2005). While in the presence of children, regardless of age, this is unmistakable. Indeed, the importance of play in a child's cognitive, emotional, and social development is without question and consistently visible in the literature (Bellack & Fleming, 1986; Petrillo & Sanger, 1980). The works of Axline (1969) and Landreth (1991) further identify play as a means of coping and therapeutic processing. Simply watching and listening to children engaged in play and developmentally appropriate activities verifies the importance of such activity not only in their social and emotional growth and development but also more specifically in their learning and understanding of the world around them. This is no different in the environment of health care.

Professionals in the field of pediatrics have begun to recognize that play, toys, and games can become successful mechanisms and tools of education related to medical issues. Although extensive research is lacking, many, including Thompson (1981, 1985, 1995) and Gaynard et al. (1990), have long identified the importance of play and development in health care. Additionally, the American Academy of Pediatrics (2006) in their most recent *Policy Statement on Child Life Services* notes that medical play specifically may offer insight into the patient's concerns and levels of understanding of the healthcare events. Medical play, as well as general play, can provide wonderful and important insight on the understanding of the developing child and can be particularly successful when teaching. Kathleen McCue (1988) identifies this form of play as generally enjoyable activity that involves a medical theme. It can be further classified into four categories: role rehearsal/role reversal, where the child actively performs or rehearses medical interventions on dolls or stuffed animals; medical fantasy play, which has a medical theme but no medical toys or equipment are used; indirect play, which involves more educational "tools" such as games, puzzles, and books; and finally, medical art. Such play allows opportunities to cope with both the physical and emotional stressors of health care, as well as act as mechanisms to increase understanding. In fact, playful distraction has even been documented to decrease the perception of discomfort during medical interventions (Sparks, 2001). (However, medical play and preparation are not synonymous. Bolig, Yolton, and Nissen [1991] and Goldberger, Gaynard, and Wolfer [1990] clarify that play can be used as one of several means to education and assist the child with coping.)

In the focus of play as an educational tool, however, one must first and foremost identify and understand key developmental milestones in childhood. This can then assist both professionals and parents alike in determining the most successful mechanisms of play to use in educational endeavors.

INFANT/TODDLER DEVELOPMENT

Play and games serve a vital role in the learning process for infants and toddlers. Whether at home or in a healthcare setting, parents/guardians can use play and games to teach and encourage "normal" development; however, to understand fully what and why specific play and games are used with infants, one must have an understanding of typical infant and toddler development.

From the moment an infant is born, he or she experiences the world through their senses, including touch, smell, sight, sound, and taste. Piaget considered these first 2 years of life to be the Sensorimotor Stage (Cole & Cole, 1997); therefore, the environment and how one adapts to the environment affect infant/toddler development.

Throughout the first 2 years of life, an infant is gaining muscle control and coordination, sucking, grasping, reaching, sitting, crawling, and walking. The latter part of the first year of life brings about a fundamental change in infants' relationships with their environment called locomotion (Cole & Cole, 1997). During this time, infants/toddlers begin to explore the world around them, becoming more independent and mobile.

As an infant's relationship changes with their environment, so does their ability to understand and communicate with people around him or her. At this age, there is an increased recognition of familiar faces and environments, which can often be observed in an increased emotional bond, called attachment. In addition, many times infants show signs of separation anxiety and stranger anxiety to these familiar faces (parents/guardians) and environment (home). Erikson stated that if an infant's basic needs are met, an infant is learning to trust others during the trust versus mistrust stage (Cole & Cole, 1997).

The way an infant communicates with people and the environment they are surrounded by changes as they age. At first, an infant reacts with physical responses such as tensing of muscles, facial expressions, change of breathing patterns, and crying. With time and experience, an infant is able to use other forms of communication such as grunting, babbling, and words. Although there is limited ability for an infant to communicate verbally, he or she understands much more than he or she can express through language (Cole & Cole, 1997). An infant's receptive language is often 6 months ahead of verbal language. For instance, infants can often follow commands such as "clap your hands" before they can say a word such as "clap."

A toddler continues to develop and gain mastery over his or her gross- and fine-motor skills. In addition, toddlers are becoming more independent working on bladder and bowel control. According to Erickson, a toddler is in the autonomy versus shame and doubt (Cole & Cole, 1997). When caregivers provide support, as well as a safe place for children to become independent and develop problem-solving skills, a child becomes autonomous. An unfamiliar environment, such as a hospital, provides challenges for parents and caregivers to encourage and facilitate autonomy.

Although a toddler begins to gain a better understanding of himself or herself, they often cannot distinguish their point of view from that of others (Cole & Cole, 1997). With this said, a toddler's favorite two words are often "no" and "mine." An increased sense of independence can often be observed in an unwillingness to make any sort of compromise. Although there is continued development of language, toddlers' receptive language is still typically 6 months ahead of verbal language. Toddlers often follow commands or requests spoken to them but often take a longer time to use phrases and sentences to communicate back (Cole & Cole, 1997). In other words, a toddler is able to understand and follow a command such as "bring me your sippy cup" quicker than he or she is able to respond back with words.

LEARNING THROUGH PLAY

As discussed earlier, a child's job is to play. Play facilitates learning through exposing a child to new experiences and new possibilities (Hughes, 1995). Whether at home or in the hospital, play is a vital tool to help all infants and toddlers develop. According to Piaget's theory, play does more than merely reflect a child's level of cognitive development; it also contributes to that development (Hughes, 1995). The environment must be adapted no matter where the child is to encourage and provide play opportunities.

The way children play differs depending on the age that they are at. Play progresses through stages that mirror children's psychosocial development. Children create model situations that help them master the demands of reality through play (Johnson, Christie, & Yawkey, 1999). Depending on what "reality" faces the individual infant/toddler, play and toys can be adapted to make it optimal for the infant/toddler to learn. By adapting the play and toys, infants/toddlers can therefore act out what they are experiencing, learn ways to work through it, and express and cope with what they are facing.

Parents/guardians and family members serve a vital role in infant/toddler play. Often, the opportunities for play and play materials are provided by the adults, including what toys a parent places in a crib and what toys are in a child's room and/or home. Play materials such as black and white pictures and brightly colored objects help to provide visual stimulation and are developmentally appropriate for an infant/toddler. This, in turn, gives an infant/toddler something to fix and follow on, as well as reach for and grab for. As an infant/toddler develops and reaches landmarks, a parent/guardian can help to encourage progression and development. For instance, make a game of "can you reach for the puppet"; with this, a parent/guardian can start with the puppet close to the infant/toddler's hand and then eventually bring it further and further away, past the infant/toddler's midline, and eventually out in front of the body so that the infant/toddler rolls, crawls, and walks to get it. This game provides the child with a visual object to fix and follow, in addition to reaching and grasping, using gross- and fine-motor skills. Healthcare providers can help to facilitate this play with infants/toddlers when in a healthcare setting.

Cause and effect toys such as musical instruments and pop-up toys are favorites of this age group. Other favorites include gross motor toys such as push/pull toys and balls of all sizes. Toddlers often repeat an action with these toys over and over again, mastering the toy; however, their attention spans are quite limited, and thus, they typically move from one toy to another quickly after repeating the action a few times. These early interactions provide a foundation for social development and social play development in particular (Hughes, 1995). For instance, an infant/toddler may observe a parent pushing a button on a toy and as a result something pops up. The infant/toddler then may attempt this for themselves. After completing the task, the infant/toddler may look to the adult for approval (i.e., smiling and clapping hands). This sequence may be repeated several times.

Case Study 12-1

After being a passenger in a car that was involved in a pretty significant accident, 22-month-old Katie was resistant to get back into a car, particularly when her mother was intended to be the driver. It was clear that this toddler associated her mother driving a car with an unpleasant experience. Katie's primary care physician suggested that the family go out and buy two small toy cars for her to play with and to try and find a car that resembled the car that she was riding in at the time of the accident. Katie's parents were able to find a small, matchbox-sized station wagon along with another car that was close in color to the other car involved in the accident. Katie began to play with the cars and would crash them together after which she would pick them up and state, "All better." After a couple of days of this play, Katie was able to work through her negative association with being in a car and became a willing passenger again.

Through this play, parents/guardians strengthen the bond and attachment with their infant/toddler. By adapting an infant/toddler's environment to meet the needs of a child, the parent/guardian can help to provide opportunities for continuing growth and development. These developmentally appropriate materials and interactions often help to normalize the environment for an infant/toddler when in the hospital, thereby allowing an opportunity for continued growth and development physically, cognitively, socially, and emotionally. Whether at home or in a healthcare setting, pictures, bright-colored objects, cause-and-effect toys, and familiar sounds can help to adapt an environment to meet the needs to the individual child.

MEDICAL PLAY FOR INFANTS AND TODDLERS

As noted previously, infants and toddlers learn in a physical manner through their senses. With this said, it is important for infants and toddlers to be introduced and involved in medical play. Medical play allows for exploration and self-expression of different healthcare equipment through rehearsal/role reversal medical play, medical fantasy play, indirect medical play, and medically related art (McCue, 1988). A child can explore and manipulate common medical materials as both plastic toys as well as real equipment (McCue, 1988). For example, a Fisher-Price doctor's bag with plastic stethoscope, syringe, blood pressure cuff, and real stethoscope, thermometer, gloves, band-aids, and tape are materials that can aid in teaching. By giving an infant/toddler an opportunity to mouth, teeth, smell, and hold these materials, he or she becomes familiar with them, gaining a sense of mastery and trust. It is beneficial to observe and take note of what and how an infant/toddler reacts to such medical equipment. A toddler may act out a previous personal experience or something that he or she has seen and give a shot to a teddy bear over and over again. This would be an opportune time for observation and teaching, as parents/guardians might observe a toddler playing with a teddy bear and say, "You have been a bad teddy bear, and now you have to have a shot." This would provide the opportunity to let the child know that shots are to help keep your body healthy. They are not given if you are a bad boy or girl, clearing up misconceptions that the toddler may have. Building blocks, doll houses, cars and trucks, and play animals can all serve a role in a medical play scenario (McCue, 1988). Movies and books that talk about going to the doctor and germs can also help to introduce health care, doctors, and hospitals to all infants and toddlers. By taking the time to read a book about going to the doctor, a parent/guardian can prepare a child for a visit.

Parents/guardians know their child the best, and thus, it is important to ask them what their child's likes and dislikes are and what soothes and comforts their infant/toddler. In addition, parents can help to provide insight into what tools they think will be most useful for their infant/toddler to encourage and promote development, mastery, and learning. Play is vital for all infants and toddlers, especially those that are involved in health care and hospitals.

PRESCHOOL DEVELOPMENT

The Preschool group encompasses normally developing children from the approximate age of 3 to 5 years. Preschoolers have active imaginations and have a difficult time separating reality from fantasy, making them particularly vulnerable to the effects of health care and hospitalization. Preschoolers, more than any other developmental age, tend to have many misconceptions about medical equipment and procedures. They are also still very egocentric, and their thoughts are very self-focused; thus, to a preschooler, illness or hospitalization can be thought of as a punishment for something that they have done (Thompson & Stanford, 1981).

Although these facts make them particularly vulnerable, it also makes them good candidates for healthcare teaching. Preschool age children have had enough personal experience to understand simple life concepts and are now entering the phase of their development in which they learn to apply and build on them.

According to Erik Erikson's Theory of Psychosocial Development, children at this age are in a stage called Initiative versus Guilt. They begin to assert themselves more frequently when they reach preschool age. They begin to plan, make up games, and initiate activities with others. It is important to provide opportunities for play and exploration, and thus, children feel comfortable developing this sense of initiative. Some ways to enhance these opportunities are to create play environments that make children feel safe to take risks. Creating activities without many rules or criticism will prevent creating a sense of failure that could lead to feelings of guilt. It is important to feature the process over the final product and to be encouraging throughout. With these points in mind, it is a good idea to make the activities group- and cooperation-based rather than individual tasks (Trawick-Smith, 2006).

According to Piaget's theory of cognitive development, preschool children fall into the stage of preoperational thought. They are developing the ability to manipulate images and symbols, especially language. They are able to use symbolism with objects and play things as well. A block can symbolize a car or a plane in play activities (Thompson & Stanford, 1981). When teaching, this can be helpful in planning play activities. Keep in mind that although preschoolers can use symbolism and have an increased knowledge of the external body, they have a limited concept of the internal body. Their ideas about causal relationships may be underdeveloped at this stage and so the concepts of illness may be challenging for them to understand.

PLAY AND THE PRESCHOOLER

As previously stated, play is the work of childhood. Play is essential to all types of development: cognitive, physical, and emotional. Preschoolers are no exception. They want to touch, taste, smell, hear, and test things for themselves. They are eager to learn and they learn best by experiencing and doing.

During play, a preschooler picks up, manipulates, and studies objects of all types. He or she learns shapes, colors, sizes, and textures and how parts of an object fit the whole. In time, a preschooler learns to formulate plans, develop strategies, and exercise his or her assessment skills in problem solving because of play. Play also helps the teacher assess what a child's understanding is and what the child is interested in.

One of the most significant ways preschoolers play is called pretend play. When children pretend, they remember past experiences or situations and replay them. Pretend play helps children get ready for life by rehearsing roles. It allows them to begin to understand information that they have received by acting it out. Many of these pretend play sessions include role-playing grown-up jobs such as, doctor, nurse, fireman, or teacher. In their role playing, children are clearly the ones in charge, and the play gives them opportunities to use many of their developing skills such as eye–hand coordination, language building, and large motor skills.

Pretend play and role rehearsal can also help a child gain mastery of an environment that can be threatening or strange to them. They can overcome fears of unpleasant experiences. This is particularly true of healthcare situations in which they are commonly asked to be passive (Thompson & Stanford, 1981). Holding still for examinations, immunizations, and procedures is one example. Many preschoolers enjoy medical play with real or toy medical equipment and often a doll or stuffed animal. It can give children a nonthreatening way to normalize medical equipment and to express their own fears and/or curiosities about medical procedures. Because of the magical thinking of this age group, be available to answer questions and clear up misconceptions that come up during play activities.

Case Study 12-2

Understanding the importance of preparation and education in health care, many members of the medical team had chatted about an upcoming surgery with Bobby, an energetic preschooler. When simply asked whether he had any questions regarding his kidney operation, Bobby would simply smile and respond with a "no." Not long before the scheduled surgery, Bobby engaged in medical play with the child life specialist. Bobby eagerly pulled out every piece of the medical play kit and went to work on the doll. Occasionally, one could hear him say something about the kidneys. Again, he was asked whether he understood the operation. He just smiled and nodded. He was further questioned: "Well, where are your kidneys? Can you point to them?" Again, he smiled, nodded, looked down and touched his *knees*. "Here they are—my kid knees!" Preschoolers perceive words concretely, thus leading to the misunderstanding. Through play and active clarification, Bobby was reassured that this operation would not be on his "kid knees" nor is it done on our "adult knees"— for that matter! Rather, Bobby was shown a doll with a bandage on its lower back to redirect and correct the understandable mistake.

TEACHING PRESCHOOLERS THROUGH PLAY AND GAMES

When teaching preschoolers it is very important to be concrete. They are not skilled in abstract thinking so giving very clear instructions and explanations is key. Using very descriptive sensory details is also helpful (i.e., how something will feel, smell, taste, and look). When discussing healthcare issues related to specific body parts, use clear identification of the body parts involved and those that will not be involved. The use of props, models, and pictures that children can manipulate and handle is encouraged.

Preschoolers learn the most when they are active; therefore, limit large periods of lecture-style teaching. It is also very important to this age group that they feel successful at the tasks that they are working on. Thus, one must plan activities with reachable goals and successes throughout while providing positive reinforcement.

Pretend play is an activity that is beneficial and enjoyable for preschool age children. The following are some other play activities that preschoolers both enjoy and should be developmentally able to participate in:

- *Basic art activities.* Preschoolers will enjoy expressive art activities using basic art materials. The focus should be on the process not the product. Activities may be messy, as art for preschoolers is all about experimentation and learning. Preschoolers can learn while completing the art activity.
- *Board games.* Because of the fact that preschoolers need encouragement and the feeling of success, board games should be simple and not competitive. Competitive games or games of strategy are especially difficult for younger children, who are not developmentally able to follow the game rules. Create informal games where children can all play together and help one another. When planning a health promotion or teaching activity by adapting a board game, choose games that are simple, visually exciting and sturdy, with pieces that are easy for a young child to grasp. Candyland, Don't Break the Ice, Guess Who, and Monopoly Junior work well.
- *Music.* The steady rhythms of song and the act of singing itself help the brain to remember. Although this is clear in the short term, it can also translate to long-term memory (e.g., *The Clean Up Song* for use in reinforcing the concept of cooperation in clean up). For preschoolers, the more emotion in a song, the stronger the memory will be. Learning is strongly influenced by emotion. When adapting songs for use in teaching activities, its helpful to use familiar tunes and to substitute the new health promotion lyrics, creating the theme you want.

DEVELOPMENT OF THE SCHOOL-AGED CHILD

Children between the ages of 6 and 12 years are identified by Erikson as being in the stage of Industry versus Inferiority. They truly enjoy mastering new skills and do so actively. They learn by doing and are quite conscious of how this appears to others, particularly peers. Role models and heroes are also very significant at this age. Thus, these children are extremely observant of the people around them. Children in this stage of development are able to engage in subject-based conversations with both adults and peers as they can use language appropriately. Piaget refers to this period of time between 7 and 11 years as the Concrete Operational stage where thought is more logical, flexible, and organized. Piaget uses the term "horizontal decalage" to describe the child's gradual mastery of logical concepts—concepts they are far better able to understand and used during adolescence (Berk, 1998). Cognitively, they are able to reason and make generalizations, as well as process and decipher information. They understand relationships between events and experiences and thus the process and consequences of interactions and behaviors.

Although this period of middle childhood, which is highlighted with increasing cognitive capacities, would appear to be an ideal time to incorporate education regarding health and healthy lifestyles, barriers may also exist. In general, children of middle childhood, as well as those in adolescence, feel "good." Thus, health and health-related topics may not appear personally as an important goal. Children in this stage of development and teenagers to some extent also lack the time perspective of adults. They simply live for the present. Additionally, there exists much contradictory information regarding health for the developing child. Friends and media, particularly advertising, can lead to confusion and often conflicting information.

Progressing along the developmental continuum, the older school-aged child grows cognitively, striving for additional information. They are more curious and knowledge driven. They want the facts—the what, why, where, when, and how of all events. This is particularly true of just how this may affect them. Understanding this will be extremely helpful to the health-care practitioner engaging in education encounters with this age group. This drive solidifies and becomes more structured and organized as the child approaches the teenage years.

Case Study 12-3

During a workshop for 5- to 7-year-old children with severe food allergies, medical play time was offered to the kids in hopes of normalizing some of the medical equipment they would encounter in relationship to their doctor visits and their condition. Fisher-Price toy medical kits were set on a large blanket on the floor along with various "real" medical items such as band-aids, gauze, and Epi-Pen trainers (without the needle). The kids rehearsed medical procedures and doctor visits on dolls that were provided. All of the children gravitated to the Epi-Pen trainers, despite the myriad of other medical toys to play with. With no prompting from staff, the kids repeatedly pretended the dolls were exposed to foods that they were allergic to and needed treatment.

During the next workshop, staff added toy food to the play area as well. Many of the kids would say their dolls were afraid of eating peanuts, and then they would hold a peanut close to the doll and recreate anaphylactic shock in the dolls. The children played doctor, carefully giving the dolls Epi-Pen "shots" and making them better. The playtime gave staff a great insight into the children's fears and how they imagined things going if they were exposed to an allergen. Staff could then use this play session as a jumping off point for the teaching and activities later in the workshop. If used at the end of the workshop, the play session offers a great opportunity for the children to practice positive skills. It also can be used as a tool for staff to evaluate learning.

DEVELOPMENT OF THE ADOLESCENT

Erikson classifies this period of 12 to 18 years as Identity versus Role Confusion. This is a stage of intense self-evaluation. Body image and real or imagined physical differences as compared with peers is of the utmost importance. Likewise, there is an increased awareness of sexual identity and one's individual role in society. Piaget further describes this stage as that of Formal Operational thought—the capacity for abstract thinking. More specifically, those in this stage can generally exhibit the ability to reflect on a given problem, consider possible means of solution, and predict what may then occur—essentially testing whether such a solution/conclusion could indeed be correct. This is known as hypotheticodeductive reasoning. These children would also be capable of propositional thought where they can consider the actual validity of verbal statements without actual, concrete, real-world situations (Berk, 1998).

In addition to their cognitive development, one must also recognize important factors of the social development of the teenager. First, the influence of peers can particularly create additional challenges to the successful education of the adolescent. In decision making, the teen may be drawn to follow the suggestions of peers rather than that of the adult, regardless of validity of the information presented. This, combined with issues of privacy, the general need for control and increased independence from family may all complicate an already developmentally commanding period. Possible strained trusting relationships with adults and/or authority figures can also impact teaching; however, this teaching need not be as challenging as one may anticipate.

The use of play strategies, games, and social interaction may indeed be the mechanism for success. This is particularly true of children already in the hospital and/or healthcare environment. Whether new to the experience due to an acute episode or a veteran to healthcare interventions (as is the case with chronic illness), a child may additionally exhibit regressive behaviors caused by stress, fear, and/or general uncertainty. Thus, many strategies and tools applicable to the school-aged child may also be effective with the adolescent—with some modifications.

WHY PLAY?

Teaching during this developmental stage of ongoing growth of cognitive processing can effectively incorporate more information than in earlier stages. Active participation, more actual, factual teaching tools, and conversation can lead to greater understanding for school-age children and teens. Therapeutic and/or medical play can be engaging and act as conduits of information (Rollins et al., 2005). Medical play, particularly role rehearsal/role reversal, as well as indirect medical play can be very effective methods of delivering education to this age group (Bolig, Yolton, & Nissen, 1991). During this stage of development, such play will incorporate more actual equipment and information. The cloth dolls popular with the younger ages can still be effective; however, more elaborate, anatomically correct tools may be more appropriate. For example, *Zadii* dolls, although no longer manufactured, are still available in established hospital play/child life programs. Also available for this type of teaching are *Legacy* dolls (www.legacyproductsinc.com) and *Claudia* dolls (www.claudiaskids.com). These allow for hands-on, active participation to learning. Unlike general dolls, Legacy dolls can be custom made to incorporate an extensive list of medical devices, including IV and G-tube sites. The Claudia dolls include overlying templates that may be superimposed onto the doll, explaining the body organs and corresponding function.

Additionally, Parten's social categorization of play (Thompson, 1981) identifies children within this phase of development as being capable of actively and successfully engaging in a wide range of games requiring rules and interaction with peers. Health-themed games such as Hospital Bingo and Adventure Park, which are also examples of indirect medical play (Boling, 1988), provide avenues of education and peer and/or family socialization. Hospital Bingo is played like general bingo with hospital-themed items and people in place of numbers. The board game Adventure Park allows participants to communicate about chronic illness and strategies to cope with this illness through play. Even the classic game Operation, which would be developmentally inappropriate with younger children generally dominated by magical thinking, may serve teens as a tool of education and communication with parents and other adults. The use of health-themed games, books, and movies can be nonthreatening methods to educate older children regarding procedures, diagnoses, and general health experiences (**Table 12-1**).

Table 12-1 Play and Toy Resources for Learning

Web and computer-based resources

- www.claudiaskids.com
- www.legacyproductsinc.com
- www.shadowbuddies.org
- www.starlight.org

Books

- Child Life Council. (1998). Activity recipe book. Rockville, MD: CLC.
- Hart, R., Mather, P., Slack, J., & Powell, M. (1992). Therapeutic play activities for hospitalized children. Boston: Mosby Year Book.
- Kim Gosslin series.
- Tillman, K. G. (1990). How to survive teaching health: games, activities, and worksheets for grades 4–12. West Nyack, NY: Parker Publishing Company.

Games and toys

- Medical kit, Fisher-Price
- Candyland, Hasbro
- Adventure Park, Phizer Co.
- Hospital Bingo, Johns Hopkins Hospital

Movies

- Arthur Goes to the Doctor
- Elmo Visits the Doctor
- Bill Nye, the Science Guy
- The Magic School Bus: Inside Ralphie
- Osmosis Jones

Additionally, there exists a wide range of activities, including arts and crafts, which can be very successful in the health-based education of the school-aged child (Hart et al., 1992).

With advances in technology, multimedia, and computer-based games have also become increasingly more popular and perhaps more regularly used in comparison with their counterpart, the board game. Recent articles have documented both enthusiasm and success with such programs (Hazzard, Celano, Collins, & Markov, 2002; Krishna, Balas, Francisco, & Konig, 2006). Evidence of increased knowledge, coping, and compliance has been witnessed in children with medical conditions. These include educational programs developed by both professional medical and educational organizations, as well as materials available to the general public. Hasbro

Interactive has created a CD-ROM version of Operation that is readily available. For more specific education of medical conditions, the Starbright organization has created a series of educational titles. This includes Quest for the Code for asthma education and the Explorer Series. The later reviews interventions such as IVs, and bone marrow aspirations, as well as the illnesses of cystic fibrosis, sickle cell, and kidney disease. Most recently an action-packed game ReMission was created specifically for teens with cancer.

CONCLUSION

Play and games serve a vital role in the learning process for all ages; however, to understand fully what and why specific play and games are used, one must have a basic understanding of typical development. With this basic knowledge of child development, parents and other healthcare professionals can use developmentally appropriate play to help children learn and understand what is happening. In addition, play and games allow children to have the opportunity to express any feelings and/or misconceptions that they have in a way that is familiar to them.

It is vital to look at the world through a child's eyes to understand where they are coming from and how they view what is going on around them. Developmentally appropriate play and games enhance teaching and allow a person to connect with a child at the child's level. By doing this, one can begin to build a relationship of trust and understanding that only enhances direct patient care to improve outcomes.

"Just Playing"

When I'm building in the block room,
Please don't say I'm "Just Playing."
For, you see, I'm learning as I play;
About balance and shapes.

When I'm getting all dressed up,
Setting the table, caring for the babies,
Don't get the idea I'm "Just Playing."
For, you see, I'm learning as I play,
I may be a mother or a father someday.

When you see me up to my elbows in paint,
Or standing at an easel, or molding and shaping clay,
Please don't let me hear you say, "He is Just Playing."
For, you see, I'm learning as I play.

I'm expressing myself and being creative,
I may be an artist or an inventor someday.

When you see me sitting in a chair
"Reading" to an imaginary audience,
Please don't laugh and think I'm "Just Playing."
For, you see, I'm learning as I play.
I may be a teacher someday.

When you see me combing the bushes for bugs,
Or packing my pockets with choice things I find,
Don't pass it off as "Just Play."
For, you see, I'm learning as I play.
I may be a scientist someday.

When you see me engrossed in a puzzle,
Or some "plaything" at my school,
Please don't feel the time is wasted in "Play."
For, you see, I'm learning as I play.
I'm learning to solve problems and concentrate.
I may be in business someday.

When you see me cooking or tasting foods,
Please don't think that because I enjoy it, it is "Just Play."
I'm learning to follow directions and see differences.
I may be a chef someday.

When you see me learning to skip, hop, run, and move my body,
Please don't say I'm "Just Playing."
For, you see, I'm learning as I play.
I'm learning how my body works.
I may be a doctor, nurse, or athlete someday.

When you ask me what I've done at school today,
And I say, "I Just Played."
Please don't misunderstand me.
For, you see, I'm learning as I play.
I'm learning to enjoy and be successful in my work.
I'm preparing for tomorrow.
Today, I'm a child and my work is play.

—Anita Wadley
Gateways to Learning
Edmond, Oklahoma

REFERENCES

American Academy of Pediatrics. (2006). Child life services. *Pediatrics, 118*(4), 1757–1763.

Axline, V. M. (1969). *Play therapy.* New York, NY: Ballantine Books.

Bellack, J., & Fleming, J. (1986). Theoretical and practical aspects of play: a universal need. In C. Fore & E. Poster (Eds.), *Meeting psychosocial needs of children and families in healthcare.* Washington, DC: Association for the Care of Children's Health.

Berk, L. E. (1998). *Development through the lifespan.* Needham Heights, MA: Allyn & Bacon.

Bolig, R., Yolton, K., & Nissen, H. (1991). Medical play and preparation: questions and issues. *Children's Health Care, 20*(4), 225–229.

Cole, M., & Cole, S. (1997). *The development of children* (3rd ed.). New York: W.H. Freeman.

Fore, C., & Poster, E. (Eds.). (1986). *Meeting psychosocial needs of children and families in health care.* Washington, DC: Association for the Care of Children's Health.

Gaynard, L., Wolfer, J., Goldberger, J., Thompson, R., Redburn, L., & Laidley, L. (1990). *Psychosocial care of children in hospitals: a clinical practice manual.* Bethesda, MD: Association for the Care of Children's Health.

Goldberger, J., Gaynard, L., & Wolfer, J. (1990). Helping children cope with health-care procedures. *Contemporary Pediatrics, 7*(3), 141–162.

Hart, R., Mather, P., Slack, J., & Powell, M. (1992). *Therapeutic play activities for hospitalized children.* Boston: Mosby-Year Book.

Hazzard, A., Celano, M., Collins, M., & Markov, Y. (2002). Effects of STARBRIGHT world on knowledge, social support, and coping in hospitalized children with sickle cell disease and asthma. *Children's Health Care, 31*(1), 69–86.

Hughes, F. (1995). *Children, play and development* (2nd ed.). Boston: Allyn & Bacon.

Johnson, J., Christie, J., & Yawkey, T. (1999). *Play and early childhood development* (2nd ed.). New York: Longman.

Krishna, S., Balas, E. A., Francisco, B. D., & Konig, P. (2006). Effective and sustainable multimedia education for children with asthma: a randomized controlled trial. *Children's Health Care, 35*(1), 75–90.

Landreth, G. (1991). *Play therapy: the art of the relationship.* Muncie, IN: Accelerated Development.

McCue, K. (1988). Medical play: an expanded perspective. *Children's Health Care, 16*(3), 157–161.

Petrillo, M., & Sanger, S. (1980). *Emotional care of hospitalized children: an environmental approach.* Philadelphia: Lippincott.

Rollins, J. A., Bolig, R., & Mahan, C. C. (2005). *Meeting children's psychosocial needs across the health-care continuum.* Austin, TX: Pro-Ed.

Sparks, L. (2001). Taking the "ouch" out of injections for children: using distraction to decrease pain. *MCN, 26*(2), 72–78.

Thompson, R. H. (1985). *Psychosocial research in pediatric hospitalization and healthcare: a review of the literature*. Springfield, IL: Charles C Thomas.

Thompson, R. (1995). Documenting the value of play for hospitalized children: the challenge in playing the game. *The ACCH Advocate, 2*(1), 11–19.

Thompson, R. H., & Stanford, G. (1981). *Child life in hospitals: theory and practice*. Springfield, IL: Charles C Thomas.

Trawick-Smith, J. (2006). *Early childhood development: a multicultural perspective*. Upper Saddle River, NJ: Pearson Education.

Chapter 13

Teaching Tools

Taryn J. Pittman

INTRODUCTION

The previous chapters focused on interactive teaching with individuals and groups and teaching on the fly. This chapter focuses on teaching tools that can be used to help you achieve your educational objectives. Keep in mind that teaching tools are not a replacement for a teacher; they are to be used to enhance or reinforce the educational interaction. Ideally, a discussion or return demonstration should always accompany or follow the educational interaction to verify that learning has occurred.

Teaching tools provide the visual, auditory, and tactile components that are essential for learning. Some tools also tap into the person's emotional involvement, which is an important component for changing behavior and attitude. In general, teaching tools serve several purposes that include providing variety of content delivery that taps into each person's individual learning style, clarifying abstract or complex concepts, and making otherwise complicated explanations understandable (Babcock & Miller, 1994).

Over the past decade, the increase of computer-based and electronic health education media has expanded the pool of resources that are available for educating patients. Your challenge is to select the appropriate teaching tool that will meet patients' individual learning style and achieve the educational learning objective identified for the patient.

WRITTEN MATERIALS

Written materials are generally the most widely used type of teaching tool. Written materials come in many forms, including handouts, brochures, booklets, pamphlets, schedules, pathways, and notebooks. Written materials may also be included, along with other teaching media in the form of a toolkit.

Sources for written materials vary and include purchasing directly from a commercial vendor, licensing of an online consumer health or patient education document system, printing materials from consumer health sources on the Internet, or developing your own. Regardless of the source, it has been shown that patients prefer written materials that are clear and written in lay language (Andrus & Roth, 2002). Patients also prefer materials that are tailored or customized to their particular learning needs. Tailored print materials have been "better remembered, read, and perceived as relevant and/or credible" (Skinner et al., 1999). Tailored materials have also been shown to have significant effects on knowledge retention, self-confidence, increased utility and sharing of information with others, and increased compliance with plan of care and follow-up (Jones et al., 1999; Pavic et al., 2007; Sockrider et al., 2006).

COMMERCIAL PRINT MATERIALS

A variety of commercial vendors produce and sell health education materials. These materials are usually written in lay language, are attractive, and use colorful graphics to enhance content. In addition to evaluating the suitability of the material (see Suitability Assessment of Materials [SAM] scale), additional things to consider when selecting materials from a commercial vendor include

- *Cost.* Does the vendor offer a discount? Most commercial vendors offer some type of price incentive if materials are ordered in large quantities.
- *Ordering.* Is there a system in place for tracking inventory and ordering materials in a timely manner?
- *Storage and distribution.* Is there adequate storage space for large quantities of print materials? What type of system is in place to streamline stocking and distribution of materials?

ELECTRONIC HEALTH EDUCATION DOCUMENT SYSTEMS

Electronic health education document systems eliminate the need for storing and distributing written materials. Access is available on every computer desktop. The database of material is usually generic in nature and written in lay language. Most of these systems allow for some degree of customization of information either through direct content editing or a fill-in-the-blank feature. Many of these systems offer material in English and Spanish as well as other languages. It has only been in recent years that vendors have started to incorporate graphics into these document systems, which has greatly enhanced the content.

Newer health education document technologies are now available that allow clinicians to develop information brochures that customize material for individual patients regardless of the complexity of their medical condition. These automated systems have been tested through applying methods of artificial intelligence and computational linguistics to tailor information to individual patient's learning needs (DiMarco et al., 2006).

In addition to applying the SAM scale, things to consider when purchasing or implementing an electronic health education document system include the following:

- *Content editing.* Are there resources and staff available to edit and customize content? Will content be edited and managed by a central group or department, or will it be decentralized and editing rights will be given to different clinicians based on their medical specialty?
- *Liability.* What are the liability issues with using health education document systems? Most vendors assume liability for the content they license; however, after content is edited by an organization, the organization assumes liability for the new content created.
- *Translation.* Is the material available in different languages? What plan is in place to update the Spanish version of a document if the English version is edited?
- *Updating of materials.* How is the database of material updated? Most vendors have a system in place to periodically update the original content. Any edited content (English or other language) made by the organization needs to be updated by staff.
- *Access to computers.* Do staff members have open and easy access to computers and the document system? Are printers readily available?
- *Training.* Are staff trained on how to use the system?

HEALTH INFORMATION ON THE INTERNET

There is a vast array of health information that clinicians and consumers can access on the Internet. Before using any written health material from a website, it is recommended that the website be evaluated to ensure the information is reliable and comes from a quality source.

In addition to applying the SAM scale, these tips from the U.S. National Library of Medicine and the National Institutes of Health (2007) "MedlinePlus Guide to Healthy Web Surfing" should be considered when evaluating written health information from any online source (www.nlm.nih.gov/medlineplus/healthywebsurfing.html).

- *Source of the site or sponsoring organization.* Use recognized authorities. Look at the "about us" page to see who runs the site. Note whether the site is sponsored by an individual or by a recognized health association such as the federal government, a nonprofit institution, a professional organization, a health system, or a commercial organization. Websites should also have a "contact us" link for those who need to contact the organization or Webmaster.
- *Quality and expertise.* Does the website have an editorial board? Is the information reviewed before it is posted? Do board members have expertise in their subject areas? Is there a process for selecting and approving information on the site? This information can usually be found under the "about us" link.
- *Beware of quackery.* Does the site make health claims that are too good to be true? Is the site gimmicky and trying to sell something? Beware of claims that one remedy will cure all problems. If skeptical, check more than one site.
- *Evidence based.* Does the site rely on medical research and not on opinion? Is the author identified? If there are testimonials or case histories, look for contact information such as an e-mail or phone number.
- *Current information.* How current is information? Look for latest information by checking the dates on documents and the date of when the website was last updated. Click on a few links on the site, and if there are a lot of dead end links, the site may not be kept up-to-date.
- *Beware of bias.* Who is providing funding for the site? Is the site being supported by public funds and donations or by commercial advertising? For example, if the information about treating depression recommends one drug by name, see whether the pharmaceutical company who makes the drug is sponsoring the website. If it does, then check another source of information.

After a reliable Internet site has been identified for health information, it can be bookmarked and used consistently to access written health materials. Many health associations and organizations are adding new features to their websites to enhance the learning experience. These features include video streaming such as the surgical videos available at MedlinePlus (http://www.nlm.nih.gov/medlineplus/surgeryvideos.html), interactive health tutorials using slide presentations at MedlinePlus (http://www.nlm.nih.gov/medlineplus/tutorial.html), and interactive health monitoring tools such as SugarStats (2007) an online blood sugar, carbohydrate counting, medication, and physical activity tracking site (http://www.sugarstats.com/). Some sites also offer interactive education programs that provide customized health information based on health assessment data that the patient enters. An example of this is the American Heart Association's (2007) online heart disease education program called Heart Profilers® (http://www.americanheart.org/presenter.jhtml?identifier=3000416).

DEVELOPING YOUR OWN MATERIALS

One of the greatest benefits of developing written health education material from scratch is that content can be very precise and specific to a particular patient population. It can be easily updated, and it can be specific to the clinical practice of the organization. With that said, there is a lot of thoughtful planning, time, and resource allocation that needs to be considered in order to produce a quality piece of written material.

The following guidelines adapted from the National Institutes of Health Plain Language Initiative (2003) (http://execsec.od.nih.gov/plainlang/guidelines/index.html) may be helpful when developing a piece of written material for the lay public.

Target Audience

- Consider the person or groups of people who will be receiving the information. Look at the age, gender, and culture of the population.
- Consider the literacy level of the group. The average American adult reads at an eighth-grade level (Andrus & Roth, 2002), and the material should be written in lay language to reflect this.
- If possible, include a member of your target audience in the planning and writing of the material.

Objectives (What the Learner Needs to Know or Do)

- Determine what information must be covered in the material. A good way to find out about this is to ask your target audience.
- Try to keep the content to a minimum of five to seven concepts. Do not overwhelm the reader with reams of information.

Content

- *Use active voice.* For example, say, "Take your medicines with meals," instead of using passive voice, "Your medicines should be taken with meals." A clue that a sentence is passive is the use of the verb "to be" or the use of the word "by." For example, "the prescription was written by your doctor" is passive voice. "Your doctor wrote the prescription" is active voice.
- *Use a positive voice.* For example, a positive voice would say, "Please send us your payment so your monthly subscription can continue." A negative voice would say, "If you don't send us a payment, we will cancel your subscription."
- *Use common words.* Stick with an "easy" vocabulary. The rule of thumb is the more syllables in a word, the harder it will be to read.

Hard	Easy
Physician	*Doctor*
Examine	*Look*
Utilize	*Use*
Frequently	*Often*
Majority	*Most*
Accompanied	*With*

- *Give help for medical terms.* Some difficult medical terms may need to be used in the document. If possible, try to define the term or to provide a phonetic spelling of the word to assist with pronunciation. Give examples to explain medical concepts or uncommon words. For example, "a large prostate gland can squeeze the urethra, like when you pinch a straw."
- *Use short sentences.* The rule is to use 15 to 20 words per sentence. Sentences that are lengthy, use a lot of commas, and contain multisyllabic words may be harder to read and understand. Sentences that are simple, use active voice, and use positive rather than negative words are more apt to engage the reader.
- *Include interaction if possible.* Give the reader a place to interact with the document. For example, provide extra space to write in a blood pressure or blood sugar number, or include a check list to mark the three actions the person will take to lower his or her blood pressure.

Layout and Typography

- *Margins and white space.* Use adequate margins and plenty of white space to break up the text. One way to test for white space is to hold the document out at arm's length and squint your eyes. If you see more dark space than white space, then you probably have too much text and not enough white space in your document.

- *Title.* The title should be clear and related to the content and purpose of the document.
- *Headings.* Use headings and subheadings to organize the information and guide the reader. Headings are usually one font size larger than the text and should be in bold. A question and answer format, used as a heading, can be an engaging and helpful way to guide the reader through the document.
- *Graphics.* The use of graphics is an excellent way to enhance a point and replace a lot of text on the page (a picture speaks a thousand words). Make sure that the graphic is appropriate, culturally sensitive, includes a caption, and is on the same page as the text describing it.
- *Font.* In general, 12 to 14 point font size is the best to use. It is also helpful to only use one or two different fonts within any document. Use lower case lettering and avoid ALL CAPS.
- *Bullets.* Use bullets to break up or chunk text into smaller segments of information. Bullets are useful and provide clarity when relating information such as a sequence of steps in a procedure or a list of signs and symptoms for a medical diagnosis.

FIELD TESTING

Have a small sample of the target audience evaluate (field test) the written document before finalizing and printing. This can be done through individual interview or by using a focus group. The key is to keep the evaluation simple and limited to a fairly small number of people. It might be helpful to develop a checklist of questions to use as a guide during the evaluation. Things to evaluate include the following:

- What is the overall look and appeal of the material? Would a person pick it up and read it?
- Does the title adequately communicate the purpose of the material?
- Is the material easy to read? Are there any difficult words or concepts that are hard to understand?
- Are graphics used appropriately? Do they enhance the content?
- Does the content tell the reader what he or she needs to know, and would he or she use the information?

- Is there any content missing?
- What is the overall impression of the material?

Testing the Suitability of Materials Using the SAM Scale

Doak, Doak, and Root (1996) published a quick and easy six-step process to evaluate the suitability of written materials when a field test is either not feasible or the writer does not have access or time to interview the target audience. The SAM scale (used with permission by Len Doak) was designed for use with print material but can also be applied to video and audio tape instructions.

For each type of material evaluated, the SAM scale looks at six general categories that include content, literacy demand, graphics, layout and typography, learning stimulation and motivation, and cultural appropriateness. There are between two to five factors within each general category that are assigned a score that reflects the grade of superior, adequate, not suitable, or not applicable. A total of 22 factors are evaluated for a maximum of 44 points.

To use SAM, follow these six steps:

1. Read through the SAM factor list and evaluation criteria.
2. Read the material you wish to evaluate.
3. For short instructions, evaluate the entire piece. For long instructions, select samples to evaluate.
4. Evaluate and score each of the 22 SAM factors. For some material, one or more of the 22 SAM factors may not apply.
5. Calculate total suitability score. Add up the total score for all factors evaluated, and enter on the score sheet next to "Total SAM Score." The maximum possible score is 44 points (100%). Calculate the percentage score. For example, if the total score for the material is 34, the percent score is 34 of 44, or 77%. To account for SAM factors that do not apply (N/A), subtract 2 points from the 44 total. Using the previous example, if you arrive at a score of 34 points but had one N/A factor, subtract 2 points from 44 to a revised maximum of 42. The revised percentage rating would become 34 of 42, or 81%. To interpret the final SAM percentage rating, use the following guideline.

   a. A percentage rating of 70% to 100% is superior material.
   b. A percentage rating of 40% to 69% is adequate material.
   c. A percentage rating of 0% to 39% is not suitable material.
6. Identify deficiencies in the material and what action to take for correction.

SAM EVALUATION CRITERIA (USED WITH PERMISSION)

1. Content
    a. *Purpose.* Does the reader clearly understand the purpose of the piece?
        i. *Superior.* Purpose is explicitly stated in title, or cover illustration, or introduction.
        ii. *Adequate.* Purpose is not explicit. It is implied, or multiple purposes are stated.
        iii. *Not suitable.* No purpose is stated in the title, cover illustration, or introduction.
    b. *Content topics.* Is the content geared toward helping the reader solve a health problem (rather than learning a series of medical facts)?
        i. *Superior.* Thrust of the material is application of knowledge/skills aimed at desirable reader behavior.
        ii. *Adequate.* At least 40% of content topics focus on desirable behaviors or actions.
        iii. *Not suitable.* Nearly all topics are focused on nonbehavior facts.
    c. *Scope.* Is the scope of the material limited to purpose or objectives? Is it limited to what the reader can reasonably learn in the time allowed?
        i. *Superior.* Scope is limited to essential information directly related to the purpose and can be learned in time allowed.
        ii. *Adequate.* Scope is expanded beyond the purpose; no more than 40% is nonessential information. Key points can be learned in time allowed.
        iii. *Not suitable.* Scope is far out of proportion to the purpose and time allowed.
    d. *Summary and review.* Is there a review of key points of the instruction in other words, examples, or visuals?
        i. *Superior.* A summary is included and retells the key messages in different words and examples.
        ii. *Adequate.* Some key ideas are reviewed.
        iii. *Not suitable.* No summary or review is included.
2. Literacy demand
    a. *Reading grade level (using Fry formula).* The text reading level needs to be determined. Reading formulas provide a reasonably accurate measure of reading difficulty.
        i. *Superior.* Fifth-grade level or lower.
        ii. *Adequate.* Sixth-, seventh-, or eighth-grade level.
        iii. *Not suitable.* Ninth-grade level and above.

b. *Writing style.* Is the material written in conversational style with active voice? Is the material free from embedded information, the long or multiple phrases included in a sentence?

    i. *Superior.* Both factors present (mostly conversational style and active voice and simple sentences used with few embedded sentences).

    ii. *Adequate.* Approximately 50% of the text uses conversational style and active voice. Less than half the sentences have embedded information.

    iii. *Not suitable.* Passive voice throughout. Over half the sentences have extensive embedded information.

c. *Vocabulary.* Are common, explicit words used? Are technical terms or concepts explained? Are imagery words used as appropriate for content (e.g., using runny nose versus excess mucus)?

    i. *Superior.* All three factors are met (common words used, technical/concepts explained, imagery words used as appropriate).

    ii. *Adequate.* Common words frequently used, technical/concepts sometimes explained, imagery sometimes explained.

    iii. *Not suitable.* Uncommon words are frequently used. Technical/concepts are not explained, and there is extensive use of jargon.

d. *In sentence construction, the context is given before new information.* Is the context given first in a sentence before the new information? For example, "To find out what's wrong with you (the context first), the doctor will take a sample of your blood for lab tests" (new information).

    i. *Superior.* Consistently provides context before providing new information.

    ii. *Adequate.* Provides context before new information about 50% of time.

    iii. *Not suitable.* Context is provided last, or no context is provided.

e. *Learning enhancement by advance organizers (road signs).* Are headers or topic captions used to tell the reader what is coming up next?

    i. *Superior.* Nearly all topics are preceded by an advance organizer (a statement that tells what is coming next).

    ii. *Adequate.* About 50% of the topics are preceded by advance organizers.

    iii. *Not suitable.* Few or no advance organizers are used.

3. Graphics (illustrations, lists, tables, charts, and graphs)
   a. *Cover graphic.* Is the cover graphic friendly, attracts attention, and clearly portrays the purpose of the material?
      i. *Superior.* The cover graphic is friendly, attracts attention, and clearly portrays the purpose of the material.
      ii. *Adequate.* The cover graphic has one or two of the superior criteria.
      iii. *Not suitable.* The cover graphic has none of the superior criteria.
   b. *Type of Illustrations.* Are illustrations simple (line drawings or sketches), appropriate for age group, and likely to be familiar to the viewer?
      i. *Superior.* Illustrations are simple, age appropriate, and familiar to viewer.
      ii. *Adequate.* One of the superior factors is missing.
      iii. *Not suitable.* All of the superior factors are missing.
   c. *Relevance of illustrations.* Do the illustrations tell the key points clearly with little or no distractions (unneeded color, elaborate borders, busy background, etc.)?
      i. *Superior.* Illustrations present key messages visually so the reader can grasp the key ideas. No distractions.
      ii. *Adequate.* Illustrations have some distractions or there is insufficient use of illustrations.
      iii. *Not suitable.* There are either (1) confusing or technical illustrations or (2) no illustrations, or (3) an overload of illustrations.
   d. *Graphics:* lists, tables, graphs, charts, geometric forms. Are graphics accompanied by clear explanations and directions for use?
      i. *Superior.* Step-by-step directions, with an example, are provided that will build comprehension and self-efficacy.
      ii. *Adequate.* "How-to" directions are too brief for reader to understand and use the graphic without additional counseling.
      iii. *Not suitable.* Graphics are presented without explanation.
4. Layout and typography
   a. *Layout.* Is the layout appropriate?
      i. *Superior.* At least five of the following eight factors are present:
         1. Illustrations are on the same page adjacent to the related text.
         2. Layout and sequence of information are consistent, making it easy for the reader to predict the flow of information.

3. Visual cuing devices (shading, boxes, and arrows) are used to direct attention to specific points or key content.
4. Adequate white space is used to reduce appearance of clutter.
5. Use of color supports. It is not distracting to the message. Viewers need not learn color codes to understand and use the message.
6. Line length is 30 to 50 characters and spaces.
7. There is high contrast between type and paper.
8. Paper has nongloss or low-gloss surface.

ii. *Adequate*. At least three of the superior factors are present.
iii. *Not suitable*. (1) Two or less factors are present and (2) looks uninviting or hard to read.

b. *Typography*. Is the type font in an appropriate upper and lower case and the size at least 12 point?
   i. *Superior*. The following four factors are present:
      1. Text type is in uppercase and lowercase serif (best) or sans serif.
      2. Type size is at least 12 point.
      3. Typographic cues (bold, size, color) emphasize key points.
      4. No ALL CAPS for long headers or running text.
   ii. *Adequate*. Two of the superior factors are preset.
   iii. *Not suitable*. One or none of the superior factors are present or six or more type styles and sizes are used on a page.

5. Learning stimulation and motivation
   a. *Interaction included in text and/or graphic*. Is there opportunity for interaction in the document? For example, are readers asked to solve a problem or make a choice?
      i. *Superior*. Problems or questions presented for reader response.
      ii. *Adequate*. Question and answer format used to discuss problems and solutions.
      iii. *Not suitable*. No interactive learning stimulation provided.
   b. *Desired behavior patterns are modeled and shown in specific terms.* Does the instruction model a specific behavior or skill or just provide technical information? For example, modeling a behavior or skill when teaching someone about nutrition would emphasize how to change eating patterns, which foods to shop for, tips on cooking, or how to read a food label. An example of providing technical infor-

mation on nutrition is indicating that carbohydrates have 4 calories per gram.

    i. *Superior.* Instruction models specific behaviors or skills.

    ii. *Adequate.* Information is a mix of technical and behavior/skills.

    iii. *Not suitable.* Information is presented in nonspecific or category terms (technical).

c. *Motivation.* Are complex topics divided into smaller parts? People are more motivated to learn when they believe the tasks/behaviors are doable.

    i. *Superior.* Complex topics are subdivided into small parts so that the reader may experience small successes in understanding or problem solving, leading to self-efficacy.

    ii. *Adequate.* Some topics are subdivided to improve readers' self-efficacy.

    iii. *Not suitable.* No subdivision of material is provided to create opportunities for small successes.

6. Cultural appropriateness

a. *Cultural match*: logic, language, experience. Does the material content adequately match the logic, language, and experience of the culture it targets. For example, if you write a nutritional brochure telling readers to eat asparagus and romaine lettuce, you need to make sure that these vegetables are usually eaten by people in that culture and are available in their neighborhood markets.

    i. *Superior.* Central concepts/ideas of the material appear to be culturally similar to the logic, language, and experience of the target culture.

    ii. *Adequate.* There is a match in logic, language, and experience for 50% of the central concepts.

    iii. *Not suitable.* Clearly a cultural mismatch in logic, language, and experience.

b. *Cultural image and examples:* Are cultural images and examples presented in realistic and positive ways?

    i. *Superior.* Images and examples present the culture in positive ways.

    ii. *Adequate.* Neutral presentation of cultural images or food.

    iii. *Not suitable.* Negative image such as exaggerated or caricatured cultural characteristics, actions, or examples.

Please see **Figure 13-1.**

2 points for superior rating
1 point for adequate rating
0 points for not suitable rating
N/A if the factor does not apply to this material

FACTOR TO BE RATED	SCORE	COMMENTS
1. CONTENT		
(a) Purpose is evident		
(b) Content about behaviors		
(c) Scope is limited		
(d) Summary or review included		
2. LITERACY DEMAND		
(a) Reading grade level		
(b) Writing style, active voice		
(c) Vocabulary uses common words		
(d) Context is given first		
(e) Learning aids via "road signs"		
3. GRAPHICS		
(a) Cover graphic shows purpose		
(b) Type of graphics		
(c) Relevance of illustrations		
(d) List, tables, etc. explained		
(e) Captions used for graphics		
4. LAYOUTS AND TYPOGRAPHY		
(a) Layout factors		
(b) Typography		
(c) Subheads ("chunking") used		
5. LEARNING STIMULATION, MOTIVATION		
(a) Interaction used		
(b) Behaviors are modeled and specific		
(c) Motivation, self-efficacy		
6. CULTURAL APPROPRIATENESS		
(a) Match in logic, language, experience		
(b) Cultural image and examples		

Total SAM score: _____

Total possible score: _____ , Percent score:_____ %

Figure 13-1 SAM scoring sheet.
Source: Used with permission from Doak, Doak, and Root (1996).

EDUCATION NOTEBOOK

Education notebooks have become a popular choice for clinicians who teach patients with complex and potentially protracted health conditions. The notebook can be used as a tool to improve patient education as well as continuity of care (Siebens & Randall, 2005). Patients who have chronic health issues or who may require extended rehabilitation for an injury or complex surgical procedure usually receive educational materials from different disciplines at each point in their continuum of care. The notebook concept provides a centralized place to house all of the educational materials a patient receives. Notebooks can be divided into different sections by clinical discipline or by content subject. Clear plastic sleeves or folder tabs help keep information organized and easy to access. Material can be added or deleted as need to meet the patient's individual learning needs.

The physical therapy, vascular nursing, and patient education department at the Massachusetts General Hospital collaborated on an education notebook for patients needing post amputation care. The notebook is divided into sections that includes an introduction page, general instructions for the patients after amputation, instructions for postoperative wound care, material on coping with amputation, a review on prosthesis selection and management, along with a directory of local prosthetists and pedorthists, information on phantom pain, and a note page for the patient to write questions or additional information. A business card sleeve was added so patients could quickly file any cards they received. Several clear plastic sleeves are included in the notebook so that additional educational materials, such as medication information, can be added. The back pocket of the notebook contains additional reading material from the Amputee Coalition of America. Overall, the notebook has been very well received. Patients like having one place to put information and found the materials very helpful during their recovery and rehabilitation. Clinicians like the interdisciplinary nature of the notebook and the ability to adapt it to patient educational needs.

TOOLKITS

Education toolkits are another modality that clinicians can use to educate a specific patient population. Toolkits are generally made up of various forms of print material or a combination of print materials and other forms of media (models, medical equipment, etc.) to enhance the learning experience. The use of educational toolkits has been shown to enhance learning and to improve self-management, morbidity, and quality of life (Juilliere et al., 2006; Tearl & Hertzog, 2007).

Toolkit development ideally requires both clinician and patient input to ensure that it is an acceptable and useful resource for both. The WAKEUP study (Ways of Addressing Knowledge Education and Understanding in Prediabetes) was conducted to determine the most effective way to develop a toolkit and the key messages that needed to be included about prediabetes that would address the information needs of patients and clinicians. The toolkit developed contained print material in various formats that covered general information about prediabetes, a food diary to list food intake, an activity chart for patients to write down goals about increasing their activity level, and a note card reviewing what a blood glucose test means. The toolkit also contained print information for clinicians that included a general overview of prediabetes that mirrored the information given to the patient and a desktop quick reference guide for easy access to information. The encouraging results of the study showed that the toolkit was a useful resource for both patients and clinicians (Evans et al., 2007).

MEDICATION SCHEDULES AND WALLET CARDS

Medication schedules and medication wallet cards are gaining wide recognition as being a useful tool in light of the medication safety initiatives being undertaken by many national organizations such as the Joint Commission for Accreditation of Healthcare Organizations, the U.S. Institute of Medicine and the Agency for Healthcare Research and Quality.

Medication schedules have been shown to enhance patient knowledge of their medications, increase compliance with taking medications, and decrease the incidence of patient-generated medication errors (Esposito, 1995; Manning et al., 2007; Raynor, Booth, & Blenkinsopp, 1993).

Tips on developing a medication schedule include the following:

- Keep the format simple.
- Provide a space on top of the document for the person's name.
- Set up the schedule as a grid.
- At a minimum, the column headings should include the following:
  - Name of the medication
  - Dose
  - Time of day to take
- Additional column headings can include the following:
  - Purpose of the medication
  - What to watch for/cautions
  - Color of pill
  - Sample of the pill

Medication wallet cards serve as a portable medication schedule that can be easily carried in the wallet and taken to each appointment or visit to the pharmacy. The same principles for developing a medication schedule apply when creating a medication wallet card; however, because of the portable nature of the card, additional patient information such as allergies, emergency contact, healthcare proxy, and so forth may be practical to include. This valuable information can be quickly accessed in the event of an emergency. Medication wallet cards that print out onto an 8.5 × 11 paper can be easily folded up and slipped into a wallet. A small waterproof sleeve, similar to what is used with a credit card, can also be used to protect the medication wallet card (**Figure 13-2**).

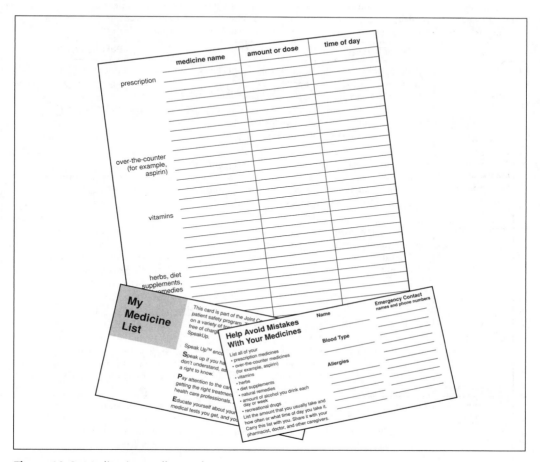

Figure 13-2 Medication wallet card.

PATIENT EDUCATION PATHWAYS

Patient education pathways (or patient care pathways) are interdisciplinary teaching tools that are modeled after the original clinical or critical pathway resource utilization tool used by many clinicians to manage a patient's stay in the hospital (**Figure 13-3**). Patient education pathways are similar in format to clinical pathways but differ in purposes and goals. The primary purpose of a patient education pathway is to provide comprehensive and consistent information in order to educate the patient effectively (Clarke, 2002). Patient education pathways have been shown to increase knowledge, enhance self-care behaviors, and decrease anxiety (Clarke, 2002; Terry, 2001).

Patient Care Pathway—Cardiac Surgery

As a patient you are the most important part of our team. We believe that knowing what to expect during your hospital stay can help lessen your anxiety and speed your recovery from surgery. The Patient Care Pathway is a road map of what most patients can expect during their hospital stay. Due to individual needs the pathway may vary from patient to patient and some patientsí care may differ from that specified on the path.

	Day of Surgery	Post-op Day 1	Post-op Day 2
Goals/ Knowledge of Cardiac Surgery Pathway	• Wake up from anesthesia • Have breathing tube removed • Have other tubes and wires removed as ordered	• Transfer from CSICU to Room 8 • Start to eat and drink • Get back to usual weight • Get out of bed • Good pain contol	• Increase activity • Demonstrate knowledge of discharge packet • Decrease need for extra oxygen
Tests & Treatments: Saline Lock, Blood Glucose, Urinary cath	• Blood drawn per protocol • Keep blood sugar less than 150	• Monitor cardiac rhythm and telemetry • Monitor fluid intake and output • Daily weight	• Blood tests • Blood glucose monitoring • Daily weight • Telemetry
Medications	• IV medication, then switch to medicines by mouth • Oxygen 4–6L	• Oxygen 4–6L • Pain medications • Anticoagulants (aspirin or Coumadin) • IV antibiotics • Cardiac medications • Insulin if needed	• IV antibiotics will be stopped • Insulin or oral hypoglycemic if needed • Vitamins and iron supplements. Decrease oxygen: 2 liters • Pain medication as needed
Activities	• Bed rest overnight • Change position every 2 hours	• Get out of bed for dinner • Bed bath • Walk or stand with assistance • Use incentive spirometer (IS) and perform cough and deep breathing exercises with help	• Get out of bed for all meals • Wash up at sink • Walk in hallway with assistance • Work with Physical Therapy if needed • Perform IS and coughing exercises every hour
Education	• Patient and family oriented to Cardiac Surgical Intensive Care Unit (CSICU)	• Get oriented to Room 8 • Review the Patient Care Pathway with your nurse A: Diabetic B. Afib • Review cardiac diet • Receive discharge packet • Start medication teaching	• Review the discharge packet • Learn about importance of walking after surgery and how to protect breast bone
Diet: Fluid restriction on 1500cc/day	• Progress to ice chips	• Increase as tolerated • Fluid restriction to 1.5 Liters	• Low sodium diet • Fluid restriction • No concentrated sweets
Communication	• Family contacted after surgery • Visiting hours per CSICU policy	• Your family may come visit • Cellular phone use okay • Receive family brochure • Wireless in Patient/Family Learning Center	• The cardiac surgical team of doctors, physician assistants, nurses, therapists and case managers will review your case, medications and discharge needs each morning • A case manager will evaluate your discharge needs and discuss with you and your family

Post-op Day 3	Post-op Day 4	Post-op Day 5
• Increase independence with activities • Demonstrate knowledge of activity do's and don'ts • Discontinue use of oxygen • Review medications	• Demonstrate knowledge of discharge packet • Be able to name purpose for each medication • Know and understand importance of a cardiac diet	**Day of Discharge!** • Go home and have a speedy, safe and healthy recovery *or* • Go to rehab and build up your strength so you may also have a quick recovery
• Removal of temporary pacing wires • Blood tests • Daily weight • Telemetry	• Blood tests • EKG • Daily weight • Chest x-ray • Telemetry	• Saline lock removed • Telemetry removed
• Laxative/suppository if needed • Oxygen will be stopped • Start medication taken at home if ordered by doctor	• Cardiac medications will be adjusted as necessary	• Prescriptions will be given to you *or* • Instructions about your meds will be sent to rehab • IV anticoagulation may be started on some patients
• Walk 250 feet in hall 4 times with supervision • Shower with assistance • Continue to use IS every hour	• Walk 500 feet 4 times per day • Up/Down stairs with supervision • Continue to use IS every hour	• You should now be independent in all personal care activities *or* • Work with your therapist and nurses to become more independent

• Learn about medications and their purpose
• Review cardiac diet (low fat/low sodium)
• Meet with a dietician if needed
	• Review all discharge material with the nurse and your family
	• Watch discharge video
		• Review/sign discharge paperwork, receive a copy
		• You should know about:
		  • Medications
		  • Diet/activity
		  • Follow-up appointments
		  • Blood work schedule if needed

• Low sodium diet • Fluid restriction • No concentrated sweets	• Low sodium diet • Fluid restriction • No concentrated sweets	• Resume pre-surgery diet if weight within 2 lbs of pre-op
• Meet with Social Worker if you need help with coping • Meet with Smoking Cessation Counselor if needed • Continue to work with case manager, nurses and your family on discharge plan and needs	• The cardiac team will continue to see you each day and discuss your plan of care	• A discharge note will be sent to referring physician, and if needed to rehab and VNA

Figure 13-3 Cardiac patient care pathways.
Source: Used with permission from Massachusetts General Hospital Heart Center and Partners Healthcare System.

Tips on designing a patient education pathway include the following:

- Use landscape page setup to provide more space.
- Use 8.5 × 11 size paper. Larger paper can be used, but the document will need to be folded.
- Set up the page as a grid-like chart.
- Place title of pathway on top.
- Use horizontal grid columns to list time line (e.g., pre-op, day of surgery, post-op day 1, post-op day 2, day of discharge, and after discharge).
- Use vertical grid to list elements of patient care (e.g., assessment, diet, tests, treatments, medications, activity, teaching needs, and discharge planning).
- Use a bulleted format to list interventions that correspond to the patient care element and time frame.
- Use lay language and write bullets at an eighth-grade reading level or below.
- Include a disclaimer at the bottom of the pathway that addresses use of the information (e.g., this document is intended as a guideline for educational purposes. Each patient is an individual and responses may vary. If you have any questions, please talk to your nurse or doctor).

DEMONSTRATION MATERIALS

Demonstration materials include a mix of written media such as posters, bulletin boards, story boards, chalkboards, whiteboards, and flipcharts and nonwritten media such as displays, models, and medical equipment. These materials primarily stimulate the sense of vision and touch and are primarily useful for cognitive learning and skills acquisition (Bastable, 2003).

Posters

Posters are a great tool for summarizing and simplifying information (London, 1999). With the addition of a powerful graphic or photo, a poster can convey a lot of important information in a small amount of space. Posters make self-paced individual learning possible and can be used as an independent source of information or combined with other teaching tools. Posters can reach a large audience if displayed in a public space and have multiple uses that can include marketing a public health awareness campaign, showing a sequence of steps in a medical procedure, or demonstrating a correct behavior or practice. Posters should be displayed for a set period of time and then removed. Overuse, or continued exposure, can lead to inattention or boredom on the viewer's part.

Tips on designing an education poster (Bach, McDaniel, & Poole, 1994; Duchin & Sherwood, 1990) include the following:

- Use attractive color combinations that grab people's attention.
- Use a simple composition: Do not crowd the poster with wording. Use succinct language to highlight important information points or concepts.
- Use short and concise text. Narrow down important points (bullets can be used).
- Use no more than 10 words in the title.
- Use appropriate spacing and balance.
- Use large enough font to be able to read text at a reasonable distance (about 4 to 6 feet).
- Use flush left, ragged right text justification.
- Use a logical sequence to display information. Concepts should flow from one to another.
- Use upper- and lower-case lettering. Avoid ALL CAPS.
- Field test the poster with the target patient population.

DISPLAYS, BULLETIN BOARDS, AND STORY BOARDS

Displays are used as a visual way to convey a message to the learner. Displays can be a combination of several teaching tools, including written materials, models, graphics, or video. A display can be a useful tool to teach patients concepts such as the correct serving size of a particular food group. A food pyramid display can be very effective in showing patients not only the types of foods that are included in each food group, but also the correct portion size as well. Written material displays can also be an effective way to draw in the learner if a particular health topic is of interest. Many organizations use the National Institutes of Health annual health observance calendar to identify topics of interest when creating a display (http://www.healthfinder.gov/library/nho/nho.asp).

Bulletin boards are visual tools that are frequently found in more informal settings. Bulletin boards provide a central location to post written information or to relate a message through pictures and graphics. When designing a bulletin board, color and creativity will go a long way in capturing the learners' interest.

Story boards are a visual tool that uses pictures and written content to explain a sequence of events or to tell a story. Story boards provide concise and consistent information to patients through using well planned and designed graphics and messaging to achieve an educational objective. A

PowerPoint program can be used to create slides that can then be printed and organized in a story board format. This has been found to be an effective technique in developing and distributing consistent patient education across a healthcare system (Kisak & Conrad, 2004).

Chalkboards, Whiteboards, and Flipcharts

Chalkboards or whiteboards are available in most classrooms and are an excellent tool to use when working with a group to capture spontaneous thoughts and ideas. An instructor can use the board for a drawing, diagram, or to note brainstorming ideas that are generated by the class. When using a board, it is easy to add or erase information, and the board can be used to organize information such as listing the pros and cons of a topic. Using a chalkboard or whiteboard is an effective way of reinforcing learning as the student can see their ideas written down, discussed, and reinforced.

Flipcharts are another tool that can be used interactively with a class to capture thoughts and ideas, or it can be used in preparation for a class to provide written content on a topic. Flipcharts are a great tool to use when a small group exercise is planned to brainstorm an idea or to plan out a project. Each page of the flipchart can be taped to the wall so that everyone in the class can see the ideas generated by each group. After a discussion, a review of the written notes on a flipchart will reinforce learning.

Models

Models are three-dimensional educational tools that replicate the features and substance of an original object. Models provide an interactive way for the learner to apply knowledge or practice a skill (Bastable, 2003). Models can be used in several ways, including (1) as a tool for the teacher to use in demonstrating a skill or procedure and the learner then repeats the demonstration such as using a manikin to learn cardiopulmonary resuscitation or using a breast model to learn self breast exam and (2) as a tool for self-directed learning such as a learner using a labeled model of the brain to learn anatomical landmarks and function or a learner taking apart a model of abdominal organs to see how the digestive tract is interconnected.

Models can be expensive, but the value of having an actual life-like replica to practice on is invaluable. One group of clinicians at an academic medical center acquired a hospital-based grant to develop a tracheostomy care teaching toolkit for nurses and respiratory therapists to use when teaching trach care to patients. The kit contains a model of the head and neck with a tracheostomy stoma. Staff members use the model to demonstrate the correct technique for trach care and then have the patient demonstrate the skill. Written materials are included in the toolkit and are used to reinforce learning. Staff and patients alike have commented that it is much easier to demonstrate this complex skill on a model rather than having the patient face a mirror and attempt to perform their own trach care. By using the model first, skill transfer is easier to manage when the patient has to perform the skill independently.

Medical equipment and supplies serve as excellent educational tools or models when teaching a skill. For example, a diabetic patient learning to self-administer insulin needs to use a real syringe in order to master the skill. He or she would also need to practice on a blood glucometer in order to learn the correct procedure.

Dolls can be useful educational models particularly for the pediatric population. A soft, anatomically accurate doll can be used to teach children about their body in a nonthreatening way. Some dolls come with teaching templates to highlight different parts of the anatomy so that children can interact with the dolls to learn the position and function of different body organs.

Audiovisual Materials

Through the boom in technological advances over the past decade, audiovisual materials have changed the landscape in which patient education is provided. These valuable teaching tools support and enrich the educational process by stimulating the learner's visual and auditory senses, add variety to the educational experience, and directly impact knowledge retention (Bastable, 2003). Sources of audiovisual materials vary and include projected media, video, audio, telecommunications, and computer formats.

Projected Audiovisuals

Projected audiovisual materials include slides and overhead transparencies. The traditional photograph slide of years past has been replaced with the ubiquitous use of PowerPoint software. Appropriate equipment is needed to view either format, a slide carousel and projector for the older format, and a computer with LCD projector for the more modern format. Either format requires a screen, and a darkened room is needed for best viewing.

Slides are an inexpensive and portable way to convey information. Slides can be updated easily and add a visual aspect to the instructor's verbal lecture. Slides are an effective medium to deliver a message to a small or large group and can also be used for individual self-directed learning. The National Institutes of Health website (www.MedlinePlus.gov) offers interactive tutorials on a variety of health topics to individuals using slideshows with sound and pictures. Each slide in the tutorial has easy-to-read written content, colorful graphics, and a voice-over that guides the learner through the content.

PowerPoint slide presentations have grown in popularity and use. Slide presentations can be programmed to include sound, video clips, and a variety of media enhancements. PowerPoint has the capacity to convey ideas and support the speaker's remarks in a concise manner. One word of caution relates to the potential overuse of PowerPoint slides within an educational session. The "death by PowerPoint" mantra can frequently be heard when learners are inundated with nothing but PowerPoint slide presentations during a workshop or a day-long conference. It is important to use a variety of educational tools to continue to stimulate the learner and create an enriched learning environment.

Tips on developing and delivering PowerPoint slides presentations include the following:

- Remember that you are creating slides to support your spoken presentation; the audience has come to hear you talk, not to just read slides.
- *Keep it simple.* Use single words or phrases rather than sentences or paragraphs (remember that slides are not a script).
- *Use only one or two graphics per slide* (be careful of using complex tables or graphs that many cannot see from the back of the room).
- *Use bullets*—no more than six per slide.
- *Enhance readability.* Use normal case (not all caps), and punctuate sparingly.
- Use slide headings that are to the point and meaningful.
- Use appropriate colors that are not too bright and allow for good contrast between the text and background. Use consistent coloring.
- *Limit the number of slides.* A rule of thumb is one slide per 1 to 2 minutes.
- Use of sound, animation, and other effects to emphasize a major point can enrich a presentation, but do not let them become distracting. Remember that it is the content that makes the presentation interesting.
- Leave a blank slide in your presentation if you plan to pause for discussion or have a question and answer period.

- *Provide handouts* of the slide presentation so learners can take notes (recommend three slides per page).
- *Pause as you move from one slide to the next.* Provide an overview of the slide before getting into specific content.

Overhead Transparencies

Overhead transparencies can be used to teach both small and large groups within a classroom. Equipment that is needed includes an overhead projector and a screen or blank wall. Remember to carry a spare projector bulb with you in case the one in the machine burns out. Clean the glass on the projector before giving a class.

Transparencies can be created by using a marker to write or draw content, or a photocopy machine can be used to copy content or graphics. A fully lit or dimly lit room is preferred when using overhead transparencies and should prove acceptable in order to read content if a dark marker is used. Overhead transparencies seem to be falling out of favor to the more versatile slide medium, but there are some advantages to using an overhead transparency, including low cost, easy access, and usefulness when highlighting key points in a discussion.

Video and DVD

Videotape (VHS) and the digital videodisc (DVD) are broadly used in health education. Both are extremely popular teaching tools next to the use of written materials. Video media has been shown to be a practical tool in that once the initial investment has been made to purchase a video recorder, television monitor, and videotapes, the video can be shown again to many patients. Video assures a standard level of teaching and consistent content that is not subject to the instructor's interpretation or bias, and video may have greater individual impact on patient learning than traditional reading or lecture-oriented formats because of its general mass appeal to people who love to watch television and movies. Past studies of using the video format showed that is was more effective than traditional methods of patient education in creating short-term knowledge but offered no advantages in improving long-term knowledge retention. Video content that contained role-modeling behavior along with instruction proved to have significant impact on decreasing anxiety in patients (Gagliano, 1988).

VHS quality, however, has been shown to decrease over time. The newer DVD technology, which has been shown to be more durable, allows for longer storage and use. DVD players seem to be replacing videocassette recorders (VCRs) in most households. A patient and family learning center at an academic medical center recognized that DVD format was preferred by 80% of the patients who had video content mailed to them.

DVDs are easy to make and copy. Several vendors now sell low-cost individual DVDs for patients to take home so that they can view the material at their own pace. Healthcare organizations can purchase these in bulk.

Video content can be found in healthcare organizations in the form of an individual VHS or DVD movie, housed on a closed circuit-television system, or copied into a video streaming format and seen on the Internet. Video content can also be downloaded from the Internet onto an individual's iPod or MP3 player and viewed at home.

Maintaining a library of individual VHS or DVD movies poses challenges. A television with a VCR or DVD player needs to be accessible and available for an individual or group who view the video. A system needs to be in place to manage video content, circulation, and storage.

Closed-circuit television systems either come with their own video library or can be set up using videos already purchased by the organization. Keep in mind that copyright permission is needed from the vendor or organization where the video was purchased before it can be copied onto the closed circuit system. An updated list of video titles and a brief description of each video should be accessible to patients and staff alike. Closed-circuit television systems usually offer a choice of showing video content on a regular schedule or making it accessible on demand. An on-demand system has the advantage of the patient being able to access the video when he or she is ready to learn. Regularly scheduled programming may be easier for staff to remember and set up for patients. A mix of both delivery systems may be an optimal solution.

Video streaming technology allows for broad video viewing outside of the organization by making the video content available on the Internet. This may also involve obtaining copyright permission unless the video was produced in-house. Many households have computer and Internet access, but be mindful of those patient populations who do not. You may want to set up an alternative method of video delivery for those who do not have access to a computer or who are not savvy on navigating the Internet.

Regardless of the format, the decision around using video media usually boils down to whether to purchase the video or create your own. Vendors and organizations that produce and sell health videos can charge between $100 and $250 each. Creating your own video can also be expensive and time consuming. You will need to conduct a cost analysis to determine the best way to go. If a decision is made to produce your own video, the following tips may be helpful (Williams, Wogin, & Hodge, 1998):

- Create concept or idea, and then draft a proposal.
- Determine a budget, and obtain approval of funding needed.
- Seek internal/external professional production assistance from a video maker.
- Review references/existing products or videos of external video maker.
- With funding secured, contract for desired services.
- Finalize script using content and professional video experts and potential viewers and stakeholders as reviewers.
- Determine shooting schedule, cast, necessary props, and equipment.
- Content expert and video maker collaborate to film/produce the video.
- Review/revise/approve rough "edit."
- Order necessary number of copies.
- Distribute video or program for closed-circuit television.

Audio Media

Audio media is an effective education tool for those patient populations who are vision impaired, have poor literacy, or have a preferred auditory learning style (London, 1999). Audio media can be played on a tape player (audiocassette, CD player, or iPod/MP3 player), recorded on a phone message, heard over a public address system, or heard over the radio. Audio media requires some type of equipment to communicate the audio message, but most are now portable and convenient, although some can be fairly expensive. People can literally take their tape player, telephone, or radio with them wherever they go. Technology has impacted the field of audio media. The audiotape may still be a useful tool in some settings, but other popular audio formats such as the compact disc (CD) and digital sound found in Pod/MP3 technology is widespread.

Therapeutic music programs are available in CD, and several national health organizations offer health-related audio and video podcasts that can be downloaded onto an iPod/MP3 player. Some disadvantages of using audio media are that there is no opportunity for interactive feedback, and it cannot be used for hearing-impaired individuals.

Audiocassette tapes may still be a good option for some, as they are inexpensive, easy to create, and can be customized for the individual patient's learning need. Doak, Doak, and Root (1996) offer detailed instruction on how to develop an audiotape.

Telephones and cell phones can be used as effective patient education tools. Telephone inquiries can be initiated by the learner such as calling a health advice line, or telephones can be used as a tool by healthcare providers who want to convey information or instruction to a patient.

Cell phones, in particular, have gained wide popularity as a tool to convey health information. Several telecommunications vendors now offer health information applications as part of a cell phone purchase plan. Consumers can get access to first-aid information, a symptom checker database, health videos, and health alerts (http://www.medicalnewstoday.com). Cell phones have also been successfully used through the text-messaging feature with adolescent patients to improve self-efficacy and adherence to diabetes treatment plans (Franklin, Waller, Pagliari, & Greene, 2006).

Radio and public address systems can be an effective educational tool, particularly in low-literacy populations. The National Assessment of Adult Literacy published in 2006 revealed that people with low literacy received a lot of information about health issues from radio and television (http://nces.ed.gov/pubs2006/2006483_1.pdf).

Radio has mass appeal and is typically used for more pleasurable pursuits such as music and sports. It can, however, be an effective media to air public health and community service announcements, medical talk shows, and health messaging sound bites.

Multimedia

Multimedia instruction is typically delivered via written text, figures, sounds, animations, and video clips all recorded onto a video CD format. Multimedia programming has been shown to increase patient's motivation to learn and promote learning effectiveness in patients who receive patient-controlled analgesia (Yeh, Yang, Chen, & Tsou, 2007). It has also been shown to statistically better functional activity and self-efficacy and reduce the hospital length of stay in patients receiving total hip replacements (Yeh, Chen, & Liu, 2004). A video compact disc (VCD) player is needed to view educational multimedia programs, and learners can repeat entire lessons as needed or select a specific program section to review.

Shared Decision-Making Tools

Shared decision-making tools, or decision aids, are gaining increased exposure as a helpful educational tool for clinicians to use to assist patients with making treatment and health management decisions. Today's patients are being asked to assume an increasing level of responsibility for self-management of their health. Decision aids help educate patients and empower them to become equal partners along with their healthcare providers in the decision-making process. Decision aids come in the form of informational booklets, scripted telephone counseling, decision boards, educational videotapes, interactive videodiscs, computer programs, and Internet websites (Myers & Kunkel, 2000).

The Ottawa Health Research Institute (2007) in Ottawa, Canada has led the way in decision aid research and development (http://decisionaid.ohri.ca). Written patient decision aids can be found at the Institute's website, as well as links to decision aid development and implementation toolkits. Decision aid algorithms can also be found on consumer health websites such as WebMD (http://www.webmd.com) or the American Heart Association "Heart Profilers®" site (http://www.americanheart.org/presenter.jhtml?identifier=3000416).

Regardless of the format, the Ottawa Health Research Institute recommends that decision aids should be used as a tool to prepare people to discuss their options with their healthcare provider by

- Informing them about the health condition, options, and possible outcomes of options using the latest quality-related scientific evidence.
- Creating realistic expectations by using diagrams that show best scientific data/estimates of what happens to people like them.
- Clarifying the personal value or importance of the benefits and risks or side effects of options.
- Guiding people to deliberate about options and to communicate on a personal worksheet their (1) knowledge of options, (2) personal values, (3) current leaning toward options, (4) unresolved decisional needs, and (5) next steps.
- Using plain language written at an eighth-grade level or below.

SUMMARY

This chapter focused on the variety of teaching tools that are at your disposal. Guidance was provided on how to best use the media to meet a variety of individual learning needs and styles. Tips on developing and evaluating teaching tools were reviewed and additional resources provided. More detailed information about technology in learning is covered in Chapter 14, and games and simulations are covered in Chapter 12.

REFERENCES

American Heart Association. (2007). *Heart profilers®*. Retrieved July 10, 2007, from http://www.americanheart.org/presenter.jhtml?identifier=3000416.

Andrus, M. R., & Ross, M. T. (2002). Health literacy: a review. *Pharmacotherapy*, 22(3), 282–302.

Babcock, D. E., & Miller, M. A. (1994). *Client education theory & practice*. St. Louis: Mosby.

Bach, C. A., McDaniel, R. W., & Poole, M. J. (1994). Posters: innovative and cost-effective tools for staff development. *Journal of Nursing Staff Development*, 10(2), 71–74.

Bastable, S. (2003). *Nurse as educator: principles of teaching and learning for nursing practice* (2nd ed.). Boston: Jones & Bartlett.

Clarke, L. (2002). Pathways for head and neck surgery: a patient-education tool. *Clinical Journal of Oncology Nursing*, 6(2), 78–82.

DiMarco, C., Bray, P., Covvey, H. D., Cowan, D. D., Di Ciccio, V., & Eng, M., et al. (2006). Authoring and generation of individualized patient education materials. *AMIA Symposium Proceedings*, 195–199.

Doak, C. C., Doak, L. G., & Root, J. H. (1996). *Teaching patients with low literacy skills* (2nd ed.). Philadelphia: Lippincott.

Duchin, S., & Sherwood, G. (1990). Posters as an educational strategy. *Journal of Continuing Education in Nursing*, 21(5), 205–208.

Esposito, L. (1995). The effects of medication education on adherence to medication regimens in an elderly population. *Journal of Advance Nursing*, 21(5), 935–943.

Evans, P. H., Greaves, C., Winder, R., Fearn-Smith, J., & Campbell, J. L. (2007). Development of an educational "toolkit" for health professionals and their patients with prediabetes: the WAKEUP Study (Ways of Addressing Knowledge Education and Understanding in Pre-diabetes). *Diabetic Medicine*, 24, 770–777.

Franklin, V. L., Waller, A., Pagliari, C., & Greene, S. A. (2006). A randomized controlled trial of Sweet Talk, a text-messaging system to support young people with diabetes. *Diabetic Medicine*, 23(12), 1332–1338.

Gagliano, M. E. (1988). A literature review on the efficacy of video in patient education. *Journal of Medical Education*, 63, 785–792.

Joint Commission for Accreditation of Healthcare Organizations. *Speak up: help avoid mistakes with your medicines: My medicine list card*. Retrieved June 15, 2007, from http://www.jointcommission.org/PatientSafety/SpeakUp/speak_up_med_mistakes.htm.

Jones, R., Pearson, J., McGregor, S., Cawsey A. J., Barrett, A., & Craig, N., et al. (1999). Randomized trial of personalized computer based information for cancer patients. *British Medical Journal*, 319(7219), 1241–1247.

Juilliere, Y., Trochu, J. N., Jourdain, P., Roncalli, J., Gravoueille, E., & Guibert, H., et al. (2006). Creation of standardized tools for therapeutic education specifically dedicated to chronic heart failure patients: the French I-CARE project. *International Journal of Cardiology*, 113, 355–363.

Kisak, A. Z., & Conrad, K. J. (2004). Using technology to develop and distribute patient education storyboards across a health system. *Oncology Nursing Forum, 31*(1), 131–135.

London, F. (1999). *No time to teach? A nurse's guide to patient and family education.* Philadelphia: Lippincott.

Manning, D. M., O'Meara, J. G., Williams, A. R., Rahman, A., Tammel, K. J., & Myhre, D., et al. (2007). 3D: a tool for medicine discharge education. *Quality and safety in health care, 16,* 71–76.

Myers, R. E., & Kunkel, J. S. (2000). Preparatory education for informed decision making in prostate cancer early detection. *Seminars in Urologic Oncology, 18*(3), 172–177.

Ottawa Health Research Institute (OHRI). *Patient decision aids.* Retrieved June 28, 2007, from http://decisionaid.ohri.ca/methods.html.

Pavic, D., Schell, M. J., Dancel, R. D., Sultana, S., Lin, L., Sejpal, S. V., & Pisano, E. D. (2007). Comparison of three methods to increase knowledge about breast cancer and breast cancer screening in screening mammography patients. *Academic Radiology, 14*(5), 553–560.

Raynor, D. K., Booth, T. G., & Blenkinsopp, A. (1993). Effects of computer generated reminder charts on patients' compliance with drug regimens. *British Medical Journal, 306*(6886), 1158–1161.

Siebens, H., & Randall, P. (2005). The patient care notebook: from pilot phase to successful hospital wide dissemination. *Journal on Quality and Patient Safety, 31*(7), 398–405.

Skinner, C. S., Campbell, M. K., Rimer, B. K., Curry, S., & Prochaska, J. O. (1999). How effective is tailored print communication. *Annals of Behavioral Medicine, 21*(4), 290–298.

Sockrider, M. M., Abramson, S., Brooks, E., Caviness, C., Pilney, S., Koerner, C., & Macias, C. G. (2006). Delivering tailored asthma family education in a pediatric emergency department setting: a pilot study. *Pediatrics, 117*(4), S135–S144.

SugarStats: simple and free online blood sugar tracking. Retrieved July 10, 2007, from http://www.sugarstats.com.

Tearl, D. K., & Hertzog, J. H. (2007). Home discharge of technology-dependent children: evaluation of a respiratory-therapist driven family education program. *Respiratory Care, 52*(2), 171–176.

Terry, L. (2001). Educational care path for the endoscopic patient. *Gastroenterology Nursing, 24*(1), 34–37.

U.S. National Center for Education Statistics. (2006). *National assessment of adult literacy.* Retrieved July 20, 2007, from http://nces.ed.gov/pubs2006/2006483_1.pdf.

U.S. National Institutes of Health. (2003). *The plain language initiative: guidelines for using plain language at NIH.* Retrieved July 20, 2007, from http://execsec.od.nih.gov/plainlang/guidelines/index.html.

U.S. National Library of Medicine & National Institutes of Health. (2006). *Medline plus guide to healthy web surfing*. Retrieved July 20, 2007, from http://www.nlm.nih.gov/medlineplus/healthywebsurfing.html.

U.S. National Library of Medicine & National Institutes of Health. (2007). *Medline plus interactive health tutorials*. Retrieved July 20, 2007, from http://www.nlm.nih.gov/medlineplus/tutorial.html.

U.S. National Library of Medicine & National Institutes of Health. (2007). *Medline plus videos of surgical procedures*. Retrieved July 20, 2007, from http://www.nlm.nih.gov/medlineplus/surgeryvideos.html.

Williams, N. H., Wolgin, F., & Hodge, C. S. (1998). Creating an educational videotape. *Journal of Nursing Staff Development, 14*(6), 261–265.

Yeh, M. L., Chen, H. H., & Liu, P. H. (2005). Effects of multimedia with printed nursing guide in education on self-efficacy and functional activity and hospitalization in patients with hip replacement. *Patient Education and Counseling, 57,* 217–224.

Yeh, M. L., Yang, H. J., Chen, H. H., & Tsou, M. Y. (February 20, 2007). Using a patient-controlled analgesia multimedia intervention for improving analgesia quality. *Journal of Clinical Nursing* (Epub ahead of print).

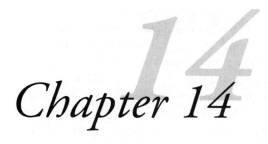

Chapter 14

Technology in Learning

Madalaine Pugliese & Karen Janowski

INTRODUCTION

We are living in a time of exponential change. Technology is transforming every aspect of society, exposing us to a rich information landscape filled with technologic advancements. A shift from text-based material and wired technology to digital, wireless tools impacts the acquisition of knowledge (Stoop & Berg, 2004). Traditional methods of the past, from dialing rotary phones to converse with others to traveling to the library gaining access to the storehouse of information, seem archaic to the current generation of children attending school in the 21st century. Every facet of daily life, including banking (ATMs, online banking), shopping (self-checkouts, online stores), and even political campaigns (YouTube debates, candidate blogs), is impacted by the digital revolution.

Many people immediately turn to the Internet when they research any imaginable topic. This is true for both patients and health educators. Nevertheless, before we can teach patients, we must become comfortable and familiar with the resources themselves. In Chapter 5, we discussed how to conduct an effective Internet search for accurate health-related information. How much do you need to know about how technology works? Not a great deal. For example, we do not know everything under the hood of our cars, but we are still able to use them to transport ourselves from place to place. In a similar fashion, we can advocate for technology tool use to educate our patients without having to know exactly how the tools work; however, the more you know about how to use today's most powerful and empowering tools, the better you can guide patients to take advantage of the most effective ways to access information in support of proper health care. This chapter is designed to define and offer specific examples of 21st century technology tools and strategies that might help to improve patients' understanding and knowledge about their own medical conditions resulting in optimal health outcomes. Building on that skill, we can use technology to disseminate information in powerful 21st century ways. Using tools of the Read/Write Web, also called Web 2.0 or social software, will allow us to collect and share information in meaningful ways. Additionally, other free technology options as well as commercially available tools are discussed. Taken together, these tools will promote health education and understanding for all patients.

THE READ/WRITE WEB OR WEB 2.0: INTERNET-BASED TOOLS THAT SUPPORT PATIENT LEARNING

A wealth of materials provides flexible, multisensory approaches that improve patient's understanding. Web 2.0, also called the Read/Write Web, is a fairly recent phenomenon that has not been sufficiently explored by healthcare providers. A literature review reveals little application of social software tools and strategies into healthcare education. A few articles demonstrate how Web 2.0 tools are changing medicine and nursing and transforming medical education. For example, Skiba (2006) describes how social networking tools provide collaborative networking opportunities for nursing students. She writes, "Imagine their potential to foster discovery learning, interdisciplinary learning, and collaborative learning with schools across the globe." In another article, Skiba (2007) describes how the use of content creation tools allows nursing students to turn from passive learners to active, engaged learners. She further reports on a number of nursing promotional videos posted on video hosting sites such as YouTube (http://youtube.com); these ideas transform the recruitment process. Finally, she reports that a medical practice in Britain has produced a number of health education videos on such topics as flu vaccinations, blood sugar testing, and cervical screening and posted them on YouTube.

Giustini (2006) reports on the popularity of podcasts and videocasts in medical schools and describes how Web 2.0 tools are used to facilitate journal searches and access to current medical information. He believes that content creation tools such as wikis may "be the answer to the world's inequities of information access in medicine." Boulos and Wheeler (2007) describe how Web 2.0 tools "represent a quite revolutionary way of managing and repurposing/remixing online information and knowledge repositories, including clinical and research information, in comparison with the traditional Web 1.0 model." He cautions the need to evaluate and research "best practice" models carefully using these technologies. Finally, another article by Boulos, Hetherington, and Wheeler (2007) discusses the role of Second Life, an online three-dimensional virtual world technology that offers an additional method to extend medical education instruction beyond the four walls of the classroom and which emphasizes social interaction in an alternative online virtual format.

To understand better how these Web 2.0 tools may benefit patients, it is important that we understand what we mean by Web 2.0 or the Read/Write Web. Wikipedia (http://en.wikipedia.org/wiki/Web_2 retrieved 12/06/07) defines it as follows:

> A perceived second generation of web-based communities and hosted services—such as social-networking sites, wikis, and folksonomies—which aim to facilitate creativity, collaboration, and sharing between users. . . . Web 2.0 websites allow users to do more than just retrieve information. They can build on the interactive facilities of "Web 1.0" to provide "Network as platform" computing, allowing users to run software-applications entirely through a browser. Users can own the data on a Web 2.0 site and exercise control over that data.

Although even this definition of Web 2.0 is somewhat obscure, most people agree that it is now possible to create content online quickly and access it freely and easily. This is an incredibly powerful capability that significantly expands the choices that are available to health educators as they strive to promote patient understanding. For example, instead of merely providing a patient brochure or pamphlet to increase patient understanding about a disease process or a home regimen, an online, interactive brochure can be created and accessed by a patient at home, whenever and as often as they need to access it. Printed text offers a static, inflexible presentation, but technology-assisted instruction is dynamic and interactive. Web 1.0 offered a static presentation, whereas Web 2.0 is dynamic and interactive.

Some patients may not have access to the Internet at home and will depend on traditional printed materials and verbal directions; however, for those who have access to a computer or any Internet-enabled mobile device anywhere, including at a family member's or friend's home or at a public library or other public facility, it is still possible for them to access social software websites. As

Brock and Smith (2007) found, technology-assisted instruction can be a convenient and powerful method for delivering patient education. Patients will not need to know how Web 2.0 tools work as long as they are able to access the provided link; therefore, no additional patient education is necessary.

Health educators can take advantage of the interactivity of computer-based healthcare information to facilitate learning and patient understanding. Ellaway (2007) identified the factors that support the adoption of technology techniques in e-learning and e-teaching with implications for health educators. She referred to two different models of technology adoption and use but specifically recommended that "rather than passively awaiting change, we should be better informed and prepared to share the nature of 21st century healthcare education, particularly its technology-mediated components." Evans and Gibbons (2007) found that adding interactivity into a computer-based software activity for undergraduate students enhanced the learning process.

> This result is consistent with the hypothesis that interactive systems facilitate deep learning by actively engaging the learner in the learning process. This suggests that educational designers who seek to foster deep learning (as opposed to mere factual recall) should adopt the incorporation of interactivity as a design principle. (p. 1147)

The pages that follow present technologies that are available as of the publication date of this book. Use these categories of technologies to explore further on your own. We begin by exploring some of the Web 2.0 tools (**Table 14-1**).

Table 14-1 Web 2.0/Read/Write Web Technologies

Online collaboration tools	Google docs and spreadsheets
	Zoho writer
Social bookmarking tools	Del.icio.us
	Furl
Wikis	Wikispaces
	PBWiki
	WetPaint
Podcasts	
Multimedia technology tools	Cellphones
	Cameras
	Digital camcorders
Multimedia technologies	Google presentation
	Slideshare
	VoiceThread

ONLINE COLLABORATION TOOLS

Sometimes health educators need to collaborate while producing health-related materials. Free, online collaboration tools such as Google Docs (http://docs.google.com) or Zoho (http://zoho.com) make online collaboration convenient and easy. Documents and presentations can be simultaneously created, shared, and edited, facilitating the creation process. The two authors of this chapter used Google Docs for collaborating in their writing. Health educators may decide to use this option when multiple authors work collaboratively from any location to produce patient material.

Social Bookmarking

Social bookmarking is "a way for Internet users to store, organize, share and search bookmarks of web pages. In a social bookmarking system, users save links to web pages that they want to remember and/or share." Social bookmarking tools include websites such as http://del.icio.us or http://www.furl.net/. Health educators can create a thematic list of online resources and share the social bookmarking link with their patients for home access. The social bookmarking account link will allow individuals to explore the resources that are saved within that particular topic area and will guide patients as they search the Internet.

Wikis

Wikis allow authorized users to create, edit, and link web pages easily and in a collaborative manner. It can also be thought of as collaborative knowledge building. The most well-known example of a wiki is Wikipedia, an online collaborative encyclopedia that as of November 2007 was one of the ten most visited Internet websites in the world (http://en.wikipedia.org). Wikis can serve as a repository for information that can be accessed anywhere. Easily upload patient materials to a wiki for access anywhere. Information can include text, graphics or images, video, podcast, and/or interactive links to other resources. When text is in a digital format, it is flexible and can be adjusted for size, and a voice can be attached to it to read aloud to bypass literacy, vision, or learning issues. Wikis offer an interactive solution for health education instruction that benefits many patients. The most popular wiki creation sites are http://pbwiki.com, http://wikispaces.com, and http://wetpaint.com.

Health educators may choose to create a wiki that will serve as the host site for all created educational materials. Brochures, videos, podcasts, and other Web 2.0 technologies can be embedded within the wiki. Wikis are invaluable tools that promote patient learning in a digital format.

Blogs

Blogs are websites in which "entries are written in chronological order and commonly displayed in reverse chronological order. A typical blog combines text, images, and links to other blogs, web pages, and other media related to its topic" (http://en.wikipedia.org).

The major differences between wikis and blogs are twofold: first, the visual presentation of the blog is such that blog posts are in chronological order; second, the authors can seek feedback, and readers are able to leave comments to a blog post, to which the author of the blog can respond. As with wikis, text is now in digital format so that patients are able to easily attach a voice to the text to hear the playback as often as necessary. They can also leave questions in the comments section to which the blog author(s) can respond as well as other readers who have a similar interest or need. It is possible to moderate comments before publishing, which is an important content control feature.

Health educators may choose to use blogs for online patient support. Patients may share experiences, ask questions, or seek out support relative to specific health issues.

Podcasts

Wikipedia defines a podcast as "a collection of digital media files which is distributed over the Internet using syndication feeds for playback on portable media players and personal computers." Healthcare professionals can record their verbal instructions using a recording device or using the record feature built into laptop or desktop computers and then upload the recording and upload to a patient education website or wiki so that patients are able to access the podcast for later review. If audio editing is necessary, download Audacity (http://audacity.sourceforge.net), a free audio editing tool that allows the educator to make changes to the audio recording, when necessary. One might also consider developing a videocast, which would include audio combined with video recordings that are uploaded and accessible using computer technology.

Multimedia Technology

The importance of offering multimedia technology, which combines audio with video recordings, to promote learning cannot be overstated. Several methods exist to create and access digital video to reinforce patient education. Cell phones and digital cameras both offer the capability to create brief digital videos for later review by a patient. For a better quality final product, use a digital video recorder to create the video. As mentioned in Chapter 5, the Flip Video is an inexpensive, portable, easy-to-use video camcorder. The recorded video can be uploaded to a number of video sites such as Google Video or YouTube or can be embedded within a blog or wiki.

A health educator can capture pictures during demonstrations using a cell phone or a digital camera. Images can then be embedded within a blog or wiki or can be uploaded to an online social slide presentation site such as Google Presentation (http://docs.google.com), Slideshare (http://www .slideshare.net/), or VoiceThread (http://voicethread.com). Slidecasting software available at the Slideshare website makes it possible to add audio to an online presentation. A VoiceThread is an online multimedia album that can hold essentially any type of media (images, documents, and videos) and allows people to leave comments or ask recorded questions. A VoiceThread allows group conversations to be collected and shared in one place from anywhere in the world. VoiceThread includes the ability to create a multimedia presentation with a drawing tool for emphasis on particular parts of the video or image. Again, this social software tool taps into all learning styles, is easily created and customized for the patient, and can be accessed from any computer or Internet-enabled mobile device anywhere. Health educators may choose to use VoiceThread technology for a variety of purposes. VoiceThread may be helpful as a means to easily post recorded demonstrations of patient exercises, patient precautions, or important information for new parents. The health educator is able to record his or her voice and use the drawing tool for additional emphasis. Patients can also leave comments or questions to offer support to others who are accessing the VoiceThread.

The advantages of using social software tools such as blogs or wikis are numerous. These tools tap into multisensory learning, which combines auditory and visual material. It is much easier to create, edit, and publish healthcare information using online tools than to create paper brochures or flyers, and there is no additional cost if the hardware needed to create the information online is already available. Furthermore, the information is immediately available after it has been created or uploaded to the Internet. Patients can easily retrieve the information for "just-in-time" learning for review and repetition as often as they need it. They can hear it read to them or watch it repeatedly to clarify any lack of understanding. If a video has been created and uploaded to a website, by accessing the video, patients have the opportunity to have a visual representation of the information so that they do not have to rely solely on their memory. There are tutorials online for many of these social software tools. See the resources at the end of this chapter for specific links.

PORTABLE RESOURCES

Personal Digital Assistants

The personal digital assistant (PDA) or handheld computer offers a number of different features, such as a calculator, organizer, and calendar. It is also possible to send/receive e-mails, make digital recordings, retrieve information from the Internet, access word processing capabilities, or play digital media such as television programs.

PDAs offer a handheld solution to access the social software tools mentioned previously here that makes it possible for the user to listen to podcasts or access video casts or other multimedia materials from anywhere, at anytime. This portability is important because the retrieved information reinforces instruction when it is needed.

Brock and Smith (2007) evaluated the effectiveness of using a PDA to display digital videos for patient education in a clinical setting. They concluded that "technology-assisted education using a digital video delivered via PDA is a convenient and potentially powerful way to deliver health messages." They further discovered that patients in the study reported satisfaction with using the device to obtain health information regardless of their literacy levels. The use of this tool is largely unexplored, but it offers a portable solution to the standard static patient brochure that has limited accessibility for many patients. Providing patients with loaner PDAs equipped with created content offers a low-cost interactive alternative to support patient education for those who do not have access to a computer.

Wii

The Wii by Nintendo is a video game system that has gained popularity among people of all ages since its release at the end of 2006 because of its specialized wireless Wii remote, which is a handheld pointing device. The Wii has been used in rehabilitation facilities throughout the country to promote motor recovery and patient health. At this point, it has not been used for patient education but has been used to promote improved motor functioning combined with a sense of fun.

WEBSITE ACCESSIBILITY

When health educators create patient content online, it is important that they consider how accessible the material is to all patients. An excellent website that promotes best practices for web developers or Web 2.0 content creators is http://juicystudio.com/index.php. This site offers a number of hosted services to ensure web accessibility which are accessed under "Quality Assurance>Local Tools." These services provide invaluable support to help identify issues that may prevent patients from independently retrieving information from websites, blogs, or wikis. One in particular that will be of benefit to health educators is the Readability Test link, which analyzes the readability level of a web page. To test the readability of a blog, wiki, or other websites, insert the URL, and click "Calculate Readability." The readability level will be quickly determined, and if the level is too high, adjustments can be made to improve readability.

TECHNOLOGIES TO SUPPORT SPECIFIC PATIENT LEARNING CHALLENGES

In Chapter 5, we introduced you to some background information about assistive technology tools. Building on that information, we can now speak more specifically about how the technologies introduced can facilitate patient learning. Here we learn how to activate some of the built-in accessibility features that are available in both the Macintosh and Windows operating systems. We also discuss some commercially available products that support unique learning needs. Although specific technologies are here identified, understand that there are often a range of options to consider in each category, each offering unique features that may better match a patient's specific needs.

Auditory Support

We know that text-to-speech converts visually digital text into auditory synthesized speech. Patients who may be diagnosed with a learning disability or cognitive challenge may struggle with reading text. These patients can benefit from knowing how to use these tools so that they can independently review digital text information by turning the text into spoken words.

The Macintosh operating system offers a user-friendly way for computer users to hear selected text anytime they wish. When using any application, the menu under the name of the application will offer a services command. After selecting text to be read aloud, the user can hear the selected text by activating the speech command inside the services menu. Additionally, using the system preferences, specifically the speech controls, a user can click on the text-to-speech tab to define keys that will read any text that they select anywhere on their computer while using any application. Using the speech controls, they can also select any voice on their computer to perform the reading. The user can also activate "talking alerts" so that they can hear any dialog boxes that might pop up while they are working and better understand their work environment. The Macintosh also offers a free dictionary application that can be made to read aloud. Finally, a translation widget, found in the built-in application called dashboard, allows the user to enter a text in one language that can be translated into another language.

Regarding text-to-speech, the Windows operating system works a bit differently as it relies on the addition of Microsoft Office 2002 or later to provide text-to-speech. It will read only text that is in Microsoft Word or in an outgoing message in Outlook. Fortunately, it is possible to copy and paste material from the Internet to hear it read aloud in Microsoft Word. Instead, there are additional free options including "WordTalk," a free tool that often proves extremely useful (http://www.wordtalk.org.uk/):

> WordTalk is a free plug-in developed for use with all versions of Microsoft Word (from Word 97 upward), which can help people with reading difficulties use Microsoft Word more effectively. It will speak the text of the document and will highlight it as it goes. It contains a talking dictionary to help decide which word spelling is most appropriate. It sits neatly in your toolbar and is highly configurable, allowing you to adjust the highlight colors, the voice and the speed of the speech.

Free Online Resources That Offer Text-to-Speech

When patients need to access information online, they can use any of these free text-to-speech online resources to overcome reading issues. Each tool offers unique benefits and features, and it will be personal preference which ones to recommend to patients.

CLiCk,Speak (http://clickspeak.clcworld.net/) is an easy-to-use text-to-speech (TTS) tool that can be downloaded as an extension application when using Firefox as the web browser of choice with any platform—Macintosh, Windows, or Linux. CLiCk,Speak is designed for sighted users who need TTS support. This tool is recommended when patients use Firefox as their web browser for its ease of use. After it is downloaded, it will appear as a toolbar underneath the web address bar near the top of the screen.

Accessibar (http://accessibar.mozdev.org/) is another toolbar extension for Firefox that provides online TTS, in addition to the integration of a text-to-speech reader, which can read out loud the browser's user interface as well as web page content. Accessibar offers additional features that make it slightly more complicated for patients. After download, it too appears as a toolbar underneath the web address bar.

Fire Vox (http://firevox.clcworld.net/) is an open-source, browser extension for the Firefox web browser. It is designed for users who are visually impaired and offers screen reading support in addition to TTS.

Spoken Text (http://spokentext.net/) converts e-mails and web pages automatically into an audio format.

Natural Reader (http://www.naturalreaders.com/) offers TTS when text is highlighted and copied into the NaturalReader window. It can also convert any written text into audio files such as MP3 or WAV for a CD or MP3 player. After downloading and installing Natural Reader to your hard drive, it will appear as an application or program. The free version requires the patient to copy text into the Natural Reader program and use the tools within the application itself.

Talklets (http://talklets.com/) is available to website creators to embed TTS within the web page, blog, or wiki. This is the easiest program for any patients to use, as it does not require them to download or install anything to their hard drive. Instead, the online content creator embeds the Talklets within their website so that visitors can listen to highlighted text.

Additional Free and Readily Available Technologies to Consider

As already said, there are technologies to consider in support of any education or learning challenge. As various challenges are addressed, this section first discusses free utilities that are built into computer operating systems. Often, many people are surprised by how many adjustments are available that might be the perfect modification to empower a patient; however, sometimes a commercial assistive device or specialty software program might be needed in order to make an accommodation beyond what is available for free. Ideas for commercial products follow the free built-in solutions for each learning challenge. The goal is to ensure full access to health education information for any patient, encouraging self-advocacy and fostering independence.

Picture or Color Label Support

The Macintosh operating system permits the use of colored labels that might help to differentiate documents and folders or even icons. On the desktop or finder level, select the label icon with one click. Under File, select Get Info. Click on an expansion triangle next to general if it is closed. Or press the control key while clicking on the label icon, and select one of the system colors. Pictures or specific icons can help a user to identify better the contents of a folder. To add or change a picture on a folder, first copy the picture or icon that you wish to use. Next, select with one click the folder or file that you wish to replace. Select Get Info from the File Menu, or press command + I to open the info window. Click the icon in the upper left corner of the info window to select it. Press command + V to replace the existing icon with the one you are pasting in.

Replacing or adding a picture or icon in the Windows Vista operating system works in a similar way. First, select the icon with one right-click on the file or folder that you wish to replace. From the context menu that opens when you click, select Properties and then customize and finally change icon. If working in the Windows XP operating system, select the icon using the same right-click, then select from the menu the customize command, followed by selecting the choose picture option.

For Picture Schedule Support

Detailed home care or a complicated medication schedule might be simplified or broken down into manageable chunks of information by providing a picture-supported schedule. For most people, auditory information is short-lived. Visual information can remain long enough for a person to see, study, and consider it (Kamp & McErlean, 2006). When a visual representation is available, a person can review it again and again to understand better and/or remember the information. Visual tools help in processing language, organizing thinking, and remembering information (Buti, 2007). Visual schedule systems provide consistent cues about daily activities. They provide a structure that helps to anticipate what will happen next, reduce anxiety by providing a vision of daily activities, and facilitate transitions. They are especially important for people who have difficulties with the understanding of oral language and instructions. The consistency provided by a visual schedule is critical in establishing accuracy and independence (Kamp & McErlean, 2006). For example, when a patient has a complicated combination of medications that must be taken on varying schedules, this can be a stressful and confusing situation. After the patent goes home, a picture supported schedule could be the perfect personalized home care tool. The picture schedule could show the image of the medication, also labeled with the name in text in order to make sure that the medication is properly identified when removed from the prescription bottle. Each picture of each medication could be aligned in a sequence and placed next to a picture of a clock that indicates the proper time to take each medication. This sort of picture supported schedule could be exactly and understandably what's needed for a patient who might be confused about which medication to take and when.

Commercially Available Technologies

For Converting Print to Digital Text

If print information is not in a digital form, the use of a scanner and optical character recognition (OCR) software can literally convert a needed flier into a digital file. Although commercially available OCR software such as OmniPage (ScanSoft division of Nuance, Inc.) could be used, there are software programs that are especially designed with features that provide unique TTS and vocabulary support for users with special learning needs (Parette et al., 2005).

Kurzweil 3000 by Cambium Learning Technologies, Inc. (http://www .kurzweiledu.com) is reading, writing, and learning software for any struggling reader, including individuals with learning difficulties such as dyslexia, attention deficit disorder, or those who are English Language Learners. Healthcare professionals or patients might scan and prepare documents and use a comprehensive set of reading, writing, and learning tools. Having a library of patient instructions in text format would permit a patient to use the information within the application, applying use of support tools for vocabulary, such as definitions and language translations. Adjustable auditory feedback provides for better comprehension and fluency when reading important information.

Read and Write Gold (TextHelp at http://www.texthelp.com) software gives added support to people who need enhancement with reading, writing, and learning through a variety of useful tools. This tool is similar to the Kurzweil software previously mentioned but is added here in support of those who may have access to this alternative, which is an equivalent-featured option. Scanned documents can be manipulated using robust study skills features, document summary capabilities, and other very helpful TTS and vocabulary support features. The mobile version of Read and Write GOLD comes on a portable device and contains all of the files required to run with no installation necessary. Users plug the key ring-sized device into the USB port of any computer running Windows Vista, 2000, or XP and they can use the tool when and where they need it with no restrictions.

For Picture Support in Reading and Writing

Specialized software can be used to support or enhance text with pictures or universal symbols to accompany print. Imagine the text for patient instructions supported with pictures throughout that provide graphic interpretation for important information.

Picture It (Slater Software, http://www.slatersoftware.com) uses over 6,000 literacy support pictures as a way you can supplement text in support of literacy and language understanding. You can adapt materials for patients with mild to severe language support needs.

Pix Writer (Slater Software, http://www.slatersoftware.com) uses over 3,000 literacy support pictures, text, and speech to make a writing environment that supports users of all ages and abilities. Patients could select pictures that serve as labels on buttons to write words, sentences, and descriptions of symptoms. Picture It software makes it easy and fast to add pictures to text. Use it to create a picture-rich environment. Just type the words or instructions for your patients, and the software will add in the symbol from the built-in library. Any activity or instructions can be adapted using Picture It because materials can be presented at a level that the individual reader can understand with the help of thousands of Literacy Support Pictures. Healthcare providers could make vocabulary word banks to target a patient's ability level in either English or Spanish.

Clicker5 (Crick Software, http://www.cricksoft.com/us) is a multimedia tool that lets you write using entire words, phrases, and pictures by clicking on cells or by typing on the keyboard in the talking word processor. For example, you might build patient instructions by typing words, phrases, and pictures. Patients can hear words spoken by the computer as you write and hear completed sentences spoken back as they might write to you. This works much like other similar tools described in this chapter. We mention so many options in order to be as thorough as possible in case you have access to one tool but not another.

For Picture Schedule Support

Use picture-supported schedules to organize and structure daily or repetitive activities. For home use, a picture card schedule can portray an entire day's activities or detail the mini steps of one important task, such as a physical therapy exercise. A picture schedule can list mini schedules, such as what things need to be done when you change a dressing or bandage. Often, the more stress caused by a situation, the more structure might be needed when providing follow-up information. High-stress situations require a more detailed breakdown using sequential pictures. Each routine can become a learn-by-doing task in sequential order. Many people need schedules only temporarily to learn certain sequences. Other routines will always need to be presented in a visual format. The goal is to create an environment where each person can operate successfully and as independently as possible.

Boardmaker by Mayer-Johnson, Inc. (http://www.mayer-johnson.com) lets you create printed symbol-based educational materials and communication boards with picture communication symbols and other pictures and graphics in 42 languages. Boardmaker is known as an important tool for creating printed materials such as schedules, communication boards, and other educational materials. Practitioners can create symbol-supported materials using over 300 templates.

Patients Who Need Support to Speak

Although computer operating systems offer built-in text-to-speech, this is not a powerful enough solution to facilitate effective communication; therefore, two categories of commercially produced products are discussed: (1) software that helps you create print communication boards and (2) augmentative communication (AAC) devices.

Numerous options exist for selecting an AAC device. A light-tech tool might be a battery-operated button and can speak one simple, but very important message. A high-tech device might be a portable computer running an intricate communication symbol-based software program that speaks any message designed by the user.

Print Communication Boards

As described previously, Boardmaker (Mayer-Johnson, Inc.) provides templates for one to create printed symbol-based educational materials and communication boards with picture communication symbols and other pictures and graphics in forty-two languages. Boardmaker is considered an important tool for creating printed materials such as schedules, communication boards, and other educational materials. Practitioners can create in advance a series of symbol-supported materials using over 300 templates.

ACC

Sometimes printed communication boards are sufficient for immediate and simple conversations; however, there are times that a conversation might need to be more dynamic or interactive. Using devices might open up a conversation beyond the topics that were designed into a static print display, thus permitting a different question or topic of discussion. Numerous choices of light-tech battery-operated devices as well as computer-based high-tech dynamic display devices are available in today's market. These devices are typically used in combination and generally prescribed by ACC specialists. They can sometimes be funded through medical insurance or federal reimbursement programs provided through legislation.

EVALUATING COMMUNICATIONS DEVICES

The following tips are general guidelines to help individuals evaluate communication devices. While every person is different, these tips will apply to almost all users of communication aids (Learning Independence through Computers Resource Center, 2006).

1. Look for solutions that are easy to use. Computerized dynamic display screens allow individuals to compose messages using familiar methods, which eliminates memorization of complicated codes and increases speed.

2. Choose portable devices. Portability allows nonspeaking individuals to take their "voices" anywhere.

3. Consider flexible devices. Look for devices that offer a variety of access options.

4. Require excellent voice quality. Sound projection and quality are obviously important. See whether the voice output can be personalized.

5. Look for a device that "grows" with the user. Think about an individual's needs a few years down the road. Can vocabulary be added and used quickly? Can the person use vocabulary independently?

6. Choose durable, reliable devices. Can the device withstand the stress of daily usage? Look for reliability. Make sure the battery life lasts long enough to meet a user's needs.

Patients Who Need Support to See

The screen reader provides synthesized speech translation of any content found on the screen for users who are blind or visually impaired. Both the Macintosh and Windows operating systems offer a free built-in screen reader.

VoiceOver on the Macintosh can be activated and customized from within the universal access system preferences.

Narrator on a Windows computer can be found in the start menu. Look for accessibility accessories in the programs menu.

Although more robust features can be found in commercially available products, both of these resources provide a wonderful place to start for computer users who are blind or have low vision.

Many other built-in features can be adjusted to accommodate vision beyond these screen readers. In Windows, the control panels permit the adjustment of screen resolution in the display controls, and the desktop can be personalized using the appearance controls. The size of the cursor can be adjusted using the mouse control panel.

In the Macintosh, these same features can be adjusted in the system preferences using the same names. The size of icons and folders can be adjusted using the view menu in the Macintosh finder and in the appearance control panel in Windows. The size of the task bar can be dragged when the pointer changes to a double-headed arrow near the edge. The dock can be adjusted using doc preferences in the Apple menu, and the size of the cursor can be adjusted in the universal access system preference.

Finally, users who have low-vision will find a zoom feature in both Windows and Macintosh operating systems. In Windows Vista, go to control panels, then ease of access, and finally, optimize visual display. There you will find a command to turn on the magnifier. In Windows XP, the magnifier is an accessibility accessory in the programs menu. On the Macintosh, the zoom feature is found in the universal access system preference.

Commercially Published Screen Reader

Jaws (Freedom Scientific, Inc. http://www.freedomscientific.com/index.html) is screen reading software for Windows computer users. Using text-to-speech and a significant number of user keyboard command controls, this software works with applications as well as on system level navigation. In a case study section within this chapter you meet Jeanette B, an expert Jaws user. As soon as her laptop starts up, so does the Jaws application, immediately permitting her to hear everything that is happening as she uses all of the rest of her standard software. Jeanette uses many of the same software applications as anyone else, including Microsoft Word, Internet Explorer, and PowerPoint. Because she is also running Jaws, she can use the keyboard navigation commands to have the computer read the contents on her screen and also announce navigation commands being used at the same time. This sort of work environment might seem technically challenging to some; however, blind computer users can receive support in learning how to use these tools through state commissions for the blind and vocational rehabilitation programs.

Commercially Published Zoom or Enlarging Software

MAGic (also available from Freedom Scientific, Inc.) is software for Windows computer users that combines powerful magnification with synthesized speech. Magnify your screen view from 1 to 16 times the original size while hearing text spoken aloud.

Patients Who Need Support to Hear

There are some useful controls that turn auditory cues into visual alerts and are built into computer operating systems. Visual cues can be activated to replace alert sounds using the accessibility control panel in Windows or the universal access system preferences in the Macintosh OS. In both operating systems, the user has the option of completely overriding any auditory alert sounds. Alert sounds typically warn the user of something important to which they must respond. For example, a computer might provide an alert sound when the printer is out of paper or when there is a break in the Internet connectivity. If the user is unable to hear this alert sound, the accessibility controls allow the user to turn on a visual flash alert instead. This then permits the user to know when the computer requires attention using a different sensory alert.

Amplification Systems

LightSPEED Technologies, Inc. (http://www.lightspeed-tek.com) makes specialized microphones, amplifiers, and speakers to provide listening enhancement. LightSPEED makes a variety of personal FM systems with high speech intelligibility, some especially useful for people with cochlear implants and with mild to moderate hearing loss.

Flashing Visual Timers

Time Tracker Visual Timer & Clock (Learning Resources, Inc., available commercially) is a lighted electronic timer that flashes a visual to alert people that it is time to complete a task. You can easily program visual and/or sound effects that indicate when time is running out.

Captioned Videos

You can locate a significant number of captioning services by using your Internet search skills. You can locate video that has been captioned already.

Harkle.com (http://www.harkle.com/) searches the Internet so that people can find web video and audio that is already closed-captioned or subtitled. Topics range from news and entertainment to science, health, and technology. The website provides up-to-date links to quality captioning that works in most web media players like Flash, Windows Media, QuickTime, and RealPlayer.

Computer-Based Sign Language Interpreters

iCommunicator by Interactive Solutions, Inc. (http://www.myicommunicator.com/) converts the spoken word into text, sign language, or computer-based speech in real time. The American Sign Language (ASL) signs in English word order (subject + verb + object) to enhance the connection with spoken, written, and signed words, resulting in better understanding. A dictionary and thesaurus translate definitions or guide internet searches to locate more information on specific words and phrases.

ASL Animations by Vcom3D, Inc. (http://www.vcom3d.com) help people learn word meanings and make connections between English text and American Sign Language. The Vcommunicator software product suite includes Vcommunicator Studio, Gesture Builder, and Vcommunicator Mobile. The stand-alone Studio and Gesture Builder authoring tools allow you to create three-dimensional characters and animations featuring embedded multicultural and contextual behaviors. Write your own patient instructions and use these characters to illustrate your treatment plan, including sign language and close captioned instructions. Your media are exportable to a variety of applications and mobile devices. Content can be created to maximize the extensive capabilities of handheld devices such as iPods and PDAs. The possibilities are endless when creating a library of accessible multimedia examples in support of patient education. Video animations can be used with other applications such as PowerPoint and on web pages. Virtual human technology provides three-dimensional animated characters that communicate through body language (including gesture or sign language), facial expression, and lip-synched speech.

Patients Who Need Motor Support

Computer users with motor challenges might find numerous built-in computer operating system features to provide for significant support. In Windows Vista, the control panel called ease of access lets you adjust sticky keys to avoid simultaneous keystrokes or the need to use two hands. See Chapter 5 for additional information and an example of sticky keys at work.

Use filter keys in Windows and slow keys on the Macintosh to slow down the acceptance rate when keys are pressed. Adjusting the key acceptance rate is extremely helpful for users who may experience a hand tremor, thus inadvertently press a key by accident while on their way to select a different key. Resting slightly longer on a key would tell the computer to actually accept this key as a keystroke. Lightly bumping a key along the way, but not resting on the key, means that the computer would ignore the inadvertent key press. This adjustment is also helpful for users who experience an eye/hand coordination challenge. Activate mouse keys to permit you to move the mouse using the numeric keypad on your keyboard instead of a standard mouse. Similar adjustments are found in the Macintosh system universal access system preferences.

Both operating systems offer an on-screen keyboard. In Windows XP the on-screen keyboard is a desk accessory from the programs menu. In Windows Vista the on-screen keyboard is activated by pressing the Windows logo key on the keyboard. In the Macintosh the on-screen keyboard is found in the keyboard system preferences, international menu. Check the keyboard viewer, and then select it from the menu bar. An on-screen keyboard sends a selected key into any open application wherever the insertion cursor is located. This means that the computer accepts any key selected with a mouse, or mouse alternative such as a track ball, rather than typed on the regular keyboard.

Speech recognition is the ability to speak directly into any text-based program (such as a word processing or e-mail program) using a headset to convert spoken language into text. Speech recognition technology is more robust in Windows, although some voice command and control navigations are available in the speech system preference on the Macintosh. In Windows Vista, you find the speech recognition controls in the ease of access control panel. In Windows XP, you can find this feature only if Microsoft Office XP or Office 2003 is installed. Admittedly, this feature does not necessarily promote health education, but health educators may find it easier to create patient materials using speech recognition rather than inputting text using traditional keyboarding methods. They may find efficiency increases when using speech recognition technology.

Commercially Produced Adaptive Access Devices

An enormous range of commercially produced adaptive access devices are available in today's market. Access devices are typically organized and considered from within a continuum offering light tech options first and then more complicated high-tech options when needed. An assistive technology specialist typically prescribes these devices as a result of a detailed and specific assessment protocol. Providers in the assistive technology community are as diverse as any. They are educators, therapists, and clinicians from many perspectives, assistive technology specialists, administrators, advocates, parents, and a small group of publishers (Schaff & Jeffs, 2005). Although no national repository of assistive technology providers currently exists, it may be possible to locate local providers by contacting the assistive technology advisory council within each state. The state councils are required as part of the Assistive Technology Act of 1998 as well as the reauthorization in 2004. Assistive technology providers are zealous professionals who are devoted to the idea of using technology to improve the lives of individuals with special needs (Wing, 2006).

The Internet offers a wealth of information about these access devices. Up-to-date and unbiased information can be found through a subscription to Solutions, an online database service published by Closing the Gap (http://closingthegap.com/ctg2/solutions/about.lasso). Solutions subscribers can search an online database to find products by feature match. Information is available about cost and sources for purchase. In addition to this comprehensive online searchable database of products, Solutions also provides subscribers with the online version of the *Closing the Gap* newspaper and its articles archives. The newspaper includes articles written by assistive technology providers, along with the articles from product developers.

Case Study 14-1

Amanda Baggs on Autism

Source: Wikipedia, the free encyclopedia. Retrieved on November 23, 2007, from http://en.wikipedia.org/wiki/Amanda_Baggs

Amanda Baggs (born 1980) is an autism rights activist. In January 2007, she published a video on YouTube describing her experience as an autistic person entitled "In My Language" that became the subject of several articles on CNN. She also guest blogged about her video on Anderson Cooper's blog and answered questions from the audience via e-mail.

About her video, Amanda Baggs writes this:

> My viewpoint in the video is that of an autistic person. But the message is far broader than autistic people. It is about what kinds of communication and language and people we consider real and which ones we do not. It applies to people with severe cognitive or physical disabilities, autistic people, signing deaf people, the kid in school who finds she is not taken seriously as a student because she does not know a lot of

English, and even the cat who gets treated like a living stuffed animal and not a creature with her own thoughts to communicate. It applies to anybody who gets written off because their communication is too unusual.

Related websites about Amanda include the following:

Abedin, S. Video reveals world of autistic woman. CNN, Anderson Cooper blog, 21 February 2007. Retrieved on November 27, 2007, from http://www.cnn.com/CNN/Programs/anderson.cooper.360/blog/2007/02/video-reveals-world-of-autistic-woman.html.

Amanda Baggs answers your questions. CNN, Anderson Cooper blog, 22 February 2007. Retrieved on November 27, 2007, from http://www.cnn.com/CNN/Programs/anderson.cooper.360/blog/2007/02/amanda-baggs-answers-your-questions.html.

Baggs, A. In my language. YouTube. Retrieved on November 27, 2007, from http://youtube.com/watch?v=JnylM1hI2jc.

Cooper, A. Why we should listen to "unusual" voices. CNN, Anderson Cooper blog, February 21, 2007. Retrieved on November 27, 2007, from http://www.cnn.com/CNN/Programs/anderson.cooper.360/blog/2007/02/why-we-should-listen-to-unusual-voices.html.

Gajilan, A. C. Living with autism in a world made for others. CNN, February 22, 2007. Retrieved on November 27, 2007, from http://www.cnn.com/2007/HEALTH/02/21/autism.amanda/index.html.

Gupta, S. Behind the veil of autism. CNN, 20 February 2007. Retrieved on November 27, 2007, from http://www.cnn.com/HEALTH/blogs/paging.dr.gupta/2007/02/behind-veil-of-autism.html.

Case Study 14-2

Jeanette B. on Sensory Disability

Hello! My name is Jeanette B. I'm the paper-pushing office chick at Simmons College in Boston, MA. My diagnosis considered low-partial blind. I have what some say is a wonderful sense of humor and one prosthetic eyeball that has fallen on many a bar floor while the other is pretty much worthless.

I have my BS from Bowling Green State University in Human Development and Family Studies and Women's Studies and am an East Boston native. Don't ask me why I ended up in the cornfields of Ohio for college. I don't have a really good answer.

My personal tools that I use are the following:

Low-tech aids

- 20/20 paper, which is a set of stencil-like guides for writing checks and signing credit card slips, along with other formats.
- 20/20 pen with black ink and extra-bold tip
- Large-print checkbook

- Traction tape to place on stairs to provide a guide for my foot to feel as I approach
- A talking book tape player from National Library Service

High-tech tools

- I use a PC laptop loaded with software such as Kurzweill Text Reader, Zoomtext enlarger, Jaws Screen Reader, and Bookport Utility tools.
- Bookport is a portable book reading device that consists of a small unit with a keypad and earbuds. Content is loaded on compact flash cards.
- PACmate is an accessible pocket PC.
- I use websites such as Recordings for Blind and Bookshare.org to find anything I'd like to read.
- Senseview is a portable pocket closed-circuit television (CCTV) to enlarge print.
- I also have a stationary CCTV to enlarge print. A CCTV has a camera pointing down on an area where I can put any piece of print. There are adjustments that permit me to enlarge the print, change the visual contrast, or adjust the way that the print appears so that I might be able to see it better. It's a nice new model, does split screen, and has a calculator and all that jazz, but it's on my desk at work and at home.

Folks are welcome to take a field trip to my office to see these tools; I always love showing off the fun stuff I use.

Whenever I go to medical appointments, I am generally not happy with the manner in which I am supported in my needs for understanding the important information presented to me. It is generally in print, a medium that I cannot use without my tools. Because healthcare professionals are unable to provide me with these translations, this is something I must unhappily do on my own.

Case Study 14-3

Michael Phillips on Physical Disability

I'm Michael Phillips, a journalist and artist from Tampa, FL. When Mac OS X first arrived, I was most excited but also a tad nervous. I have Spinal Muscular Atrophy and rely on a single switch and scanning to access my Mac. Then I was introduced to SwitchXS software that provides full emulation of mouse and keyboard. People with very limited limb movement typically use keyboard and mouse emulation for computer access. For example, a user who is quadriplegic due to an accident or living with a neuromotor disease such as amyotrophic lateral sclerosis (ALS) or spinal muscular atrophy (SMA) might enjoy full access because of this tool. Emulation software provides virtually complete access to all standard applications for people who can only use one or more reliable muscle in order to activate a switch. The software offers full mouse and keyboard emulation by means of a so-called scanning mode. With each click on the switch the user selects an action, such as "move the cursor up" or "type B," from a "scanning" menu.

With SwitchXS, I can do everything I want to do in OS X. For instance, I'm a Mac journalist, mostly focusing on game reviews and interviews. I also wrote the chapters on card and board games, role-playing games, and online games for Peachpit's *Macintosh Bible*. By using keyboard and mouse emulation, I can play and review games such as Massive Assault, Neverwinter Nights, Shadowbane, Myst IV Revelation, Star Wars: Knights of the Old Republic, and World of Warcraft with ease. Of course, after I play a game, I have to write about it, but that's not a problem thanks to my assistive technology tools. SwitchXS works seamlessly with Microsoft Word and also allows me to use high-end creative applications, such as Adobe Photoshop, Illustrator, and GoLive. SwitchXS can deftly handle every application that I need to use.

I use the Internet and my adaptive access devices to research my own medical information. I am an intelligent individual who can read and write, but not without my access tools. My doctors and family all understand and appreciate these access devices as much as I do.

Thanks to SwitchXS, I can use the newest technology. I can use the applications I want to use, all while using Apple's latest hardware and Mac OS X. Without SwitchXS, I wouldn't be able to use my laptop. SwitchXS is the way!

Meet me and read more about the technology I use at www.assistiveware.com/community.php.

CONCLUSION

Hopefully this information helps readers appreciate the value of technology-assisted instruction in all areas of patient education. We have described a multitude of free and commercially available resources. Free solutions can be found inside every computer on today's market. The Internet offers a wealth of tools that promote health education and which make it accessible to all. Commercial publishers offer more robust, full-featured products. These are sometimes better able to be customized for particular patient needs or specialized populations. The value of providing patient healthcare materials in a variety of formats is easily accomplished and cannot be over-emphasized.

WEB RESOURCES

Amanda Baggs
From Wikipedia, the free encyclopedia
Retrieved from Wikipedia on November 23, 2007
http://en.wikipedia.org/wiki/Amanda_Baggs

Web 2.0 http://en.wikipedia.org/wiki/Web_2, retrieved December 6, 2007.

Web 2.0 Tutorials

Social Bookmarking—Watch a 3-minute tutorial here: Social Bookmarking in Plain English at http://www.commoncraft.com/bookmarking-plain-english.

Blogs—Watch a 3-minute tutorial here: Blogs in Plain English at http://www.commoncraft.com/blogs.

Wikis—Watch a 3-minute tutorial here: Wikis in Plain English at http://www.commoncraft.com/video-wikis-plain-english.

How to Podcast—http://www.how-to-podcast-tutorial.com/index.htm.

VoiceThread—http://voicethread.com/about/featuring/.

Slidecasting—Watch a 2-minute tutorial here: http://www.slideshare.net/jboutelle/slidecasting-101.

REFERENCES

Boulos, M. N. K., & Wheeler, S. (2007). The emerging web 2.0 social software: an enabling suite of sociable technologies in health and health care education. *Health Information & Libraries Journal, 24*(1), 2–23.

Boulos, M. N. K., Hetherington, L., & Wheeler, S. (2007). Second life: an overview of the potential of 3-D virtual worlds in medical and health education. *Health Information & Libraries Journal, 24*(4), 233–245.

Brock, T. P., & Smith, S. R. (2007). Using digital videos displayed on personal digital assistants (PDAs) to enhance patient education in clinical settings. *International Journal of Medical Informatics, 76*(11), 829–835.

Buti, M. (2007). Editorial feature: Let's get visual. *Closing the Gap* (April/May).

Ellaway, R. (2007). eMedical teacher. *Medical Teacher, 29*(4), 420–421.

Evans, C., & Gibbons, N. J. (2007). The interactivity effect in multimedia learning. *Computers & Education, 49*(4), 1147–1160.

Giustini, D. (2006). How Web 2.0 is changing medicine. *British Medical Journal, 333*(7582), 1283–1284.

Kamp, L., & McErlean, T. (2006). Visual schedule systems. *LATI Region 3 Newsletter, 1*(6), 3.

Learning Independence through Computers. Six Tips for Choosing AugCom Devices. Retrieved on November 23, 2007, from http://www.linc.org/ataugcom.html.

Parette, H., Huer, M., VanBiervliet, A. (2005). Cultural research in special education technology. In D. Edyburn, K. Higgins, & R. Boone (Eds.), *Handbook of special education technology research and practice* (pp. 81, 98). Whitefish Bay, WI: Knowledge by Design.

Schaff, G. C. & Jeffs, J. (2005). Physical access in today's schools: empowerment through assistive technology. In D. Edyburn, K. Higgins, & R. Boone (Eds.),

Handbook of special education technology research and practice (pp. 355–377). Whitefish Bay, WI: Knowledge by Design.

Skiba, D. J. (2006). Web 2.0: next great thing or just marketing hype? *Nursing Education Perspectives, 27*(4), 212–214.

Skiba, D. J. (2007). Nursing education 2.0: YouTube. *Nursing Education Perspectives, 28*(3), 156–157.

Stoop, A. P., van't Riet, A., & Berg, M. (2004). Using information technology for patient education: realizing surplus value? *Patient education and counseling, 54*(2), 187–195.

Wing, A. (2006). Assistive technology: a remarkable community of collaboration. *Closing the Gap 4*(6), 4–5, 14.

15

Chapter 15

Searching the Literature: Resources and Research Methods

Vivienne B. Piroli

INTRODUCTION

One of the greatest challenges facing health educators and patients alike is dealing with the ever-increasing volume of information relating to health and wellness. From government-sponsored campaigns to drug and insurance companies, there is freely available information for health professionals and consumers dropping into real and virtual mailboxes daily. The prevalence of web-based health information has been a boon to the curious, but also a concern for the professional because of its lack of mediation and verification. Reliance on the Internet as a health information resource continues to grow at rapid rates. Successive Harris Polls indicate the increase in this trend. In 2005, 117 million U.S. adults had searched online for health information. By 2007, this had increased by 37%, to 160 million (Harris Interactive, 2007). The pollsters at Harris Interactive refer to these individuals as "cyberchondriacs" (Harris Interactive, 2007). This title alone should be worrying clinicians and health professionals. Coupled with the fact that

85 million Americans rarely evaluate the health information they find online (Pew Internet, 2006), this emphasizes the need for intervention and behavioral changes. Health professionals should actively seek to make health literacy part of the patient's treatment plan (Sihota & Lennard, 2004). Reaching this goal involves encouraging patients to become active and informed partners in their health information needs. To do this, health professionals need to be comfortable advocating resources that are reliable and geared toward consumer health topics. Bridging the gap between what consumers need and the level of information professionals are typically exposed to is not as great as it might first appear. Indeed, that challenge is representative of the larger issue faced by professionals and patients alike where the rate and volume of health data production "expands faster than our capability to access, receive, filter, accept, integrate, manage and use information" (Salim & Choo Ming, 2004). At the Consensus Conference on Undergraduate Public Health Education in Boston, MA on November 7–8 2006, "Conference attendees agreed that undergraduate public health education can help produce an educated citizenry that is better prepared to cope with public health challenges from acquired immunodeficiency syndrome to aging, avian influenza, and health-care costs" (Council of Colleges of Arts & Sciences, 2007). A working group at a nursing symposium on diabetes self-management identified an increased knowledge of how research is done and is encouraging more research as fundamental to positive outcomes for patient self-care (Lewis, 2007).

CURRENT ISSUES IN HEALTH INFORMATION ACCESS AND RETRIEVAL

Encouraging patients toward health literacy implies that health promoters have achieved this fluency too. Even with a solid foundation in evidence-based practice (EBP), many professionals still have difficulty merging an inquiry-based approach with their professional practice. The barriers to making EBP a practice norm are cited as the culture of the workplace and lack of time (Morris & Maynard, 2007); nevertheless, for many professionals and practitioners, one of the greatest barriers to self-efficacy and advanced practice is the act of conducting research. A recent study indicated that of 270 physical therapists surveyed most were interested in learning about EBP; nevertheless, 50% of the group believed they should not bear responsibility for conducting the necessary literature reviews (Salbach, Jaglal, & Korner-Bitensky et al., 2007). The same study concluded that access to web-based resources alone was insufficient to encourage practitioners to conduct their own research. Additional motivation often in the form of licensure renewal or the need for continuing education units is more successful in getting practitioners to examine the literature and remain current with professional standards and trends (Landers, McWhorter, & Krum et al., 2005).

There are attempts in some practice areas to move beyond simply identifying the need for EBP. Taking a proactive approach, clinicians are encouraging consultation with research literature by fostering an atmosphere where questioning stated practices is welcomed and expected. One nursing manager comments, "Seeking the most current research evidence is the gold standard to move nursing forward as a scientifically-based profession" (Minnesota Nursing Accent, 2007). This shift in practice culture is significant, as it marks participation in activities such as conference attendance, research studies, and publishing as priorities rather than professional extras. The EBP approach is not just about self-improvement and professional edification; central to this way of learning and practice is the inherent goal of sharing findings and teaching one's colleagues. This leads to better patient outcomes and a greater sense of professional fulfillment (Weston, Estrada, & Carrington, 2007).

Research studies are finding positive links between patient health and the degree to which active self-efficacy is encouraged by the health professional and adopted by the patient. In health promotion, the Transtheoretical Model is often used to move patients through a series of changes to the point where they will adapt and maintain behaviors that will minimize their health risks (Highstein, O'Toole, & Shetty et al., 2007). The success of this model relies in part on collaboration between the patient and caregiver. One study in particular noted that Resources and Supports for Self-Management, coupled with the Transtheoretical Model, was more successful when the emphasis was placed on teaching patients how to manage their conditions and not just instructing them on what to do (Davis, O'Toole, & Brownson et al., 2007).

Health promotion and health literacy are part of the overall trend of lifelong learning. This approach to learning underscores the expectation that practitioners and patients alike have a responsibility for being critically informed. Navigating the web or reading literature from a database may seem unnecessarily complex, and spending time on it may be difficult to justify. Critically evaluating information may seem daunting to patients when an article describes their condition in clinical language; nevertheless, a basic introduction to the tenets of health literacy can be empowering and potentially life-saving (Meadows, 2006).

RESEARCH METHODS AND TECHNIQUES

Most searchers would like to be able to find necessary information as easily as they search Google; however, the wealth of results from a Google search is in no way related to their usefulness to the searcher. Selectivity and relevancy in results require a searcher to have a strategy for uncovering the most useful and appropriate results. Discipline specific databases related to health and medicine are more likely to have usable content over general web-based search engines. Because they are discipline specific, the user can expect a certain quality from the content as it has been vetted before being included. Quality assurance is certainly welcome when dealing with health-related topics. After a searcher has decided where to search for their information need, the next step is to become adept in executing the search. The following strategies discuss methods used by information professionals to produce the best quality results in the most efficient manner.

WORDY SEARCHES

The greatest inclination when searching for information is to enter an entire phrase or sentence into the search box. This would be a convenient approach except for the fact that it credits the database with greater intelligence than it really possesses. Breaking the topic into its requisite parts is likely to lead to a better result. The search "effects of spiritual interventions on women with cancer" is unlikely to be successful for several reasons. First, it is expressed as a lengthy phrase, and the database will work hard to find results in which all the search words are expressed exactly and in that same order. Additionally, it includes words such as "of," "on," and "with." These common and unspecific terms are known as stop words and are filtered out of the search; thus, including them is a redundant effort. Taking the same phrase and extracting the specific and relevant keywords and concepts are likely to return better results. The key ideas here are "spirituality," "women," "cancer." The database will look for results that match these individual words and not as a phrase.

A useful technique for determining suitable search terms is to devise a Keyword Grid (**Table 15-1**). This involves identifying the most relevant terms, listing each, and then coming up with synonyms for each of the terms.

Table 15-1 Keyword Grid

spirituality	religion	faith
women	female	adult
cancer	neoplasms	tumors

The Keyword Grid is a flexible instrument. It can extend as necessary, and the terms can be exactly synonymous with the original words or can incorporate broader and narrower ideas. The extended combinations of search possibilities are its greatest strength. This expands the opportunities for finding useful and usable information.

Keywords are an excellent way to commence searching. Keywords are natural language search terms that try to find a match on the major fields within records in a database. Subject searching can enhance that experience. Subject searches are more selective and use controlled vocabulary. This means that individual concepts are tagged or described using predefined terms. This improves the indexing feature of a database and makes it easy to retrieve all of the given information on a particular topic. This is how the Yellow Pages and blogs work. Many bloggers will tag their posts using consistent headings. This makes it easier to follow threads and retrieve multiple postings on a given topic.

Large databases such as Medline use extensive controlled vocabularies. Medline is known as MeSH (Medical Subject Heading). Each record in the database can be tagged with multiple MeSH terms that accurately and consistently describe the content within the article being indexed. Because these taxonomies tend not to rely on natural language, choosing a correct subject heading could easily become a guessing game. To manage this, many online databases now include thesauri features. This allows the user to enter their term and find the equivalent word or phrase used to describe that concept in the database. Searching the term "cancer" in the thesaurus of CINAHL (Cumulative Index to Nursing and Allied Health Literature) will direct the searcher to use the term "neoplasms." Another reason subject searches are so precise is because they find matches only in the subject field of each record. They have a more limited search area but are primed to return results with the highest degree of relevance.

MAKING CONNECTIONS

The Keyword Grid in Table 15-1 is a good example of the complexities of most searches. Rarely do we look for information just on spirituality or cancer alone. Most searches try to find very specific pieces of information related to a condition or context. The ability to manipulate search terms allows the searcher greater flexibility. Databases and search engines are programmed to respond to searches entered with connecting words. These connectors typically are "AND," "OR," and "NOT." They are sometimes referred to as Boolean operators, as they function in the same way as the algebraic expressions of the same name. Connecting multiple search terms with "AND" can lead to a lengthy search string but will return a list of results where all your search terms are present. Using "OR" will return results where one or the other or both of your search terms are present. This connector works best when you are searching words that are synonymous, "treatment OR therapy." The operator "NOT" is particularly useful when you want to exclude a term that might be commonly associated with the concept you are trying to research. Searching for "heart disease NOT congenital" will be more likely to return results dealing with heart disease caused by environmental factors rather than information on those born with congenital heart disease. In general, using connectors with your search terms will control the result list in a way that makes it more relevant with a higher degree of usable information.

SETTING LIMITS

Using select keywords and connectors is no guarantee to get a manageable result set. A typical search can return hundreds of thousands of results. Even in a discipline specific database such as Medline or CINAHL, that number can still be in the hundreds. Limiters are controls you can apply to focus a search and reduce irrelevant results. In general, limiters will allow you to select results based on criteria such as format, dates of publication, peer review, and language. In specialized databases, there are additional limiters available, such as age-related, gender, clinical trials, research, and publication type. The use and range of limiters varies from one database to the next. The built-in help screens are worth consulting to determine the control values of the limiters offered in any given database.

GOOGLE

Google is one of the most popular choices for searchers when trying to satisfy an information need (Google Operating System Blogspot, 2007). By judging Google on its popularity alone, we cannot conclude that all users are searching effectively or efficiently; however, it is a helpful tool and more so when searchers incorporate a few simple search techniques.

Searching in the main Google search engine can be improved by using the features in the advanced search screens, as well as being knowledgeable about Google's search syntax. Google accepts some of the Boolean connectors and formats discussed earlier. It ignores many common stop words. If a stop word is essential to the search, place a "+" in front of the word. Similarly to exclude a term from the search results put a "−" in front of the word. The Boolean operator "OR" is recognized when it is in uppercase letters. To look for a synonymous word in a search term simply put a "~" before the word. Searchers can also limit by criteria such as language or domain name to refine results further. To find results using an exact phrase, simply place the phrase in quotation marks and search.

Additional features can help control and manipulate searches. Users can opt for one of the Google topic specific subsearches, such as using Google Scholar. Google Scholar limits its content to academic and scholarly papers, theses, conference publications, and presentations. It covers many disciplines and is wide ranging. For health and medical data, it will often include the PubMed ID (PMID) number to assist in finding the citation in PubMed databases. Some papers are presented in their entirety, but the vast majority offers just a citation. Google Scholar is a select set of scholarly resources, and therefore, its content tends to be more reliable. As with any information source, results should always be critically evaluated.

FOUND IT, WANT IT

Often, users perform a search that uncovers the "perfect" site, only to find that partial content or brief citations are all that are available to read. Many organizations limit their premium content to members only. Lack of access is frustrating but not insurmountable. Health professionals who subscribe to journals in their field can usually activate an online subscription to web content at little or no extra cost. Public libraries are another good resource. Many will provide databases with full text content on a wide variety of topics, including health. They are likely to subscribe to print periodicals that are of interest to the general community, which will undoubtedly cover many aspects of health and wellness. In addition, most libraries will offer interlibrary loan services. For a low or no fee, the home library will request books or articles from other libraries for their own patrons to use. Also, many college and university libraries welcome members of the public and will allow them to use materials in their library. Borrowing privileges are usually extended only to current members of the institution and alumni; however, some academic libraries will issue privileges to nonaffiliated users for a reasonable fee.

WEB RESOURCES

The following list of resources is a sampling of web-based health information. It is meant to offer starting points for those interested in health research. Many sites offer information and statistical data that are useful to the health professional or clinician. Other sites have a stronger focus on consumer health issues and are well suited to the needs of patients and their families. All types of information have to be evaluated for their authority, coverage, objectivity, accuracy, and currency. The following resources have intrinsic controls that provide some degree of validation in the information that they provide. On a larger level, there are currently two organizations that act as watchdogs for health information on the web: Health on the Net Foundation and Operation Cure-All (Health on the Net Foundation http://www.hon.ch; Operation Cure-All, http://www.operationcureall.com/, FTC & FDA news and information). The Health on the Net Foundation supports users by offering a quality assurance award to sites that meet its criteria for excellence. Operation Cure-All aims to make consumers aware of health fraud.

Comprehensive Sites

Medline Plus

http://medlineplus.gov/

This is the online presence of the National Institutes of Health. It is wide ranging in scope providing information on health topics, drug information, clinical trials, and interactive tutorials. Many of the features on this site are also available in Spanish.

InteliHealth

http://www.intelihealth.com/IH/ihtIH/WSIHW000/408/408.html

This site is sponsored by the Aetna insurance company. Its content is provided in conjunction with Harvard Medical School. It offers an A–Z list on diseases and conditions, as well as advice on fitness, nutrition, and weight management. There are interactive tools, quizzes, and assessments.

Health A–Z Your Family Health Site

http://www.healthatoz.com/healthatoz/Atoz/clients/haz/general/custom/default.jsp

Here the A–Z entries have expert authored entries with the dates of the most recent revisions listed. The site includes a Personal Health Center with tools to manage weight loss and smoking cessation. One of the outstanding features of this site is its nurse chat. A registered nurse is available 24/7 to handle all manner of health questions in a live chat environment.

MayoClinic.com

http://www.mayoclinic.com/

This is the site of the Mayo Foundation for Medical Education and Research. It has the ability to be customized to the user's preferences using its "My Health Interests" section. It provides health decision guides that walk users through diagnostic trees.

HealthCentral
http://www.healthcentral.com/

This is run by MD Choice Inc., founded by Dr. Dean Edell. It uses a very simple navigation system of topic tags. It simply aims to answer questions, suggest a course of action, and offer advice.

WebMD Health
http://www.webmd.com/

Most of the content on this site is free. Membership provides access to personalized services including newsletters and e-mail updates. Some of the more interesting features include video clips with topics such as a fridge makeover and facelift without going to sleep. The site offers a symptom checker and a top 12 health topic section.

Portals

About.com—Health and Fitness
http://www.about.com/health/

This is a well-organized directory where health topics are easily accessible. In some cases, there are overviews and critical evaluations of the sites listed.

Internet Public Library—IPL
http://www.ipl.org/div/subject/browse/hea00.00.00/

IPL wants to go beyond just providing a list of sources and offer a measure of public service in its offerings. The site is well put together. The topics are specific, and all the sites are evaluated. Users can search individual collections or all of IPL. It also offers an advanced search capability.

Infomine—Scholarly Internet Resource Collection
http://infomine.ucr.edu/

Infomine is geared for faculty, students, and researchers at the university level. It offers links to databases, e-journals, books, library catalogs, articles, and directories. Consumer health is found in the biological, agricultural, medical topic area.

Librarians' Index to the Internet
http://search.lii.org/index.jsp?more=SubTopic4

LII is an annotated subject directory evaluated by librarians. The content sites are chosen for their usefulness to public library patrons. The boldface type indicates topics have additional subdivisions.

Government Sites

Centers for Disease Control and Prevention (CDC)
http://www.cdc.gov/

This site represents some of the work done by the CDC. It offers good statistical data, growth charts, and health-management tools. The site includes information on birth defects, disabilities, emergency preparedness and response, environmental health, health promotion, and traveler's health. The content is also available in Spanish.

Clinical Trials
http://clinicaltrials.gov/

Information here is regularly updated and details federally and privately supported clinical research in human volunteers. The site describes the purpose and scope of the trials, as well as who can participate and the contact details. Searchers can look up a specific trial by condition, sponsor, status, or peer writings.

Go Local
http://www.nlm.nih.gov/medlineplus/golocalcontacts.html

The Go Local sites are a National Library of Medicine/National Institutes of Health initiative to target resources at a state-wide level. They act primarily as service directories. Visual maps allow users to click on the relevant geographic area. Search results are listed alphabetically with the number of providers given in parentheses. Contact details and referrals are one level down.

Healthfinder
http://www.healthfinder.gov/

This is the Department of Health and Human Service's web presence. It includes a health library; a section on wellness, diseases, and conditions; and links to medical dictionaries.

National Cancer Institute
http://www.cancer.gov/

This is available in English and Spanish and lists common types of cancer, treatment options, as well as information on causes, prevention, and screening.

National Center for Health Statistics
http://www.cdc.gov/nchs/

This is a unit of the CDC. Their purpose is to collect and disseminate information on vital statistics. This is the place to go when trying to locate statistical information on births, deaths, marriages, and divorces.

National Institute of Mental Health
http://www.nimh.nih.gov/

This is one of the units of the National Institutes of Health. Here searchers will find links to information about specific mental diseases from anxiety disorders to schizophrenia. It offers definitions and overviews, signs, symptoms, and treatments. This site offers links back to the PubMed and Clinical Trials sites.

Professional Association Sites

American Medical Association (AMA)
http://www.ama-assn.org/

This site offers background on the AMA. There is access to patient information, links to medical specialties, as well as state medical association sites. It contains Physician Select, where users can retrieve information on all the licensed physicians in the United States.

Familydoctor.org—American Academy of Family Physicians
http://familydoctor.org/online/famdocen/home.html

Here users will find a variety of information on everything from health tips to tools and calculators. The site is visually appealing and easy to navigate and has a Spanish language version. There is an A–Z guide as well as thematically arranged topics such as men, women, seniors, and healthy living. There is also a symptom finder with appropriate remediation.

American Academy of Pediatrics
http://www.aap.org/

The AAP site provides helpful information for parents on children's health growth and development. This is a good place to look for additional resources on topics such as immunizations and car safety seats.

American Dental Association
http://www.ada.org/

This is a consumer health site with information and resources to help individuals with their dental care. Also included are games and puzzles to prepare children for dental visits.

American Dietetic Association
http://www.eatright.org/cps/rde/xchg/ada/hs.xsl/index.html

There are two distinct sections to this site. One is focused on health and nutrition topics, and the other is the member-only site. This is a good place to go to read releases on the latest research pertaining to diet and nutrition.

Diseases and Health Conditions

Alzheimer's Association

http://www.alz.org/index.asp

This is a useful site for individuals diagnosed with the disease and their caregivers. There is information on the warning signs, diagnosis, stages, and treatments. The site offers links to local chapters and support groups as well an index to information in foreign languages.

American Cancer Association

http://www.cancer.org/docroot/home/index.asp

Here is a site designed specifically for patients and cancer survivors along with those who are interested in prevention and early detection. Interactive tools let users explore treatment options. This site links to the Clinical Trials website.

American Diabetes Association

http://www.diabetes.org/home.jsp

The site is designed for those with diabetes or who are at risk for the disease. It gives an overview of diabetes and its risk factors as well as classifying it by type 1, type 2, and gestational. There are summaries of the latest research studies as well as tips, recipes, and suggestions for living with the disease. A Spanish version of the site is available.

American Heart Association

http://www.americanheart.org/presenter.jhtml?identifier=1200000

This site provides information on the warning signs of heart disease and other related conditions. It covers information on diet and nutrition along with fitness and exercise. There are links to the Heart and Stroke Encyclopedia as well as to the American Stroke Association.

American Lung Association

http://www.lungusa.org/site/pp.asp?c=dvLUK9O0E&b=22542

This site notes that the American Lung Association dates from 1904 and is the oldest voluntary health organization. It advocates against smoking and air pollution. There is information on specific diseases, treatment, and prevention, as well as support for patients.

Drug Information

Food and Drug Administration (FDA)

http://www.fda.gov/

This is the primary site for information related to public health and the safety of food, drugs, medical devices, and cosmetics. There are links to specific products regulated by the FDA. The site also includes the Orange Book, which tells users the therapeutic equivalents and generics that can replace a brand name drug. The FDA online consumer magazine gives information about new drugs to the market as well as health and safety issues.

People's Pharmacy
http://www.peoplespharmacy.com/index.asp

This site is designed especially for the lay person. The articles explain topics in easily understandable language. There is information on frequently prescribed drugs as well as home remedies.

HerbMed
http://www.herbmed.org/

This is an interactive database of herbal remedies. It is meant to be an information resource for processionals. Up to 40 herbs are freely accessible after which there is a fee per access.

Alternative and Complementary Medicine

Alternative Medicine Homepage
http://www.pitt.edu/~cbw/altm.html

This website is maintained by a medical librarian at the University of Pittsburg. It provides links to resources about alternative medicine. Organized like a directory, it is quite simple to navigate.

MedlinePlus—Alternative Medicine
http://www.nlm.nih.gov/medlineplus/complementaryandalternativemedicine.html

This is one of the health topic pages from the main MedlinePlus website. It is arranged for ease of use, and the content is oriented toward consumers. There are links to complementary and alternative medicine topics such as acupuncture, chiropractic, and herbal medicines.

CAM on PubMed
http://nccam.nih.gov/camonpubmed/

This is a database rather than just a website. The content is geared toward health professionals. All searches in this database are automatically limited to complementary and alternative medicine topics and link to citations in PubMed.

Alternative Medicine Foundation
http://www.amfoundation.org/

This is a nonprofit organization founded in 1998. Their goal is to provide reliable information to consumers and healthcare professionals. The site gives extensive information about alternative medicine. They are behind the development of the HerbMed site.

Diet and Nutrition

Food and Nutrition Information
http://www.eatright.org/cps/rde/xchg/ada/hs.xsl/nutrition.html

This is produced by the American Dietetic Association and provides the latest information on food management and safety, as well as a wide array of nutrition topics. It offers annual reviews of popular diets and has links to international organizations and government initiatives.

Food and Nutrition Information Center
http://www.nal.usda.gov/fnic/topics_a-z.shtml

This site is part of the National Agriculture Library. It is designed to appeal to a wide range of users from consumers to health professionals and educators, as well as government personnel. It is arranged in a directory format.

Food Safety
http://www.foodsafety.gov/

The focus of this comprehensive site is on food safety and deals with topics on food-borne pathogens and offers links to programs on food safety. There are also more links to the federal and state agencies concerned with food safety.

Nutrition.gov
http://www.nutrition.gov/nal_display/index.php?info_center=11&tax_level=1

Here users can access content to food and nutrition information. The site is suitable for consumers and health professionals. Topics include nutrition and healthy eating, physical activity, and food safety.

Age and Gender Related

NIH Senior Health.gov
http://nihseniorhealth.gov/

This was developed by the National Institute on Aging, the National Library of Medicine, and the National Institutes of Health. In an attempt to be accessible to its target users, it is possible to change site design features such as text size, contrast, and speech options. Content is offered in question and answer format with common topics presented in alphabetical order.

ElderCare Online

http://www.ec-online.net/

This is a resource for information and support for patients and caregivers. Topics focus on Alzheimer's disease, dementia. There is a strong emphasis on caregivers taking adequate care of themselves as well as their charges.

Not for Men Only: The Male Health Center

http://www.malehealthcenter.com/

Founded in 1989 by a urologist, this site is dedicated to men's health. It offers information on symptoms of diseases and conditions along with treatments. There are also sections on health and wellness topics.

National Women's Health Information Center

http://www.4women.gov/

This is the Department of Health and Human Services Office on Women's Health website. It offers a wide array of topic areas from girls' health to body image and from HIV/AIDS to men's health issues from the viewpoint of what women should know.

REFERENCES

About.com: health. (2008). Retrieved January 28, 2008, from http://www.about.com/health/.

ADA.org: welcome to the American dental association web site. (2008). Retrieved January 28, 2008, from http://www.ada.org/.

Alternative Medicine Foundation, Inc., Bethesda, MD—welcome. (2008). Retrieved January 28, 2008, from http://www.amfoundation.org/.

The alternative medicine homepage. (2008). Retrieved January 28, 2008, from http://www.pitt.edu/~cbw/altm.html.

Alzheimer's Association: home. (2008). Retrieved January 28, 2008, from http://www.alz.org/index.asp.

American Academy of Pediatrics. (2008). Retrieved January 28, 2008, from http://www.aap.org/.

American Cancer Society: information and resources for cancer: breast, colon, prostate, lung and other forms. (2008). Retrieved January 28, 2008, from http://www.cancer.org/docroot/home/index.asp.

American Diabetes Association. (2008). Retrieved January 28, 2008, from http://www.diabetes.org/home.jsp.

American Dietetic Association. (2008). Retrieved January 28, 2008, from http://www.eatright.org/cps/rde/xchg/ada/hs.xsl/index.html.

American Heart Association. (2008). Retrieved January 28, 2008, from http://www.americanheart.org/presenter.jhtml?identifier=1200000.

American Lung Association. (2008). Retrieved January 28, 2008, from http://www.lungusa.org/site/pp.asp?c=dvLUK9O0E&b=22542.

American Medical Association. (2008). Retrieved January 28, 2008, from http://www.ama-assn.org/.

Centers for Disease Control and Prevention. (2008). Retrieved January 28, 2008, from http://www.cdc.gov/.

Clinical Trials: home. (2008). Retrieved January 28, 2008, from http://clinicaltrials.gov/.

Council of Colleges of Arts & Sciences. (2007). Recommendations for public health curriculum—consensus conference on undergraduate public health education, November 2006. *Morbidity & Mortality Weekly Report, 56*(41), 1085–1086.

Davis, K. L., O'Toole, M. L., Brownson, C. A., Llanos, P., & Fisher, E. B. (2007). Teaching how, not what: the contributions of community health workers to diabetes self-management. *The Diabetes Educator, 33*(6), 208S–215S

ElderCare Online: information, education, and support for elderly and Alzheimer's caregivers. (2008). Retrieved January 28, 2008, from http://www.ec-online.net/.

Familydoctor.org. (2008). Retrieved January 28, 2008, from http://familydoctor.org/online/famdocen/home.html.

Food and Drug Administration. (2008). Retrieved January 28, 2008, from http://www.fda.gov/.

Food and nutrition information. (2008). Retrieved January 28, 2008, from http://www.eatright.org/cps/rde/xchg/ada/hs.xsl/nutrition.html.

Food and Nutrition Information Center: topics A–Z. (2008). Retrieved January 28, 2008, from http://www.nal.usda.gov/fnic/topics_a-z.shtml.

Google Operating System Blogspot. (2007). Google's popularity increases. Retrieved January 24, 2008, from http://googlesystem.blogspot.com/2007/01/googles-popularity-increases.html.

Harris Interactive. (2007). Harris Interactive—The Harris Poll—Harris Poll shows number of "cyberchondriacs"—adults who have ever gone online for health information increases to an estimated 160 million nationwide. Retrieved January 15, 2008, from http://www.harrisinteractive.com/harris_poll/index.asp?PID=792.

Healthcentral.com—trusted, reliable and up to date health information. (2008). Retrieved January 28, 2008, from http://www.healthcentral.com/.

Healthfinder.gov—your guide to reliable health information. (2008). Retrieved January 28, 2008, from http://www.healthfinder.gov/.

Health information, health articles, health tips and online medical advice for healthy living: home—www.HealthAtoZ.com. (2008). Retrieved January 28, 2008, from http://www.healthatoz.com/healthatoz/Atoz/clients/haz/general/custom/default.jsp.

Health on the Net Foundation. (2008). Retrieved January 28, 2008, from http://www.hon.ch/.

HerbMed. (2008). Retrieved January 28, 2008, from http://www.herbmed.org/.

Highstein, G. R., O'Toole, M. L., Shetty, G., Brownson, C. A., & Fisher, E. B. (2007). Use of the transtheoretical model to enhance resources and supports for diabetes self-management: lessons from the Robert Wood Johnson Foundation diabetes initiative. *The Diabetes Educator, 33*(6), 193S–200S.

InteliHealth. (2008). Retrieved January 28, 2008, from http://www.intelihealth.com/IH/ihtIH/WSIHW000/408/408.html.

Internet public library: health and medical sciences. (2008). Retrieved January 28, 2008, from http://www.ipl.org/div/subject/browse/hea00.00.00/.

Landers, M. R., McWhorter, J. W., Krum, L. L., & Glovinsky, D. (2005). Mandatory continuing education in physical therapy: survey of physical therapists in states with and states without a mandate. *Physical Therapy, 85*(9), 861–871.

Lewis, L. (2007). Discussion and recommendations: Improving diabetes self-management. *American Journal of Nursing, 107*(Suppl), 70–73.

Librarians' Internet index. (2008). Retrieved January 28, 2008, from http://search.lii.org/index.jsp?more=SubTopic4.

Male Health Center. (2008). Retrieved January 28, 2008, from http://www.malehealthcenter.com/.

Mayo Clinic medical information and tools for healthy living. (2008). Retrieved January 28, 2008, from http://www.mayoclinic.com/.

Meadows, M. (2006). Outreach program to teach safe medicine use to middle school children. *FDA Consumer, 40*(6), 9–10.

MedlinePlus: complementary and alternative medicine. (2008). Retrieved January 28, 2008, from http://www.nlm.nih.gov/medlineplus/complementaryandalternativemedicine.html.

MedlinePlus: go local contacts. (2008). Retrieved January 28, 2008, from http://www.nlm.nih.gov/medlineplus/golocalcontacts.html.

MedlinePlus: health information from the national library of medicine. (2008). Retrieved January 28, 2008, from http://medlineplus.gov/.

Minnesota Nursing Accent. (2007). Building a culture of inquiry. *Minnesota Nursing Accent, 79*(1), 1–2.

Morris, J., & Maynard, V. (2007). The value of an evidence based practice module to skill development. *Nurse Education Today, 27*(6), 534–541.

National Cancer Institute. (2008). Retrieved January 28, 2008, from http://www.cancer.gov/.

National Center for Health Statistics. (2008). Retrieved January 28, 2008, from http://www.cdc.gov/nchs/.

National Women's Health Information Center—1-800-994-9662. (2008). Retrieved January 28, 2008, from http://www.4women.gov/.

NCCAM and the National Library of Medicine. (2007). CAM on PubMed. (2008). Retrieved January 28, 2008, from http://nccam.nih.gov/camonpubmed/.

NIH Senior Health: health information for older adults. (2008). Retrieved January 28, 2008, from http://nihseniorhealth.gov/.

NIMH. (2008). Retrieved January 28, 2008, from http://www.nimh.nih.gov/.

Nutrition.gov. (2008). Retrieved January 28, 2008, from http://www.nutrition.gov/nal_display/index.php?info_center=11&tax_level=1.

Operation Cure-All: FTC & FDA news and information. (2008). Retrieved January 28, 2008, from http://www.operationcureall.com/.

People's Pharmacy. (2008). Retrieved January 28, 2008, from http://www.peoplespharmacy.com/index.asp.

Pew Internet: online health search. (2006). Retrieved January 15, 2008, from http://www.pewinternet.org/PPF/r/190/report_display.asp.

Salbach, N. M., Jaglal, S. B., Korner-Bitensky, N., Rappolt, S., Davis, D., & Duncan, P. W. (2007). Practitioner and organizational barriers to evidence-based practice of physical therapists for people with stroke. *Physical Therapy, 87*(10), 1284–1305.

Salim, J., & Choo Ming, D. (2004). Information skills: perspectives and alternatives in search strategies. *Malaysian Journal of Library & Information Science, 9*(2), 79–94.

Sihota, S., & Lennard, L. (2008). Health literacy: being able to make the most of health. Retrieved January 28, 2008, from http://66.102.1.104/scholar?hl=en&lr=&q=cache:fAIzLp8wKY8J:www.ncc.org.uk/nccpdf/poldocs/NCC064_health_literacy.pdf+.

WebMD: better information, better health. (2008). Retrieved January 28, 2008, from http://www.webmd.com/.

Welcome to INFOMINE: scholarly internet resource collections. (2008). Retrieved January 28, 2008, from http://infomine.ucr.edu/.

Weston, M. J., Estrada, N. A., & Carrington, J. (2007). Reaping benefits from intellectual capital. *Nursing Administration Quarterly, 31*(1), 6–12.

www.FoodSafety.gov: gateway to government food safety information. (2008). Retrieved January 28, 2008, from http://www.foodsafety.gov/.

Section *III*

Specific Conditions and Health Education

Much of healthcare practice has become specialized, as providers are required to recognize and respond to the specific needs of patients and their families. The remaining chapters address a variety of different systems disorders and specific conditions.

The chapters in this section build from the foundational elements found in Section I and the methods provided in Section II, to focus on the challenges of providing health education for a variety of specific impairments and conditions. The section begins with discussions of personal wellness, behavioral change, and health promotion, as these interests are common to all patients and communities.

Each of the following chapters provides an overview of the unique needs of one specific patient population and provides suggestions and resources for addressing those needs. The case studies provided in each chapter, provide evidence of the foundational concepts and theories explored in Section I as well as applications of a variety of the teaching methods presented in Section II. In the health professions literature, it is rare to hear about ineffective teaching and how or why things went wrong. In these chapters, both positive *and* negative teaching experiences are discussed and analyzed to demonstrate how positive teaching can be accomplished and encouraged and how negative teaching experiences can either be avoided or turned into positive ones.

The information and examples in the chapters in this final section confirm and may perhaps enlighten the work of practitioners experienced with each condition. Clinicians new to practice in any of these areas will welcome this introduction to the educational needs of patients and their families. The examples of instruction are supported by established educational theory and illustrated by authentic case studies. They will provide a valuable resource as they engage the reader in teaching in their specialty area.

Chapter 16

Health Promotion and Wellness

James S. Huddleston

> *The greatest discovery of my generation is that human beings, by changing the inner attitudes of their minds, can change the outer aspects of their lives.*
>
> —William James

INTRODUCTION

Remarkable progress has been made over the course of the last century in the health status of the U.S. population. Life expectancy from birth has increased nearly 30 years in that time period, a remarkable and unprecedented accomplishment. Because of that success, there seems to be a shift in emphasis from quantity to quality of life. No longer concerned with just surviving, we are more interested in learning what constitutes a healthy life and a healthy society and feel more empowered to take control of our health fate.

It is just such an attitude of empowerment that prompted *Healthy People*, the Surgeon General's first report on health promotion and disease prevention in 1979. It established a paradigm for health improvement and measurable health goals to be accomplished by 1990 (U.S. Department of Health, Education, and Welfare, 1979). Ambitious in scope, it set national goals of reducing premature deaths and preserving independence in the elderly. Some progress was made in working toward the goals and subsequently led to the future generations of *Healthy People*. Healthy People 2000 (U.S. Department of Health and Human Service [DHHS], 1990) was another ambitious 10-year strategy for improving the health of the general population by 2000. Healthy People 2010 (http://www.healthypeople.gov) builds on the vision that began with Healthy People over 20 years ago, setting out focus areas and objectives emphasizing improvements in health status, risk reduction, prevention awareness, and delivery of health services, culminating in two far-reaching goals:

• Increased quality and years of healthy life
• Elimination of health disparities

Each goal is important and they are not mutually exclusive. The first goal addresses the issues of maintaining good life quality while living longer with chronic disease and maximizing quality of life for those who don't achieve longevity. The second goal addresses problems related to differences in access to care and treatment based on gender, race, and socioeconomic status. Health disparities are linked to longevity and quality-of-life issues. Research demonstrates that black men and women receive less invasive and less expensive interventions for heart disease than white men and women (Canto, Allison, & Keefe, 2000). These data reflect the racial disparity in health care in this country and its contribution to the shorter life span of blacks compared with that of whites (Greiner & Edelman, 2006).

The *Midcourse Review Executive Summary of Healthy People 2010* (U.S. DHHS, 2000), in conjunction with the HealthierUS initiative (http://www.healthierus.gov), identifies several initiatives to help achieve these goals: an emphasis on the four "pillars" of physical fitness, nutrition, prevention, and making healthy choices; and support for community-based programs focused on reducing the burden of chronic disease. The inclusion of an emphasis on prevention is a welcome paradigm shift in the delivery of health care and recognizes that the risk of many diseases and health conditions can be attenuated through preventive actions and healthy behavior change. The resulting culture of wellness decreases the debilitation and cost of negative health events. The initiatives seek to promote prevention on an individual, clinical, and community level.

A review of progress toward goals in the Healthy People initiative indicates that we are making progress across the health continuum—from the individual to the community to the nation as a whole. Infant mortality is down significantly, as are death rates for coronary heart disease and stroke; substance abuse is leveling off; however, other health indicators reveal that we still have a lot of work to do. Diabetes is on the rise and is strongly associated with the 50% increase in adult obesity over the past 20 years and the 40% of adults who engage in no leisure time activity. Smoking among adolescents has shown an increase, and HIV/AIDS continues to be a serious health concern, especially among women and communities of other races. An underlying theme in this review is that there is a reciprocal relationship between individual and community health. The health of each significantly affects the other, and together, they determine the overall health of the nation. Meeting the challenge of becoming a healthier people requires the involvement of all levels of society—from government agencies to policy makers, community leaders, business executives, healthcare providers, and the individual. This chapter emphasizes the interaction of the healthcare provider and the individual in promoting health and wellness.

THE THREE-LEGGED STOOL

The last several decades have seen tremendous advances in medical technology, surgical techniques, and pharmaceuticals. Most Americans would probably agree that we have the most technologically advanced, comprehensive, successful healthcare system in the world. It is interesting that there are at least 18 countries with populations of more than 1 million that have life expectancies greater than the United States for both men and women (U.S. DHHS, 2000). In addition, years of healthy life, that time spent free of chronic or acute limitations, has not increased to the same degree as life expectancy, indicating that although people are living longer, the quality of those years is negatively affected by chronic conditions. American's healthy life expectancy ranks 22 out of 23 industrialized countries, better only than the Czech Republic; however, despite this poor reflection on the U.S. healthcare system, we spend twice as much per person on health care as the other industrialized nations (Abramson, 2004).

The significant missing ingredient in our recipe for improving the health status of people is self-care: empowering individuals to assume more responsibility for their own health. Healthy People 2010 recognizes this need and has set a goal of helping individuals gain the knowledge, motivation, and opportunities that they need to make informed decisions about their health. In addition, the Agency for Healthcare Research and Quality has developed a new

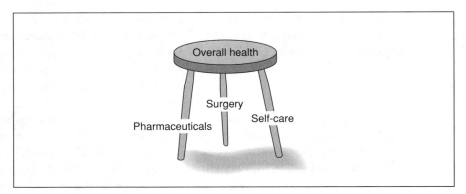

Figure 16-1 The three-legged stool.

public awareness campaign in conjunction with the Ad Council to encourage patients to take a more active role in their health care (Clancy, 2007).

Herbert Benson, MD, President Emeritus of the Benson Henry Institute for Mind/Body Medicine at Massachusetts General Hospital envisioned "Overall Health" as a three-legged stool (**Figure 16-1**), with self-care considered as important a component as surgery and reliance on medications. Take away self-care, the balance is disrupted and health suffers (**Figure 16-2**).

Disease may be defined as functional or structural disturbances resulting from failed adaptation to stress and stimuli. It reflects a state of imbalance and a failure to survive and create a higher quality of life. Health is more

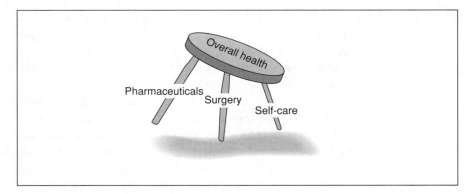

Figure 16-2 Unbalanced three-legged stool.

than just the absence of disease. It can be defined as a state of physical, mental, and social functioning that realizes a person's potential and reflects a state of homeostasis, balance, equilibrium, stability, and resilience (Greiner & Edelman, 2006). The individual has an awareness of what he or she needs in order to move toward their highest health potential across the biopsychosocial/spiritual spectrum. Mind/body medicine uses a variety of techniques to enhance the mind's ability to affect body function and symptoms (National Center for Complementary and Alternative Medicine, 2005). Grounded in evidence-based research, it integrates modern scientific medicine, psychology, nutrition, exercise, and behavior change to enhance the natural healing capacities of the mind and body (self-care). The goal is to facilitate the individual's ability to monitor and take care of his or her own health and to decrease dependence on the healthcare system.

Case Study 16-1

Sally is a 48-year-old female who came to the Cardiac Wellness Program (CWP) at the Benson-Henry Institute, with a chief complaint of chest pain and episodes of syncope. A cardiac workup was negative, and she was felt to have coronary vasospasm secondary to anxiety. Her cardiac risk profile included hypertension, obesity (body mass index, 34), low levels of physical activity, and stress (anxiety). Underlying this more recent complaint was chronic back pain, secondary to degenerative joint disease and spinal stenosis. After years of multiple surgeries, epidurals and nerve blocks, treatment at pain clinics, physical therapy, and acupuncture, she reported being told that, besides medication manipulation, there was nothing else that could be done for her pain. On a pain scale of 1 (least) to 10 (most), Sally rated her pain 5 to 10 for both discomfort and interference (with daily activities), usually in the 8 to 10 range. She saw herself leading a fulfilling life as wife and mother (two daughters in their 20s, one with Down syndrome and the other with obsessive compulsive disorder) but was frustrated that her pain interfered with her ability to do usual daily activities. She tended to see her days in all or nothing terms: good days and bad days. On her good days she would try to make up for lost time and opportunities, doing too much physical activity, and resulting in more bad days, which she generally spent in bed; however, she also saw herself as spiritual and optimistic and expressed a strong desire to improve her health potential. Her motivation for coming to the program was to gain more control over her health and physical functioning by developing stronger coping mechanisms, losing weight, and developing comfortable exercise/physical activity habits.

The core components of the CWP include exercise, nutrition counseling, and stress management (relaxation response and cognitive therapy). The emphasis is on helping patients gain knowledge, develop skills, and shift their habits of thinking to support long-term behavior change and self-care, in conjunction with surgery and medications as necessary. Self-care was the key component to improving Sally's quality of life. Through her participation in the program, she experienced a significant shift in how she saw herself with chronic pain, realizing that she had more control over the choices she made regarding healthy lifestyle practices. As she developed an awareness of what she needed (to feel better), she was able to let go of a number of self-defeating patterns of thinking that blocked her from making improvements.

> "What I want is what I've not got, but what I need is all around me."
>
> Dave Matthews in the song *Jimi Thing*

For example, she was initially horrified at the suggestion of using a Rollator (rolling walker with seat) for ambulating long distances because "that was for old people." When she opened up to its potential, it made a tremendous difference in her ability to perform normal daily activities in and out of the house. In addition, through her practice of meditation and yoga, she was able to move out of "black and white" "all or nothing thinking" and begin to appreciate the subtleties of shades of gray. Instead of a "bad day" resulting in the loss of an entire day, she would rest for an hour or so, re-evaluate how she felt, and then make a decision on activities for the rest of the day. She lost 17 pounds over 3 months and developed regular exercise and meditation practices. Her blood pressure decreased significantly, and she had no further complaints of chest discomfort. Her pain rating for back discomfort did not change, but the interference rating dropped to 1 to 2 on the 10-point scale; however, the true measure of improvement was the increased participation in her life in areas that she had given up: cooking for her family, taking her daughter to doctor's visits, going to the gym to exercise, and socializing with family and friends. Sally now feels like she has her life back, something that could not be achieved with surgery and medications. She experienced a degree of healing, a process of integration and balance of all parts of one's self at deep levels of inner knowing and self-awareness, with each part having equal importance and value. (Dossey & Keegan, 2005)

HEALTH PROMOTION

In addition to the major advances in medical technologies, the last half century has also seen a deeper understanding of the factors that influence our susceptibilities and predispositions to disease (McGinnis, 2003). Five major health domains have been identified that interact with relative degrees of influence to impact current life expectancies of Americans (**Table 16-1**).

For example, even though genetics influences a predisposition to health or disease, gene expression is affected by environmental exposures or behavioral choices. In turn, these behavioral choices are affected by social circumstances (McGinnis, 2003). Behavior patterns represent the single most controllable factor influencing our health prospects, accounting for 40 to

Table 16-1 Major Health Domains

Genetic and gestational endowment	30%
Social circumstances	15%
Environmental conditions	5%
Behavior	40%
Medical care	10%

Source: McGinnis, Williams-Russo, and Knickman (2002). Reprinted with permission from Project Hope/Health Affairs Journal.

50% of early deaths among Americans (McGinnis, 2003). Consistent data over the years indicate that 50% of all deaths are likely related to unhealthy lifestyle practices such as smoking, alcohol use, sedentary lifestyle, dietary indiscretions, and maladaptive coping mechanisms (McGinnis & Foege, 1993; U.S. Department of Health, Education, and Welfare, 1979).

Data from the Nurses Health Study (Stampfer, Hu, & Manson et al., 2000) indicate that women who exercise regularly, eat a healthy diet, don't smoke, maintain a proper body weight and drink alcohol moderately have less than 20% the risk of developing heart disease as women who do not subscribe to these lifestyle behaviors. A recent study looking at the decrease in U.S. deaths from coronary disease between 1980 and 2000 also provides evidence for the influence of behavior on health outcomes. Although half of the decline in deaths from coronary disease may be attributable to evidence-based medical therapies, approximately half is also due to reductions in major risk factors (cholesterol, blood pressure, smoking, and physical inactivity); however, the positive influence of risk factor modification is muted by increases in body mass index and the prevalence of type 2 diabetes, both of which are also under the influence of behavior (Ford et al., 2007). Other data extrapolated from the Nurses Health Study (Hu et al., 2003) indicate that both the incidence in obesity and type 2 diabetes are significantly influenced by activity levels: every 2 hour/day increment in television watching is associated with a 23% increase in obesity and a 14% increase in risk of diabetes. In contrast, every 1 hour/day of brisk walking is associated with a 24% reduction in obesity and a 34% reduction in risk of diabetes. It is estimated that 30% of new cases of obesity and 43% of new cases of diabetes could be prevented by watching television less than 10 hours per week and brisk walking at least 30 minutes per day. In addition, data from the Diabetes Prevention Program Research Group (2002) indicates that the effectiveness of lifestyle interventions on decreasing the incidence of type 2 diabetes has been found to be even greater than treatment with an antihyperglycemic agent such as Metformin. The lifestyle choices we make and the behaviors we adopt have the potential to seriously affect our overall health.

Over the past 30 years, the health literature reflects an awareness of the benefits of healthy lifestyle choices and stress management for health promotion and chronic disease prevention. A healthy lifestyle has been defined as the combined effect on health risks and health status of all of those behaviors over which an individual has control (Walker, Sechrist, & Pender, 1987). It combines elements of health protection (prevention), which decreases the individual's chances of encountering illness, and health promotion, which is a positive approach to living that leads individuals toward well-being, not because it will help avoid disease but because it is satisfying and enjoyable (Walker et al., 1987). How individuals view health may influence their willingness to pursue healthy behaviors. Having a personal definition of health as the presence of wellness, including conceptions such as functioning as expected and desired, being flexible with change, and adjusting to life stressors, as opposed to defining health as the absence of illness or symptoms, may increase the likelihood of participating in healthy lifestyles (Pullen, Walker, & Fiandt, 2001).

HEALTHY LIFESTYLE PARADIGMS

Different paradigms of what constitutes a healthy lifestyle have been proposed. Healthy People 2010 identifies 10 health indicators that have the greatest potential to shape the health of the nation (**Table 16-2**).

Improvement in many of these indicators implies collaboration on an individual, community, and national level. Other paradigms propose a network of healthy behaviors that can help patients achieve consistent improve-

---

Table 16-2 Leading Health Indicators

- Physical activity
- Overweight and obesity
- Tobacco use
- Substance abuse
- Responsible sexual behavior
- Mental health
- Injury and violence
- Environmental quality
- Immunization
- Access to health care

Source: Healthy People 2010.

ment in their health. Although the emphasis is on the individual, the relevance of family and community relationships is also indicated.

The circle is an ancient symbol of wholeness. In a holistic (whole-istic) approach to health, one could visualize the components of a healthy lifestyle forming a circle, all intersecting and of equal importance. Two different versions have appeared in the literature, and although they contain similar components, their orientations are slightly different. Together, however, they represent a departure from the biomedically oriented segmented model of what comprises a healthy life in the tables above, encompassing instead a more comprehensive biopsychosocial/spiritual model.

The first model comes from the fitness literature and establishes six dimensions of wellness that could be visualized as spokes of a wheel (**Figure 16-3**).

1. The *physical* dimension suggests regular participation in physical activity, healthy eating, and positive lifestyle choices.
2. The *emotional* dimension involves awareness and acceptance of both positive and negative emotions, developing mind/body awareness through a relaxation/meditation practice, and good communication skills.

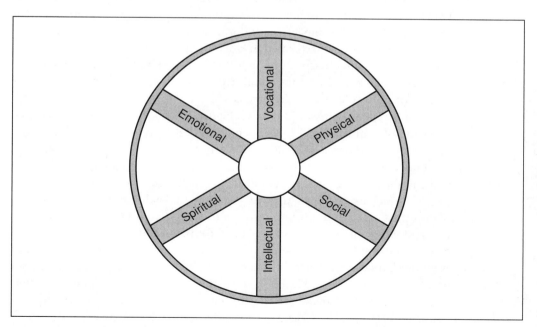

Figure 16-3 Six dimensions of wellness.
Source: Adapted from Armbruster and Gladwin (2001).

3. The *intellectual* dimension challenges the mind to increase knowledge and creativity.

4. The *spiritual* dimension involves a reflection on seeking meaning and purpose in life, understanding and feeling a connectedness to self and others, and focusing on personal values.

5. The *social* dimension suggests maintaining and nuturing healthy relationships with family and the community, at work, and in the healthcare environment.

6. The *vocational* dimension relates to the pursuit of personal interests and growth through work or volunteer activities (Armbruster & Gladwin, 2001; Geithner, Albert, & Vincent, 2007).

Although each individual dimension serves as a vital cog in the wheel of health, they do not exist in isolation and the strength of their overlap creates a state of personal balance and wellness. For example, a meditation practice helps the individual achieve emotional stability and spiritual awareness. Tai Chi and Yoga have significant physical benefits in terms of strength, endurance, flexibility, and balance, but also can be an important component of a meditation practice. Regular exercise has significant cognitive and stress management benefits, influencing both the intellectual and cognitive dimensions, in addition to impact on endurance, strength, and flexibility. All of these activities can be performed in isolation and also in a social group environment, enhancing a sense of connectedness to self and others. A sense of personal balance and rhythm comes from incorporating elements of all six dimensions into lifestyle choices.

The Circle of Human Potentials (**Figure 16-4**) also incorporates a holistic vision of health, but with an orientation that emphasizes the relationship between spirit and choice in lifestyle behavior.

Our continually evolving spiritual development guides the choices we make in the physical, mental, emotional, and relationship dimensions of our lives, helping us to move toward our highest health potential. All areas within the circle are important parts of the self that are constantly interacting, and when one part is not developed to its full potential, then the health of the whole suffers. Life is a biodance, and our bodies are in a constant state of change. In order to move toward our highest health potential, we need to continuously assess our strengths and weaknesses and with that awareness choose to make the changes necessary to move toward health and wholeness (Dossey & Keegan, 2005). To improve that awareness, a self-assessment tool has been developed to help us more clearly identify our cur-

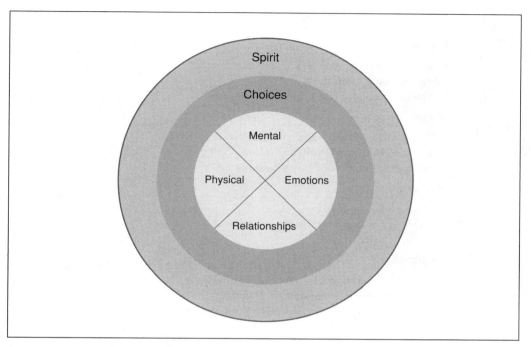

Figure 16-4 Circle of Human Potentials.
Source: Dossey and Keegan (2005). Reprinted with permission from Jones and Bartlett Publishers, Inc.

rent position in each of the six areas (Keegan & Dossey, 2004). Individuals taking the self-assessment questionnaire are asked how strongly they see themselves in relation to different aspects of each potential area. Scores are then generated that give an indication of practicing good life patterns that reflect health and balance (higher score) or being out of balance with life stressors and not taking care of oneself (lower score). **Table 16-3** provides samples of topics for scoring.

Assessing our human potential increases our awareness of what we need to improve our health. With awareness of our mind–body–spirit relationships, we have more control over the lifestyle choices we make.

A useful clinical tool for looking at lifestyle behaviors is the Health-Promoting Lifestyle Profile (HPLP) developed by Walker et al. (1987). It identifies six dimensions of a health-promoting lifestyle, including spiritual growth, health responsibility, interpersonal support, and stress management,

Table 16-3 Self-Assessments Topics

Physical

- Exercise three to five times a week for 20 minutes.
- Eat nutritious foods daily.
- Practice meditation daily.

Mental

- Am open and receptive to new ideas and life patterns.
- Enjoy developing new skills and talents.
- Ask for suggestions and help when I need it.

Emotions

- Have a nonjudgmental attitude.
- Listen to and respect the feelings of others.
- Listen to inner self-talk.

Relationships

- Create and participate in satisfying relationships.
- Have a balance between work and family life.
- Am open and honest with people without fearing the consequences.

Choices

- Manage my time to meet my personal goals.
- Take on no more new tasks than I can successfully handle.
- Can accept circumstances that are beyond my control.

Spirit

- Know at some level a connection with the universe.
- Know how to create balance and feel a sense of connectedness.
- Know that life is important and I make a difference.

Source: Adapted from Keegan and Dossey (2004).

along with exercise and nutrition. In a sense, it reflects an individual's desire to change behavior because he or she wants to, not because he or she has to—a move toward realizing his or her highest health potential as opposed to a move away from the risk of disease. The behavior is grounded in self-awareness, well-being, and personal fulfillment. Similar in scope to the circle paradigm, it incorporates measures of feeling good about self and life, having a sense of purpose, paying attention to and accepting responsibility for one's own health, being educated about health, accessing social support and managing life's stressors, doing regular exercise, and making healthy nutrition choices. The HPLP II (Walker & Hill-Polerecky, unpublished manuscript) is a revised 52-item questionnaire that employs a 4-point rating scale, from 1 = never to 4 = routinely, and continues to measure the frequency of each of the six dimensions. The questionnaire can be given pre- and post-intervention (i.e., a program like the CWP at the Benson-Henry Institute) to determine program outcome data relative to the shifts in an individual's participation in health-promoting behaviors. Permission for use of the instrument can be obtained through the University of Nebraska Medical Center College of Nursing and once granted includes copies of the instrument and scoring instructions (contact Susan Noble Walker, EdD, RN, 600 South 42nd Street, Omaha, NE 68198-5330).

Case Study 16-2

Bob is a 60 year old with a long history of heart disease; his first myocardial infarction was in 1994, and his second myocardial infarction and three-vessel coronary artery bypass graft were in January 2002. When he came to the CWP in January of 2007, he still had hypertension despite medications, and he was still smoking. He had quit at the time of his coronary artery bypass graft but had started smoking again a couple years after. He considered himself an alcoholic, recently sober, going to AA. Six months before coming to the CWP he had started psychotherapy as he began to realize that he was not happy and felt stuck in old habits. His approach to life had always been to control and change other people and his environment to make himself happy, and he self-medicated (alcohol) to numb his response to stress. As he described himself, "I'm a kid from the projects; what do I know about emotions and self-awareness?" Through therapy he began to explore the relationship between emotions and behavior. He began to realize that he could not change others, only himself, and that his happiness depended on increasing self-awareness and self-change. His therapist suggested he come to the CWP for further support in gaining self awareness and changing behaviors. Bob was already exercising fairly regularly, but was interested in the social support of the group, stress management, and nutrition. Just before beginning the group, he started taking an antidepressant, and he identified the day he would quit smoking as the day he started the program.

An indication of the significant change Bob made in the program is reflected in his pre- and postprogram HPLP II scores:

	Pre	Post
Spiritual growth	1.67	4.00
Health responsibility	1.78	3.67
Exercise	2.75	3.50
Nutrition	2.44	3.78
Social support	2.22	3.89
Stress management	1.75	4.00

Bob felt strongly that daily elicitation of the relaxation response (meditation CD and breath focus), and challenging his negative thinking (cognitive restructuring) really helped to increase his self-awareness and keep him in the present, focusing on what he needed for self-care. The significant increase in his scores certainly reflects a greater sense of self-care and personal responsibility for his health. He felt confident leaving the program that he would remain smoke and alcohol free, while continuing with meditation, exercise, and healthy eating. Not bad for a kid from the projects!

COMPONENTS OF A HEALTHY LIFESTYLE

Exercise and nutrition have been consistently recognized as playing a major role in promoting health and decreasing the incidence of morbidity and mortality from chronic disease: heart disease, diabetes, cancer, and obesity. They appear in all of the paradigms of health noted previously.

"If exercise could be put in a pill, it would be the most widely prescribed medicine in the world."

Dr. Robert N. Butler, National Institute on Aging

Much has been written on what to do for exercise and what to eat, but the basic recommendations for these two self-care practices to insure good health benefits are actually quite simple:

- *Exercise/physical activity.* All adults should accumulate at least 30 minutes of moderately brisk physical activity most or all days of the week (daily activities—housework and yard work, organized exercise, and sports and recreation) to gain a basic health benefit; 45 to 90 minutes (60 minutes on average), or roughly 10,000 steps per day, for weight maintenance/weight loss. For cardiovascular fitness, the recommendation is 20 to 60 minutes of moderate to high-intensity endurance exercise for three to five times per week. Exercise for muscular strength and flexibility, two other components of fitness, is also recommended two to three times per week in order to preserve performance of every day tasks, prevent injury, and avoid disability (Howley, Bassett, & Thompson, 2005; Institute of Medicine, 2002; Pate et al., 1995; Thompson, Rakow & Perdue, 2004; U.S. DHHS, 2000).
- *Nutrition.* All standard diet recommendations seem to be converging with an emphasis on lots of fruits and vegetables, whole-grain products, nuts and seeds, lean sources of protein, non-fat or low-fat dairy products, healthy

fats (monounsaturated fats and sources of omega 3 fatty acids); limited sources of sweets, processed foods, and saturated and trans-fats (Ard et al., 2000; Dietary Guidelines Advisory Committee, 2004; Willett, 2001).

Managing life's stressors is also beginning to appreciate significant recognition as a cornerstone of a balanced, healthy lifestyle. Studies demonstrate links between chronic stress and indices of poor health, including risk factors for heart disease, onset of myocardial infarction, and compromised immune function (Epel et al., 2004; Kubzansky, 2007; McEwen, 1998). Mind/body practices such as cognitive therapy (Wells-Federman, Stuart-Shor, & Webster, 2001), accessing social support (Frasure-Smith et al., 2000; Pengilly & Dowd, 2000), meditation practices (Bonadonna, 2003; Oman, Hedberg, & Thorensen, 2006), and spirituality (Burkhardt & Nagai-Jacobson, 2005; Kass et al., 1991) have all been shown to counter the negative health effects of stress and have a positive effect on health outcomes. Exercise (Lawlor & Hopker, 2001; Scully et al., 1998) and nutrition (Nieman, 2006) are also important players in modifying the negative effects of stress. The mind/body exercise practices of yoga, tai chi, and pilates are especially effective in providing health benefits across the biopsychosocial/spiritual continuum (Brown & Gerberg, 2005; LaForge, 2005). Not only do they help to increase strength, flexibility, endurance, and balance, but they also strengthen the mind/body connection and self-awareness, thereby helping individuals transition to healthier life choices. With increased awareness comes a sense of control; having more control leads to an ability to make healthier choices.

> "Yoga goes to the roots of a poor lifestyle, and when presented in a comprehensive manner, tends to convince the patient that a good lifestyle is not only healthier, but also more enjoyable than a poor lifestyle. If patients introduce lifestyle changes because they want to, rather than because they have to, the changes are less likely to be stressful."
>
> Deepak Chopra

AGING GRACEFULLY

Impacting the aging process is an area of interest in health promotion and disease prevention. We are concerned with living longer and living better. There is an association between health-promoting lifestyle practices and survival and health status in later years, suggesting that lifestyle may influence quality as well as length of life. Unhealthy practices and chronic diseases such as smoking, physical inactivity, hypertension, and obesity have been shown to result in a loss of life expectancy anywhere from 2 to 8 years (Franco et al., 2005; Nieman, 2007). In a prospective population study of over 20,000 men and women, the combined effect of four health behaviors (not smoking, physical activity, moderate alcohol intake and consumption of at least five fruits and vegetables per day) compared to zero health behaviors, predicted a fourfold difference in mortality, equivalent to fourteen years in chronological age (Khaw et al., 2008).

What about stress? Does it also influence the aging process? It has often been observed that people who suffer from significant life stressors look haggard and older than their chronological age. Both internal and external stress may play a role in the aging process.

Oxidation is a natural physiologic process that takes place as we breathe at rest and during physical activity. A consequence of oxidation is the formation of unstable oxygen particles called free radicals. Over time, the damage caused by free radicals promotes chronic disease and accelerates aging, especially in people who are obese, smoke, and consume low levels of fruits and vegetables. Fortunately, even though aerobic exercise produces oxidative stress, it also stimulates improved antioxidant defenses; the more physically fit you are, the stronger your antioxidant defenses. The effectiveness of exercise as an antioxidant therapy is so strong that it can help counter the negative effects of oxidative stress on heart disease and aging (Kojda & Hambrecht, 2005; Nieman, 2007). In addition, the foods we consume also play a role in providing defense against oxidative stress. Diets rich in fruits and vegetables, whole grains, and nuts and seeds provide an abundance of antioxidants and phytochemicals that have health-protective effects and may also help prevent chronic disease and premature aging (Nieman, 2007; Powers, DeRuisseau, & Quindry, 2004).

A link between psychological stress and aging may also have been found. Telomeres are protective caps at the end of chromosomes in cells. Chromosomes carry genetic information and the telomeres protect the ends of chromosomes from fraying (like the tips on the end of shoelaces). Telomerase is an enzyme that helps to rebuild telomeres and protects the chromosomes when they get worn down. As we age, the telomeres slowly wear down. Laboratory studies have shown that psychological stress ages cells, as measured by the shortening of the telomeres. Epel at al. (2004) demonstrated that women with the highest levels of perceived stress (care giving mothers of chronically ill children) have telomeres shorter on average, which correlates with 1 decade of additional aging, compared with women with lower levels of perceived stress. A sedentary lifestyle may also accelerate the aging process. In a study by Cherkas et al. (2008), the difference in telomere length between most and least physically active individuals, suggests that inactive individuals may be biologically ten years older than those who are more active. In addition, low telomerase activity has been found to be associated with a cardiovascular disease risk profile that resembles the profile of metabolic syndrome (poor lipid profile, high systolic blood pressure, high fasting glucose, abdominal obesity, and smoking) (Epel et al., 2006). There is a bidirectional mind–body connection, and the lifestyle practices we choose to employ can have a significant impact on our overall health and how we move through the aging process. For websites and resources that provide extensive information on the benefits and recommendations for practice of various lifestyle interventions, please see Appendix 16-1.

SUMMARY

Although one of the major achievements of our healthcare system in the last century is the recognition of risk factors in the etiology of disease, prevention seems to rank below intervention within the medical system hierarchy. The orientation of our healthcare system is more toward an emphasis on treating disease rather than maintaining or promoting health. Insurance companies are more inclined to cover the costs of expensive interventions and medications than nutrition counseling and fitness programs; physician counseling on healthy lifestyle behaviors is inconsistent and questionably effective, often because of lack of time and lack of confidence in the effectiveness of counseling, and patients often lack the motivation and/or knowledge necessary to initiate and sustain behavior change (Bartlett, 2003; Eden et al., 2002; Ribeiro, Martins, & Carvalho, 2007). Most individuals view their primary care physician as their primary source of healthcare information, but if physicians are not providing counseling on healthy behaviors, patients may think that it really must not be that important (Bartlett, 2003). It is recommended that doctors and healthcare professionals include such counseling as part of medical visits (Healthy People 2010). In addition, we live in an environment that is not conducive to supporting good health. We are bombarded with advertisements for fast and processed foods. We have industrialized most of the physical activity out of our lives, and we seem to have forgotten how to relax; even when we go on vacation, the expectation is that we are accessible to work and home 24/7 with our laptops, Blackberries, and cell phones;

however, these are barriers that can be overcome. HealthierUS and Healthy People 2010 have established prevention and making healthy choices as two of the pillars (along with nutrition and physical fitness) to help people live longer and healthier lives. It is this attitude of prevention and fostering healthy lifestyle behaviors that we as healthcare professionals can bring to our interactions with patients to help shift their attitudes about taking responsibility for their own health. The more individuals begin to appreciate the benefits of self-care, the faster the population as a whole will move toward a healthcare philosophy of prevention and wellness, but engaging individuals to think in terms of prevention and making lifestyle choices that will improve their health and decrease their risk of disease is not easy. The following chapter focuses on the process of behavior change that facilitates the shift into self-care and movement toward the individual's highest health potential.

REFERENCES

Abramson, J. (2004). *Overdosed America*. New York: Harper Collins.

Ard, J. D., Svetkey, L. P., LaChance, P., & Bray, G. (2000). Lowering blood pressure using a dietary pattern: a review of the dietary approaches to stop hypertension (DASH) trial. *Journal of Clinical Hypertension, 2*, 387–391.

Armbruster, B., & Gladwin, L. A. (2001). More than fitness for older adults. *ACSMs Health and Fitness Journal, 5*, 6–12.

Bartlett, S. J. (2003). Motivating patients toward weight loss: practical strategies for addressing overweight and obesity. *Physician and Sportsmedicine, 31*, 29–36, 47–48.

Bonadonna, R. (2003). Meditation's impact on chronic illness. *Holistic Nursing Practice, 17*, 309–319.

Brown, R. P., & Gerbarg, P. L. (2005). Sudarshan Kriya yogic breathing in the treatment of stress, anxiety and depression: Part II—clinical applications and guidelines. *Journal of Complementary Medicine, 11*, 711–717.

Burkhardt, M. A., & Nagai-Jacobson, M. G. (2005). Spirituality and health. In B. M. Dossey, L. Keegan, & C. E. Guzzetta (Eds.), *Holistic nursing: a handbook for practice* (pp. 137–172). Sudbury, MA: Jones and Bartlett.

Canto, J. G., Allison, J. J., & Keefe, C. I. (2000). Relation of race and sex to the use of reperfusion therapy in Medicare beneficiaries with acute myocardial infarction. *New England Journal of Medicine, 342*, 1094–1100.

Cherkas, L. F., Hunkin, J. L., Kato, B. S., Richards, J. B., Gardner, J. P., & Surdulescu, G. L., et al. (2008). The association between physical activity in leisure time and leukocyte telomere length. *Archives of Internal Medicine, 168*, 154–158.

Clancy, C. (2007). How do we involve patients in their own healthcare decisions? *Medscape General Medicine, 9*(4), 46. Retrieved November 30, 2007, from http://www.medscape.com/viewarticle/565951.

Diabetes Prevention Program Research Group. (2002). Reduction in the incidence of type II diabetes with lifestyle intervention or metformin. *New England Journal of Medicine, 346,* 393–403.

Dietary Guidelines Advisory Committee. (2005). *Backgrounder 2005 dietary guidelines advisory committee report.* Retrieved November 29, 2004, from http://www.health.gov/dietaryguidelines/dga2005/Backgrounder.htm.

Dossey, B. M., & Keegan, L. (2005). Self-assessments: facilitating healing in self and others. In B. M. Dossey, L. Keegan, & C. E. Guzzetta (Eds.), *Holistic nursing: a handbook for practice* (pp. 379–393). Sudbury, MA: Jones and Bartlett.

Eden, K. B., Orleans, C. T., Mulrow, C. D., Pender, N. J., & Teutsch, S. M. (2002). Does counseling by clinicians improve physical activity? A summary of the evidence for the U.S. preventive services task force. *Annals of Internal Medicine, 137,* 205–207.

Epel, E. S., Blackburn, E. H., Lin, J., Dhabhar, F. S., Adler, N. E., & Morrow, J. D., et al. (2004). Accelerated telomere shortening in response to life stress. *Proceedings of the National Academy of Sciences of the United States of America, 101,* 17312–17315.

Epel, E. S., Lin, J., Wilhelm, F. H., Wolkowitz, O. M., Cawthon, R., & Adler, N. E., et al. (2006). Cell aging in relation to stress arousal and cardiovascular disease risk factors. *Psychoneuroendocrinology, 31,* 277–287.

Ford, E. S., Ajani, U. A., Croft, J. B., Critchley, J. A., Labarthe, D. R., & Kottke, T. E., et al. (2007). Explaining the decrease in U.S. deaths from coronary disease, 1980–2000. *New England Journal of Medicine, 356,* 2388–2398.

Franco, O., Peeters, A., Bonneux, L., & de Laet, C. (2005). Blood pressure in adulthood and life expectancy with cardiovascular disease in men and women. *Hypertension, 46,* 280–286.

Frasure-Smith, N., Lesperance, F., Gravel, G., Masson, A., Martin, J., & Talajic, M., et al. (2000). Social support, depression, and mortality during the first year after myocardial infarction. *Circulation, 101,* 1919–1924.

Geithner, C. A., Albert, J. F., & Vincent, B. S. (2007). Personal balance: its importance and how to achieve it. *ACSMs Health and Fitness Journal, 11,* 7–14.

Greiner, P. A., & Edelman, C. L. (2006). Health defined: objectives for promotion and prevention. In C. L. Edelman & C. L. Mandle (Eds.), *Health promotion throughout the life span* (pp. 3–22). St. Louis: Mosby.

Howley, E. T., Bassett, D. R., & Thompson, D. L. (2005). Get them moving: balancing weight with physical activity, part II. *ACSMs Health and Fitness Journal, 9,* 19–24.

Hu, F. B., Li, T. Y., Colditz, G. A., Willett, W. C., & Manson, J. E. (2003). Television watching and other sedentary behaviors in relation to risk of obesity and type II diabetes mellitus in women. *Journal of the American Medical Association, 289,* 1785–1791.

Institute of Medicine. (2002). *Dietary reference intakes for energy, carbohydrate, fiber, fat, fatty acids, cholesterol, protein, and amino acids.* Washington, DC: National Academies Press.

Kass, J., Friedman, R., Lesserman, J., Zuttermeister, P. C., & Benson, H. (1991). Health outcomes and a new index of spiritual experience. *Journal for the Scientific Study of Religion, 30,* 203–211.

Keegan, L., & Dossey, B. M. (2004). *Self-care: a program to improve your life.* Port Angeles, WA: Holistic Nursing Consultants.

Khaw, K-T., Wareham, N., Bingham, S., Welch, A., Luben, R., & Day, N. (2008). Combined impact of health behaviours and mortality in men and women: the EPIC-Norfolk prospective population study. *PLoS Medicine, 5,* 0001–0008.

Kojda, G., & Hambrecht, R. (2005). Molecular mechanisms of vascular adaptation to exercise: physical activity as an effective anti-oxidant therapy? *Cardiovascular Research, 67,* 187–197.

Kubzansky, L. D. (2007). Sick at heart: the pathophysiology of negative emotions. *Cleveland Clinic Journal of Medicine, 74,* S67–S72.

LaForge, R. (2005). Aligning mind and body: exploring the disciplines of mindful exercise. *ACSMs Health and Fitness Journal, 9,* 7–14.

Lawlor, D. A., & Hopker, S. W. (2001). The effectiveness of exercise as an intervention in the management of depression: systematic review and meta regression analysis of randomized controlled studies. *British Medical Journal, 322,* 763–767.

McEwen, B. S. (1998). Protective and damaging effects of stress mediators. *New England Journal of Medicine, 338,* 171–179.

McGinnis, J. M. (2003). A vision for health in our new century. *American Journal of Health Promotion, 18,* 146–149.

McGinnis, J. M., & Foege, W. (1993). Actual causes of death in the U.S. *Journal of the American Medical Association, 270,* 2207–2211.

McGinnis, J. M., Williams-Russo, P., & Knickman, J. R. (2002). The case for more active policy attention to health promotion. *Health Affairs, 21,* 78–93.

National Center for Complementary and Alternative Medicine. (2005). *What is complementary and alternative medicine (CAM).* Retrieved May 23, 2008, from http://nccam.nih.gov/health/whatiscam/.

Nieman, D. C. (2006). Nutritional strategies to counter stress to the immune system. *ACSMs Health and Fitness Journal, 10*(6), 15–20.

Nieman, D. C. (2007). You asked for it: question authority. *ACSMs Health and Fitness Journal, 11*(4), 5–6.

Oman, D., Hedberg, J., & Thorensen, C. (2006). Passage meditation reduces perceived stress in health professionals: a randomized controlled trial. *Journaling of Consulting and Clinical Psychology, 74,* 714–719.

Pate, R. R., Pratt, M., Blair, S. N., Haskell, W. L., Macera, C. A., & Bouchard, C., et al. (1995). Physical activity and public health. *Journal of the American Medical Association, 273,* 402–407.

Pengilly, J. W., & Dowd, E. T. (2000). Hardiness and social support as moderators of stress. *Journal of Clinical Psychology, 56,* 813–820.

Powers, S. K., DeRuisseau, K. C., & Quindry, J. (2004). Dietary anti-oxidants and exercise. *Journal of Sports Medicine, 22,* 81–94.

Pullen, C., Walker, S. N., & Fiandt, K. (2001). Determinants of health-promoting lifestyle behaviors in rural older women. *Family and Community Health, 24,* 49–72.

Ribeiro, M. A., Martins, A., & Carvalho, C. (2007). The role of physician counseling in improving adherence to physical activity among the general population. *Sao Paulo Medical Journal, 125,* 115–121.

Scully, D., Kremer, J., Meade, M., Graham, R., & Dudgeon, K. (1998). Physical exercise and psychological well-being: a critical review. *British Journal of Sports Medicine, 32,* 111–120.

Stampfer, M. J., Hu, F. B., Manson, J. E., Rimm, E. B., & Willett, W. C. (2000). Primary prevention of coronary heart disease in women through diet and lifestyle. *New England Journal of Medicine, 343,* 16–22.

Thompson, D. L., Rakow, J., & Perdue, S. M. (2004). Relationship between accumulated walking and body composition in middle-aged women. *Medicine and Science in Sports and Exercise, 36,* 911–914.

U.S. Department of Health and Human Services. (1990). *Healthy People 2000: national health promotion and disease prevention objectives.* Washington, DC: U.S. Department of Health and Human Services.

U.S. Department of Health and Human Services. (2000). *Healthy People 2010: understanding and improving health.* Washington, DC: U.S. Department of Health and Human Services.

U.S. Department of Health, Education, and Welfare. (1979). *Healthy People: The Surgeon General's report on health promotion and disease prevention.* Washington, DC: Public Health Service. PHS Publication 79-55071.

Walker, S. N., Sechrist, K. R., & Pender, N. J. (1987). The health-promoting lifestyle profile: development and psychometric characteristics. *Nursing Research, 36,* 76–81.

Wells-Federman, C., Stuart-Shor, E., & Webster, A. (2001). Cognitive therapy: applications for health promotion, disease prevention, and disease management. *Nursing Clinics of North America, 36,* 93–113.

Willett, W. C. (2001). *Eat, drink and be healthy.* New York: Free Press.

APPENDIX 16-1

RESOURCE LIST

Exercise

http://www.nhlbi.nih.gov/health/public/heart/obesity/phy_active.htm

http://www.acefitness.org (American Council on Exercise)

http://www.nlm.gov/medlineplus/exerciseandphysicalfitness.html

http://www.mayoclinic.com/health/exercise/HQ01676

http://www.womenshealth.gov/faq/exercise.htm (from USDHHS)

http://www.diabetes.org/weightloss-and-exercise/exercise/overview.jsp

http://www.strongwomen.com

Exercise: a guide from the national institute of aging. Publication #NIH 98-4258; 800-222-2225: http://www.nia.nih.gov.

Nutrition

http://www.tcme.org/downloads/principles_handout_1_22.pdf

http://www.health.gov/dietaryguidelines/dga2005/recommendations.htm

http://mypyramid.gov

http://www.nhlbi/nih.gove/health/public/heart/hbp/dash/new-dash.pdf (DASH diet)

http://www.oldwayspt.org (Mediterranean diet and pyramid)

Willett, W. C. (2001). *Eat, drink, and be healthy.* New York: Free Press (includes Healthy Eating Pyramid).

http://www.health.harvard.edu/books/Eat_Drink_and_Be_Healthy.htm

http://www.ewg.org (organic vs. conventional)

Center for Science in the Public Interest. *Nutrition action health letter.* 1875 Connecticut Ave., N.W., Suite 300, Washington, DC, 20009.

www.cspinet.org.

Relaxation Response/Meditation

Van Dixhoorn, J., & White, A. (2005). Relaxation therapy for rehabilitation and prevention in ischemic heart disease: a systematic review and meta-analysis. *European Journal of Cardiovascular Prevention and Rehabilitation, 12,* 193–202.

Fontana, D. (1999). *Learn to meditate: a practical guide to self-discovery and fulfillment.* San Francisco: Chronicle Books.

Roche, L. (1998). *Meditation made easy.* San Francisco: Harper Collins.

Benson, H. (1975). *The relaxation response.* New York: William Morrow.

Yoga/Tai Chi

www.yogajournal.com

http://americanyogaassociation.org

Cook, J. Not all yoga is created equal. Retrieved May 23, 2008, from http://yogajournal.com/newtoyoga/165.cfm

Shaw, B. (2001). *Beth Shaw's YogaFit*. Champaign, IL: Human Kinetics.

Anderson, S., & Sovik, R. (2000) *Yoga: mastering the basics*. Honesdale, PA: The Himalayan Institute.

http://nccam.nih.gov/health/taichi

http://www.mayoclinic.com/health/tai-chi/SA00087

Li, J. X., Hong, Y., & Chan, K. M. (2001). Tai chi: physiological characteristics and beneficial effects on health. *British Journal of Sports Medicine, 35,* 148–156.

Chewning, B., Yu, T., & Johnson, J. (March/April, May/June 2000). Tai Chi (parts I and II; ancient exercise for contemporary life, and effects on health). *ACSMs Health and Fitness Journal, 4,* 17–19, 21–26; 28.

Rones, R. (2007). *Sunrise tai chi: simplified tai chi for health and longevity.* Boston: YMMA Publication Center.

Spiritual

http://spiritualityandpractice.com

http://spiritualityhealth.com/newsh/item/home/item_216.html

Burkhardt, M. A., & Nagai-Jacobson, M. G. (2005). Spirituality and health. In B. M. Dossey, L. Keegan, & C. E. Guzzetta (Eds.), *Holistic nursing: a handbook for practice* (pp. 137–172). Sudbury, MA: Jones and Bartlett.

Psychosocial

Underwood, A. The good heart. Retrieved May 23, 2008, from http://www.msnbc.msn.com/id/9467735/site/newsweek/print/1/displaymode/1098.

Rozanski, A., Blumenthal, J. A., Davidson, K. W., Saab, P. G., & Kubzansky, L. (2005). The epidemiology, pathophysiology, and management of psychosocial risk factors in cardiac practice: the emerging field of behavioral cardiology. *Journal of the American College of Cardiology, 45,* 637–651.

Kabat-Zinn, J. (1994). *Wherever you go there you are: mindfulness meditation in everyday life.* New York: Hyperion.

Burns, D. (1993). *Ten days to self-esteem: the leader's manual.* New York: William Morrow.

Burns, D. (1999). *The feeling good handbook.* New York: Plume (Penguin Group).

Meichenbaum, D. (1993). Changing conceptions of cognitive behavior modifications: retrospect and prospect. *Journal of Clinical Psychology, 61,* 202–204.

Meichenbaum, D. (1999). *Cognitive behavior modification: an integrative approach.* New York: Perseus Press.

Beck, J. (2007). *The Beck diet solution.* Birmingham, Alabama: Oxmoor House.

Frederickson, B. L. (2004). The broaden-and-build theory of positive emotions. *Philosophical Transactions of the Royal Society of London, Series B, 359,* 1367–1377.

Other General Sources

www.americanheart.org/presenter.jhtml?identifier=1200009

www.healthierus.gov

Casey, A., & Benson, H. (2004). *Mind your heart: a mind/body approach to stress management, exercise and nutrition for heart health.* New York: Free Press.

Casey, A., & Benson, H. (2006). *The Harvard Medical School guide to lowering your blood pressure.* New York: McGraw-Hill.

Chapter 17

Health Promotion
and Behavior Change

James S. Huddleston

> *Habit is a habit and not to be flung out of a window by any man, but coaxed*
> *downstairs a step at a time.*
>
> —Mark Twain

INTRODUCTION

In the previous chapter, we discussed health promotion and wellness and
how self-care impacts the health of the individual. In a medical culture that
emphasizes treating illness rather than preventing illness, it is often difficult
to facilitate a paradigm shift in which individuals assume more responsibility for their own health and begin to make the change to more healthful
behaviors. Changing behaviors is complex and challenging. Habits develop
over time under the influence of beliefs, attitudes, and life experiences, and
it takes time and commitment to change those behaviors so that they
become ingrained as part of self-identity. Although this chapter deals most
specifically with individual behavior change, individuals do not exist in isolation, and their interaction with the environment and community play a

role in the success of that change. The behavior change process may involve elements of behavioral theory (goal setting and reinforcement), constructivism (cognitive approach to learning and reflection on life experiences, attitudes, and beliefs), readiness to change, and social ecology (shared social and cultural influences of family, friends, community, institutions, and public policy) (Lund, Carruth, Moody, & Logan, 2005). As healthcare providers effecting behavior change, we need to provide knowledge, help develop skills, facilitate attitude shifts, and create positive therapeutic relationships. It is within a successful therapeutic relationship that a plan of action for change, which best fits into the life of the patient, can be mutually established.

Case Study 17-1

Sam is a 50-year-old dairy farmer. He is married and has an 18-year-old son. Family and work life center around the farm; social activities generally involve other farm families. The family's dietary habits lean heavily toward dairy and animal products high in saturated fats. At a recent health screening, Sam was found to have a BMI of more than 30 (obesity), a waist circumference of more than 40 inches, a total cholesterol of 248, and hypertension. He also acknowledged high stress levels from working long hours and economic concerns. Sam was aware that his profile increased his risk of heart disease, and although he was willing to take an antihypertension medication, he was not motivated to change activity or eating habits; however, Sam's wife Janet expressed concern over both Sam's and their son Ted's risk (overweight with high cholesterol) and was more open to exploring avenues of change. Although instructing Sam to change his diet and increase his daily activity might seem like the best plan to decrease his risk, this was not the best plan for Sam. Mutual goal setting would not be effective because he was not ready to change; however, providing educational material about the benefits and risks of certain behaviors would help raise his awareness and begin to provoke some self-assessment. Janet provided good support and was open to suggestions on modifying the family's eating habits. Over time, Sam became more invested in the possibility of making some changes, but it was a slow process, as he had to reflect on his beliefs and attitudes about his farm lifestyle and eating habits that seemed comfortable after all of this time. In meeting with his healthcare team at the local health clinic, he acknowledged that he would need a lot of structure to help him make changes. Specific goals related to weight loss (1 to 2 pounds a week) through dietary changes and increasing physical activity were set, along with rewards (a dessert of his choice if he met his weekly goal) and consequences (no dessert) for positive and negative reinforcement. Friends also provided some support. Wives in the community shared recipe modifications (successes and failures), and the health clinic provided educational seminars on heart health-related topics at the various social organization meetings in town. It would be interesting to see what the long-term outcome for Sam and his family would be, but it is evident that his success depends on his own behaviors, his willingness to reflect on his values and beliefs, his readiness to change and the social supports available to him.

Adapted from Lund et al., 2005.

FACILITATING BEHAVIOR CHANGE

The case of Sam is a good example of the complexity in facilitating behavior change. It reflects the evidence that individuals are more successful making lifestyle changes with the ongoing support of healthcare providers and/or community programs that provide ongoing support, than with counseling performed in physician offices (Eden et al., 2002). Counseling for disease prevention and health promotion is a complex process that incorporates different theoretical perspectives, techniques, and behaviors. It involves skill and motivation on the part of both the practitioner and the patient. It is a real challenge for healthcare providers to motivate and facilitate behavior change. Our role must include an understanding of the interpersonal skills that can be used to motivate individuals toward optimal health (Shinitzky & Kub, 2001). We need to shift away from being the authoritative expert who simply provides information and instruction to a client toward being a facilitator of health behavior change. Combining educational and behavioral strategies to increase client's knowledge and improve adherence to prevention or therapeutic regimes has been shown to have a higher success rate than educational strategies alone (Burke & Fair, 2003; National Cancer Institute, 2005).

It is generally accepted that health behavior change is a critical component in health and well-being, and there is growing evidence that similar factors also play an important role in rehabilitation outcomes (Chen, Neufeld, Feely, & Skinner, 1999). Besides the behavior of the healthcare provider, several other themes are prevalent in the rehabilitation literature related to health behavior change:

1. *Prevention* relates to behaviors that lead to health promotion and well-being and the primary prevention of disease, disorder, and injury.
2. *Early detection* involves behaviors related to addressing health issues possibly already present.
3. *Self-management* reflects the concepts of monitoring behaviors associated with a chronic health condition or disability; softening the impact of

long-term disease, and disability and impairments, and minimizing suffering and maximizing years of useful life.

4. *Treatment adherence* relates to the effectiveness of the provider/patient interface, based on patient readiness to change, and an intervention developed to match patient intention, thereby increasing its impact and effectiveness (Nieuwenhuijsen, Zemper, Miner, & Epstein, 2006).

These themes compare favorably with the integration of health behavior change factors discussed earlier: interpersonal, intrapersonal, community, and policy. There is an important role for the rehabilitation specialist along the disease prevention–health promotion–rehabilitation continuum (Frey, Szalda-Petree, Traci, & Seekins, 2001; Martin & Fell, 1999). Healing, in the truest sense of the word, depends on the recognition and acceptance of this role.

Case Study 17-2

The case of Mr. John R. is a good example of the continuum between health promotion and rehabilitation. John is a 29-year-old black male who was referred to physical therapy after his third visit to urgent care in the past 9 months complaining of neck and right shoulder pain. Similar to his other appearances in urgent care, he was only interested in getting another prescription of NSAIDS for his pain, but reluctantly agreed to therapy, when the nurse practitioner strongly suggested that he needed to treat the cause of his pain and not just the symptoms. His past medical history includes hypertension, overweight, sedentary lifestyle, current smoker and a family history of CAD.

At his initial evaluation, John appeared tired, slouching in his chair, with rounded shoulders and forward head posture. He shared that he works in the high tech industry, doing a lot of computer work. He has worked a lot of overtime the past 3 weeks because of project deadlines and an upcoming performance review. During this time, the pain in his neck and shoulder has worsened, especially with reaching for items on shelves or behind him. He also shared that he has been separated from his wife for the past year and rarely saw his two children and other family members, even though they all lived locally. His diet consists of "fast food on the run," and he does minimal physical activity. He sleeps about 6 hours per night with one or two early morning awakenings.

It is evident that John's chief complaint is neck and shoulder pain and physical therapy evaluation and treatment will help alleviate his pain and improve function in the short term; however, if the therapeutic interaction and intervention stops there, what is the likelihood of long term success and healing? Based on the holistic models of health discussed in the previous chapter, John's life is out of balance. Consequently, not only does he face a reoccurrence of his pain, but he also is putting himself at risk for significant health problems. How can we as healthcare providers help to increase his awareness of the need to change behaviors, move him along the continuum of readiness to change, and facilitate the change process?

Unsuccessful Provider/Client Exchange

PT: John, from what you have told me about your pain, what do you think might have contributed to it?

John: Probably all of the work I have been doing on the computer. I thought that just taking some pain medication would solve the problem, but as we have talked during the evaluation I can see that how I use my body at work probably has a lot to do with it.

PT: That's true, and we will spend some time doing some exercises to help with posture and will also take a look at your work station to make it physically easier for you to do your job, but you know, based on your history of pain, I think your lifestyle is contributing to your problem.

John: What do you mean "my lifestyle"?

PT: Well, you seem to be under a lot of stress and if you stopped smoking, started exercising and eating better, and taking some time to relax during the day you would feel a lot better.

John: I don't think so. None of that has anything to do with my shoulder pain.

Rationale

John is unaware of his need to change and is not ready to change. His resistance increases as the provider tries to push him into change. It is true that he would benefit from changing behaviors, but the judgmental, confrontational tone of the provider prevents them from engaging in problem-solving opportunities together. It is easy to feel overwhelmed when multiple areas for change are targeted simultaneously.

Successful Provider/Client Exchange

PT: John, based on your pain symptoms and the pressures at work, I wonder if all of the stress is contributing to the reoccurrences of your pain and your general fatigue level. You might want to think about the potential impact of so much stress on your overall health.

John: I never really gave it much thought. Things are pretty crazy right now, and I don't feel like I have time for anything but work; so you might be right.

PT: Would you be interested in maybe learning a few small activities that you could easily build into your day that might help decrease the stress?

John: Well, maybe one or two, but you know I don't have much free time. If I had more energy during the day, it might be easier.

PT: What do you think would help you feel more energetic?

John: I used to be pretty active and when I was doing more exercise I slept a lot better, and I didn't seem to feel as tired or stressed during the day.

PT: Both exercise and practicing relaxation techniques can help improve sleep and decrease stress. You have mentioned how important work is to you, and we have identified that both exercise and relaxation could help you to work more effectively. If you could begin to work on one of these areas, which would you choose?

John: I have some experience with exercise so that might be easier to start with.

PT: Great, let's talk about some easy ways you can begin to build some exercise into your day.

Rationale

In this scenario, the PT demonstrates genuine interest in John and engages him in a partnership in making treatment decisions. In this patient-centered interaction, the PT actively listens to John, respects his values and beliefs, and helps guide him into an increased awareness about his lifestyle and its impact on his health. Even though the therapist may have ideas on what the best course of treatment might be, allowing option development without judgment is crucial to successful negotiation and moving the patient along in his openness to change. Limiting the number of targeted changes initially increases the potential for success as the patient builds skill and confidence.

As previously noted, changes in lifestyle are often easy to initiate but difficult to sustain. People often initiate change with much enthusiasm, but then relapse after some improvement. Others approach change with much less enthusiasm. It is estimated that less than 20% of the population is prepared to actively change behaviors at any given time (Prochaska, Norcross, & DiClemente, 1994). Many models/theories have evolved over the past 50 years to help us better understand the process of initiating and maintaining health behavior changes. Personal health behavior really began to attract attention in the 1960s with the release of the Surgeon General's report on smoking and health. The U.S.-based Behavior Change Consortium, consisting of 15 universities and institutes, has investigated the effectiveness of health behavior change interventions in improving various health behaviors. The testing of various theories has demonstrated that there is no single quick fix solution leading to change. No one single theory of health behavior change explains the process and no one intervention technique results in positive outcomes; instead, elements from a combination of theories and interventions are most useful for the needs of patients and practitioners (Nieuwenhuijsen et al., 2006; Ory, Jordan, & Bazzarre, 2002).

HEALTH BELIEF MODEL

This model of behavior change identifies three factors that significantly influence a person's motivation to change: health attitudes, beliefs, and social support. The motivation to change comes from the belief in the efficacy of an action to reduce the perceived health threat and that the reward and benefit for changing outweighs the perceived barriers such as costs, risks, and regimen complexity. Influential elements in the decision-making process include the following (Prochaska, DiClemente, & Norcross, 1992):

- General beliefs regarding health
- Willingness to seek healthcare advice
- Openness to accepting and faith in the safety and efficacy of proposed recommendations
- Perceived vulnerability and risk of illness if no change occurs
- Concern for how the new behavior might change social relationships

The Health Belief Model (HBM) emphasizes the personal context of decision making. It focuses on the beliefs, expectations, and perceptions of the patient and not the provider. To help the patient through the change process, the provider needs to put aside personal beliefs and match interventions to the patient's coping styles. For example, if the patient has negative health beliefs and attitudes, but good social support, the provider may want to take advantage of the social support network by enlisting the assistance of family members, or encouraging participation in group programs, to help increase awareness and facilitate healthy behavior choices. Behavior modification techniques, such as diary keeping and setting small goals and rewards, are helpful for increasing cues and consequences of maintaining or shifting certain behaviors. Alternatively, if the client has positive health beliefs and attitudes, but little or inadequate social support, interventions may put more emphasis on participation with community or self-help groups. Cognitive activities such as meditation, problem solving, and goal setting may help strengthen personal confidence and awareness (Gaydos, 2005). Studies indicate that family and friends are viewed by clients as important sources of information (Pullen et al., 2001) and that community programs provide ongoing social support (Task Force on Community Preventive Services, 2001).

THEORY OF REASONED ACTION/THEORY OF PLANNED BEHAVIOR

Developed by Ajzen and Fishbein (1980), this theory focuses on the concept that an individual's intention to perform a behavior, grounded in values and expectations, is the most important determinant of consequent actions. It also includes the influence of the beliefs of significant others on the individual. If a person has a positive attitude toward the outcome of a behavior and it is supported by significant others, it is more likely they will engage in the behavior change in order to meet their own expectations and the expectations of the "others." The opposite is also true; negative expectations lead to low motivation and outcomes. Motivation to change is also influenced by the perception of how difficult it is to perform a behavior and the sense of control and confidence the person has in handling the perceived difficulty (Brown, 1999a).

HEALTH LOCUS OF CONTROL

Locus of control relates to the belief of an individual that certain health outcomes are the result of their own actions (internal) or the result of forces independent of themselves (external). With an internal locus of control, the individual is motivated to change behaviors by a personal core desire. With an external locus of control, the individual is motivated by the suggestion of powerful others (significant other, doctor) or feel powerless to influence their own health by the belief that any outcome is determined by fate, luck or chance (Brown, 1999b). In a national telephone survey study on cardiovascular disease and women (Mosca et al., 2006), the second most common reason for not taking action to lower cardiovascular risk was the feeling that God or a higher power determines health. Many individuals view their doctor as their primary source of healthcare information, and when they are not counseled on weight loss and physical activity, they often interpret this to mean that healthy behavior is not important (Bartlett, 2003). Patients often enroll in cardiac rehabilitation programs at the urging of their physician or their significant other, or the fear generated from a recent cardiac event (heart attack, stent placement, open heart surgery). If they have not identified some internal motivation that inspires readiness to change, they have little chance of adhering long term to health behaviors that will improve their cardiovascular health.

Successful change is most likely to occur when the patient's motivation is internally derived and consistent with their own values, beliefs, and needs.

TRANSTHEORETICAL MODEL OF BEHAVIOR CHANGE

The Transtheoretical Model of Behavior Change (TTM) has been applied to many health behaviors since it was introduced as a multiple-stage behavior change model in the 1980s. Most of the early research focused on smoking cessation, but the model has been applied to the termination of health risking behaviors including alcoholism, drug abuse, and gambling, as well as the adaptation of health promoting behaviors, including weight loss, exercise, and condom use (DiClemente & Prochaska, 1998). The model has also been applied to the rehabilitation setting, including the management of chronic pain (Biller, Arnstein, Caudill, Federman, & Guberman, 2000) and the promotion of health and well being (Martin & Fell, 1999). This model integrates various constructs of behavior change and suggests that people move through a series of stages in their attempts to change behaviors. Health promotion programs tend to be action oriented, assuming that anyone coming into the program is ready for immediate behavior change and will adopt healthy behaviors in a timely fashion. The TTM suggests that action is only one part of change and that people follow a predictable course on the way to change.

The TTM has two major dimensions: stages of change (**Table 17-1**), which indicate when people change based on their attitudes, intentions and behaviors, and the processes of change (**Table 17-2**), which are the behavioral and cognitive activities engaged in when changing behavior (Prochaska et al., 1992).

Progression from stage to stage is often not linear, but instead, individuals move through stages in a cyclical manner. They may progress from precontemplation into action, but then when faced with influential barriers, relapse back to a previous stage. Similar patterns of cycling through stages may occur several times before change is successful. Some individuals may

Table 17-1 Stages of Change

Precontemplation	indicates that the individual is not ready to change or denies the need to change. He or she is not thinking about change and has no intention to change in the near future, usually 6 months. An individual in this stage does not want information and may get defensive when confronted.
Contemplation	suggests thinking about change, but not yet committed. There is intention to change in the next 6 months.
Preparation	involves getting ready to change, but the individual needs motivation and guidance with setting goals. There is intention to change in the near future, usually 1 month.
Action	demonstrates a readiness to actively engage in behavior change or modification, and the individual needs reinforcement for consistent behavior over a 6-month period.
Maintenance	involves focusing on stabilizing the behavior and avoiding relapse—sustaining behavior for 6 months or more until there is no temptation to return to the former behavior.
Termination	is the ultimate goal. The former behavior does not pose a threat, and the individual has confidence there will not be a relapse.

Source: Adapted from Prochaska et al. (1992); Shinitzky and Kub (2001).

Table 17-2 Processes of Change

Cognitive Processes	
Consciousness-raising	seeks new information, understanding, and feedback about the problem behavior.
Dramatic relief	involves the emotional reaction or experiences related to the behavior.
Environmental re-evaluation	is the assessment of how the behavior affects the physical environment and other people.
Self re-evaluation	is the assessment of personal values related to the behavior.
Social liberation	involves an awareness and acceptance of healthier, alternative lifestyles.

Behavioral Processes	
Counter conditioning	is a process that substitutes new behaviors for the problem behavior.
Helping relationships	involves accepting and using the support from others during attempts to change behavior.
Reinforcement management	reinforces positive behaviors by establishing rewards when goals are met.
Self-liberation	reflects choice and commitment in changing behavior, including a belief in the ability to change.
Stimulus control	removes cues for unhealthy habits while adding prompts for healthy choices.

Source: Adapted from Prochaska et al. (1992); Marcus, Banspach, Lefebvre, Rossi, Carleton, and Abrams (1992); Fahrenwald and Walker (2003).

move through the stages fairly rapidly; others may progress more slowly or stay stuck in a stage for a period of time (**Box 17-1**).

BOX 17-1

When we first met Mr. John R. in Case Study 17-2 he was in precontemplation. With the help of his physical therapist, he moved into contemplation as he began to think about the possibility of changing his exercise behavior. The process moved into preparation with goal setting, and on to action when John began to act on his goals. Interestingly, however, he remained in precontemplation with several other behaviors: dietary habits, engaging social support, and smoking.

PROCESSES OF CHANGE

Ten processes of change (Table 17-2) have been identified that help facilitate movement through the stages of change. Five of these stages are cognitive or experiential processes. Applied at the earlier stages of change (precontemplation, contemplation, and preparation), these processes are associated with an individual's emotions, values, and cognitions. The behavioral processes of change are most important when initiating and performing the behavior in the later stages of the change process (action and maintenance) (**Box 17-2**).

BOX 17-2

Bob, whom we met earlier in the previous chapter, joined a cardiac rehabilitation program after his first cardiac event; however, despite the encouragement of his physician and the ongoing threat of heart disease progression, he was not ready to change behaviors. After some initial attempts at smoking cessation and exercise, he dropped out of rehabilitation and reverted back to old behaviors. He had several other spirals through the stages after his second myocardial infarction and coronary artery bypass graft but still seemed unable to progress into maintenance and termination. By the time he came to our clinic, he had used several of the cognitive and behavioral processes to bring him to a stage of action readiness (refer to Table 17-2). Continuing to use counter conditioning, helping relationships, self-liberation, and stimulus control, as well as ongoing self-reevaluation, he was confident he would continue to move from action into maintenance and on to termination.

PROMOTING CHANGE

The process of behavior change can be promoted when the individual receives individualized education and counseling strategies to match his or her stage of readiness. Providing written materials about the benefits and risks of unhealthy behaviors might be appropriate for someone in precontemplation in order to raise consciousness and provoke self-evaluation, but goal setting would not be effective as the person is not ready and does not intend to change; however, goal setting would be appropriate for helping someone move from preparation into action (Fahrenwald & Walker, 2003). An exercise study by Marcus et al. (1992), looked at the effectiveness of written materials, targeted to specific stages of readiness in helping individuals adopt exercise behaviors. Written documents such as, "What's in it for you?" (contemplation) and "Ready for action" (preparation), were found to help move 30% of contemplators and 60% of preparators into the action stage. Even if not all of the subjects moved into action, progressing from even just one stage to the next should be looked at as a success in the change process. Fahrenwald and Walker (2003) looked to see how WIC (Women, Infants, and Children Program) mothers used the processes of change in attempting to change exercise behaviors. Even though the TTM model postulates that the five cognitive processes are used most at the contemplation and precontemplation stages, WIC mothers in the preparation stage used the five cognitive processes the most. Counter conditioning and self-liberation are considered key in the first 6 months of a new behavior, but this study also showed that they are important in maintenance. For some behaviors such as exercise, there may be a need for use of all the processes to maintain behavior over time.

CONSTRUCTS FOR CHANGE

Despite the differentiation of the various behavior change theories discussed previously here, there are several constructs that reflect a commonality among the different theories and are clinically important for patients moving through the stages of change:

Decisional balance refers to the process of identifying and weighing the pros (anticipated gains) against the cons (anticipated losses or costs) of adopting or changing a problem behavior. As the pros increase and the cons decrease, a person will move forward from contemplation into preparation and action

(Marcus, Eaton, Rossi, & Harlow, 1994; Spencer, Adams, Malone, Roy, & Yost, 2006). As we know from the earlier case study, Bob had a difficult time stopping drinking and smoking. All of his socialization revolved around a circle of friends who enjoyed time together at the bars. He was afraid that if he stopped smoking and drinking he would lose his friends; the cons outweighed the pros. After he began to realize that his health was more important and that his true friends would support him in the change process, the pros outweighed the cons, and he was able to move into preparation and action.

Self-efficacy comes out of Bandura's Social Cognitive Theory (1977), which argues that health behavior is influenced by the interactive, reciprocal relationship among the person, behaviors, and the social environment. It is the degree of confidence a person has that he or she can perform a certain behavior and overcome any barriers that may impede progress; if successful, there is a positive health benefit to be gained. Self-efficacy is not concerned with performance skills, but rather the perception of being able to perform certain tasks or behaviors. It has been shown to predict exercise behavior (Dallow & Anderson, 2003), and with respect to the rehabilitation environment, researchers have found that individuals with strong self-efficacy perceive their disabilities as less severe and report them less often compared to individuals with low self-efficacy (Seeman, Unger, McAvay, & Mendes de Leon, 1999). Enhancement of self-efficacy in relation to a new behavior increases the chances for successful behavior change (Holloway & Watson, 2002). Increases in self-efficacy are experienced through four primary sources:

- *Performance attainment* involves learning and achieving proficiency through the personal experience of participating in the task or behavior. Although success generally leads to increased self-efficacy and failure leads to a decrease, future success can be enhanced when patients are encouraged to view "failures" as learning experiences from which one can learn and develop new strategies.
- *Vicarious experience* relates to learning through the observation of others (appropriate models) in a social environment that supports the desired behavior. Healthcare providers can serve as models, but models in the living environment of the patient also must be considered when attempting to change behaviors.
- *Verbal persuasion* reflects the importance of communication in attempting to increase an individual's sense of ability and skill for a certain task

or behavior. Trusting the source of information with respect to skill and expertise is a significant influence on perceived self-efficacy.

- *Physiological feedback* can influence perception of performance. Awareness of uncomfortable or unpleasant sensations may bias feelings toward failure; in contrast, the absence of such sensations, especially with the experience of successfully performing a perceived challenging task, may increase physical self-efficacy (Holloway & Watson, 2002).

Social Support has been identified as an element of one of the change processes: helping relationships. Individuals who identify positive social supports are more likely to choose healthy behaviors and demonstrate good stress hardiness. Research shows that social support in the medical setting has a positive effect on both the health of the individual as well as the quality of the health care itself (Frasure-Smith et al., 2000). Social support includes emotional support, material support, and all resources provided by other persons, including family, friends, healthcare team, and community organizations (Pengilly & Dowd, 2000). Both the number of supports and the quality of those supports are important. Support groups, educational classes, clinical programs, website chat rooms, and exercise facilities all provide valuable support. Organizations such as the American Heart Association, the Arthritis Foundation, and the American Cancer Society are wonderful sources of information and support for individuals, families, and healthcare providers. Perhaps most important of all is that individuals have supports that allow them to discuss the change process, who listen without judgment, and who can feel and understand their emotions and point of view (empathy).

Relapse Prevention is an integral part of the behavior change stages. Relapse is more common than linear progression through the stages and reflects the cyclical nature of the change process. Although relapse is the recurrence of a behavior (or symptom) after a period of improvement, it is not a failure; instead, it is part of the learning process that eventually leads to more permanent change. It is important to distinguish between a lapse and a relapse. A lapse is a single event, the re-emergence of a habit (having a cigarette at a social event or stopping exercise routine when on vacation) that may or may not lead to a relapse (back to smoking a pack a day or not exercising for 3 months), the more permanent return of an unhealthy habit. Providers need to emphasize with patients that a lapse is normal and should be expected. This helps to avoid feelings of discouragement and loss of self-esteem. It also helps patients avoid getting stuck in the "saint or sinner syndrome," bogged down by "all or nothing thinking," in which they see themselves as total successes or failures. Hopefully, lapses can be viewed as a learning experience, helping patients to understand the barriers and high risk situations that affect their decision making. A high-risk situation is any situation (including the emotional reaction to it) that poses a threat to a personal sense of control and increases the risk of relapse. Psychological and situational factors that are associated with 75% of all relapses include the following:

- Negative emotional states (35%) such as anger, frustration, anxiety, boredom, or depression
- Interpersonal conflicts (20%) that involve difficult interactions with family, friends or work relationships
- Social pressure (20%) that influences behavior choices through verbal persuasion or physical exposure to the unhealthy behavior (Marlatt & Gordon, 1985).

Providers can assist patients to recognize their high risk situations and help them set goals and problem solve with effective countering tactics. This leads to increased self-efficacy and helps avoid the probability of a relapse.

The process of collaborative problem solving and negotiation between provider and patient is necessary to establish mutually acceptable goals and treatment plans. Although knowledge about the problem behavior or medical/physical condition, and treatment recommendations are important, the patient's motivation is also a critical element. Providers are more likely to facilitate change in the patient's behavior by understanding the patient's values and beliefs, based on culture, past experiences, and support systems. This reflects a biopsychosocial/spiritual model of care with a core element of helping individuals assume responsibility for their own health.

MOTIVATIONAL INTERVIEWING

Motivational interviewing (MI) is a framework of provider–patient interaction that facilitates the movement of the patient along the behavior change continuum. Developed by Miller and Rollnick (1991), it suggests that the role of the healthcare provider is to assist patients into a stage of action necessary to improve health status outcomes. MI involves developing a therapeutic relationship, based on mutual commitment, nonjudging acceptance, and a sense of safety and trust. Providers need to know not just the patient's problem behavior or disability (biomedical), but their experience of that diagnosis (biopsychosocial/spiritual) (Jensen, Lorish, & Shepard, 2002). The framework of MI helps the patient explore the origins of lack of motivation or ambivalence toward change, helping the patient move along the change continuum (Mears & Kilpatrick, 2008). The core elements of MI that promote motivation for behavior change include the following:

- *Empathy* reflects listening to patient concerns with a non-authoritarian and non-judgmental attitude, helping the patient reach his or her goals rather than impose goals.
- *Rolling with resistance* relates to supporting efforts to change by being patient and creative, avoiding argument and confrontation, as the patient works through barriers.
- *Enhancing self-efficacy* encourages realistic goals and the ability to deal with lapses and setbacks, thereby increasing patient confidence and self-belief.
- *Developing discrepancies* helps the patient gain a clear view of the difference between current and desired behavior, as reflected by his or her personal values and goals, and intentions and reasons to change (Miller & Rollnick, 2002).

The art of MI is a dance between provider and patient, avoiding confrontation and minimizing patient defensiveness. Instead, the two parties negotiate common ground in order to determine not the best treatment for the client, but the best treatment that the client is willing to follow and that fits most comfortably into his or her life (Jensen et al., 2002). The patient–practitioner collaborative model is outlined in **Figure 17-1**.

Ultimately, the role of the provider is to help patients take control of their lives because they are the ones responsible for making the behavioral changes; but before they can experience control, they need to experience awareness. Through mind/body interventions, such as eliciting the relaxation response (RR), cognitive restructuring (CR), and goal setting, patients can build awareness that allows them to bring mind, body, and emotion under control. With control comes the ability to make choices about health behaviors.

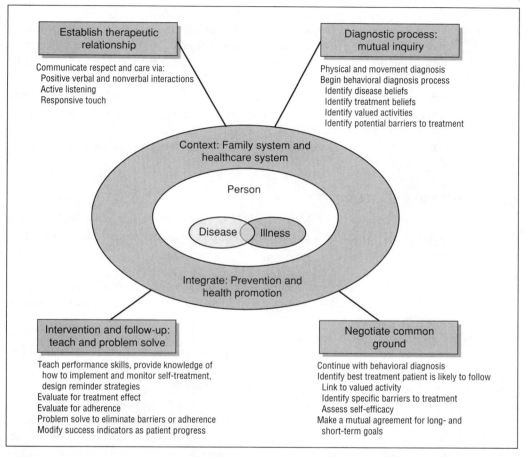

Figure 17-1 Patient–practitioner collaborative model (Jensen et al., 2002, reprinted with permission).

MIND/BODY INTERVENTIONS

Dealing with emotional factors is a large component of the collaborative practice model. It is difficult to change behaviors when caught up in the stress of everyday life or inhibited by negative emotional states. Stress could be defined as any experience that disrupts homeostasis, thereby requiring change or adaptation. From an individual perspective, it is the perception of a threat to physical or psychological well-being, and the perception that the individual cannot cope (Wells-Federman & Mandle, 2002). Stress has been shown to cause or exacerbate many of the leading health problems in the United States (U.S. Department of Health and Human Services, 2000); consequently, helping individuals find more effective ways to cope with stress is important for promoting health. Stress management has been shown to be an effective intervention for health promotion, disease prevention, and symptom management. Some stress management strategies such as CR, RR, goal setting, self-monitoring, and problem solving have long been part of community programs such as Alcoholics Anonymous and Weight Watchers, which help people modify health risking behaviors (Wells-Federman & Mandle, 2002).

COGNITIVE RESTRUCTURING

Based on the work of Aaron Beck (1991), cognitive restructuring (CR) is a conceptual model for a short-term, talk therapy, intervention that is based on two premises:

- Much of our stress and emotional suffering comes from the way we think.
- The thoughts that cause stress are usually negative, unrealistic, illogical, or exaggerated.

Our behaviors are an extension of how we think and feel. CR is a series of strategies that helps people recognize their sabotaging, negative thoughts, challenge them, and replace them with more helpful, rational responses. It teaches people to recognize that negative thinking often causes emotional distress and that these patterns of thinking are related to their values, beliefs, and past experiences. As they learn how to challenge and reframe their inaccurate and unhelpful thinking, they begin to feel better emotionally, reduce the negative health effects of stress, and behave in more productive ways to help them establish and reach their health goals (Stuart & Wells-Federman, 2005).

It takes time to change a mind-set that took years to develop, and the process of developing skills to challenge sabotaging thoughts and increase self-confidence is often a roller coaster of doubt and frustration. We cannot always control negative thinking, but we can choose how we want to respond to those thoughts. The four-step paradigm of CR is a useful tool to help individuals develop the skills to manage stress and increase their ability to choose more healthful behaviors. In stressful situations or when overcome with thoughts that may sabotage healthy choices, the individual is instructed to

- *Stop:* a self-instruction that breaks the cycle of escalating negative thoughts and allows them to
- *Take a breath*, which releases physical tension, elicits RR, and creates a "time out" so that the person can
- *Reflect* and take a look at their thoughts and ask "What am I thinking?" "Are these thoughts true?" "Is this way of thinking helpful?" "Am I jumping to conclusions, or making it worse than it really is?" Challenging the thoughts allows the person to
- *Choose* a more realistic, rational response that gives them a fighting chance in overcoming the sabotaging thoughts and making a healthier choice (Stuart & Wells-Federman, 2005).

A new self-help book by Judith Beck, *The Beck Diet Solution* (2007), is based on the principles of cognitive therapy. The book doesn't tell us what to eat, but it teaches us how to eat, how to motivate ourselves, how to create time and energy for healthy eating, how to problem solve, and how to challenge our thoughts about eating that always seem to sabotage our best intentions. It teaches us how to exercise and strengthen our "resistance muscle" so when overcome with sabotaging thoughts we have the power to choose a healthier response. The instructions and guidelines outlined in the book may be too restrictive for some who wish to change their eating habits and lose weight, but they provide a very structured framework of support for those who have repeatedly tried and failed to lose weight. For a more comprehensive review of cognitive therapy and its clinical applications, see resources by David Burns (1993, 1999) and Donald Meichenbaum (1993, 1999) in Appendix 16-1.

THE POSITIVE PERSPECTIVE

The field of positive psychology adds another element to the promotion of health behaviors. Positive emotions about the past, present and future, including satisfaction, contentment, fulfillment, gratitude, forgiveness, appreciation, hope, optimism, trust, faith, and confidence, buffer depression and other negative emotional states and counteract the detrimental effects of negative emotions on physiology, attention, and creativity. When combined with an open attitude of interest for choosing how to move forward with behavior change, focusing on the positive leads to an upward spiral of well-being (Seligman, Rashid, & Parks, 2006). When stuck in a negative emotion such as anger or frustration, it is often helpful to shift appraisal of the situation to gratitude or appreciation, to help counteract the negative effects. Similarly, finding meaning in a situation that is uncomfortable or unpleasant, but out of one's control, helps the individual move beyond the limitations of the negative perspectives, giving back some sense of control.

The approach of positive psychology dovetails nicely with the health promoting lifestyle discussed in the previous chapter; as opposed to moving away from disease and disability, the focus is on moving toward health (Walker, Sechrist, & Pender, 1987). It is also reflective of a new theoretical approach to health promotion and behavior change, Appreciative Inquiry (AI), an organizational development process that focuses on the positive and creative as a force for an improved future (Moore & Charvat, 2007). Although more widely known as a business model, it has application to the health field. Whereas the problem-solving approach (moving away from problem behaviors) focuses on identifying the problem, considering solutions, and treating the problem, AI is based on the positive psychology of supporting positive change, building on strengths, generating energy, and encouraging creativity. It does not deny problems, but does support the view that behavior change may be more effective when individuals focus on strengths rather than on problems (Moore & Charvat, 2007). The hopeful goal is to create a patient–provider relationship that promotes mutual trust and sharing and opens the patient to new possibilities for a healthful future. As healthcare professionals look for effective ways to help patients manage stress and make health behavior changes, focusing on the strengths and hopes of the patient is as important as helping them overcome problems that put their health at risk.

THE RELAXATION RESPONSE

Elicitation of the relaxation response (RR) is another effective tool for managing stress and increasing awareness. Based on studies of practices of Transcendental Meditation (TM) practitioners, Benson, Beary, and Carol (1974) described the RR as the physiological opposite of the stress (fight or flight) response. It is a physical state of deep rest that engenders a change in brain physiology necessary for stable mood. The long-term physiological effect is a decrease in central nervous system arousal, with a decrease in musculoskeletal system, sympathetic nervous system, and psychoneuroendocrine system arousal (Hoffman et al., 1982). In addition to the physiological changes, psychological changes such as improved mood and a decrease in health risking behaviors also occur. With regular RR practice, individuals also develop a spiritual perspective that can engender a shift in values and beliefs that help facilitate symptom management, personal growth, and health promotion (Kass et al., 1991; Wells-Federman & Mandle, 2002).

Many techniques are used to elicit the RR, the common elements being a focus to hold attention in the present moment, and a nonjudging attitude of interest, such that the practitioner is open to the learning inherent in the experience. Meditation, a technique commonly used to elicit the RR, is the practice of becoming aware, of paying attention in the moment. It is also the practice of inward contemplation during which the mind settles into reflection on a specific object, quality (gratitude, appreciation), or question/issue of personal significance. Although there are many different meditation practices, there are two general approaches: the concentrative form, in which there is a specific focus (word, sound, breath, or visualization), and mindfulness meditation, which involves an awareness of the internal (observing heart beat or watching the breath) and external environment (walking, eating, or observing nature). The approaches can be practiced alone or in combination as in some Buddhist meditation practices (Delmonte, 1989; Ott, 2004). With experience, the practitioner may progress from using a more concrete focus (breath or word) to observing thoughts and emotions. With respect to decreasing the effects of stress and chronic disease and promoting health, a literature review by Bonadonna (2003) reports that meditation has been shown to reduce anxiety and depression, decrease pain, increase mood and self-esteem, decrease stress, and reduce the use of healthcare resources. Research suggests that TM may be a valuable treatment modality for modulating the physiological response to stress and modifying risk factors of coronary heart disease (Paul-Labrador et al., 2006).

When there is increased self-awareness, there is potential for long-term behavior change. One quality of registrants of the National Weight Control Registry (lost at least 30 pounds and kept off for at least a year) is an increased sense of self-awareness and self-esteem. They seem to incorporate some meditative element into their lives, a little "self-time" that allows them to redefine themselves with healthier habits (Mithers, 2007). Although long-term exercisers start the change process by making exercise a priority, the most powerful influences motivating them to continue exercise are experiential feelings that include a sense of well-being, having more energy, enjoyment, and feeling more alert and relaxed (Stone & Klein, 2004). The effects of meditation are not only beneficial for the patient, but also for the healthcare provider. Oman, Hedberg, and Thorensen (2006) showed that meditation helps reduce stress and improves mental health in healthcare providers, as they demonstrate better decision making and develop stronger, more satisfying relationships with their patients. Developing an RR/meditation practice provides time away from the worries, concerns, and stress of everyday life, and opens the potential for more creative thinking and new possibilities.

GOAL SETTING

Goal setting is another valuable health promoting strategy. When based on the individual's values and beliefs, an action plan for change can be an effective stress management strategy as well as a foundation for facilitating behavior change. Goal setting is a mutual, dynamic process within the patient–practitioner relationship. The practitioner serves as coach, respecting the individual's input, and using values clarification and decisional balance to help match the individual's goals to what they identify as valuable and meaningful. Setting specific goals leads to more successful outcomes compared with no goals or vague ones. Keeping goals simple and small in number is helpful if clients struggle with change or are trying to change multiple behaviors. Breaking down long-term goals into shorter term goals may provide more opportunity for review and feedback, as does writing goals in a mutually agreed on health contract. Self-monitoring in the form of weekly diaries helps to keep patients focused on their healthful activities. It is a key strategy for increasing awareness of behavior. Although the self-monitoring activity may actually change the behavior, its use for increasing awareness is of prime importance (Bartlett, 2003; Burke & Fair, 2003). Successfully meeting short-term goals enhances self-efficacy, self-esteem, and performance satisfaction and increases adherence to continuing the behavior change process (Burke & Fair, 2003). Goals should be specific, concrete, measurable, and achievable. SMART goals provide a framework for defining successful goal setting.

Specific—detailed, easily described
Measurable—allows for self-monitoring and concrete end points
Achievable—realistic, challenging, leads to self-efficacy
Relevant—related to values and personal orientation
Timely—includes a time frame for completion or re-evaluation
(Geithner, Albert, & Vincent, 2007; Kaye & Kim, 1998)

For example:

Ineffective goal: I will cut back on fat intake in order to lose weight.
Effective goal: LTG: I will lose 20 pounds in 6 months
                STG: I will lose 0.5 to 1 pound/week by

- Exercising 30–40 minutes, 5–7 times/week
- Decreasing my calorie intake by 250 calories/week (switching to low-fat or nonfat dairy; eating high-fiber cereals instead of high-fat breakfast foods).

Combining the practice of mindfulness with goal setting involves a paradigm shift in which the focus becomes the process instead of the outcome. After the goals are set, the focus becomes the learning experience of each step along the path toward achieving the goal. This approach is helpful as self-awareness and self-observation are enhanced, and the dichotomy of success or failure is eliminated; there is much to be learned in the experience itself. After all, "you don't dance to get to the other side of the floor" (Alan Watts).

HEALTHCARE DISPARITIES

Eliminating disparities in health care is one of the two main goals of Healthy People 2010. Part of the problem is not fully knowing the underlying causes; however, shorter lives are the price that black, Hispanic, American Indian, and Native Alaskan populations pay for inadequate health care, poor living conditions, and high psychologic stress (Sankar et al., 2004). A study by Bach, Pham, Schrag, Tate, and Hargraves (2004) reveals that there is a difference in the quality of health care and the training of physicians (and their access to clinical resources) who tend to treat black versus white patients. In addition, many healthcare providers feel that they lack the preparation and guidance to understand and respond effectively to the cultural and linguistic needs of culturally diverse patients. The Office of Minority Health (2005) reports that there is a lack of comprehensive cultural and linguistic standards; however, the results of the Healthy Directions—Small Business study, which looked at promoting behavior change among working class, multiethnic workers, demonstrates that interventions targeted to the worksite level and addressing multiple cultures and low literacy levels can be effective (Sorensen et al., 2005). In addition, AI has been proposed as an effective behavior change process for socioeconomically disadvantaged individuals. Because it focuses on individuals' strengths, hopes, and a positive vision of the future, it helps elevate them above the problems and negative life events that hinder behavior change (Moore & Chavat, 2007). This process may have application to improving cultural competence in health care, as it encourages the provider to understand the patient's experience of the illness/problem within the personal and cultural context of his or her life.

Case Study 17-3

Mary is a 71-year-old black woman with coronary artery disease (CAD) and multiple risk factors (HTN, hyperlipidemia, obesity, glucose intolerance, and sedentary) who was referred to our CWP by her physician. Although she vocalized a readiness to make dietary, activity, and stress-management changes and set initial goals in each area, she had difficulty adhering to her health contract. Each week we had a discussion about her difficulty motivating herself to exercise; she was aware of her risks and the benefits of exercise but had no internal locus, no core desire or motivation. Growing up she had never been encouraged to exercise, and she just never saw herself as an active person beyond the usual daily physical activity of raising a family. Several weeks into the program we had a discussion about what was valuable and meaningful to her, and she shared with me that her faith and church community were important and that she had just become the guardian for her 6-year-old granddaughter. Mary was distressed that she could not comfortably play with her granddaughter, as she became easily short winded with activity. When asked what she thought might help her improve her tolerance for playing with her granddaughter, she discovered her internal motivation to exercise. It had nothing to do with the recommendations of her healthcare providers, and it was not related to a fear of further heart complications; however, it had everything to do with wanting to be a more active part of her granddaughter's life. Together we set a goal of attending exercise classes that were held in the church activity room twice a week and walking in the local park with two of her friends from church on 2 other days. By focusing on her strengths, values, and beliefs, instead of her health problems, Mary was able to identify a core desire of internal locus that enabled her to begin to change her exercise behavior. An outcome of improved health most likely will still occur, but the process will be more meaningful and fulfilling to Mary.

SUMMARY

Whether the objective is to alter addictive behaviors, modify heart disease risk factors, change sexual behavior to decrease risk of sexually transmitted diseases, or improve adherence to rehabilitation treatment plans, the principles of behavior change are consistent. Effective patient–practitioner relationships and group support programs help individuals to identify their motivation to change to move toward their highest health potential. Individuals need imagination and self-awareness for motivation to answer this question: "What do I really need?" They also need discipline and determination. To begin the behavior change process, sometimes they just need to make it a priority, but when they begin to experience the benefits of the change and recognize their need to maintain the changes, then maintenance shifts to termination; the behavior becomes part of their self-identity. **Table 17-3** summarizes elements that facilitate successful individual behavior change.

As previously indicated, successful behavior change involves a dance between the patient and the practitioner. Developing a therapeutic relationship based on mutual trust and respect is vital for the change process. Practi-

Table 17-3 Individual Behavior Change

- Perceive the need to change.
- Make it a priority.
- Gather information.
- Evaluate that benefits outweigh the costs.
- Determine internal locus of control/core desire.
- Set SMART goals.
- Increase self-efficacy.
- Minimize self-judgment/criticism.
- Focus on the process/appreciate the outcome.

tioners need to be culturally sensitive, listen to the patient's story, and understand their point of view. **Table 17-4** outlines guidelines for a successful practitioner/patient interface.

The last bullet point in Table 17-4 is one worth emphasizing. Although this chapter has focused on individual health promotion and behavior change, people do not exist in isolation. The health of the population in general and individuals in specific depends on positive change on the community and national levels. Fortunately, we are starting to see some progress. Most communities have no smoking bans in public areas, including restau-

Table 17-4 Practitioner Guidelines

- Consider the patient's perspective; listen with acceptance and understanding.
- Form a collaborative relationship based on negotiation.
- Individualize treatment/goals based on patient values.
- Minimize confrontation; eliminate judgment and labeling.
- Avoid lecturing; limit the potential for alienation and feelings of disapproval.
- Ride the wave of resistance; anticipate lapses.
- Build self-efficacy; promote hope and confidence and personal responsibility.
- Brainstorm; encourage new ways of thinking and challenge old paradigms.
- Be a role model; walk the talk.
- Repeat everything.
- Do not give up.
- Enlist family support.
- Make use of the community.

Source: Adapted from Shinitzky and Kub (2001); Jensen et al. (2002).

rants and bars. Some cities are banning trans fats from food in restaurants. Many schools are starting to divest themselves of contracts with junk food and soft drink vendors. Healthy People 2010 urges providers to partner with community organizations to better serve the needs of individuals, such as providing health screenings and medication reviews at senior housing organizations and senior centers. As evidenced in the case study of Mary (mentioned previously), faith communities can also play a significant role in health promotion and behavior change support, as they provide an environment that equalizes shared health information across all socioeconomic and gender/race barriers.

The Robert Woods Foundation helps to bridge the gap between the community and the national level by supporting the National Blueprint Project (http://www.agingblueprint.org), a project that provides different physical activity programs for older adults (Greiner & Edelman, 2006). Several other developments at the national level will hopefully lead to significant increases in the resources available to healthcare policymakers and practitioners. A reorganization of the Centers for Disease Control has changed its focus to public health and health promotion, especially the obesity epidemic. The passage of IMPACT (Improved Nutrition and Physical Activity Act) by the Senate in 2004 is designed to provide new funding to practitioners for fitness and nutrition programs through communities, schools, and work sites (Spencer et al., 2006). The health of the population depends on the continued efforts to shift the focus of health care from intervention to prevention and to empower individuals to assume more responsibility for their own health in order to move toward their highest health potential.

REFERENCES

Ajzen, I., & Fishbein, M. (1980). *Understanding attitudes and predicting social behavior.* Englewood Cliffs, NJ: Prentice Hall.

Bach, P. B., Pham, H. H., Schrag, D., Tate, R. C., & Hargraves, J. L. (2004). Primary care physicians who treat blacks and whites. *New England Journal of Medicine, 351,* 575–584.

Bandura, A. (1977). Self-efficacy: toward a unifying theory of behavior change. *Psychology Review, 84,* 191–215.

Bartlett, S. J. (2003). Motivating patients toward weight loss: practical strategies for addressing overweight and obesity. *Physician and Sportsmedicine, 31,* 29–36, 47–48.

Beck, A. (1991). Cognitive therapy: a 30 year retrospective. *American Psychologist, 46,* 368–375.

Beck, J. (2007). *The Beck diet solution.* Birmingham, AL: Oxmoor House.

Benson, H., Beary, J. F., & Carol, M. P. (1974). The relaxation response. *Psychiatry,* *37,* 37–46.

Biller, N., Arnstein, P., Caudill, M. A., Federman, C. W., & Guberman, C. (2000). Predicting completion of a cognitive behavioral pain management program by initial measures of a chronic pain patient's readiness for change. *Clinical Journal of Pain, 16,* 325–359.

Bonadonna, R. (2003). Meditation's impact on chronic illness. *Holistic Nursing Practice, 17,* 309–319.

Brown, K. M. (1999a). *Theory of reasoned action/theory of planned behavior.* Retrieved September 27, 2002, from http://hsc.usf.edu/~kmbrown/TRA_TPB.htm.

Brown, K. M. (1999b). *Health locus of control.* Retrieved September 27, 2002, from http://hsc.usf.edu/~kmbrown/Locus_of_Control_Overview.htm.

Burke, L. E., & Fair, J. (2003). Skill sets and attributes of health care providers who deliver behavioral interventions. *Journal of Cardiovascular Nursing, 18,* 256–266.

Chen, C. Y., Neufeld, P. S., Feely, C. A., & Skinner, C. S. (1999). Factors influencing compliance with home exercise programs among patients with upper-extremity impairment. *The American Journal of Occupational Therapy, 53,* 171–180.

Dallow, C. B., & Anderson, J. (2003). Using self-efficacy and a transtheoretical model to develop a physical activity intervention for obese women. *American Journal of Health Promotion, 17,* 373–381.

Delmonte, M. M. (1989). Meditation, the unconscious, and psychosomatic disorders. *International Journal of Psychosomatics, 36*(1–4), 45–52.

DiClemente, C., & Prochaska, J. (1998). Toward a comprehensive transtheoretical model of change. In W. R. Miller & N. Healther (Eds.), *Treating addictive behaviors* (pp. 3–24). New York: Plenum Press.

Eden, K. B., Orleans, C. T., Mulrow, C. D., Pender, N. J., & Teutsch, S. M. (2002). Does counseling by clinicians improve physical activity? A summary of the evidence for the U.S. preventive services task force. *Annals of Internal Medicine, 137,* 205–207.

Fahrenwald, N. L., & Walker, S. N. (2003). Application of the transtheoretical model of behavior change to the physical activity behavior of WIC mothers. *Public Health Nursing, 20,* 307–317.

Frasure-Smith, N., Lesperance, F., Gravel, G., Masson, A., Martin, J., Talajic, M., & Bourassa, M. G. (2000). Social support, depression, and mortality during the first year after myocardial infarction. *Circulation, 101,* 1919–1924.

Frey, L., Szalda-Petree, S., Traci, M. A., & Seekins, T. (2001). Prevention of secondary health conditions in adults with developmental disabilities: a review of the literature. *Disability and Rehabilitation, 23,* 361–369.

Gaydos, H. L. B. (2005). The art of holistic nursing and the human health experience. In B. M. Dossey, L. Keegan, & C. E. Guzzetta (Eds.), *Holistic nursing: a handbook for practice* (pp. 57–76). Sudbury, MA: Jones and Bartlett.

Geithner, C. A., Albert, J. F., & Vincent, B. S. (2007). Personal balance: it's importance and how to achieve it. *ACSM's Health and Fitness Journal, 11,* 7–14.

Greiner, P. A., & Edelman, C. L. (2006). Health defined: objectives for promotion and prevention. In C. L. Edelman & C. L. Mandle (Eds.), *Health promotion throughout the life span* (pp. 3–22). St. Louis, MO: Mosby.

Hoffman, J. W., Benson, H., Arns, P. A., Stainbrook, G. L., Landsberg, L., Young, J. B., & Gill, A. (1982). Reduced sympathetic nervous system responsivity associated with the relaxation response. *Science, 215,* 190–192.

Holloway, A., & Watson, H. E. (2002). Role of self-efficacy and behaviour change. *International Journal of Nursing Practice, 8,* 106–115.

Jensen, G. M., Lorish, C. D., Shepard, K. F. (2002). Understanding and influencing patient receptivity to change: the patient–practitioner collaborative model. In K. F. Shepard & G. M. Jensen (Eds.), *Handbook of teaching for physical therapists* (pp. 329–350). Philadelphia, PA: Elsevier Health Sciences.

Kass, J., Friedman, R., Lesserman, J., Zuttermeister, P. C., & Benson, H. (1991). Health outcomes and a new index of spiritual experience. *Journal for the Scientific Study of Religion, 30,* 203–211.

Kaye, S., & Kim, I. (1998). Time management: decide what you want to accomplish, how to get there, and what to do first. *Chemical Engineering, 105,* 137–140.

Lund, C. H., Carruth, A. K., Moody, K. B., & Logan, C. A. (2005). Theoretical approaches to motivating change: a farm family case example. *American Journal of Health Education, 36,* 279–285.

Marcus, B. H., Banspach, S. W., Lefebvre, R. C., Rossi, J. S., Carleton, R. A., & Abrams, D. B. (1992). Using the stages of change model to increase the adoption of physical activity among community participants. *American Journal of Health Promotion, 6,* 424–429.

Marcus, B. H., Eaton, C. A., Rossi, J. S., & Harlow, L. L. (1994). Self-efficacy, decision-making, and stages of change: an integrative model of physical exercise. *Journal of Applied Social Psychology, 24,* 489–509.

Marlatt, G. A., & Gordon, J. R. (1985). *Relapse prevention: maintenance strategies in the treatment of addictive disorders.* New York: Guilford Press.

Martin, P. C., & Fell, D. W. (1999). Beyond treatment: patient education for health promotion and disease prevention. *Journal of Physical Therapy Education, 13,* 49–56.

Mears, J., & Kilpatrick, M. (2008). Applying theory to make a difference in adoption and adherence. *ACSM's Health and Fitness Journal, 12,* 20–26.

Miller, W., & Rollnick, S. (1991). *Motivational interviewing: preparing people for change.* New York: Guilford Press.

Miller, W., & Rollnick, S. (2002). *Motivational interviewing.* New York: Guilford Press.

Mithers, C. (2007). Weight loss is all in your head. Retrieved July 23, 2007, from http://www.cnn.com/2007/living/personal/06/29/in.your.head/index.html.

Moore, S. M., & Charvat, J. (2007). Promoting health behavior change using appreciative inquiry. *Family and Community Health, 30,* S64–S74.

Mosca, L., Mochari, H., Christian, A., Berra, K., Taubert, K., Mills, T., Burdick, K. A., & Simpson, S. L. (2006). National study of women's awareness, preventive action, and barriers to cardiovascular health. *Circulation, 113,* 525–534.

National Cancer Institute. (2005). *Theory at a glance: a guide for health promotion* (2nd ed.). Retrieved from http://www.cancer.gov/aboutnci/oc/theory-at-a-glance.

Nieuwenhuijsen, E. R., Semper, E., Miner, K. R., & Epstein, M. (2006). Health behavior change models and theories: contributions to rehabilitation. *Disability and Rehabilitation, 28,* 245–256.

Office of Minority Health, USDHHS. (2005). *Assuring cultural competence in health care.* Retrieved October 13, 2005, from http://www.omhrc.gov/clas/po.htm.

Oman, D., Hedberg, J., & Thorensen, C. (2006). Passage meditation reduces perceived stress in health professionals: a randomized controlled trial. *Journaling of Consulting and Clinical Psychology, 74,* 714–719.

Ory, M. G., Jordan, P. J., & Bazzarre, T. (2002). The behavior change consortium: setting the stage for a new century of health behavior-change research. *Health Education Research Theory and Practice, 17,* 500–511.

Ott, M. (2004). Mindfulness meditation: a path of transformation and healing. *Journal of Psychosocial Nursing & Mental Health Services, 42*(7), 22–29.

Paul-Labrador, M., Polk, D., Dwyer, J. H., Velasquez, I., Nidich, S., Rainforth, M., Schneider, R., & Merz, N. B. (2006). Effects of a randomized controlled trial of transcendental meditation on components of the metabolic syndrome in subjects with coronary heart disease. *Archives of Internal Medicine, 166,* 1218–1224.

Pengilly, J. W., & Dowd, E. T. (2000). Hardiness and social support as moderators of stress. *Journal of Clinical Psychology, 56,* 813–820.

Prochaska, J. O., DiClemente, C. C., & Norcross, J. C. (1992). In search of how people change. *American Psychologist, 47,* 1102–1114.

Prochaska, J., Norcross, J., & DiClemente, C. (1994). *Changing for good.* New York: William Morrow.

Pullen, C., Walker, S. N., & Fiandt, K. (2001). Determinants of health-promoting lifestyle behaviors in rural older women. *Family and Community Health, 24,* 49–72.

Sankar, P., Cho, M. K., Condit, C. M., Hunt, L. M., Koenig, B., Marshall, P., Lee, S. S., & Spicer, P. (2004). Genetic research and health disparities. *Journal of the American Medical Association, 291,* 2985–2989.

Seeman, T. E., Unger, J. B., McAvay, G., & Mendes de Leon, C. F. (1999). Self-efficacy beliefs and perceived declines in functional ability: MacArthur studies of successful aging. *Journal of Gerontology, 54B,* 214–222.

Seligman, M. E. P., Rashid, T., & Parks, A. C. (2006). Positive psychotherapy. *American Psychologist, 61,* 774–788.

Shinitzky, H. E., & Kub, J. (2001). The art of motivating behavior change: the use of motivational interviewing to promote health. *Public Health Nursing, 18,* 178–185.

Sorensen, G., Barbeau, E., Stoddard, A. M., Hunt, M. K., Kaphingst, K., & Wallace, L. (2005). Promoting behavior change among working-class, multiethnic workers: results of the healthy directions-small business study. *American Journal of Public Health, 95,* 1389–1395.

Spencer, L., Adams, T. B., Malone, S., Roy, L., & Yost, E. (2006). Applying the transtheoretical model to exercise: a systematic and comprehensive review of the literature. *Health Promotion Practice, 7,* 428–443.

Stone, W. J., & Klein, D. A. (2004). Long-term exercisers: what can we learn from them? *ACSM's Health and Fitness Journal, 8,* 11–14.

Stuart, E., & Wells-Federman, C. L. (2005). Cognitive therapy. In B. M. Dossey, L. Keegan, & C. E. Guzzetta (Eds.), *Holistic nursing: a handbook for practice* (pp. 397–426). Sudbury, MA: Jones and Bartlett.

Task Force on Community Preventive Services. (2001). Increasing physical activity: a report on recommendations of the Task Force on Community Preventive Services. *Morbidity and Mortality Weekly Report, 50,* 1–14.

U.S. Department of Health and Human Services. (2000). *Healthy People 2010: understanding and improving health.* Washington, DC: Author.

Walker, S. N., Sechrist, K. R., & Pender, N. J. (1987). The health-promoting lifestyle profile: development and psychometric characteristics. *Nursing Research, 36,* 76–81.

Wells-Federman, C. L., & Mandle, C. L. (2002). Stress management. In C. L. Edelman & C. L. Mandle (Eds.), *Health promotion throughout the lifespan* (pp. 353–374). St. Louis: Mosby.

Chapter 18

Community Approaches to Health Promotion

Jean Oulund Peteet

INTRODUCTION

Previous chapters have emphasized changing the health of individuals; this chapter focuses on changing health in groups of individuals, communities, and broader populations. We discuss the different settings where community health promotion might occur, explore several behavioral and social science theoretical models that can assist clinicians in developing programs, discuss the evidence for effectiveness of community-based approaches and challenges to developing programs, and throughout the chapter use this case example to apply theory and concepts.

Case Study 18-1

Sophia, a 62-year-old single woman, lives and works in a city employed as an administrative assistant in the Hancock Insurance Company. She experiences a heart attack, receives treatment, and begins an outpatient cardiac rehabilitation program. She is motivated, participates in every session, and on completion of the program is taught how to continue on an exercise program that includes walking on her own. On returning for a 1-month clinic follow-up, she notes that neighborhood crime and safety concerns are keeping her from walking. How could a community health education and promotion approach address Sophia's situation?

DEFINING COMMUNITY

Community, in the context of health promotion, can have many meanings (Green & Kreuter, 1999; Sharpe, 2003). Community can be defined as a structural area with geographic and political boundaries or functionally where community members share characteristics (within a faith community, a school, or a group of individuals with a similar health problem). Community organization is also a term that will be used and is the process through which communities identify common problems and intervention methods to reach shared goals (McKenzie & Smeltzer, 1997).

Community-based approaches (King, 1998) can focus on the following:

- *Specific subgroups of individuals*—people with chronic disease, smokers
- *Community institutions*—organizations such as schools, worksites, healthcare settings
- *Community-wide settings*—comprehensive, integrated approaches that target people in a community to reduce risk (high blood pressure, obesity)
- *Legislation*—policy and environmental changes that reduce barriers for health behavior change

What are some of the differences between approaching a change in health for an individual and changing the health of a community? Let us use the example of obesity. In an individual approach, your goal would be to change individual behavior, perhaps through counseling, an individual exercise program, and/or a supervised exercise class. In a community approach, you might include these strategies but would also include a social support group for weight loss (subgroup of individuals), a worksite weight loss program (organization), improved parks and walking trails (environmental), and/or legislation to provide more nutritional information on packaged food (policy).

SUPPORT FOR COMMUNITY-BASED APPROACHES

Community-based approaches have been used in public health since the late 1800s and have evolved from interventions imposed on the community (e.g., water purification and sewage disposal) to programs that include community participation to meet recognized needs, such as neighborhood watch programs to reduce crime (Gilliland & Taylor, as cited in Raczynski & DiClemente, 1999). The rationale for community approaches is that people cannot be isolated from their social environment and programs that create change in broader community structures, processes, and policies can support individual health behavior change (Baker & Brownson, 1998; Best et al., 2003).

Some early community-based approaches occurred in the mid 1980s when the Centers for Disease Control (CDC) adopted the Planned Approach to Community Health (PATCH) (Kreuter, 1992) and Community Chronic Disease Prevention programs (Luepker et al., 1996; Schooler, Farquhar, Fortmann, & Flora, 1997). These strategies centered on creating a volunteer community network to promote health promotion activities. Community preventive services have become an integral part of the U.S. national strategy to improve the health of the nation (USDHHS, 2001). An example of a community prevention program is the Bootheel Heart Health Project, a community-based risk-reduction program for cardiovascular disease that included annual heart healthy festivals, a "High Blood Pressure Sunday" in which ministers included heart disease education in the sermon, local school poster contests, and a weekly newspaper heart healthy column (Brownson et al., 1996).

Successful community approaches pay attention to the context of the health problem being addressed. Communities may differ widely in social characteristics, political influences, and cultural traditions, and health promotion within communities requires community members with different ideas, values, and priorities to work together to solve community-wide health problems (Stokols, 1992). When a community- or population-based approach is successful, Rose (1992) maintains that the whole distribution of exposure levels is shifted, and everyone then experiences a lower risk.

THEORIES AND CONCEPTS TO SUPPORT COMMUNITY APPROACHES

Commonly used theories and concepts important to community health behavior change are:

- Diffusion of Innovations Theory
- Stage Theory
- Organizational Development (OD) Theory
- Social Marketing
- Community Organizational Concepts

To illustrate how community-based theories and organizational concepts are relevant to a program developed for specific subgroups of people, we now return to the case example of Sophia who is not able to participate in a walking program because of neighborhood safety concerns. Sophia's case demonstrates how community-based theories and organizational concepts are relevant to a program developed for specific subgroups of people, a worksite, and a comprehensive community-wide setting.

First, we develop a community intervention to help Sophia and others like her (i.e., a specific subgroup of people who have experienced a cardiac event and have completed cardiac rehabilitation).

> The health professionals in the outpatient cardiac rehabilitation program are concerned that many patients like Sophia have difficulty continuing to exercise once discharged from the program. They survey discharged patients who have not continued with exercise to determine barriers that have prevented them from exercising. Based on survey results and through a literature search, they decide to adapt an in-home video exercise program developed by Jette et al. (1999) for patients who complete the cardiac rehabilitation program.

The Diffusion of Innovations Theory focuses on how new ideas or innovations can become disseminated and adopted. A home-based video exercise program is the new idea that we want patients to adopt. Diffusion requires not only strategies at the individual level but may require the use of both formal communication (e.g., television, print, and radio), as well as informal communication, such as family support and friends. The concept of using a home-based video exercise program needs to be communicated through various channels over time and among the members of a social system. Rogers' theory of how new ideas are dispersed and adopted has five predictable characteristics (Rogers, 1983). **Table 18-1** shows how these characteristics are relevant in developing the home-based video exercise program.

The diffusion of an idea also depends on communication channels. In this case, as well as others, communication will be more effective when, for example, healthcare professionals explain and demonstrate the video to patients and emphasize the importance of exercise to family members or friends who can support the patient. A buddy system might be developed so two patients could be paired to support each other in exercise.

Another element in diffusion of innovation is time. People are often at different stages of individual decision making about new ideas; they may be in the precontemplation, contemplation, preparation, action, or maintenance phase (or in other words, not yet thinking about accepting a new idea, think-

Table 18-1 Diffusion of Innovations Theory and Application

Characteristic	Definition: The Idea	Application to a Program in Which People Would Use a Home Video Exercise Program
Relative advantage	Better than what was there before	The barrier of safety would be removed so that people could exercise without having to leave their homes.
Compatibility	Fits with the needs, values, habits of the intended audience	The video is culturally relevant with respect to the ethnicity of people demonstrating the exercises and the music selected to accompany the exercises.
Complexity	Easy to use	Individuals can use the exercise any time of the day within a safe setting. The video equipment is provided at no or low cost and is simple to use.
Trialability	Can be tried before being adopted (e.g., test driving a car before buying)	People can check the video out for a trial use before committing to use it on a regular basis
Observability	Provides visible results	Video would include testimonials from people who successfully followed the video exercise program

ing about accepting it, taking steps to implement a new idea, actually implementing a new idea or making the new idea part of their lives) (Prochaska, Norcross, & DiClemente, 1994). The number of people who adopt a new idea can be plotted against time on a graph and will result in a predictable S-shaped curve (Rogers, 1995).

Figure 18-1 illustrates how initially, only a few individuals adopt the idea (action) after which the curve climbs as more individuals adopt. The curve levels off when most have adopted. The curve is also characteristic of many product life cycles.

To move patients along this curve, health professionals might ask a person who is actively making changes in his or her life to talk with a person who is still unsure about making changes.

The final element in diffusion is the social system. Social norms and opinion leadership will influence diffusion. For example, we cannot assume that this group of patients who have had a cardiac event will automatically

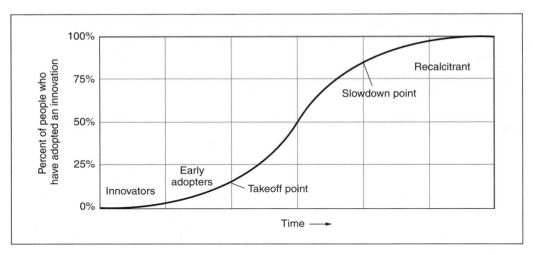

Figure 18-1 Typical adoption rate of innovations.
Source: Reprinted with permission by Schutt (2001). This figure summarizes the work by Rogers (1983).

adopt the home video exercise program. If the social norm in the community is for older people to sit and rest rather than be active, diffusion will be slow. The program will flourish, however, if opinion leaders such as former patients, family members, and health professionals encourage and support patients to participate.

Paying attention to the characteristics of innovations can improve the potential for adoption and dissemination of new ideas. Innovations in industries, including health care, often disseminate slowly, if at all. Increased attention to these characteristics of diffusion and careful plans to disseminate new ideas and programs can promote promising health promotion programs (Berwick, 2003; Caburnay, Kreuter, & Donlin, 2001).

ORGANIZATIONAL STAGE THEORY AND ORGANIZATIONAL DEVELOPMENT

Another type of community approach, a worksite program, could be developed to support Sophia's progress with her exercise program.

Sophia works in the Hancock Insurance Company that allows employees a 1-hour lunch break, although if there is extra work, employees are expected to forgo a break and eat while they work. Hancock executives are already discussing the idea of a worksite exercise program as a possible strategy to be competitive with other large firms who are offering a similar benefit and because Hancock hopes to reduce employee health insurance premiums.

Theories important to developing this program would be diffusion of innovation, already discussed, and organizational stage theory and OD. What changes must occur in the Hancock organization in order to introduce the change of a worksite exercise program? Organizational stage theory holds that organizations go through predictable stages as they introduce change (Lewin, 1951). The process is complex; both individual organizational members and the organization as a whole needs to move through stages of change for the organization to change. Lewin's early work was developed into an organizational change model that included seven stages (Beyer & Trice, 1978). An abbreviated version of the stages (Glanz, Lewis, & Rimer, 2002) is presented in **Table 18-2**.

Even when change is well supported by best practice and the literature, a gap can occur between the evidence and the actual institutional change of a health practice or behavior (Grol & Wensing, 2004). For example, employees who want to exercise on their own may resist the change because they

Table 18-2 Stage Theory

Definitions	Application to Developing a Worksite Program
Stage 1: Awareness	
Problems are recognized, defined, and analyzed	Employer uses employee focus groups and a needs assessment to determine the need for a worksite exercise program.
Stage 2: Adoption	
Initiation of action in which a policy or plan is developed and resources are identified for the chosen change	Employer creates a task force that includes employees, health professionals, and management who work together to develop a lunchtime program that has exercise equipment, is supervised by a health professional, and is provided at a minimal cost to the employee.
Stage 3: Implementation	
Change is implemented, and role changes occur.	Employer begins lunchtime exercise program. Works with its health insurer carrier to offer decreased premiums for employees who participate. Management changes expectation that employees work through lunch.
Stage 4: Institutionalization	
Change becomes a recognized part of the organization.	Employer adds lunchtime exercise as a benefit for all employees.

feel that it is unfair if the employer only offers an insurance discount for employees who attend the worksite program or the organization may resist the change if there is no evidence that it will help to reduce its health insurance premiums.

A common problem in organizational change is that stages are omitted. For example, the Hancock organization might initiate a program without identifying all of the resources needed or not develop a mechanism to assure that the program can continue and as a result be unable to implement the program as it had originally intended.

OD can be used to help the organization improve the likelihood of successfully implementing an organizational change. OD is defined as "a system-wide application and transfer of behavioral science knowledge to the planned development, improvement, and reinforcement of the strategies, structures, and processes that lead to organization effectiveness" (Cummings & Worley, 2005).

OD focuses on identifying problems that prevent an organization from functioning. This theory has its roots in sensitivity training used by management in the 1940s and 1950s. Over time, OD has changed to focus less on individuals and more on work group relationships (Organ & Bateman, 1986). An organization might use an outside consultant to "diagnose" organizational problems and present a plan for change by addressing the concepts of organizational climate, culture, and capacity (Brown & Covey, 1987, cited in Woodman & Pasmore, 1987).

In diagnosing an organizational problem, the climate, culture, and capacity of the organization should be considered. Organizational climate can be thought of as the organization's personality. Organizational culture is the shared beliefs of people in an organization, and organizational capacity is the organization's ability to produce and maintain services and operations.

Organizations "stuck" in one stage can use organization development to identify obstacles in aspects of culture, climate, and capacity and change them to move to the next stage. Changes at the community and organizational levels are likely to be successful when the problem is accurately identified (OD) and organizational change is introduced following all four steps of organizational change (stage theory) (see Table 18-2).

In our case example, the Hancock organization might decide that its culture of expecting employees to work through lunch is an obstacle. If it is not eliminated, the worksite exercise program might not attract many employees and the program will be "stuck" (Table 18-2, stage 3), and Hancock will not be able to justify making this program part of the organization (Table 18-2, stage 4). Stage and OD theories can inform community health approaches and increase the likelihood of program success.

SOCIAL MARKETING THEORY

Next, we consider how to apply social marketing theory in a community-wide setting to make it more likely that Sophia and other people in their 60s in the community will exercise.

> A survey of a sampling of the residents in Sophia's inner city neighborhood reveals that (1) the neighborhood is not perceived as a safe environment for older people, (2) some residents are low income and/or are on fixed retirement incomes, and (3) most of the residents have more than one chronic health problem.
>
> A program is developed at the local YMCA, a facility accessible by public transportation and which has parking, where residents 60 and older can use its exercise facilities at a low cost. Participants are initially screened as to their level of fitness. Then a personalized program is developed each participant, and several times a week, a health professional with fitness training and medical expertise is present onsite to guide and progress residents in their exercise.

Social marketing theory uses concepts developed from commercial marketing to promote voluntary behavior change to improve the health of individuals and society. When applied to the implementation of behavioral change, social marketing theory focuses on satisfying the needs of consumers through the design, communication, pricing, and delivery of appropriate and competitive innovations or programs (Glanz & Rimer, 2002).

Social marketing has been used at a national level by the CDC as a theory that supports programs (e.g., that increase fruit and vegetable consumption), promote physical activity, and consider other preventive health behaviors (Coreil, Bryant, & Henderson, 2000). What defines social marketing from other public health planning is its emphasis on integrating the marketing elements of exchange theory, audience segmentation, competition, the marketing mix, consumer orientation, and continuous monitoring (Grier & Bryant, 2005) (**Table 18-3**).

Social marketing often includes education (persuading people to adopt healthy behaviors) and law or policy development (e.g., the use of coercion when society is unwilling to pay the cost of risky behaviors [e.g., drunk driving]). Social marketing also reduces barriers to change by creating an environment that encourages people to willingly make voluntary health behavior changes as opposed to involuntary exchanges (e.g., policies and laws

Table 18-3 Social Marketing Definitions and Application

Element	Definition	Application: Increasing Physical Activity of Older People Within a Community
Exchange Theory	Assumes consumers act primarily out of self-interest, and gives consumers the greatest benefit at the least cost in time, money, and psychological discomfort in changing behavior.	The campaign would be geographically close to people, mindful of their ability to pay, and set within an existing social structure, in this case, the YMCA.
Audience segmentation	May divide populations on basis of ethnicity, age, and on basis of current behavior (e.g., current exercisers versus have never exercised).	The program selects those people who have never exercised or rarely exercise and focuses on what would help them begin to exercise.
Competition	Behavioral options and services that compete with public health recommendations.	Television and people's safety and comfort sitting in their home may be the behavioral competition. The program uses the local cable channel to promote the importance of exercise and program developers go door-to-door based on census data to personally invite the residents.
Marketing mix	Product—set of benefits the desired behavior will bring	Product—may emphasize campaign as a way for older residents to have fun and become more fit and get to know neighbors
	Price—tangible and intangible	Price—residents may not value something that is entirely free, and thus, the program uses a sliding scale fee.
	Place—location	Place—YMCA is easily accessed by residents.
	Promotion—types of persuasive communication to convey the product	Promotion—use a group of residents already committed to exercise to promote the program.
Consumer orientation	Commitment to providing programs that meet consumer needs	Use of surveys and focus groups to determine people's needs
Continuous monitoring	Evaluating effectiveness	Evaluation tools developed to monitor program

imposed on people) (Rothschild, 1999). Table 18-3 illustrates how health educators could use social marketing in a community-wide campaign to increase the physical activity of Sophia and people in their 60s in an inner-city neighborhood.

CONCEPTS OF COMMUNITY CHANGE

In addition to a sound theoretical base, effective community interventions engage community members in both the design and implementation phases.

To illustrate how a community change might unfold, we continue our case example.

> In the hospital where Sophia was treated for her cardiac event and rehabilitation, health professionals are increasingly aware that many patients have health problems that could be lessened by physical activity and improved nutrition. Hospital management creates a task force of interested health personnel to begin discussions about the problem. Task force members wonder if an integrated, comprehensive community approach to improve physical activity in the entire population within the community where Sophia lives might be the best approach.

Concepts important to community change include empowerment, critical consciousness, community capacity, issue selection, and participation and relevance (Glanz & Rimer, 2002), as described in **Table 18-4**. This table describes the next steps in the process that would be needed to create an integrated community-wide change in physical activity and nutrition.

> Through broad community involvement and wide social and organizational support from law enforcement, insurers, local grocers, and so forth, a farmer's market is created in the neighborhood. Once a week, local area farmers come to the parking lot of a neighborhood grocery store. The insurance company commits to providing cash vouchers that low-income residents can use to purchase fruits and vegetables in the grocery store or farmer's market. The grocery store also benefits from now being able to purchase fruits and vegetables at a lower cost from local vendors. With the help of law enforcement and city officials, a neighborhood-watch program is implemented, and street lighting is improved. Local churches, in their weekly bulletins, promote the farmer's market, and the city hires teens to work with the parks department to improve the parks.

Sound improbable? Not so. The literature provides many examples of similar community approaches to changing health. For example, the United States Department of Agriculture awarded grants in 2007 to some 47 states to

Table 18-4 Community Organization Concepts

Element	Definition	Application to a Community-Wide Program
Empowerment	The process of gaining mastery and power over oneself/one's community to produce change and give individuals and communities the tools and the responsibility for making decisions that affect them.	Community members assume power within the task force to create change.
Community competence	The community's ability to engage in effective problem solving. It identifies problems, creates consensus, and achieves goals.	The task force is broadened to include representatives from the community, the insurance industry, law enforcement, the local community health center, the YMCA, several churches, and a private physical and occupational therapy outpatient clinic. Consensus is reached to educate the community on the importance of physical activity and good nutrition, to improve safety in local parks and to increase the availability of fresh fruits and vegetables within the community.
Participation and relevance	The work should "start where the people are" and allow community members to actively participate in identifying problems.	The task force includes community members. Focus groups are held with community members to gain their ideas.
Issue selection	The community needs to identify achievable, simple, and specific issues for action.	The community identifies physical activity and the lack of availability and high cost of fresh fruits and vegetables as issues for action.
Critical consciousness	The community needs to understand root causes of social problems from a broad social perspective.	This broad task force identifies several factors which affect the ability of its members to engage in physical activity: a diminished sense of safety and fear of crime related to poor street lighting and lack of law enforcement, widespread disrepair of sidewalks, a lack of parks, and significant unemployment. The task force identifies the lack of good supermarkets within the neighborhood as a cause of the lack of fruits and vegetables.

Source: Adapted from Glanz, Lewis, and Rimer (2002, p. 288).

start a Senior's Market Nutrition Program to give vouchers to low-income seniors 60 years of age and older to purchase fruits and vegetables at local community farmer's markets (United States Department of Agriculture, n.d.). Other community programs have focused on strategies to improve cardiovascular health (Alcalay, Alvarado, Balcazar, Newman, & Huerta, 1999; Brice & Gorey, 1996; Brownson et al., 1996; Elder, Schmid, Dower, & Hedlund, 1993; O'Loughlin, Paradis, Gray-Donald, & Renaud, 1999). The Salud Para Su Corazon program (Alcalay et al., 1999) included multimedia bilingual television, radio programs, brochures, motivational videos, and recipe booklets targeted to change health behaviors to prevent cardiovascular disease. Some community programs have also targeted prevention and physical activity for older people (Brice & Gorey, 1996; King, Rejeski, & Buchner, 1998), whereas others have offered programs in faith-based settings (Brudenell, 2003; Droege & Wenger, 1997).

What role do health professionals have in the community change approaches to health education and promotion? As part of a team, we can help identify and analyze the community or organization's health problem, identify individual, community, and organizational theories that can best inform the problem, and participate in health education and promotion using community approaches. Nurses have been integrated into community work for many years and the opportunity is emerging for other health professionals to also increase their participation in community approaches to improving health. Resources such as the Community Tool Box (http://ctb.ku.edu/) developed through the CDC (Fawcett et al., 2000) provide valuable help for developing effective community programs.

CHALLENGES IN COMMUNITY CHANGE

In spite of the progress that has been made in changing communities, there are challenges that remain. One challenge in healthcare interventions is to design methods of research and analysis that will be capable of determining the program effectiveness (DiClemente, Crosby, & Kegler, 2002; Shortell et al., 2002). Although research has shown some program elements to be effective, the length of time needed to demonstrate program effectiveness is often longer than the program's duration (Shortell et al., 2002). More research is needed to determine long-term effectiveness (Merzel & D'Afflitti, 2003).

The CDC, using an expert panel task force, reviewed the literature and classified programs on the strength of evidence for effectiveness and concluded that although evidence shows that some interventions such as community-wide campaigns and school-based physical education to increase physical activity show strong evidence, many efforts such as mass media campaigns to increase physical activity have insufficient evidence to determine effectiveness (Zara, Briss, & Harris, 2005). There is recognition at the national level that health issues require social change in the environment, social groups, and organizations to improve national health and fitness (Satcher, 1998).

Some of the limitations in determining effectiveness are the limited duration, intensity, and scope of program activities that focus on individuals rather than multiple levels of focus (e.g., environmental and policy level), the small magnitude of effect in community programs where the intervention may be less intensive, and the positive changes that may occur in both the intervention group and the control group when programs are presented that include societal changes such as smoking, diet, and exercise programs (Merzel & D'Afflitti, 2003).

Other challenges to effective programs of community change are developing culturally appropriate educational material, gaining community participation and involvement, and addressing social inequities (Stokols, 1992). To achieve these, significant resources may be needed. For example, programs for communities with people of different ethnic backgrounds require educational material that is culturally relevant to the people who live there and gaining entry into the community requires an understanding of concepts of community organization and coalitions. Programs to increase exercise in older people may necessitate social changes and policies in the housing industry, parks, and through legislation.

Another challenge is finding adequate funding for community-based health efforts. The insurance reimbursement system operates on the medical model of individual treatment, not wide-based program reimbursement. Health professionals may need to become active in advocating for change in the funding of community health projects.

Finally, getting involved in the community requires an understanding of the role health professionals and participants should have in the change process. Health professionals must first assume that people want to and can change and that those individuals should participate in making, adjusting, or controlling community changes. In the medical model, the provider is often viewed as the expert who helps make a diagnosis and establish treatment. In contrast, in the community organization model, health professionals may need to develop an increased capacity to listen to community members' perspectives on health problems and what changes are needed and accept a role in which the health professional is not considered the expert.

These challenges can be viewed as opportunities for us to be involved in health promotion research, develop health promotion programs that include environmental and policy level changes, and advocate for increased health promotion program funding.

SUMMARY

This chapter has emphasized the importance of community-based health promotion approaches that can support individual health behavior change. Several behavior and social science theoretical models have been discussed that can help us promote health at the community and organizational levels.

The health professional's role in health promotion is evolving and changing. Healthcare settings (e.g., rehabilitation facilities, private practices, and acute-care hospitals) where many health professionals work have a mission not only to improve the health of the individual, but also to provide strategies for prevention programs to enhance the health of the communities they serve. Health professionals in all disciplines have new opportunities to help meet this mission by participating in community-based efforts.

REFERENCES

Alcalay, R., Alvarado, M., Balcazar, H., Newman, E., & Huerta, E. (1999). Salud para su corazon: a community-based Latino cardiovascular disease prevention and outreach model. *Journal of Community Health, 24,* 359–378.

Baker, E. A., & Brownson, C. A. (1998). Defining characteristics of community-based health promotion programs. *Journal of Public Health Management Practice, 4,* 1–9.

Berwick, D. M. (2003). Disseminating innovations in health care. *Journal of the American Medical Association, 289,* 1969–1975.

Best, A., Stokols, D., Green, L. W., Leischow, S., Holmes, B., & Buchholz, K. (2003). An integrative framework for community partnering to translate theory into effective health promotion strategy. *American Journal of Health Promotion, 18*(2), 169–176.

Beyer, J. M., & Trice, H. M. (1978). *Implementing change: alcoholism policies in work organizations.* New York: Free Press.

Brice, G. C., & Gorey, K. M. (1996). The staywell program: maximizing elders' capacity for independent living through health promotion and disease prevention activities. *Research on Aging, 18,* 202–219.

Brown, L. D., & Covey, J. G. (1987). Development organizations and organization development: toward an expanded paradigm for organization development. In R. W. Woodman & W. A. Pasmore (Eds.), *Research in organizational change and development.* Greenwich, CT: JAI Press.

Brownson, R. C., Smith, C. A., Pratt, M., Mack, N. E., Jackson-Thompson, J., Dean, C. G., Dabney, S., & Wilkerson, J. C. (1996). Preventing cardiovascular disease through community-based risk reduction: the Bootheel Heart Healthy Project. *American Journal of Public Health, 86,* 206–213.

Brudenell, I. (2003). Parish nursing: nurturing body, mind, spirit, and community. *Public Health Nursing, 20,* 85–94.

Caburnay, C. A., Kreuter, M. W., & Donlin, M. J. (2001). Disseminating effective health promotion programs from prevention research to community organizations. *Journal of Public Health Management Practice, 7,* 81–89.

Coreil, J., Bryant, C. A., & Henderson, J. N. (2000). *Social and behavioral foundations of public health.* Thousand Oaks, CA: Sage.

Cummings, T. G., & Worley, C. G. (2005). *Organization development and change.* Mason, OH: South-Western.

DiClemente, R. J., Crosby, R. A., & Kegler, M. C. (Eds.). (2002). *Emerging theories in health promotion practice and research: strategies for improving public health.* San Francisco: Jossey-Bass, John Wiley & Sons.

Droege, T., & Wenger, A. F. (1997). *Starting point: empowering communities to improve health.* Atlanta, GA: The Interfaith Health Program, The Carter Center.

Elder, J. P., Schmid, T. L., Dower, P., & Hedlund, S. (1993). Community heart health programs: Components, rationale, and strategies for effective interventions. *Journal of Public Health Policy, 14,* 463–479.

Fawcett, S. B., Francisco, V. T., Schultz, J. A., Berkowitz, B., Wolff, T. J., & Nagy, G. (2000). The community tool box: a web-based resource for building healthier communities. *Public Health Reports, 115,* 274–278.

Gilliland, J. M., & Taylor, E. (1999). Planning community health interventions. In J. M. Raczynski & R. J. DiClemente (Eds.), *Handbook of health promotion and disease prevention* (pp. 427–439). New York: Kluwer Academic/Plenum.

Glanz, K., Lewis, F. M., & Rimer, B. K. (Eds.). (2002). *Health behavior and health education.* San Francisco: Jossey-Bass.

Green, L. W., & Kreuter, M. W. (1999). *Health promotion planning: an educational and ecological approach.* Mountain View, CA: Mayfield Publishing Company.

Grier, S., & Bryant, C. A. (2005). Social marketing in public health. *Annual Review of Public Health, 26,* 319–339.

Grol, R., & Wensing, M. (2004). What drives change? Barriers to and incentives for achieving evidence-based practice. *Medical Journal of Australia, 180,* S57–S60.

King, A. C. (1994). Community and public health approaches to the promotion of physical activity. *Medicine and Science in Sports and Exercise, 26,* 1405–1412.

King, A. C. (1998). How to promote physical activity in a community: research experiences from the US highlighting different community approaches. *Patient Education Counseling, 1*(Suppl.), S3–S12.

King, A. C., Rejeski, W. J., & Buchner, D. M. (1998). Physical activity interventions targeting older adults: a critical review and recommendations. *American Journal of Preventive Medicine, 15*(4), 316–333.

Kreuter, M. W. (1992). PATCH: its origin, basic concepts, and links to contemporary public health policy. *Journal of Health Education, 23,* 135–139.

Lewin, K. (1951). *Field theory in social science.* In K. Glanz, F. M. Lewis, & B. K. Rimer (Eds.), *Health behavior and health education.* San Francisco: Jossey-Bass Publishers.

Luepker, R. V., Rastam, L., Hannan, P. J., Murray, D. M., Gray, C., Baker, W. L., Crow, R., Jacobs Jr., D. R., Pirie, P. L., Mascioli, S. R., Mittelmark, M. B., & Blackburn, H. (1996). Community education for cardiovascular disease prevention. *American Journal of Epidemiology, 144,* 351–362.

McKenzie, J. F., & Smeltzer, J. L. (Eds.). (2001). *Planning, implementing, and evaluating health promotion programs.* Boston: Allyn and Bacon.

Merzel, C., & D'Afflitti, J. (2003). Reconsidering community-based health promotion: promise, performance, and potential. *American Journal of Public Health, 93,* 557–574.

Minkler, M., & Wallerstein, N. (2005). *Improving health through community organization and community building.* In M. Minkler (Ed.), *Community organizing and community building for health.* New Brunswick: Rutgers University Press.

O'Loughlin, J. L., Paradis, G., Gray-Donald, K., & Renaud, L. (1999). The impact of a community-based heart disease prevention program in a low-income inner-city neighborhood. *American Journal of Public Health, 89,* 1819–1826.

Organ, D. W., & Bateman, T. (1986). *Organizational behavior* (3rd ed.). Plano, TX: Business Publications.

Prochaska, J. O., Norcross, J. C., & DiClemente, C. C. (1994). *Changing for good.* New York: Avon Books.

Rogers, E. M. (1983). *Diffusions of innovations.* New York: Free Press.

Rose, G. (1992). *The strategy of preventive medicine.* Oxford, UK: Oxford University Press.

Rothschild, M. L. (1999). Carrots, sticks, and promises: a conceptual framework for the management of public health and social issue behaviors. *Journal of Marketing, 63,* 24–37.

Satcher, D. (1998). *Progress review: physical activity and fitness.* Washington, DC: Department of Health and Human Services, Public Health Service.

Schooler, C., Farquhar, J. W., Fortmann, S. P., & Flora, J. A. (1997). Synthesis of findings and issues from community prevention trials. *Annals of Epidemiology,* 7(Suppl.), S54–S68.

Schutt, R. (2001). *Inciting democracy: a practical proposal for creating a good society.* Cleveland, OH: SpringForward Press.

Sharpe, P. A. (2003). Community-based physical activity intervention. *Arthritis and Rheumatism, 49,* 455–462.

Shortell, S. M., Zukoski, A. P., Alexander, J. A., Bassoli, G. J., Conrad, D. A., & Hasnain-Wynia, R., et al. (2002). Evaluating partnerships for community health improvement: tracking the footprints. *Journal of Health Politics, Policy and Law, 27,* 49–93.

Stokols, D. (1992). Establishing and maintaining healthy environments toward a social ecology of health promotion. *American Psychologist, 47,* 6–22.

United States Department of Agriculture. (n.d.) Retrieved July 18, 2007, from http://www.fns.usda.gov/wic/SFMNP-Fact-Sheet.pdf.

USDHHS. (2001). Healthy People 2010. Retrieved May 11, 2001, from http://www.health.gov/healthypeople/.

Zara, S., Briss, P. A., & Harris, K. W. (2005). *Guide to community preventive services.* Oxford: Oxford University Press.

Chapter 19

Teaching Patients About Medications

Kathy Zaiken & Caroline S. Zeind

INTRODUCTION

Teaching patients about medications is of paramount importance in achieving positive health outcomes. It is estimated that one third to one half of patients who are taking chronic medications fail to take their medicines appropriately (Horne, 1998; Smith, 1985). The inappropriate use of medications has led to significant adverse events, including fatalities, as well as ineffective management of disease states. Managing chronic disease states has become a tremendous societal and economic burden on the U.S. healthcare system; approximately 70% of all deaths in the United States are attributed to chronic diseases (Centers for Disease Control and Prevention, 2008). In 2006, there were 37.3 million persons 65 years or older, representing 12.4% of the U.S. population; this growing population is living longer, adding to the numbers of persons with chronic diseases (U.S. Department of Health and Human Service, 2006).

In 2006, prescription drug spending reached 216.7 billion, which reflected an increase from 5.8% in 2005 to 8.5% (U.S. Department of Health and Human Service, 2006). The factors impacting this change include the increased use of prescription drugs, new indications for existing drugs, expansion of therapeutic classes of drugs, and the increased use of specialty drugs. Likewise, the use of over-the-counter (OTC) drugs in the United States has increased with more than 80 therapeutic categories on the market (Food and Drug Administration, 2008). A 2006 Institute of Medicine (IOM) report estimated that in any given week four of five adults in the United States use prescription medicines, OTC drugs, or dietary supplements, and approximately one third of adults take five or more different medications.

Although the use of prescription and OTC drugs has increased in the healthcare system, the inefficiencies within the healthcare delivery system have resulted in shortcomings in the provision of high-quality care to Americans. The 2001 IOM report "Crossing the Quality Chasm" argued that the healthcare industry has become disjointed, and has fallen short in achieving its goals to provide optimal care to all people. With the rapid advancements in science and technology, the report stated that the healthcare system has not effectively used information technology to provide safe and quality care consistently to patients. The 2006 IOM report "Preventing Medication Errors" described the problem of inadequate patient safety in the healthcare system, and promoted strategies for enhancing communication between the patient and the healthcare provider. In the proposed model, healthcare providers were challenged to take on a greater role to educate, consult with, and listen to patients. Specifically, the report emphasized that patients should be informed about the benefits and risks of their medications, contraindications, and possible side effects; it also stressed that patients should also take on a more active role in managing their illnesses, including the use of medications as an important component of their health care.

Teaching patients about medications has become increasingly challenging, as approximately 90 million people in the United States have limited health literacy skills (Neilsen-Bohlman, Panzer, & Kindig, 2004). Patients who have difficulty understanding medication directions may use incorrect doses, wrong schedules, or wrong routes of administration. Older persons in particular have difficulty with understanding when to time their medications in relation to meals (Zuccollo & Liddell, 1985). Parents who do not clearly understand medication dosing directions may give their children incorrect doses of medications that may lead to drug toxicity or treatment failure, depending on the type of dosage error. Many patients are taking more complicated regimens with the potential for drug–drug, drug–disease, and drug–food interactions. In addition, research and technology have led to advancements in drug development that has resulted in the approval of many formulations on the market requiring special instructions for proper administration. Thus, it has become increasingly important to explain to patients how to use medicines appropriately to ensure an optimal outcome.

TEACHING TECHNIQUES

Healthcare professionals are generally well trained in the professional and clinical aspects of their duties, but fewer people are skilled in interpersonal communication (Herrier, Gardner, & Meldrum, 2007; Robinson, 2004). In addition, many healthcare providers may have limited education and training in adult patient education principles and strategies (Hansen & Fischer, 1998; Robinson, 2004). This results in a significant challenge to healthcare providers who, according to the 2006 IOM report, "must communicate more with patients at every step of the way and make that communication a two-way street, listening to the patients as well as talking to them."

Thus, effective interpersonal communication skills are necessary for pharmacists and other healthcare providers to teach patients about their medications. Counseling should include both oral and written components whenever possible; visual images are also helpful. Providers must be skilled in interviewing the patient, and in asking questions that are relevant to the medications that patients are taking (Herrier et al., 2007). Appropriate open-ended questions start with "who, what, where, when, and how" and should not invoke blame or criticism. For example, it would be inappropriate to ask a patient, "Why did you skip a few days of taking your high blood pressure medicine?" A better way to approach the patient would be to use a universal statement, followed by an open-ended question, such as: "Sometimes people miss doses of their high blood pressure regimens because they feel fine and they forget to take it. What has been your experience in taking high blood pressure medications?"

It is also important for the healthcare provider to display empathetic communication skills that put patients at ease, enabling them to discuss concerns regarding medications. Likewise, the provider must use reflective responding with the patient that will illicit a sense of the patient's thoughts and feelings (Herrier et al., 2007). This approach will enable the pharmacist to cultivate an open and empathic environment that can lead to the formation of a trusting relationship with the patient. Thus, the patient is more likely to discuss information relevant to his or her medication therapy that will be useful in achieving positive outcomes for therapy management.

Clinical interviewing skills are a necessary component of teaching patients about their medications (Herrier et al., 2007). As part of the interview, the provider must obtain a thorough assessment of medication use, including the following: currently prescribed medications; past medication usage (including time period of use), and reason(s) for discontinuation; current nonprescription medications (including herbal and dietary supplements); drug allergies (including an accurate description of the allergies); adverse

Table 19-1 Key Components in Counseling Patients Regarding Medications

Counseling Components	Information to Include
Introducing the medication	• What is the trade and generic name of the medication? • What the medication is being used for? • The therapeutic class of the medication.
How to use the medication	• By what route should the patient take the medication (oral, inhalation, injection, etc.)? • Explain what form the medication is in such as a tablet, capsule, or liquid. • What is the dose of the medication in metric amounts (e.g., 10 mL) or the number of tablets or capsules taken? • Explain how often the medication should be taken. • Explain specific requirements when using the medications if applicable (e.g., take on an empty stomach, and take 30 minutes before all other medications). • Explain what actions the patient should take if they miss a dose. • Tell the patient how long they will be using the medication.
What to expect	• Explain how the medication will improve their condition, symptoms. • What beneficial effects can the patient expect to see? • Tell the patient how long it will take to see these effects.
Adverse effects	• Warn patient about common as well as severe side effects. • Provide ways for these side effects to be avoided or minimized (e.g., take with food to decrease stomach upset). • Explain what the patient should look for if an adverse effect were to occur. • Provide information about what the patient should do if they experience a side effect.
Monitoring	• Inform patient how to monitor for improvement of their condition or disease state. • Provide information regarding signs that their condition or disease state may be worsening. • Provide examples of ways the patient can self-monitor.
Storage and refills	• Provide information about the proper storage and disposal of the medication. • Explain to the patient how many refills are on the medication as well as how long their supply should last.
Interactions	• Include information about potential interactions, including drug–drug, drug–disease, drug–food, and any other contraindications.
Miscellaneous information	• Reinforce the availability of pharmacy resources and personnel.

Source: Adapted from Herrier, Gardner, and Meldrum (2007).

reactions; and lifestyle factors (e.g., nicotine, alcohol, illicit drug usage, dietary habits, occupation, and stressors). **Table 19-1** summarizes the key components of counseling patients on the medications.

Effective consultation techniques focusing on interaction between the provider and the patient have been well established. Refinements in these techniques over the years have allowed healthcare professionals to better engage patients as active participants in their medication management. Healthcare educators have made significant changes to healthcare curricula to better educate and train students to communicate with patients more effectively.

THE EVOLVING ROLE OF THE PHARMACIST IN COUNSELING

Over the past 40 years, the pharmacy profession in the United States has embraced the concept of pharmaceutical care that extends the pharmacist's professional role to include social responsibility for health care (Hepler & Strand, 1990). In addition, the clinical role of the pharmacist expanded, and pharmacists have become active in a variety of patient-centered activities, including patient counseling and teaching patients about medications (Hepler, 1985).

Legislative changes that supported healthcare reform also expanded the role of the pharmacists. The Omnibus Budget Reconciliation Act of 1990 (OBRA '90) required states to develop standards governing patient counseling for patients receiving new and refill prescriptions. More recently, the Medicare Modernization Act of 2003 led to changes in 2006 for outpatient prescription drug benefits for Medicare beneficiaries, known as Medicare Part D. In addition, the Medicare Modernization Act enables certain Medicare beneficiaries to receive medication therapy management services as part of expanded drug benefits. Pharmacists now counsel patients on the appropriate use of medications in conjunction with medication therapy management programs, as well as offer disease-prevention and wellness programs. These types of legislative changes are occurring in other parts of the world, such as the United Kingdom and Canada, thus expanding the roles and responsibilities of pharmacists in the community setting (Dyck, Deschamps, & Taylor, 2005; Noyce, 2007).

PATIENT COUNSELING AND DISEASE STATE MANAGEMENT PROGRAMS

Pharmacists counsel patients on medicines in a variety of settings and participate in disease state management programs. Community pharmacies, in particular, are located in settings that are generally convenient for patients to access, including those who may live in remote areas that are not close to a clinic. Pharmacists provide advice on OTC products, dietary supplements, and counsel patients regarding medicines, including potential adverse effects, drug–drug, drug–disease, drug–food interactions, and cost-related medication issues.

Pharmacists participate in a variety of community outreach events that are designed to teach patients and their families about the medications that they may be taking. Pharmacists also have the opportunity to emphasize to patients who are on medications the importance of monitoring for adverse effects and encourage them to take an active role in management of their disease. Pharmacists attend health fairs held in an array of settings including assisted living and nursing homes, senior centers, schools, clinics, and community pharmacies. There is an event referred to as "The Brown Bag" in which patients bring all of their medications in a brown bag to the program. The pharmacist would then check to make sure that all of the medications were compatible with each other and that none of the medications were beyond their expiration dates. The pharmacist would also meet with each person and discuss the proper use of his or her medications, side effects, and other medication-related issues as well as answer any specific questions and/or concern regarding the medications.

Nurses, physicians, and physician assistants continue to play an integral role in patient education and disease-management programs in patient care settings. An increasing number of community pharmacies now offer disease-prevention and management programs, including blood pressure and cholesterol screening, diabetes and asthma education, and weight-management programs. By offering these services, pharmacists are able to work closely with patients on optimizing medication outcomes for these particular disease states.

BARRIERS TO TEACHING PATIENTS ABOUT MEDICATIONS

Healthy People 2010 initiatives have included strategies to eliminate health disparities that would improve access to care as well as language and cultural barriers. About half of adult Americans have intermediate health literacy, indicating difficulty reading and using health information (2003 National Assessment of Adult Literacy, 2004). About 14% of adults (30 million people) have below basic health literacy, meaning that they are either nonliterate in English or cannot perform beyond the most simple and concrete health literacy tasks, such as circling a follow-up clinic appointment date on a card. Only 12% of adults demonstrated proficient health literacy, where they may have the understanding and skills needed to prevent and manage disease states. Adults that were more likely to have limited health literacy included those who were Hispanic, black, and American Indians/Alaskan Native, those with lower incomes, poorer health, limited English proficiency, and who were age 65 and older (National Assessment of Adult Literacy, 2003). These findings highlight significant barriers and challenges faced by healthcare providers in providing optimal care.

Problems pertaining to health literacy are particularly important with regards to medication information (Shrank & Avorn, 2007). A study that evaluated primary care patients found that nearly half of the patients had difficulty understanding one or more of the prescription label instructions on five common prescription drugs (Davis et al., 2006a). Various studies have found that older persons in particular have difficulty in reading and understanding drug labeling, and clearly understanding medication directions (Morrell, Park, & Poon, 1989, 1990). Another study evaluated parents' ability to understand drug labels for their children's medications, and to calculate doses for therapies (Patel, Brant, & Arocha, 2002). The results indicated that 56% of parents incorrectly calculated correct doses of cough syrup, and 68% of parents planned therapy schedules that led to incorrect dosing. Another study examined whether adult patients were able to understand and correctly interpret commonly used prescription medical warning labels (Davis et al., 2006b). The study was conducted in a primary care clinic for adults waiting for an appointment. Two hundred forty-one patients were evaluated for their ability to interpret warning stickers on the prescription bottles. The results of the study indicated that about one third of patients exhibited reading at or below the sixth-grade level (low literacy), and that those with low literacy were 3.4 times less likely to interpret prescription medication warning labels correctly (Davis et al., 2006b).

By the same token, healthcare professionals have demonstrated shortcomings in providing appropriate medication-related information to patients about their prescribed medications (Shrank & Avorn, 2007). A study evaluated audiotaped office visits of physicians communicating to patients about prescribed medicines. Physicians provided patients with instructions for medications use in only 55% of discussions, and only in approximately one third of the discussions did physicians explain adverse effects of medications prescribed and duration of therapy (Tarn et al., 2006). Pharmacist communication with patients regarding medications has also been inadequate (Svarstad,

Bultman, & Mount, 2004). The community pharmacy is usually busy; pharmacists many times are dealing with insurance coverage issues, or they are experiencing a high volume of prescriptions and medication refills as opposed to counseling patients about medications. Thus, many patients are relying primarily on written labels or on complicated package inserts that present information in difficult-to-digest form to the layman. Healthcare providers must strive to improve patient communication regarding medications (Hardin, 2005). Likewise, efforts to re-evaluate and improve written medication information to help patients safely administer and monitor their therapies are strongly warranted (Shrank & Avorn, 2007).

Cultural competency is an important component of health care, and can significantly affect patient outcomes (Vanderpool, 2005). Providers who are culturally competent are likely to communicate better with patients and provide them with the appropriate medication counseling. In order to optimize teaching methods to patients regarding medications, healthcare providers must also have an understanding and appreciation for the communities that they serve (Zweber, 2002). *Pharmaceutical Care* (as termed by Hepler and Strand) necessitates that the pharmacist tailor medication information toward the needs of the individual patient, as well as the communities that they serve. This approach includes awareness and understanding of the patient's culture and perspectives, since these factors influence decisions regarding both the patient's health and the medications that they take (Mullins et al., 2005). Those patients who have difficulty with the English language may bring English-speaking caregivers or family members who communicate well in English to serve as a translator. Many healthcare centers now have translators on staff, and increasingly medical literature for the community setting is available in different languages.

Many treatment choices are influenced by cultural beliefs. In some cultures, alternative treatments are frequently used. It is important for the provider to ask the patient about the use of complementary and alternative medicines, and to include them as part of the complete listing of the patient's medicines. This will assist the healthcare provider in making an accurate assessment regarding medications, including potential interactions and adverse effects of the patient's medicines. Information regarding complementary and alternative medicines may not be readily available to the provider, but they should evaluate evidence-based data if such exists for the non-standard product in question. There are limited data regarding the appropriate use of many natural products operating with more traditional medication. Currently, there are about 100 drug information centers (DICs) in the United

States that are affiliated with either medical centers or schools of pharmacy. These DICs generally have databases containing information on the use of natural products that can assist providers and patients to make informed decisions regarding therapies (Zeind & McCloskey, 2006). Many DICs service both healthcare providers and patients.

Patients with hearing or vision problems present further obstacles to counseling, necessitating a different set of methods for healthcare providers to assist patients in various settings. Using large-type print materials, in tandem with clear verbal instructions, can aid in alleviating barriers to understanding about medications for patients with visual and aural difficulties. (Herrier et al., 2007). It is important that providers discussing medications with patients with hearing problems select a quiet area, repeat information, and ask the patient to also repeat information.

ADHERENCE TO MEDICINES

Healthcare providers in all settings encounter patients who do not adhere to various components of their disease state management plan. The economic burden that results as a consequence of nonadherence is estimated to be at $100 billion annually in the United States (Lewis, 1997). The term "compliance" has changed to "adherence" as a way of embracing the concept of a partnership between the patient and the provider. This new terminology moves away from the negative connotation that the patient is a subservient individual who must comply with the paternalistic healthcare provider (Burkiewicz & Fit, 2007). This modification is also important because it promotes a shared responsibility of nonadherence for both the patient and provider as opposed to blaming the patient.

Pharmacists are well positioned to address medication nonadherence based on their drug expertise, as well as their easy accessibility within various patient care settings. Pharmacists have the opportunity to incorporate strategies to improve patient adherence to medications within their counseling sessions. A study conducted in England selected patients from a sample of community pharmacies. The study assessed the effects of pharmacists who gave patient-centered advice after initiation of a new medicine for a chronic condition to individuals who were 75 years or older, or who were suffering from a stroke, cardiovascular disease, asthma, diabetes, or rheumatoid arthritis (Clifford et al., 2006). The intervention used in the study was based on a theoretical basis, and was designed to elicit the patients' experiences with, and concerns about, the medicine that they were starting. The intervention group received a phone call from a pharmacist two weeks after the patient was recruited. The pharmacist providing the service had been trained in therapy regarding telephone communication skills, the types and causes of nonadherence, and the types of medicine-related problems and adherence issues that patients had experienced in a previous study (Barber et al., 2004). Four weeks after recruitment, and the completion of a postal questionnaire, a telephone interview from a researcher was conducted for both the intervention and control groups. The primary outcome measure was patient self-reported medication adherence, with nonadherence defined as a self-report of at least one dose of the new medicine having been missed within the last seven days. The number of medicine-related problems and beliefs about the medicine were secondary outcome measures. Of the 255 patients in the intervention group and the 237 in the control group, the response rates to the 4-week questionnaire were 72% (intervention) and 66% (control). At the 4-week follow-up period, of those patients who were still prescribed their medication, nonadherence was less frequent in the intervention group (9%, 16 of 185) compared with the control group (16%, 31 of 194 [$P = 0.032$]). There were also fewer problems reported at four weeks in the intervention group (23%, 43 of 185) compared with the control group (34%, 66 of 194 [$P = 0.021$]). The findings of this study demonstrate benefits from pharmacists providing patient-centered advice and information on medicines upon initiation of new medicines. Further research in the area of medication adherence as a component of patient counseling on medicines will be beneficial.

MEDICATION/PATIENT SAFETY

Counseling patients on medicines is also an important component of medication safety. Medication error databases have documented errors that were directly related to dispensing the wrong drug, the wrong dose or dosage form, or providing incorrect directions for use (Cohen & Smetzer, 2007). These errors resulted in adverse events, and in some cases fatality, and could have been prevented if the pharmacists had counseled the patient before dispensation of medications. Approximately 83% of dispensing errors can be discovered during patient counseling, and corrected before the patient leaves the pharmacy (Ukens, 1997). Numerous events, including deaths, could have been prevented if the pharmacist had counseled the patient before dispensation. It is important for the pharmacist to review the prescriber's product indication, dose, and directions for use for the patient. If the pharmacist discovers anything that appears incorrect or unusual, he or she should research the information carefully and call the prescriber if necessary.

Patient counseling thus provides the opportunity to avert patients' mistakes in medication use. Even after counseling patients, it is important to listen to the patient and to make sure that he or she understands the proper use of the medication. If a patient has low health literacy, family members may assist the individual in medication management. Many pharmacies now have counseling areas that offer some degree of privacy, which creates a comfortable environment for the patient to ask questions and bring forward concerns regarding his or her medicines. It is important to demonstrate proper medication techniques to patients, such as the correct use of an inhaler, providing feedback as they practice the technique. It is particularly important to counsel patients who have new prescriptions for high-alert medications, or for those patients who are high risk (e.g., older and pediatric patients) (Cohen & Smetzer, 2007).

SUMMARY

Teaching patients, families, and communities about medicines is an essential component of health care that requires that all healthcare providers be skilled in communication. Given the complexity of managing chronic disease states, healthcare providers must work closely together as members of the multidisciplinary healthcare team to provide optimal patient care. Providers should strive to eliminate barriers that prevent the achievement of positive patient outcomes, including those pertaining to medication therapies. Patients must have a clear understanding of their disease state and the role of the medications in treating the disease. They should also be given clear directions about their medications and encouraged to discuss their concerns as a means of promoting patient safety. Pharmacists and other healthcare providers should take an active role in assisting patients with medication adherence.

Case Study 19–1

Mrs. R is a 28-year-old recently married female who is otherwise healthy except for asthma diagnosed when she was a young girl. At a routine physical exam, she complains of worsening asthma symptoms, but she is not interested in using a daily inhaler to manage her symptoms. Her primary care provider gives her a peak flow device and a new prescription for Advair 250/50 mcg inhaler. Mrs. R agrees that

(Continues)

Case Study 19-1 (*Continued*)

she will use the inhaler and that she will begin the regimen today. One month later she is seen for an emergency visit at the primary care provider's office because of an asthma exacerbation. After discussing the factors that led to this exacerbation, she reports that she often forgets to use the Advair and does not like the funny taste in her mouth after she uses it. Her provider asks her to make an appointment with the pharmacist in the patient care center located within the local community pharmacy for further counseling.

The pharmacist provides Mrs. R with both reading material and visual aids indicating what asthma can do to your lungs, and how medications like Advair can help in managing the disease. The pharmacist uses a teaching inhaler (placebo inhaler) to demonstrate properly how to use the device, and instructs her to rinse her mouth after each use to help prevent side effects. The pharmacist then asks Mrs. R to repeat the information just provided and to practice using a placebo inhaler to ensure that she understands all of the information given. Mrs. R practices using the inhaler, and after two attempts, feels confident in her technique. The pharmacist confirms with her that she has used the teaching inhaler appropriately. The pharmacist also reviews with Mrs. R the proper use of the peak flow device and emphasizes the importance of taking the readings. Mrs. R agrees to use the Advair on a daily basis and to perform her peak flow readings at home. She leaves the pharmacy feeling much more knowledgeable and comfortable with her asthma management plan. The pharmacist also tells Mrs. R. that she can contact her if she has any further questions after she leaves the pharmacy. Upon her next visit to the pharmacy, Mrs. R states that she is feeling much better. The pharmacist also notices that Mrs. R has been adherent with her medication, as is refilling prescriptions on time.

Analysis for Case 19-1

In this patient case, Mrs. R's asthma eventually came under control as she became adherent with her asthma medication. Mrs. R's primary care provider worked in collaboration with the community pharmacist to provide medication therapy management, and the pharmacist took the time to appropriately counsel Mrs. R on her asthma medication, explaining how important it was in terms of managing her disease. Neither the primary care provider nor the pharmacist blamed Mrs. R, nor spoke to her in a condescending manner. The pharmacist spent time with Mrs. R to demonstrate the proper inhaler technique and then watched

Mrs. R practice the technique. The pharmacist also provided feedback to Mrs. R and confirmed that her technique was appropriate. By practicing the inhaler technique and repeating the information, Mrs. R gained confidence in her skills, and understood how she could minimize the adverse effects of the inhaler. Printed information reinforced this confidence, as did the offer by the pharmacist to be contacted by Mrs. R should she have further questions about her medication upon leaving the pharmacy.

Case Study 19–2

Mr. P is a 52-year-old Hispanic male with a 25-year history of smoking. He is married and lives with his wife and two sons. His first language is Spanish, and he can understand and speak only a little English, primarily conversational. His family moved to the United States from Mexico six years ago, and he works for a construction company in North Carolina. He usually comes to appointments with his son who serves as his translator. He has been seen by his physician only once in the past three years, has a history of canceling appointments, and contacts the doctor's office only when in need of medication refills. Today Mr. P arrives at the clinic with his son for an evaluation of a chronic cough with thick yellow/green mucus production. His son informs the provider that his father has been sick and feeling run down for about two months. He also states that his father is still smoking about 1.5 packs of cigarettes per day. His physician confirms bilateral wheezing suggestive of pneumonia, and notices that Mr. P is short of breath. A prescription for a Levaquin and Albuterol inhaler is called into the pharmacy by the physician. The physician does not discuss the specific medications with Mr. P because the doctor assumes that the pharmacist will go over the medications. He also does not explain the importance of the medications and how they will impact his diseases. Mr. P arrives at the pharmacy at about 10 PM without his son to pick up his prescriptions. Unfortunately, the pharmacist on duty did not speak Spanish, and the translator has gone home for the day; therefore, the pharmacist attempts to counsel Mr. P without adequate translation concerning his medications, proper use of

(Continues)

his inhaler and the importance of taking the inhaler and antibiotic as prescribed. The pharmacist realizes that Mr. P does not understand but decides to discuss the medication directions verbally without attempting to show Mr. P how to use the inhaler owing to the language barrier. Two days later Mr. P experiences difficulty breathing and is brought back to the clinic feeling worse, and in some respiratory distress.

Analysis for Case 19-2

In this case, Mr. P had experienced an asthma flare-up that required him to go back to the clinic with worsening symptoms. There are multiple factors that led to this negative health outcome. One of the primary barriers is that Mr. P primarily speaks Spanish, and could not understand the information that the pharmacist had discussed with him in English. Because the pharmacist did not speak any Spanish, the pharmacist should have checked to see whether anyone else working in the pharmacy spoke Spanish. In addition, it would have been helpful to provide Mr. P with written directions for his medications in Spanish. Any written directions should be clear and easy to understand, complemented by visual aids. This is particularly important since the patient may also have low health literacy. The pharmacy may consider purchasing a software program that provides directions in different languages for medications. In addition, the healthcare providers should recommend to Mr. P that he always bring along a family member who can translate with the provider's office and with the pharmacy. The pharmacist should also have offered to arrange an appointment with Mr. P at the next opportunity when a translator would be available, or when a family member who understands English would be available to come with Mr. P to the pharmacy. When a translator is available, the pharmacist should demonstrate the inhaler technique with Mr. P, and should also ask Mr. P to practice the technique in the pharmacist's presence. The pharmacist should assess his technique to confirm that Mr. P is using the inhaler appropriately. The pharmacist should emphasize the importance of taking the antibiotic as prescribed, and counsel Mr. P on the potential adverse effects and other medication-related issues. In addition, the pharmacist should explain the importance of completing his antibiotic regimen even if he begins to feel better.

After Mr. P returns to the pharmacy or to his doctor, he should also be counseled on smoking, which is contributing to his health problems. Once Mr. P agrees that he would be willing to try to stop smoking, the doctor, nurse, or pharmacist can work with him on decreasing his smoking, and eventually quitting, as a long-term plan. The pharmacist can also help by providing smoking cessation options that are covered by his insurance plan. His healthcare providers should also be aware of the cultural beliefs and attitudes that Mr. P may have with regards to his health. The pharmacist should make sure that he has an accurate listing of all of the prescription and OTC medications that Mr. P is taking, including complementary and alternative medicines. His healthcare providers should work with Mr. P and emphasize that if he is proactive with his health, and meets his appointments, he can prevent some of his health problems. His family members should also be encouraged to help Mr. P with both medication adherence and in his overall management of his illnesses.

WEB RESOURCES

Agency for Healthcare Research and Quality
www.ahrq.org

Centers for Disease Control and Prevention
www.cdc.org

Institute of Medicine of the National Academies
www.iom.edu

Institute for Safe Medication Practices
www.ismp.org

National Institutes of Health: Health Information
http://health.nih.gov/

U.S. Food and Drug Administration
www.fda.gov/

U.S. Department of Health and Human Services:
Drug and Food Information
www.hhs.gov/drugs/index.html

World Health Organization (Health Topics: Pharmaceutical Products)
www.who.int/topics/pharmaceutical_products/en/

REFERENCES

Barber, N., Parsons, J., Clifford, S., Darracott, R., & Horne, R. (2004). Patients' problems with new medication for chronic conditions. *Quality and Safety in Health Care, 13,* 172–175.

Burkiewicz, J. S., & Fit, K. E. (2007). Improving adherence-sharing experiences. *The Annals of Pharmacotherapy, 41,* 2058–2060.

Centers for Disease Control and Prevention. (2008). Retrieved January, 2008, from http://www.cdc.gov/nccdphp/.

Clifford, S., Barber, N., Elliot, R., Hartley, E., Horne, R. (2006). Patient-centered advice is effective in improving adherence to medicines. *Pharmacy World Science, 28,* 165–170.

Cohen, M. R., & Smetzer, J. L. (2007). Preventing dispensing errors. In M. R. Cohen (Ed.), *Medication errors* (2nd ed.). Washington, DC: American Pharmacists Association.

Davis, T. C., Wolf, M. S., Bass, P. F., Thompson, J. A., Tilson, H. H., Neuberger, M., & Parker, R. M. (2006a). Literacy and misunderstanding prescription drug labels. *Annals of Internal Medicine, 145,* 887–894.

Davis, T. C., Wolf, M. S., Bass, P. F., Middlebrooks, M., Kennen, E., Baker, D. W., Bennett, C. L., Durazo-Arvizu, R., Bocchini, A., & Savory, S. (2006b). Low literacy impairs comprehension of prescription drug warning labels. *Journal of General Internal Medicine, 21,* 847–851.

Dyck, A., Deschamps, M., & Taylor, J. (2005) Pharmacists' discussions of medication side effects: a descriptive study. *Patient Education and Counseling, 56,* 21–27.

Food and Drug Administration: Office of Non-Prescription Products. (2008). Retrieved January 2008, from http://www.fda.gov/cder/Offices/otc/default.htm.

Hallworth, R. B., & Goldberg, L.A. (1984). Geriatric patients understanding of labeling of medicines: part I. *British Journal of Pharmaceutical Practice, 6,* 6–14.

Hansen, M., & Fischer, J. C. (1998). Patient-centered teaching from theory to practice. *American Journal of Nursing, 98,* 56–60.

Hardin, L. R. (2005). Counseling patients with low literacy. *American Journal of Health-System Pharmacy, 62,* 364–365.

Hepler, C. D. (1985). Pharmacy as a clinical profession. *American Journal of Hospital Pharmacy, 42,* 1298–1306.

Hepler, C. D., & Strand, L. M. (1990). Opportunities and responsibilities in pharmaceutical care. *American Journal of Hospital Pharmacy, 47,* 533–543.

Herrier, R. N., Gardner, M. E., & Meldrum, H. (2007). Patient communication in clinical pharmacy practice. In R. Helms, D. Quan, T. Herfindal, D. R. Gourley, C. S. Zeind, J. Q. Hudson, G. K. Gourley, K. A. Bergstrom, P. M. Beringer, A. J. Olyaei, W. N. Rawls, P. D. Rogers, T. H. Self (Eds.), *Textbook of drug and disease state management* (8th ed.). Baltimore, MD: Lippincott Williams & Wilkins.

Horne, R. (1998). Adherence to medication: a review of the existing literature. In L. Myers & K. Midence (Eds.), *Adherence to treatment in medical conditions.* Amsterdam: Harwood Academic Press.

Institute of Medicine. (2001). *Crossing the quality chasm: a new health system for the 21st century.* Washington, DC: National Academies Press.

Institute of Medicine. (2004). *Health literacy: a prescription to end confusion.* Washington, DC: National Academies Press.

Institute of Medicine. (2006). *Preventing medication errors.* Washington, DC: National Academies Press.

Lewis, A. (1997). Noncompliance: a $100 billion problem. *Remington Report, 5,* 14–15.

Morrell, R. W., Park, D. C., & Poon, L. W. (1989). Quality of instructions on prescription drug labels: effects on memory and comprehension in young and old adults. *Gerontologist, 29,* 345–354.

Morrell, R. W., Park, D. C., & Poon, L. W. (1990). Effects of labeling techniques on memory and comprehension of prescription information in young and old adults. *Journal of Gerontology, 45,* 166–172.

Mullins, C. D., Blatt, L., Gbarayor, C. M., Yang, H. K., Baquet, C. (2005). Health disparities: a barrier to high-quality care. *American Journal of Health-System Pharmacy, 62,* 1873–1882.

National Assessment of Adult Literacy. (2003). The health literacy of America's adults: results from the 2003 National Assessment of Adult Literacy. Retrieved from http://nces.ed.gov/pubs2006/2006483.pdf.

Neilsen-Bohlman, L., Panzer, A. M., & Kindig, D. A. (Eds.). (2004). Health literacy: a prescription to end confusion. Washington, DC: National Academies Press.

Noyce, P. R. (2007). Providing patient care through community pharmacies in the UK: policy, practice, and research. *The Annals of Pharmacotherapy, 41,* 861–868.

Patel, V. L., Brant, T., & Arocha, J. F. (2002). Errors in interpreting quantities as procedures: the case of pharmaceutical labels. *International Journal of Medical Informatics, 65,* 193–211.

Robinson, E. T. (2004). The pharmacist as educator: implications for practice and education. *American Journal of Pharmaceutical Education, 68,* 1–4.

Shrank, W. H., & Avorn, J. (2007). Educating patients about their medications: the potential and limitations of written drug information. *Health Affairs, 26,* 731–740.

Smith, M. (1985). The cost of non-compliance and the capacity of improved compliance to reduce health care expenditures. In *Improving medication compliance.* Proceeding of a Symposium held in Washington, DC. Reston, VA: National Pharmaceutical Council, 35–44.

Svarstad, B. L., Bultman, D. C., & Mount, J. K. (2004). Patient counseling provided in community pharmacies effects of state regulation, pharmacist age, and busyness. *Journal of the American Pharmacists Association, 44,* 22–29.

Tarn, D. M., Heritage, J., Paterniti, D. A., Hays, R. D., Kravitz, R. L., Wenger, N. S. (2006). Physician communication when prescribing new medications. *Archives of Internal Medicine, 166,* 1855–1862.

Ukens, C. (1997). Deadly dispensing: an exclusive survey of Rx errors by pharmacists. *Drug Topics, 141,* 100–111.

U.S. Department of Health and Human Service. (2000). *Healthy people 2010: understanding and improving health* (2nd ed.). Washington, DC: U.S. Government Printing Office.

U.S. Department of Health and Human Services & Centers for Medicare & Medicaid Services. (2006). National Health Expenditure Data, Highlights 2006. Retrieved January 25, 2008, from http://www.cms.hhs.gov/NationalHealthExpendData/02_NationalHealthAccountHistorical.asp#TopOfPage.

Vanderpool, H. K. (2005). Report of the ASHP Ad Hoc Committee on ethnic diversity and cultural competence. *American Journal of Health-System Pharmacy, 62,* 1924–1930.

Zeind, C. S., & McCloskey, W. W. (2006). Pharmacists' role in the health care system. *Harvard Health Policy Review, 7,* 147–154.

Zuccollo, G., & Liddell, H. (1985). The elderly and the medication label: doing it better. *Ageing, 14,* 371–376.

Zweber, A. (2002). Cultural competence in pharmacy practice. *American Journal of Pharmaceutical Education, 66,* 172–176.

Chapter 20

Oral Health and Education

Aditi Puri & Mary E. Foley

INTRODUCTION

In May 2000, the U.S. Department of Health and Human Services released the first ever Surgeon General's report on oral health. Within the report, *Oral Health in America: A Report of the Surgeon General*, two major themes were highlighted: (1) "Oral health is more than healthy teeth," and (2) "oral health is integral to overall health" (U.S. Department of Health and Human Services [USDHHS], 2000). These messages, along with several major findings published within the report created a national impetus to improve oral health education, prevention, and access to care for all Americans. A year after the release of the report, the Office of the Surgeon General released a *National Call to Action to Promote Oral Health* (USDHHS, 2001). This follow-up communication called for health professionals and policymakers to partner in an effort to change perceptions of oral health and oral diseases, overcome barriers, build the science base, accelerate science transfer into practice, increase capacity of the oral health workforce, and increase collaborations. Underscored in both documents were the findings that many Americans suffer needlessly from preventable oral diseases and that oral health disparities exist among cultural, ethnic, and low-income minority groups. Furthermore, it was noted that the oral health workforce alone is insufficient to overcome these disparities and that collaboration among and across the disciplines is paramount to improving oral health and overall health and well-being. The purpose of this chapter is to raise awareness among health professionals from all disciplines of the most common oral diseases affecting children, adults, and seniors and to provide appropriate information for non–dental healthcare and education professionals regarding risk factors, early detection, education, health promotion, prevention, and disease management. Both population-based and individual strategies are discussed.

DENTAL CARIES

Dental caries is a chronic, infectious, transmissible disease caused by the bacteria known as *Mutans streptococci* (MS). The disease and bacteria are acquired most often in childhood from mothers or caretakers. Dental caries is diet dependent, progressive, and destructive (Edelstein, 2002). Similar to other chronic diseases such as heart disease, dental caries arises as the result of risk and preventive factors that become imbalanced. When risk factors such as the presence of MS, frequent ingestion of fermentable carbohydrates and diminished salivary flow outweigh preventive factors such as fluoride use, reduced bacterial count, and controlled carbohydrate diet, disease occurs.

In its early stages, the disease is "silent." During this time, the disease reveals no symptoms to the individual patient, and visual signs are barely detectable, even to the trained oral health professional. As the disease progresses, white and brown spot lesions may appear; and in its late stage, cavitation (cavities) of tooth structure results (Crall, 2006). When protective factors such as fluoride and diet control are introduced or increased, disease progression halts and may even reverse. Hence, the disease is fluoride mediated, manageable, and often reversible (Edelstein, 2002). These processes of mineral breakdown and rebuilding are known as demineralization and remineralization.

During demineralization, MS combines with fermentable carbohydrates to produce organic acids that dissolve the tooth surface, releasing calcium and phosphate from the microscopic enamel matrix of the tooth structure. When this happens, the tooth becomes more porous and weakened, similar to what is observed in bone during osteoporosis. Remineralization occurs when saliva delivers calcium and phosphate back to the outer surface of the tooth "remineralizing" the enamel matrix. Additionally, when fluoride is added, remineralization is enhanced, as the fluoride ion creates a stronger enamel matrix (Featherstone, 2006).

The disease process itself is only minimally affected by dental restoration (fillings) (Edelstein, 2002). Restoration of cavities (fillings) serves to reduce the potential for disease progression and tooth destruction; however, it does not eliminate the disease and must be accompanied with other preventive factors in order to stop progression and arrest disease. Removal of bacteria during cavity preparation and restoration eliminates the potential for further acid production and demineralization. As part of disease management and prevention, restoration must be accompanied with increases in use of fluoride and diet control.

Dental caries occurs most often (90%) on the occlusal (biting) surfaces of permanent posterior teeth (Beauchamp, 2008). Although fluoride acts most efficiently on smooth tooth surfaces, it is recommended that additional clinical strategies be implemented to prevent disease progression and cavitation on occlusal surfaces (Beauchamp, 2008). Protecting occlusal surfaces may be accomplished through the application of pit and fissure dental sealants. Dental sealants, applied to deep pits and grooves on these surfaces, have demonstrated significant decreases (86% after 1 year, 78.6% after 2 years) in dental caries incidence among adolescents at risk (Beauchamp, 2008). It is recommended that all children and adults that are at risk for dental caries have dental sealants applied to their primary or permanent posterior teeth to prevent dental caries, its progression, and potential cavitation (Beauchamp, 2008).

PERIODONTAL DISEASE

According to the American Association of Periodontology, "Periodontal disease is a chronic bacterial infection that affects the gums and bone supporting the teeth" (American Academy of Periodontology [AAP], 2006). Periodontal disease manifests itself differently in its various stages. It begins with gingivitis, which is a bacterial inflammation of the gingival or gum tissue caused by plaque biofilm. Clinical and subclinical signs of gingival inflammation include redness, swelling, heat, and pain. Professional treatment and routine oral hygiene to remove local irritants can reverse gingivitis. If left untreated, gingivitis can progress into periodontal disease.

Periodontal disease is caused by specific groups of indigenous oral bacteria that produce toxins that irritate the gum tissue. These toxins stimulate an inflammatory response in which the body turns on itself and leads to break down and destruction of bone and soft tissue that surround the teeth. When this happens, periodontal pockets or gaps are formed, separating the gums from the teeth. As the disease progresses, the periodontal pockets provide the venue for additional bacteria and irritants to collect, which increases the pocket depth and leads to further destruction of surrounding bone and tissue. Like dental caries, periodontal disease is a silent, chronic, progressive, and destructive disease that is generally asymptomatic but over time can lead to tooth loss. As the disease progresses, bleeding becomes more apparent, and teeth become mobile. In some cases, teeth are displaced, and in patients with severe periodontitis, chewing of food may become difficult because of pain from infection and tooth mobility.

All adults should have routine assessment for periodontal disease. A periodontal assessment is considered part of a comprehensive oral health assessment and examination. It should take place at all initial dental examination visits as well as all routine maintenance visits (dental recall). Included in a periodontal assessment is the visual evaluation of soft gingival tissue, as well as the periodontal probing of each tooth and the recording of "pocket" depths in six locations per tooth. Healthy gingival tissue should look pink and "hug" the tooth surface firmly, allowing little room for the insertion of a periodontal probe. As such, the periodontal probe should record pocket depths no greater than 3 mm. In the event that a periodontal pocket depth reading exceeds 3 mm, a gingival/periodontal treatment regimen should be prescribed. The type of treatment prescribed will depend on the actual pocket depth, how many teeth are involved, and whether any bleeding or mobility is observed. Dental radiographs support the assessment and identification of periodontal disease and are therefore recommended once every 5 years for clinical assessment (AAP, 2006).

Periodontal disease can be treated by surgical and nonsurgical therapy. The AAP recommends treating periodontal disease via the least invasive and most cost-effective procedures. This is often accomplished by a dental professional using a nonsurgical procedure known as scaling and root planing. Professional scaling and root planing involves cleaning periodontal pockets by careful removal of irritants such as plaque, calculus, and removal of bacterial toxins by smoothing the root surface of the tooth. In more advanced cases, this procedure is followed by local or systemic delivery of antibiotics (adjunctive therapy) and host modulation.

In the event of failure of nonsurgical therapy, surgical therapy is recommended. The four most common surgical treatments are the following: pocket-reduction procedure, regenerative procedures, crown lengthening, and soft tissue graft. The pocket-reduction procedure involves removal of disease causing bacteria by first surgically folding back the gum tissue to expose and remove the deposits; after the procedure the tissue is secured back in its original place. In regenerative procedures, gum tissue is once again surgically folded back to remove disease-causing bacteria, and then the bone and tissue can be regenerated by using membrane (filter), bone grafts, or tissue-stimulating proteins. In this scenario as well, the tissue is then replaced to its original location. Damage done by gingival (gum) recession and bone loss can be reduced by a soft tissue graft. In these cases, the soft tissue graft is laid over the soft tissue to provide additional support to the tooth within the periodontium. Crown lengthening involves increased exposure of the tooth by adjusting the gum and bone level (AAP, 2006). Most of these procedures are provided by trained periodontists; however, in less severe cases, where only localized (one or two teeth involvement) surgery is warranted, general dentists may opt to perform the procedure.

ORAL CANCER

According to Greenlee as cited in the Surgeon General's report, an estimated 30,200 Americans were diagnosed with oral cancer in the year 2000. Oral cancer is the fourth most common cancer among black males and the sixth most common cancer in U.S. males. More than 90% of these cancers are squamous cell carcinomas. The most common sites for oral cancer are tongue, lip, and floor of the mouth; the most common risk factors responsible for this disease are tobacco and alcohol. In fact, the combination of drug and alcohol is responsible for 70% to 90% of all oral pharyngeal cancers in the United States. Carcinogens found in tobacco initiate carcinogenesis; tars of tobacco smoke contain the most harmful carcinogens. Alcohol acts as a solvent that facilitates the absorption of tobacco carcinogens in the oral cavity. Other factors responsible for oral cancer are viruses (herpes simplex I, human papilloma virus, Epstein-Barr virus, and herpes simplex 8), fungus (*Candida albicans*), genetic derangement, growth factor, and loss of immunosurveillance and control. Genetic derangement is accountable for causing cancerous changes that effect the position of the gene via alteration, deletion, and breakpoint in the chromosome. Immunodeficient patients (AIDS, organ transplant, etc.) are at an increased risk of acquiring oral cancer as their immune system is incapable of providing immunosurveillance that destroys initial clones of transformed cells. In oral and pharyngeal cancers, epidermal growth factor, a marker of malignancy has been found. Moreover, one of the endocrine effects of nicotine is the stimulation of growth hormone (USDHSS, 2000).

The prevalence of oral cancer in the United States can be significantly reduced by promoting oral health screenings and knowledge of the risk factors. Premalignant changes, in the form of either white or red patches or spots, often precede the oral cancer (ADA, 2005). Oral health providers and trained health professionals from all disciplines can provide information about the risk factors and can detect the premalignant changes by looking in the mouth, assessing and referring patients with suspicious lesions to their dentists or oral surgeon for evaluation and biopsy.

ORAL HEALTH DISPARITIES AND WORKFORCE TRENDS

As noted previously, the Surgeon General reported in 2000 that significant oral health disparities exist among certain socioeconomic groups, and that many Americans live in pain because of untreated dental disease because they are unable to access preventive and treatment services (Edelstein, 2002). There are many reasons for this, and the issues are complex. Among the contributing factors noted in the Surgeon General's report are the changes in the dental workforce. Traditionally, dentists and hygienists have assumed the role of the oral health provider. Working in most cases independent of medical providers, dentists established their "cottage industry" with small dental offices widely dispersed in communities across the states. During the 60s, 70s, and early 80s, public and private dental insurance became more widely available, and most individuals had easy access to local dentists. Recent trends in the dental workforce, however, reveal that the dentist to patient ratio is declining and will continue to do so from 2000 to 2010. Within the last decade alone, six dental schools have closed, and the 54 remaining are vulnerable to being closed. To make matters worse, the ADA estimates the number of dentists retiring by 2014 will exceed the number of new dental graduates (Institute of Medicine, 1995). As a result, it is estimated that there will be a significant shortfall of dentists in the future to meet the nation's needs. Although some believe that there are already an insufficient number of dentists to provide care, the American Dental Association asserts that the "apparent shortage" is due rather to an uneven geographical distribution of dental offices (Edelstein, 2002). For low-income families, the picture is even more grim. Of the 160,000 dentists currently practicing in the United States, less than 25% participate in state public insurance programs because of poor reimbursement rates, administrative burdens, and patient failure rates leaving the nation's most vulnerable populations at an even greater risk (USDHHS, 2000).

Another recent trend affecting access to dental care is the change in the types of dental services currently being sought. The demands for tooth whitening and other cosmetic services have transformed dentistry in some arenas from an oral healthcare industry to one that is less health focused and more cosmetic based. As a result of these changes in practice, fewer preventive services are available, and many are unable to access them.

COLLABORATION WITH NON–DENTAL HEALTHCARE PROFESSIONALS

In the last decade, advances in technology, science, medicine, and dentistry have led the way toward better oral health and treatment. Services and personnel are more efficient. Evidence-based practices are improving quality and efficacy of care, and technological changes such as the electronic medical record are helping to integrate oral health with primary health care. Although dentists and hygienists are specially trained to assess oral health, identify oral diseases, and provide treatment, workforce and access issues are steering oral health care into the broader stream of health care. Advances, such as the ones aforementioned, are opening doors for improved collaboration between dental and non–dental healthcare professionals and will assist in addressing the challenges and barriers to care under the traditional paradigm.

Total patient-centered care includes the integration of oral health into primary health care. Primary non–dental healthcare providers who have a fundamental understanding of oral heath and its associated conditions and diseases and trained to assess risk and screen for oral diseases may intercept disease processes early on by educating their patients and providing anticipatory guidance. Assessing and recognizing oral health and or oral conditions and diseases during well-care visits are key in assisting the primary healthcare provider in developing educational messages, providing anticipatory guidance and making appropriate referrals. "Anticipatory guidance" is a term used by physicians that means providing guidance and guiding health behaviors in anticipation of normal development or onset of risk. It forms the framework for prevention (American Academy of Pediatric Dentistry, 2007). When health behavior recommendations or "cues to action" are made and patients understand negative and positive consequences, it is believed that they will take the recommended health action. This concept of perceived susceptibility, perceived severity, perceived benefits, and perceived personal success in taking the recommended health action is known as the Health Belief Model (Glanz, Rimer, & Lewis, 2002).

LEARNING AND BEHAVIORAL MODELS, ORAL HEALTH EDUCATION, AND ANTICIPATORY GUIDANCE

The clinician, after having assessed the disease risk and oral health status should provide anticipatory guidance. If a patient presents "healthy" with observed normal conditions, then the age or stage of development will generally determine the guidance. If, on the other hand, the patient presents with detectable signs of risk or disease, then the message, as well as the strategy to deliver the message, becomes more complex. Behavioral models such as the Health Belief Model mentioned earlier and the Stages of Change model may be used by the provider to develop and guide message delivery. For example, with regard to dental caries, the desired outcome is to prevent all stages of the disease by making patients and caretakers aware of (1) the risk and protective factors, (2) the need to balance risk and protective factors, (3) the various stages of the disease, (4) the importance of daily personal oral hygiene, and (5) the importance of routine professional oral healthcare services and by suggesting specific health-related actions to each (ADA, 2007; Crall, 2005; Featherstone, 2006); therefore, the clinician must know and understand the constructs of the disease to effectively inform and provide guidance.

Educating patients and caretakers about the risk factors, as well as protective factors that contribute to disease, is an important step in disease prevention. When individuals are aware of the risks associated with a disease and understand the preventive aspects of the disease process, they are better equipped to practice healthy preventive behaviors (Glanz et al., 2002). **Table 20-1** shows a list of risk factors for dental caries, periodontal disease, and oral cancer.

Table 20-2 shows the preventive strategies that may be incorporated into education and anticipatory guidance by healthcare professionals.

Knowing and limiting the risk factors and balancing them with protective factors can prevent and help manage the disease.

As mentioned previously, oral health education that incorporates learning and behavioral theories can play a vital role in raising awareness, educating patients, providing motivation, and eliciting change. The Humanistic Learning Theory as an educational model attempts to actualize potential for self-growth, and it is also playful, spontaneous, and creative. It encourages the educator to listen emphatically, allows freedom of choice, and respects the learner. The sources of motivation used by the educator are needs of the patient, desire for positive self-growth, and confirmation of concept. The learning procedure in this theory is impacted by internal feelings about self, ability to make wise choices, and needs to effect learning and change

Table 20-1 Risk Factors

Dental Caries	Periodontal Disease	Oral Cancer
• Frequent ingestions of fermentable carbohydrates • Putting a child to bed with a bottle • Day-long use of a sippy cup or "grazing" on beverages containing sugar (i.e., coffee, juice, soft drinks) • High levels of oral bacteria (MS) from poor oral hygiene • Insufficient fluoride exposure • Sugar-based medications; or medications that cause "dry mouth" • Untreated tooth decay • Sharing food and beverages	• High levels of oral bacteria and other irritants from poor oral hygiene • Use of tobacco products • Substance abuse • Diabetes	• Age > 40 • Male gender • African-American ethnicity • Use of tobacco products • Use of alcohol • Persistent viral infections • Fungus • Genetic derangement • Growth factor • Loss of immunosurveillance and control

Table 20-2 Preventive Strategies

Dental Caries	Periodontal Disease	Oral Cancer
• Increase the use of fluoride (i.e., fluoride toothpaste, fluoride rinses, fluoridated water, prescription supplemental tablets) • Regulate diet; control the frequency of carbohydrate ingestion • Reduce oral bacteria via tooth brushing and flossing • Use antimicrobial oral rinses • Apply dental sealants • Use xylitol products • Obtain routine dental care	• Reduce oral bacteria via tooth brushing and flossing • Use of antimicrobial oral rinses • Obtain routine dental care • Stop smoking • Limit alcohol consumption	• Stop smoking • Limit alcohol consumption • Obtain routine dental care and oral cancer screenings

(Bastable, 2003); therefore, the Humanistic Learning Theory can be used as an educational model by healthcare professionals to provide patient-centered education.

The Stages of Change model proposes that changes in behavior occur gradually over a period of time. This model describes five stages where individuals move or progress from a stage of precontemplation, through contemplation, preparation, and action, to a maintenance stage. For example, patients who smoke are at risk for oral cancer. Health professionals who recognize a person at risk should provide an oral health intervention through education and anticipatory guidance. For those patients who are uninterested in quitting, an oral health intervention may merely suggest the harm that tobacco use may bring to a person who smokes. This intervention targets the person in the precontemplation stage with the goal of moving the person into the contemplative stage of thinking about quitting; however, another individual may already recognize the health danger but may not know how to take action. In this case, the healthcare provider might provide some "tips" for quitting smoking, thereby targeting the person in the action stage (American Academy of Family Physicians, 2000).

INTERDISCIPLINARY EDUCATION

Given the changes taking place within dentistry and across the disciplines, the need to incorporate interdisciplinary education is evident. When healthcare providers know and understand oral health and disease constructs, they are better prepared to assess, inform, and guide their patients. As a result, patients who are unable to access oral healthcare services because of limited or lack of access to dental insurance but have access to medical providers will be more likely to receive information about oral health. Institutions of higher education that educate and train a variety of healthcare professionals are positioned well to offer interdisciplinary education to their students. As the healthcare industry continues to change, the authors believe that the demand for this educational approach will increase.

COMMUNICATION

Communication is a powerful tool in promoting oral health and its relationship to general health. The role of communication in the world today is not limited to providing information. Communication should have the capability of influencing and motivating the public at large, audiences, and individuals about significant health issues (Jhangiani, 2002). Communication professionals can work along with healthcare professionals to resolve issues related to decreasing oral health disparities and increasing oral health awareness by providing care and educating the population about the impact of oral health on overall health and well-being.

A study by Worden and Flynn at the University of Vermont as cited in the speech by Jhangiani indicated a 35% lower smoking rate among teens when mass media strategies were combined with school-based smoking prevention programs as compared with school-based programs alone (Jhangiani, 2002). Mass media strategies can be successfully implemented to educate the public about the link between oral and general health and the importance of routine oral healthcare services.

Interpersonal communication skills are essential for creating a patient-centered environment. Successful communication of oral health education is dependent on the communication skills of a healthcare provider. Communication involves a multilayered, complex, and dynamic process through which meaning is exchanged. Every communication has a sender and a message receiver. Communication includes sending both verbal (words) and nonverbal messages (tone of voice, verbal expression, behavior, physical setting, etc.) (Adler, 2002). Successful communicators are culturally competent, efficiently communicate and interpret verbal and nonverbal messages, and possess cultural self-awareness. Cultural self-awareness is significant, as Adler (2002) noted; Americans are least aware of their own personal cultural characteristics and are surprised when foreigners describe them. Understanding of self is the most important step in understanding others. A healthcare provider who is an efficient communicator and culturally competent successfully communicates across cultures and can motivate patients to change existing behavior and accept practices that will enhance their oral and overall health.

POPULATION-BASED PREVENTIVE SERVICES

Community Water Fluoridation

Community water fluoridation has been cited as one of the top 10 public health achievements of the 20th century, along with vaccination, motor-vehicle safety, and control of infectious diseases (CDC, 2007b). It is a population-based preventive measure proven to be one of the most cost effective means of preventing dental caries. The economic analysis of two studies conducted by the Centers for Disease Control and Prevention (CDC) found that in communities of over 20,000 inhabitants with the cost of fluoridation of approximately 50 cents per person per year, a savings of $38 in dental treatment was observed for every $1 invested in prevention (CDC, 2007a). This is important, as community water fluoridation delivers effective preventive agents to all members of a society regardless of one's socioeconomic status or ability to pay; therefore, health providers, along with advocating for fluoridation in their communities and states, should encourage all patients who live in a fluoridated community to drink fluoridated water.

School-Based Dental Sealant Programs

In recent years, the delivery of pediatric health care has moved into school-based settings with primary care services being provided by federal and state funded school-based health centers. Across the states, there exist nearly 1,700 school-based health centers serving approximately 2 million children in 44 states (National Assembly of School-Based Health Care, 2007). Because of the inability of many low-income families to access primary healthcare services in traditional office settings, these school-based healthcare sites have been established. Policymakers interested in oral health and disparities in accessing care have recognized the value of the school-based model and have collaborated with education professionals as well as school health nurses and other non–dental healthcare providers to develop similar models for the delivery of preventive oral healthcare services. School-based and school-linked dental sealant programs have demonstrated widespread use and have not only significantly increased the number of children receiving preventive services, but have also reduced the prevalence of dental disease among children at risk (CDC, 2001). Healthcare providers working with low-income children and families should assess whether their patients routinely seek professional oral healthcare services and their potential need for dental sealants. If access to a dentist is prohibitive, then the provider may assist his or her patients by investigating the existence of local school-based oral health programs.

ORAL HEALTH RESOURCES

The ADA, AAPD, American Academy of Pediatrics, AAP, American Dental Hygienists' Association, and the American Academy of Family Physicians among other professional groups have developed risk assessment tools, clinical guidelines, policies, and protocols for use by professionals as well as the public. These resources may be accessed online at the various organizations' websites. Each is unique and offers guidance in the appropriate standards of care for various oral diseases and conditions. For additional information, clinical depth, and further insight, the authors recommend that the reader investigate these professional resources.

Case Study 20–1

A 22-year-old female presents at her physician's office complaining of nausea, fatigue, and bleeding gums. After obtaining a medical history and learning that the patient had not had a menstrual period for 3 months, the physician suspects that the patient may be pregnant. In addition, the patient reports that she smokes a pack of cigarettes a day and is a social drinker. A comprehensive health assessment is made and a series of tests to confirm the diagnosis are recommended.

In an interdisciplinary model of care, a comprehensive health assessment would include an oral health assessment. In this scenario, the physician would have assessed the patient's oral health for the presence of risk factors, as well as any obvious signs of dental caries, pregnancy gingivitis, oral cancer, and periodontal disease. Depending on the findings of the assessment, the physician would provide the appropriate anticipatory guidance and referrals.

REFERENCES

Adler, N. J. (2002). Communicating across culture. In J. Szilagyi, V. True, K. Meere, & M. Seers (Eds.), *International dimensions of organizational behavior* (pp. 73–102). Canada: South-Western, a division of Thomson Learning.

American Academy of Family Physicians. (2000, March 1). *Stages of change.* Retrieved March 29, 2008, from http://www.aafp.org/afp/20000301/1409.html.

American Academy of Pediatric Dentistry. (2007). *Guidelines on periodicity of examination, preventive dental services, anticipatory guidance/counseling, and oral treatment of infants, children, and adolescents.* Retrieved March 8, 2008, from http://books.nap.edu/openbook.php?record_id=4925&page=254.

American Academy of Periodontology. (2006). *Periodontal (gum) diseases.* Retrieved January 12, 2008, from http://www.perio.org/consumer/2a.html#treatment.

American Dental Association. (2005, March 14). *Oral cancer.* Retrieved March 31, 2008, from http://www.ada.org/public/topics/cancer_oral.asp.

American Dental Association. (2006, May). *Evidence-based clinical recommendation: professionally applied topical fluoride.* Retrieved March 29, 2008, from http://www.fluoridation.com/prof/resources/pubs/jada/reports/report_fluoride.pdf.

Bastable, S. B. (2003). *Nurse as educator: principles of teaching and learning for nursing practice.* Boston: Jones and Bartlett.

Beauchamp, J., Caufield, P. W., Crall, J. J., Donly, K., Feigal, R., Gooch, B., Donly, K., Feigal, R., Ismail, A., Kohn, W., Siegal, M., & Simosen, R. (2008). Evidence-based clinical recommendations for the use of pit-and-fissure sealants. *Journal of American Dental Association, 139,* 257–267.

Centers for Disease Control and Prevention. (2001, August 1). *Impact of targeted programs in reducing racial and economic disparities in sealant prevalence among school children.* Retrieved March 31, 2008, from http://www.cdc.gov/mmwr/preview/mmwrhtml/mm5034a2.htm.

Centers for Disease Control and Prevention. (2007a, August). *Cost savings of community water fluoridation.* Retrieved January 12, 2007, from http://www.cdc.gov/fluoridation/fact_sheets/cost.htm.

Centers for Disease Control and Prevention. (2007b). *Community water fluoridation.* Retrieved March 29, 2008, from http://www.cdc.gov/fluoridation/.

Crall, J. J. (2005). *Rethinking prevention.* Paper presented at the meeting of the American Academy of Pediatric Dentistry's Prevention Symposium at Chicago.

Edelstein, B. L. (2002). Dental care consideration for young children. *Special Care Dentist, 22,* 11s–25s.

Featherstone, J. D. B. (2006). Caries prevention and reversal based on the caries balance. *Pediatric Dentistry 28*(2), 128–132.

Glanz, K., Rimer, B. K., & Lewis, F. M. (2002). *Health behavior and health education: theory, research and practice.* San Francisco: Wiley & Sons.

Institute of Medicine. (1995). Dental education at the crossroads: challenges and changes. Retrieved March 29, 2008, from http://books.nap.edu/openbook.php?record_id=4925&page=254.

Jhangiani, S. S. (2002, September 28). *Health care in America: reform through communication.* Delivered to the 8th Annual American Communication Association Convention, Georgetown University, Washington, DC.

National Assembly of School-Based Health Care. (2007, January). *Capitol Hill briefing explains school-based center's role as first responder to student crisis.* News release. Retrieved March 29, 2008, from http://www.nasbhc.org/atf/cf/%7BCD9949F2-2761-42FB-BC7A-CEE165C701D9%7D/nationalrelease1.25.pdf.

United States Department of Health and Human Services. (2000, July 27). *Oral health in America: a report of surgeon general.* Retrieved March 30, 2008, http://www2.nidcr.nih.gov/sgr/sgrohweb/execsum.htm#part4.

United States Department of Health and Human Services. (2001). *Healthy People 2010.* Retrieved March 29, 2008, from http://www.healthypeople.gov/About/history.htm.

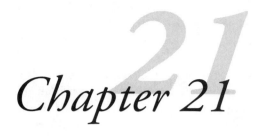

Chapter 21

Obesity, Healthy Eating, and Eating Disorders: Definitions, Education, and Treatment

Debra Wein & Lynn Foord

INTRODUCTION

Obesity and eating disorders represent opposite ends of the spectrum with regard to body weight and body composition (percent body fat). Body mass index (BMI) is one measure used to determine one's risk for mortality and other diseases. It is defined as the ratio of weight to height.

An adult BMI above 25 represents overweight, above 30 obesity, and below 19.5 an abnormally low body fat, which could be an indicator of an eating disorder. In this chapter, we discuss obesity and eating disorders, consider areas of concern surrounding each one, and explore opportunities for prevention and treatment.

OBESITY

For adults, a healthy weight is defined as the appropriate weight in relation to height. This ratio of weight to height is known as the BMI. People who are obese almost always have a large amount of body fat in relationship to their height; however, large athletes who bear lots of muscle might have a BMI over 30.0 but would not be considered overweight from the perspective of health risk. Likewise, pregnant women with a high BMI are not considered obese.

Both children and adults are at risk for obesity. Childhood obesity is a term that was not frequently heard 30 years ago, but today it is so prominent in our daily lives that many health organizations are now dedicated to the study and treatment of childhood obesity. According to the National Center for Health Statistics and Centers for Disease Control and Prevention, 4% to 7% of children and adolescents in the 1970s and 1980s were overweight. In the 1990s, this number increased to 11%, and by 2000, it had further increased to 16%. The tripling of this statistic in the last 2 decades is alarming, considering the medical and psychosocial consequences of childhood obesity. This rapid increase in childhood obesity suggests that an environmental influence is responsible, as our genetic makeup is unlikely to have changed in such a short time.

Although there are many methods used to measure an adult's body composition, the most common measure of childhood adiposity is BMI. The standard BMI ranges used for defining overweight and obesity in adults are not applicable for children and adolescents. Instead, age- and gender-specific reference growth charts were developed by the U.S. Centers for Disease Control and Prevention to be used for the pediatric population. They are available online at www.cdc.gov/growthcharts.

A child/adolescent (age 2–20) with a BMI > 85th percentile is considered "at risk for overweight." A child/adolescent with a BMI > 95th percentile is considered overweight. To understand the factors that contribute to childhood obesity, one must consider both those risk factors that can be changed and those that are nonmodifiable.

Nonmodifiable risk factors include the following:

- *Genetics.* Genetics and family environment are the most likely links between overweight parents and overweight children. Children born to overweight/obese parents are more likely to become overweight themselves.
- *Ethnicity.* Minority groups such as Native Americans, blacks, and Mexican Americans have higher rates of obesity than whites.
- *Socioeconomic status.* A lower socioeconomic status is associated with a higher prevalence of obesity.
- *Birth weight.* A higher birth weight may also be associated with childhood obesity.

There are also well-recognized risk factors for childhood obesity that can be modified. Preventing childhood obesity needs to start with teaching healthy behaviors at a young age so that these behaviors can be applied throughout life. Families are a critical link in providing the tools and serving as role models for those behaviors and need to be involved in instruction aimed at developing and maintaining healthy behaviors. In particular, behaviors involving physical activity and healthful eating are keys in preventing childhood obesity.

The following behaviors are likely to be associated with excessive energy intake for children and adults alike; each can be modified by learning and practicing changes in behavior:

- Skipping meals
- Increased consumption of sugar sweetened beverages and foods
- Limited fruit and vegetable intake
- Easy access to a variety of energy dense snacks and fast food (i.e., vending machines, school lunches, cafeterias, and fast-food restaurants)
- Fewer meals consumed at home
- Increased frequency of dining out
- Increased portion sizes
- Eating while watching television

MANAGING WEIGHT LOSS IN CHILDREN AND ADULTS

Gradual weight loss through sound nutritional strategies is justified to attain an increase in the ratio of lean to fat tissue in your body; however, many people do not choose to lose weight through this preferred gradual form of reduction. Instead, a variety of rapid weight-reduction techniques such as severe caloric restriction and fasting are often used, and as a result, lean body mass (muscle) and water are lost. The result is a decrease in one's ability to maintain a healthy weight over the long term as well as lower muscle glycogen, muscle water content, and decreased physical endurance.

Many people turn to "dieting" as a method of losing weight; however, for some people, the word *diet* conjures up visions of frustration and failure. "Going on" a diet teaches denial and sets the stage for "going off" the diet, engaging in binge eating, and developing disordered eating patterns.

On the other hand, the safest and most effective way to lose weight, and more importantly maintain the loss, is through moderate caloric restriction with an emphasis on high-carbohydrate, low-fat foods. In this way, cells are fueled with sufficient energy to function properly. The majority of our nation's health experts support a plant-based diet, which is high in carbohydrate (45% to 65% of total calories), moderate in fat (20% to 35% of total calories), and adequate in protein (10% to 35% of total calories).

The following tips can be used to help design and implement a successful weight-reduction program that will not be associated with serious dieting but instead develops a positive focus on how to eat healthfully.

- Evaluate behavior patterns for potential unhealthy habits such as skipping breakfast, nibbling all day, and munching out at night because of increased hunger.
- Pay attention to mood when eating. Food becomes dangerous when it is abused for entertainment, comfort, or stress reduction.
- Distribute estimated caloric allotment evenly throughout the day, ensuring that calories and therefore energy are available to make it through the entire day.
- Eat slowly! The brain needs 20 minutes to receive a signal of satiety.
- Eat favorite foods on a regular basis. If you deny yourself permission to eat and enjoy, you are likely to suffer from the temptation to devour; however, if you regularly consume small portions of your favorite foods, binges are less likely.
- Perform positive self-talk and exercise every day.

For those who may question the effectiveness of changing behavior as opposed to "dieting," consider the experience of so-called masters, individuals identified by the National Weight Control Registry who have lost 30 pounds or more and kept the weight off for a year or longer. The masters describe the principles of their success:

1. The masters stop seeing the way they eat as dieting. Healthy eating should be a way of life. You should not "go on" or "go off" a diet; be consistent with your choices, and weight loss will be a reality.
2. The masters survive the transition from weight loss to maintenance. As long as you have changed the word "diet" in your mind to be a way of life instead of something you go on and off, this transition should be easy.
3. The masters see the beauty of low-fat eating. Enjoying fruits and veggies are a great way to keep calories and fat in control throughout the day. These fiber and vitamin packed foods will keep hunger low and make you feel great!
4. The masters develop and enjoy new tastes in food. Trying new foods will keep you from getting bored of your new eating habits.

5. The masters develop consistency in their way of eating. It is important to have scheduled meals and snacks throughout the day. If you miss a meal or snack, this can lead to extreme hunger and overeating at the next meal time.

6. The masters keep track of what they eat. Keeping a food diary is a great way to see what you eat throughout the day. This can help you realize whether your eating habits are better or worse than you think.

7. The masters indulge themselves but spend their calories wisely. Allowing yourself treats is good to do. Just be sure that you keep treats to small amounts and only as a special occasion. Having these treats often will take away the special feeling when you do have them.

8. The masters try to listen to their bodies. It is important to know when you are truly hungry or just bored and when you are satisfied instead of stuffed. This is important in weight loss and management.

EATING DISORDERS: THE OTHER SIDE OF THE SPECTRUM

If we consider obesity and overeating to be at one end of a spectrum of eating behaviors, eating disorders would be at the opposite end. To gain an understanding of eating disorders, we begin with a discussion of what is known regarding the prevalence, warning signs, and symptoms of eating disorders. From there, we consider possible causes and consequences.

Description and Prevalence

Disordered eating can itself be viewed as a continuum. At one extreme are eating disorders such as anorexia nervosa and bulimia nervosa; at the other end is disordered eating, which is characterized by preoccupations with weight and restrictive eating. The diagnostic criteria to define anorexia nervosa, bulimia nervosa, and "eating disorders not otherwise specified" are found in the *Diagnostic and Statistical Manual of Mental Disorders*, 4th edition (American Psychiatric Association [APA], 1994) (**Tables 21-1 and 21-2**).

Anorexia nervosa is an eating disorder that can be recognized when an individual demonstrates an intense fear of gaining weight even though she is considered underweight (at least 5% below normal weight for height and age). Behaviors associated with anorexia nervosa include skipping meals or severely limiting food consumption. Warning signs for anorexia include drastic weight loss, wearing of baggy or layered clothing, excessive exercise, and avoidance of food-related social activities.

Bulimia nervosa occurs when an individual binges on large amounts of food and then attempts to rid her body of the calories that she has consumed

Table 21-1 How Eating Disorders Differ from Disordered Eating

	Disordered Eating	Eating Disorders
Essential distinction	Reaction to life situations, a habit	An illness
Psychological symptoms	Infrequent thoughts and behaviors and thoughts about body, foods, and eating that do not lead to health, social, school, and work problems	Frequent and persistent thoughts and behaviors about body, foods and eating that do lead to health, social, school, and work problems
Associated medical problems	May lead to transient weight changes or nutritional problems; rarely causes major medical complications	Can result in major medical complications leading to the need for hospitalization or even death
Treatment	Education and/or self-help group can assist; psychotherapy and nutritional counseling can be helpful but not always essential. Problem may go away without treatment	Requires specific medical and mental health treatment. Problem does not go away without treatment

Source: Adapted from the National Eating Disorders Screening Program (1996).

through vomiting, laxatives, diuretics, or excessive exercise. Warning signs for bulimia nervosa include excessive concern about weight, bathroom visits after meals (sometimes for long periods with water running constantly), strict dieting, followed by large binges, depressive mood, and increased criticism of one's body.

In addition to the criteria described in Table 21-2, look for more subtle physical signs characteristic of an individual with an eating disorder, such as a decreased pulse rate of 40 to 50 beats per minute, history of fainting, parotid swelling or "chipmunk cheeks," erosion of the tooth enamel or a large amount of dental work, and Russell's sign (finger and nail changes on the first and second digits of the dominant hand (Brandstater, 1995). One might also observe medical signals such as abnormally low white blood cell counts, mild anemia, constipation, abdominal pain, high cholesterol, low mineral levels (especially magnesium, zinc, phosphates), and elevated amylase (APA, 1994).

Although eating disorders may occur at any time in the life cycle, adolescents and young girls are the most vulnerable (Shisslak et al., 1998). Recent studies have revealed that views of one's body and concerns about body image develop well before puberty and that girls as young as 9 years old are following diets and restricting calories to lose weight (Sands, Tricker, Sherman,

Table 21-2 Warning Signs for Eating Disorders

- Intense fears of gaining weight
- Repeated comments about feeling fat
- Preoccupation with food
- Complaints of feeling cold
- Excessive exercise outside of training
- Bulky clothing
- Emaciated appearance
- Food restriction
- Leaving table soon after finishing meal
- Tooth erosion
- Dry skin
- Hair loss
- Brittle fingernails
- Lanugo (fine, downy hair on the body)
- Scarring on the back of the hand (bulimia)
- Mood swings and irritability and depression
- Amenorrhea in women

Source: APA (1994).

Armatas, & Maschette, 1997; author observations). Although eating disturbances can intensify as girls undergo puberty, it is the psychological perspective of the individual that actually determines whether the disordered eating subsides or becomes more intensified. Negative self-image, poor self-esteem, and psychopathology can enhance the disordered eating pattern (Sands et al.). Girls may become less satisfied with their shape over time as a result of interrelated factors, including familial influences and nutritional practices, developmental integrity, actual height, current weight, and peer-group influences. Body images popularized by the media can also have an influence, as well as the individual's sense of self-efficacy or control (Sands et al.).

Boys who identified themselves as gay or bisexual were also more likely to diet (35% vs. 13%), take diet pills (18% vs. 3%), and vomit or use laxatives (32% vs. 3%). These behaviors are seen increasingly in adult males and have become prevalent in bodybuilders (Andersen, Barlett, Morgan, & Brownell, 1995). Almost half (46%) of the 49 all natural bodybuilders who responded to a questionnaire reported episodes of binge eating after competitions, whereas more than three quarters (82%) reported being preoccupied with food sometimes, often, or always 1 week before competition (Andersen et al.).

Researchers are beginning to find a high incidence of subclinical eating disorders (Culnane & Deutsch, 1998; author observations) that do not exactly match the standard criteria set by the *Diagnostic and Statistical Manual of Mental Disorders*, 4th edition (APA, 1994), yet can still be harmful for athletes and young girls (Yeager, Agostini, Nattiv, & Drinkwater, 1993). Based on these findings, it becomes important to watch for and seek out not only those individuals whose behavior patterns match established criteria but also those who regularly calorie restrict, are slightly preoccupied with food, have a less than ideal body image, and possess poor attitudes about food.

Possible Causes of Eating Disorders

Eichner, Loucks, Johnson, and Nelson Steen (1997) demonstrated that psychological issues, including poor coping skills, low self-esteem, and a lack of identity as well as physical or sexual abuse can lead an individual to an eating disorder. Lunner et al. (2000) established that girls ages 13 to 16 years were more likely to diet if they perceived pressures from their parents to diet or fit a certain mold. Alternatively, those girls who were taught self-confidence and autonomy at home were less likely to diet.

The stress leading to disordered eating could stem from an intense determination to succeed at sports, in academics, or even in social situations. A closer look at certain requirements of sport reveals that athletes especially may be at risk. Although exercise provides numerous benefits to the individual who partakes in sensible and balanced activities, extreme intense physical activity can cause delayed puberty, menstrual disorders, stress fractures, and early onset of non–age-related osteoporosis (Myszkewycz & Koutedakis, 1998). Athletes involved in at-risk sports include those in which revealing clothing is the uniform, such as in ballet and other dance, figure skating, diving, and swimming; those in which performance is based on subjectivity, such as with dancers, gymnasts, divers, and synchronized swimmers; those in which weight can be a hindrance to performance, such as with distance runners, ballet dancers, figure skaters, cross-country skiers; or those in which weight classifications are built in, such as with rowing, bodybuilding, and the martial arts.

Although research reveals that those who participate in physical activity are more likely to have high self-esteem and feel more positive about their bodies than are those who do not (Biddle, 1993; Sands et al., 1997), research also describes athletes as having a higher prevalence of eating disorders than the general population (Brandstater, 1995). It seems that even though athletes maintain a high level of conditioning, they may also be very dissatisfied

Table 21-3 Factors Placing Athletes at Greater Risk of Eating Disorder

- Poor coping skills
- Lack of self-esteem
- Poor identity
- Necessity to meet inappropriate weight goals
- Pressure to succeed
- Perceived societal expectations
- Trying to fit into established norms
- Inability to deal with stress properly

with their body (Finkenberg, 1993). See **Table 21-3** for factors placing athletes at greater risk of developing an eating disorder.

Treatment

Some well-meaning individuals may wrongly try to "treat" the eating disorder by suggesting the individual resume normal eating practices, eat more, or merely stop participating in these risky behaviors, as if the suggestion could actually make it so. Clinically, however, eating disorders are considered to be a mental disorder and are often an expression of underlying emotional distress, thereby insuring that the treatment must address issues such as concerns related to food-intake patterns, food- and weight-related behaviors, body image, and weight reduction (ADA, 1994).

Outpatient treatment is adequate for most individuals working through their eating disorder; however, for some, the comprehensive support and treatment available through hospitalization becomes necessary. Typically, those with bulimia nervosa do not require hospitalization, whereas those with anorexia nervosa are more likely candidates. Decisions about hospitalization are always made on a case-by-case basis and should be made by members of a treatment team that includes doctors, registered dietitians, mental health professionals, coaches, and parents. The following issues should be considered when deciding whether to admit a patient (ADA, 1994):

- Amount of weight lost
- BMI
- Rapidity of progressive weight loss (1- to 2-pound weight loss despite concomitant psychotherapy)
- Weight less than 20% below average weight for height
- Severe metabolic disturbances

- Certain cardiac dysfunctions such as syncope
- Psychomotor retardation
- Severe depression or suicide risk
- Severe bingeing and purging (with risk of aspiration)
- Psychosis
- Family crisis
- Inability to perform normal daily functions
- A lack of response to outpatient programs

Each member of the treatment team contributes his or her special expertise to the care of the individual. A physician should be available to coordinate treatment and monitor overall progress, serving as a case manager to monitor the medical progress of the interrelated issues and insure compliance of the individual with treatment.

A registered dietitian/nutritionist is imperative to the team to provide the individual with an adequate understanding of the body's needs during growth and maturation. In their position statement on intervention in the treatment of anorexia nervosa, bulimia nervosa, and binge eating, the American Dietetic Association (ADA, 2006) outlines specific objectives that should be addressed by the nutritional counselor working with the individual with the eating disorder. The nutritionist should perform a comprehensive history in order to collect relevant information regarding the individual's history of weight changes and eating and exercise patterns as well as purging behaviors. Developing a therapeutic alliance with the patient is important to resolve food fears successfully and develop goals for weight and behavior changes. Accurate principles of food, nutrition, and weight control must be taught, and myths should be dispelled.

Over the course of nutritional treatment, the patient needs to understand the symptoms of and the body's response to starvation and normal and abnormal hunger. The patient also needs to learn about day-to-day weight fluctuations, maintaining a healthy weight range, recognizing the minimum food intake needed to stabilize weight and metabolic rate, and principles of optimal food intake for health. Examples of individuals who have successfully recovered from an eating disorder, their hunger patterns, typical food intake patterns, and total caloric intakes should be presented to the individual. Educating the family is another objective important to the successful recovery of the individual. Working with both the patient and the family, the nutritionist can offer suggestions on meal planning, nutrient needs, and strategies for dealing with inappropriate food- and weight-related behaviors.

The psychologist or mental health professional is necessary to help the individual come to terms with the problems responsible for bringing on the disorder in the first place. Decreasing stress at meal times and helping the family work toward a supportive rather than confrontational environment are important goals. As the treatment proceeds, it is possible that disturbing emotions may surface and affect the patient's ability to make changes in food intake, weight management, and healthy behaviors. During these difficult times, working with supportive and understanding professionals allows the patient to feel more comfortable about stopping and resuming therapy (APA, 1994).

Coaches, parents, athletic training staff, teachers, administrators, and physical therapists all need to be involved with the team in identifying, addressing, and helping to monitor recovery from an eating disorder. All team members must be aware of the symptoms, the risks, the consequences, and the severity of the disorder; they should also be informed about local resources that may contribute to the patient's recovery. Members of the team must also do their best to separate their personal biases and needs when determining the appropriate treatment for the patient.

All team members should be prepared to interact appropriately with patients with eating disorders, recognizing their special needs. In approaching an individual you suspect has an eating disorder, keep in mind the following guidelines (Wein, 1997):

- The best person to approach the at-risk individual will be someone who shares a solid and positive relationship with him or her.
- Approach the individual in a relaxed manner and in private. Go by yourself rather than in an intimidating group.
- Use "I statements" when sharing your thoughts with the individual. For example, say, "I am concerned about your well-being" or "I feel that . . . ." This approach is much less confrontational than "You have done this . . . ." The individual will find it harder to argue with your feelings. How can she say you are wrong? You are simply expressing your feelings.
- Explain that you are there for the individual, not against him or her. Assure the individual that no matter what he or she says you will not criticize or make him or her feel bad or embarrassed.
- Use terms like "well-being" rather than "disorder" or "sickness." Approach the individual rather than accusing him or her.
- Do not use terms such as "bingeing," "fasting," or "purging," as they may make the individual defensive.

- If you are not in the position of making a specific diagnosis, then don't. Simply ask whether the individual needs help rather than tell him or her that they have a problem or try to diagnose them.
- Do not try to gather evidence by catching the individual in the act of bingeing or purging. Sometimes even mentioning these activities may cause him or her to feel more pressure and more defensive.
- No matter the outcome, give the individual the phone number of a qualified psychologist, eating-disorder specialist, or resource organization in your area that he or she can use in the future should they decide that they want to contact someone. See the reference list at the conclusion of this chapter for organizations providing resources and referrals for eating disorders.
- Most important, let the individual know that you are there if and when he or she is ready to talk.

In addition, the following techniques and strategies should be considered when working with each new patient:

- Separate food- and weight-related behaviors from feelings and psychological issues. Having the individual appreciate the difference can help him or her to learn to separate facts and move toward a better understanding of how to get better.
- Teach the connection between food intake and health and the requirement of nutrients in food for the optimal functioning of our bodies.
- Incorporate education with behavior change. For example, teach the need for nutrients and energy before suggesting an increase in caloric intake.
- Work on small changes rather than making gross alterations in the individual's lifestyle. Discourage the individual from wanting to change everything at once. Small changes are more likely to be adapted and maintained.
- Explain that setbacks are normal and can be used as learning tools to re-sculpture responses to cues.
- Teach self-monitoring techniques such as a food diary and behavior records so that the individual can feel a sense of control over his or her treatment and choices. You can include food, exercise, and behaviors such as frequency of bingeing and/or purging as well as weight gain/fluctuation.
- Use weight and eating contracts, but avoid using these techniques if the individual becomes too over involved and if you feel that they may be counterproductive.

- Slowly increase or decrease weight to prevent the individual from feeling a loss of control and potentially cause him or her to withdraw from therapy.
- Learn to maintain a weight that is healthful. Encourage regular meal times, variety and moderation of intake, and gradual reintroduction of foods (typically those most recently excluded from the diet are best received).
- Evaluate and change your approach as necessary throughout treatment and with each individual.
- Strive, ultimately, for the individual to be comfortable in social eating situations in which he or she does not have total control.

GROUP COUNSELING: SHAPE YOUR FUTURE: A WEIGHT-MANAGEMENT PROGRAM FOR CHILDREN

The South Shore Medical Center (Norwell, MA, www.ssmedcenter.com) and Sensible Nutrition, Inc. (Hingham, MA, www.sensiblenutrition.com) have teamed up to create the Shape Your Future pediatric weight loss program. This program serves overweight and obese children and their families in the South Shore, Massachusetts area. In this program, children and their families receive 10 weeks of fitness and nutrition instruction and guidance, including an exercise program, associated with South Shore Hospital (Weymouth, MA, http://www.sshosp.org/), and nutrition education.

The courses cover a range of information including reading nutrition labels, healthful foods, and information on fat, fiber, sugar, calorie, and beverage consumption. Weekly exercise classes get children active both in and out of the pool and teach them how they can be active at home. Funds cover materials used for food demonstrations, food tasting, and exercise equipment such as pedometers and jump ropes. Participants receive healthy food samples and coupons and are encouraged to try all of the new foods presented at each event. Children and their families are provided with informative handouts and materials such as the American Dietetic Association's booklet, *If Your Child Is Overweight, A Guide for Parents*, 3rd edition, by Susan M. Kosharek, MS, RD.

The staff of Shape Your Future is comprised of physicians at the South Shore Medical Center, certified diabetes educators, nurses, an exercise physiologist, and registered dietitians. At the beginning of the program, children and their parents meet one-on-one with a registered dietitian to discuss their goals, progress, and healthful nutrition. Parents attend a Shape Your Future support group.

At the start and completion of the 10-week session, children are assessed using the American Academy of Pediatrics guidelines for a healthy weight. Each child is measured for their starting height, weight, BMI, BMI percentile, percentage body fat, and goal weight. In addition, their knowledge and behaviors relating to diet and physical activity are assessed. Children and families sign a program contract agreeing to attend the weekly nutrition and exercise classes. Families agree to be a healthy role model for their family and help their child reach his or her healthier lifestyle goals. After completion of the Shape Your Future pilot study:

- Three of 10 participants achieved their goal weight loss, as set by their physician.
- Eight of 10 participants lost weight.
- Nine of 10 participants changed their habits enough to alter their prior rate of weight gain.
- All participants lowered their percent body fat.

After the pilot sessions, the following changes were made.

- Children and parents met with the registered dietitian at the beginning and again, at the midway point.
- The program was extended to 12 weeks.
- Additional hands-on learning activities were included such as a supermarket shopping tour.

It is the goal of the staff at the Shape Your Future program to expand on this success with more sessions in the upcoming years to reduce childhood overweight and obesity in the South Shore area.

CONCLUSION

As health professionals, we have the opportunity to help individuals maximize their nutritional intake and fitness regimen by focusing them on healthy habits and lifestyles. We can teach our clients to adopt enjoyable eating and exercise behaviors to reduce disease risk and improve well-being in the long run. We can help them to think of every action as a permanent change in lifestyle habits rather than as temporary behaviors. We can be sensitive to their changes in mood and energy level—a sign that they may be pushing themselves a bit too aggressively. We can learn to reward our clients for even small successes and to deal with lapses in healthy eating by problem solving not sabotaging. We can teach them to use social support systems—friends, relatives, school staff, and support groups—to help stay on track and maintain new habits.

Referring to another health professional allows us to work together to pool knowledge and share responsibility as well as providing a model of team collaboration for our patients and clients. A cohesive treatment team must include individuals who share philosophies similar to our own about intervention, treatment, and recovery. By working together, we can increase our ability to recognize, treat, and prevent obesity and eating disorders. With our help, individuals can learn to plan a well-balanced life filled with proper amounts of food and exercise as a means of promoting a healthy weight and a positive outlook.

Case Study 21–1

Weight Loss in a Weight-Sensitive Sport

Betsy is in her first year of collegiate gymnastics living in the college dorm with another gymnast. She is training well but is anxious to lose 10 pounds from her present body mass of 119 pounds. Her body fat level has been assessed at 23% and her coach wants her to achieve a level of 20%. She is 5' 2" and is 18 years old.

Betsy wants to lose weight but needs expert advice on how to achieve this. She admits that her eating habits are often poor, especially when sharing meals with her roommate, another gymnast who does not need to watch her weight. She does not eat in the dorm cafeteria and has no access to cooking facilities; therefore, all meals are eaten out.

Betsy does not have much time to eat during the day. She eats a good breakfast but skips lunch, apart from a protein bar, to fit in extra classes before going to gymnastics practice. Practice, from 1 to 5 PM, is followed by an hour of physical therapy. She is starving by the time she eats dinner at a fast-food restaurant and continues to snack during the evening while she studies or watches television. She does not consume anything during practice and does not take any supplements. Menstrual status is reported to be normal.

Her typical eating pattern is shown in **Table 21-4**.

(Continues)

Case Study 21–1 (*Continued*)

Table 21-4 Eating Patterns

Breakfast	Lunch	Dinner	Snacks During Evening
Bowl instant, flavored oatmeal with skim milk Orange juice Coffee with cream	Power bar	Dinner at a fast-food restaurant (sub sandwich; soup and salad; chicken, rice, and vegetable; pizza; hamburger and fries)	Popcorn, fat-free chocolate cookies, pretzels, ice cream, diet pop, cheese, brownies

Considering her eating habits and her desire to lose weight, what types of nutritional intervention would you recommend?

Strategies

Betsy needs a meal plan that accommodates her daily schedule and living situation. To achieve weight loss, Betsy needs to decrease energy intake by 200 to 300 kcal/day and add an aerobic activity component to her overall training plan. Betsy is encouraged to spend 3 nights a week at the gym doing aerobic activity on the treadmill (30 to 40 minutes) instead of watching television. The following dietary suggestions may be made to Betsy.

1. Continue to choose a good breakfast, but have 1% milk in her coffee to decrease saturated fat intake.
2. Buy a sandwich (whole-wheat bread, low-fat meat, cheese, and salad) and a piece of fruit on the way to classes each morning. Eat lunch between or during class, but before practice.
3. Bring a piece of fruit or half an energy bar to eat immediately after practice while working with the physical therapist. This will curb hunger and reduce overeating at dinner. Use a sports drink during exercise.
4. Decide on three separate eating plans for dinner at various "healthier" restaurants near campus. Select specific menu items, and set an appropriate amount to be consumed and then stick to the plan.
5. Allow a snack of yogurt and fruit or pretzels at night.
6. Use a multivitamin supplement while energy intake is restricted.
7. Review the dietary plan and exercise goals with the gymnastics coach.

Case Study 21-2

Loss of Body Fat

Katie is a 17-year-old swimmer who holds many local and regional records, including the national record for 100-m backstroke. She is 5' 6" and has been swimming at the national team level for 4 years. At the age of 15, Katie has just failed to qualify for the upcoming Olympics. Although her typical training commitment is at least nine sessions a week, in recent times, her weekly training load has been reduced to four or five sessions.

Katie is referred by her coach for assistance to lose body fat. After her failed Olympic trial, Katie had reduced her training significantly and had gained weight—from a pretrial level of 130 pounds to her current weight of 150 pounds. Although she has always been stocky, she is now definitely overfat. She complains of feeling weak and out of breath. Her best time in the 100-m backstroke was 1.06.51, but she is now struggling to achieve 1.10.00. Her coach feels that she is capable of better performance, even with her curtailed program.

Before the consultation, Katie had never paid much attention to her eating habits. On training days, her eating pattern consisted of two meals and two snacks. On race day, she skipped breakfast, and ate a big lunch and maybe a snack at night. Fluid replacement was not given a high priority, although during competition she made an effort to drink more water. During competition periods she also tried to increase her carbohydrate intake by increasing her intake of vegetables and fruit (**Table 21-5**).

Table 21-5 Training Goals

Posttraining Snack	Lunch	Snack (3 PM)	Dinner
One slice pineapple Half large bread roll	Salad with lots of dressing Baked chicken thigh Orange drink	One glass juice	Fried rice, fried plantain, fried fish 1 cup pineapple juice

Considering her training goals and desire to lose body fat, what types of nutrient interventions would you recommend?

(Continues)

Case Study 21–2 (*Continued*)

Strategies

The energy deficit needed to produce a loss of body fat is achieved primarily via an increase in training level rather than a reduction in energy intake. A reorganization of macronutrient intake is desired—primarily to increase protein and carbohydrate, while moderating fat intake. Suggestions to improve nutrient intake from a similar energy intake may include the following suggestions:

1. Adjustment of the timing and volume of meals so that eating would coincide more appropriately with the training schedule. In particular, the size of the breakfast snack should be increased to promote recovery after the morning training session.
2. A reduction of fat intake, particularly fats added in cooking and food preparation. This energy should be replaced by increasing the consumption of staple foods such as bread and rice.
3. Replacement of some salads with steamed vegetables so that oily dressings could be replaced.
4. Increased intake of protein and simultaneous improvement of calcium intake by adding reduced-fat dairy foods to meals and snacks.
5. Increased intake of fresh fruit.

Case Study 21–3

Athlete with Low Energy Needs: Ballet Dancer

Joanna is a 14-year-old classical ballet dancer studying for an intermediate level ballet examination. She is about 5' 7" and is 150 pounds. She attends a one and a half hour classical ballet class four times per week and completes one class of repertoire, contemporary, and jazz ballet each Saturday. Joanna has recently moved from her local suburban dancing school to one that provides a highly regarded but rigorous dance training program.

Joanna's ballet teachers are concerned about her increasing weight, which is 15 pounds higher than when she first started at their school 9 months earlier. In addition to the weight concern, Joanna has recently become moody, tired, and less motivated.

Joanna has been dieting in an attempt to reduce weight with little success since her menstrual cycle began 18 months previously. She tried almost every diet given to her by other ballet students, but any weight loss achieved seemed to rapidly reappear. The experience of "nothing seeming to work" left Joanna convinced that her metabolism was slow and that she would never be able to lose weight (**Table 21-6**).

Table 21-6 Nutritional Plans

Breakfast	Lunch	Dinner	Snacks
Nothing or one slice whole-grain toast with jam (no butter) 1 cup tea	Green salad One apple Diet soda	Steamed chicken or fish with steamed vegetables 1 cup tea	Diet soda and if feeling really low before class a chocolate bar or two

What nutritional plan would you recommend to help her lose weight, yet maintain the energy she needs to perform well for her ballet classes?

Strategies

The following suggestions can be made to improve intake of calcium, iron, and general nutrients, control cravings, and facilitate weight loss.

1. Consume a balanced breakfast each day, which is high in fiber and includes low glycemic index carbohydrate and protein to boost satiety. Examples include a bowl of whole-grain cereal or oats with calcium-fortified milk, fresh citrus juice, or milk instead of tea (to avoid inhibition of iron absorption).
2. Include nutritious nutrient-dense snacks between meals: examples include fresh fruit, reduced-fat milk, or a slice of whole-grain bread or toast.
3. Include protein-rich foods at lunch (e.g., lean meat, poultry, seafood, or reduced-fat cheese) to boost iron and/or calcium intake. Team this with plenty of vegetables or salad to increase the feeling of fullness, and add a small serving of carbohydrates (e.g., whole-grain bread, pasta, rice, and potato) to maintain blood glucose and glycogen stores. For example, try a whole-grain roll filled with salad and lean chicken.

(Continues)

Case Study 21-3 (*Continued*)

4. Use the same principle with the evening meal, with particular focus on adding a carbohydrate serving. For example, try a lean meat or chicken with stir-fry of vegetables, served with rice or pasta.

5. Use a food diary to monitor food intake, cravings, and feelings. Allow chocolate or another treat once or twice a week to help prevent binge eating.

6. Obtain a body composition assessment to properly assess and monitor changes in body fat levels.

7. Also consider the possibility of low-impact aerobic training to preserve lean tissue (e.g., walking, cycling, swimming, or deep-water running) to help weight loss via increasing energy expenditure and strength training.

RESOURCES FOR RELIABLE NUTRITION INFORMATION

Professional Organizations

American Academy of Pediatrics

American Anorexia/Bulimia Association, www.members.aol.com/amanbu

American College of Sports Medicine, www.acsm.org

American Dietetic Association, www.eatright.org

American Institute of Nutrition

American Medical Association

American Public Health Association

American Society for Clinical Nutrition

Anorexia Nervosa and Related Eating Disorders Inc., www.anred.com

Eating Disorders Awareness and Prevention, www.members.aol.com/EDAPinc

Food and Nutrition Board

National Research Council

National Academy of Science

National Collegiate Athletic Association, www.ncaa.org

National Eating Disorders Organization, www.laureate.com

Society for Nutrition Education, www.healthfinder.gov

Sports and Cardiovascular Nutritionists (SCAN)

Computer Retrieval of Information on Scientific Projects (NIH CRISP)

National Association of Anorexia Nervosa and Associated Disorders, www.healthtouch.com

National Toxicology Program (NIEHS/NTP)

Health Information Index (NIH/HII)

National Institutes of Health

National Library of Medicine

Gatorade Sports Science Institute, Risky Dietary Supplements

RESOURCES

Cooperative Extension Publications by State

National Institute of Health

Mayo Clinic

Healthfinder

Journals

American Journal of Sports Medicine

Journal of Applied Physiology

Physician and Sports Medicine

American Journal of Clinical Nutrition

Journal of Nutrition Education

Journal of American College of Nutrition

Journal of the American Dietetic Association

Nutrition Reviews

American Society for Nutritional Sciences

Journal of the National Strength and Conditioning Association

Medicine and Science in Sports and Exercise

Newsletters

Nutrition Action Health Letter

Nutrition Science News

Tufts University Diet and Nutrition Letter

Nutrition Action

National Strength and Conditioning Association's Online Performance Training Journal

REFERENCES

American Dietetic Association. (2006, December). Position of the American Dietetic Association: nutrition intervention in the treatment of anorexia nervosa, bulimia nervosa, and other eating disorders. *Journal of the American Dietetic Association, 106*(12), 2073–2082.

American Psychiatric Association. (1994). *Diagnostic and statistical manual of mental disorders* (4th ed.). Washington, DC: Author.

Andersen, R. E., Barlett, S. J., Morgan, G. D., & Brownell, K. D. (1995). Weight loss, psychological, and nutritional patterns in competitive male body builders. *International Journal of Eating Disorders, 18,* 49–57.

Biddle, S. (1993). Children, exercise and health. *International Journal of Sport Psychology, 24,* 200–216.

Brandstater, M. E. (1995). Female athlete triad. *Western Journal of Medicine, 162,* 149–150. Retrieved May 29, 2008, from http://www.cdc.gov/nccdphp/dnpa/obesity/childhood/prevalence.htm.

Culnane, C., & Deutsch, D. (1998). Dancer disordered eating. *Journal of Dance Medicine and Science, 2,* 95–100.

Eichner, E. R., Loucks, A. B., Johnson, M., & Nelson Steen, S. (1997). The female-athlete triad. *Sports Science Exchange Roundtable #27.* Retrieved June 5, 2008, from http://www.gssiweb.com/Article_Detail.aspx?articleid=66.

Finkenberg, M. E., DiNucci, J. M., McCune, S. L., & McCune, E. D. (1993). Body esteem and enrollment in classes with different levels of physical activity. *Perceptual and Motor Skills, 76,* 783–792.

Glace, B. (2002). Food intake and electrolyte status of ultramarathoners competing in extreme heat. *Journal of the American College of Nutrition, 21,* 553–559.

Louise Burke, J. H. (2002). Effects of short term fat adaptation on metabolism and performance of prolonged exercise. *Medicine and Science in Sports and Exercise, 96,* 1492–1498.

Lunner, K., Werthem, E. H., Thompson, J. K., Paxton, S. J., McDonald, F., Halvaarson, K. S. (2000). A cross-cultural examination of weight-related teasing, body image, and eating disturbance in Swedish and Australian samples. *International Journal of Eating Disorders, 28*(4), 430–435.

Myszkewycz, L., & Koutedakis, Y. (1998). Injuries, amenorrhea and osteoporosis in active athletes: an overview. *Journal of Dance Medicine and Science, 2,* 88–94.

Rehrer, N. (2001). Fluid and electrolyte balance in ultra-endurance sport. *Sports Medicine, 31,* 701–715.

Sands, R., Tricker, J., Sherman, C., Armatas, C., & Maschette, W. (1997). Disordered eating patterns, body image, self-esteem, and physical activity in preadolescent school children. *International Journal of Eating Disorders, 21,* 159–166.

Shisslak, C. M., Crago, M., McKnight, K. M., Estes, L. S., Gray, N., & Parnaby, O. G. (1998). Potential risk factors associated with weight control behaviors in elementary and middle school girls. *Journal of the Psychosomatic Research, 44,* 301–313.

Wein, D. (1997, April). Clients with eating disorders: give the right message when you suspect clients have eating disorders. *IDEA Today,* 22–23.

Yeager, K., Agostini, R., Nattiv, A., & Drinkwater, B. (1993). The female athlete triad: disordered eating, amenorrhea and osteoporosis. *Medicine and Science in Sports and Exercise, 25,* 775–777.

Chapter 22

Parenting Education

Patricia Christensen

> *Your children are not your children.*
> *They are the sons and daughters of Life's longing for itself.*
> *They come through you but not from you,*
> *and though they are with you, yet they belong not to you.*
> —*the Prophet*

INTRODUCTION

The ultimate goal of parenting is to create an ideal environment for a child to develop into a healthy, independent, and capable adult. Creating a positive, safe, and nurturing environment for a child begins at conception or ideally before conception. A woman who practices a healthy lifestyle throughout her life has the best chance of delivering a healthy baby. Beyond the physical health of the child, as supported by the parent's lifestyle, there are other issues and concerns that directly impact the journey from infant to adult.

Among these issues are lack of resources, lack of knowledge, and the persistence of parenting patterns that tend to be reinforced and practiced throughout several previous generations. Parents tend to parent as they were parented. Breaking the negative traditions that include physical punishment and irrational expectations takes motivation, teaching, and reinforcement. Health professionals can have a profound influence on these families and can eliminate some of the negative aspects of parenting.

Many well-meaning parents fail to support their child's journey to independence because of a lack of information about child growth and development, poor parenting examples, and a lack of resources (Elster, McAnarney, & Lamb, 1983). These parents expect either too much or too little of their children and may punish a child for something that the child is incapable of understanding or performing. In addition, parents may lose sight of the ultimate goal of raising children to be independent. Either from lack of appropriate role models or misconceptions, these parents may strive to impose their wills on their children (Teti & Candelaria, 2002).

This chapter examines the issues of parenting: a tough, challenging, and hopefully, an ultimately rewarding experience. The context of the chapter is in child development and appropriate parenting behaviors. Examples of assessments, teaching methods, and scenarios are presented.

LACK OF INFORMATION ABOUT CHILD DEVELOPMENT

Conception and Pregnancy

Many people "fall into" pregnancy without adequate knowledge of what will be required throughout the prenatal and parenting time. These unintended pregnancies can range from teenagers experimenting to birth control failures to lack of motivation or discipline to prevent pregnancy. In addition, women with substance abuse problems may be disconnected from their physiology and mental status because of drug abuse. Thus, many parents are lacking in information about prenatal care, stages of pregnancies, nutrition, labor and delivery expectations, danger signs to look for, possible genetic anomalies, and parenting education; therefore, for many families, the subsequent problems of parenting begin at conception (Bugental & Goodnow, 1998).

The health professionals who face this population confront daunting tasks—mainly identifying this group and getting them into clinics and health facilities for education and preparation for childbirth and parenting. The parents who are substance abusers need counseling and treatment before the child arrives.

Most women, while faced with the forces of labor, will eventually show up at hospitals to give birth, but this is far too late to be effective in teaching and preventing complications of pregnancy and parenting. Outreach programs sponsored by clinics, hospitals, health departments, private doctors, and even law enforcement can be used to identify this population. These outreach programs need to emphasize help and support over judgment and punishment. If a pregnant woman who is an abused wife or substance abuser discloses her need to a representative of the previously mentioned establishments, she needs to know that the information will be handled in a sensitive and safe manner. Radio, television, billboards, flyers, and interviews while the parent is exposed to an agency are avenues to reach this population. Crisis-line personnel need to be alerted to this condition and make the recommended suggestions for help in pregnancies.

In contrast, the middle-class client who is well educated cannot be assumed to know all about pregnancy and parenting. Although this group has more access to information, there remain many misconceptions and wrong notions of parenting. As is discussed later, parental role models and popular media can be negative influences in the parenting styles of even educated clients (Chase-Lansdale, Wakschlage, & Brooks-Gunn, 1995; Demick, 2002).

Presented here is a list of basic information that is essential for pregnant women.

BASIC CURRICULA FOR PREGNANCY

1. Prenatal care, including schedule of visits to health professionals and clinic, should be explained why these visits are necessary.
2. Track the development of the fetus.
3. Monitor the vital signs, blood, and urine tests of the mother to look for possible complications.
4. Schedule necessary tests such as ultrasound, genetic studies, or amniocentesis as needed.
5. Communicate expectations of labor and delivery.
6. Watch for danger signs of pregnancy.
7. Begin parenting education.
8. Assess and teach about the nutrition of mother and baby. This aspect of prenatal care is discussed in depth, and an example of a teaching plan is presented later.

CHILD DEVELOPMENT

Numerous research studies have been done by such authorities as Piaget, Kohlberg, Maslow, Erickson (Lowdermilk & Perry, 2004; Papalia, Olds, & Feldman 2004; Potts & Mandleco, 2007), and others that have documented the milestones and characteristics of children through the years. The findings of these theorists are not often known by parents or used as guides to appropriate parenting (Benasich & Brooks-Gunn, 1996). Physical, psychological, social, and cognitive milestones have been established by age as a result of this thorough research (Bornstein, 2006; Garrett, Ferron, Ng'andu, Bryant, & Harbin, 1994).

Summaries of these milestones with ages are presented in **Table 22-1**. Health professionals can use these guides to help parents understand what a child can and cannot understand. In addition, these guides serve to show what children are able to perform or not at certain stages. These milestones are typical behaviors at certain times but should be individualized for each child as each child grows in a unique rate.

Infancy

The time of infancy is marked in the human by a time of almost complete helplessness. Infants are unable to care for themselves in any way; therefore, a consistent, omnipresent, loving parent or caretaker is essential. They must be fed and kept warm and safe, and diapers need to be changed and cleaned. According to Erickson, as cited in Hockenberry, Wilson, Winkelstein, and Kline (2003), this is when the infant develops trust or mistrust of the world.

Table 22-1 Age Milestones

Age Group	Psychological—Erickson	Cognitive—Piaget	Moral—Kohlberg
Infancy	Trust vs. Mistrust	Sensorimotor (birth to 2 years)	Preconventional—premoral
Toddlerhood (1–3 years)	Autonomy vs. Shame and Doubt	Preoperational thought, preconceptual phase (transductive reasoning, specific to specific)	Punishment and obedience phases, the beginning of understanding consequences for actions
Early childhood (3–6 years)	Initiative vs. Guilt	Preoperational thought, intuitive phase, transclusive reasoning	Prevential, premoral level, naïve instrumental orientation
Middle childhood (6–12 years)	Industry vs. Inferiority	Concrete operations (inductive reasoning and beginning logic)	Conventional level, good-boy, nice-girl orientation
Adolescence	Identity and Repudiation vs. Identity Confusion	Formal operations abstract thinking, can plan for the future	Postconventional or principled level. Social contract orientation. Universal ethical principles

If the infant's every need is not met in a timely manner, it can be the beginning of that child seeing the world as untrustworthy, and this can handicap the child for all his or her life (Bornstein, 2002; Sirignano & Lachman, 1985).

Many well-intentioned parents believe that an infant will be "spoiled" if picked up and cared for promptly. They believe that the child must be controlled from birth onward; however, Piaget, as cited in Hockenberry et al. (2003), theorized that the baby is incapable of understanding the need to wait for his legitimate needs. The war of wills is a fruitless and frustrating exercise.

According to Hockenberry et al. (2003), "Parenting is not an instinctual ability but a learned, acquired process" (p. 504). The prompt and loving care of persistent parenting is possible mainly through attachment that occurs between the child and parents. This attachment ideally begins in pregnancy where the mother cares for herself, anticipates with happiness the arrival of the baby, and incorporates him or her into the family unit. This all-consuming work of caring for an infant means a lack of sleep for the parents, a lack of free time, and other sacrifices. Without the proper attachment, these needs of the infant may not be met or met with anger and frustration (Emde, 2000; Papoušek & Papoušek, 2002).

Health professionals play an important role in assessing this bond/attachment (mainly through parental behaviors at the time of birth). "It has been established that the formation of attachment in the infant goes through four distinct and overlapping stages. For the first few weeks, infants respond indiscriminately to anyone. Beginning at approximately 8 to 12 weeks of age, they cry, smile, and vocalize more to the mother than anyone else and continue to respond to others" (Hockenberry et al., 2003, p. 505). There are many ways that health professionals can assess this bond progressing. Observations of behaviors include the following:

1. Enfolding the infant in the arms
2. Touching and stroking the baby's body
3. Looking directly at the baby's eyes (en face)
4. Being attuned to the baby's needs for warmth, food, and cuddling
5. Talking to the infant in a high-pitched tone
6. Wanting to hold the infant and reaching for him or her

If the parents do not exhibit these behaviors, they should be taught and modeled and monitored by health professionals so that the infant does not go home without the essential support that he or she needs to survive. Regular and frequent visits to clinics, pediatricians, nurse practitioners and others will help to monitor the growth and development of the child and parenting strategies and will ensure that the child is immunized.

Early Childhood

How often do people refer to toddlerhood as the "terrible twos" when it can be a fun and delightful time for child and parents? Some of the "terrible" part may stem from a misunderstanding about this time in a child's life when he or she is striving for some autonomy and independence. The crescendo of "no's" signals the child's wanting to assert his or her own way of exploring the world or doing things for himself. Unfortunately, some parents may interpret this as disobedience or stubbornness, and another test of wills ensues. In order to take those first independent steps from their parents, children need to venture and explore and be allowed to do more for themselves, within safe boundaries (Edwards & Liu, 2002). It is typical of toddlers to dash away from a parent to play or to explore and then come back soon for a touchstone of security. The parents who allow this independence and then reinforce the safety of their arms are nourishing a child toward being a separate being. Sometimes reminders of the ultimate goal of parenting—to make the child an independent, separate, and competent being—are necessary for parents to start to let go. Health professionals in teaching and reinforcing the developmental phases can give parents the confidence to let the child explore and be away from the parents for longer periods of time than are possible in infancy (Edwards & Liu, 2002).

The toddlers' striving for independence may bring on much frustration. Although they want to do more, such as go to a friend's house alone, put on their clothes, or tie their shoes, their inability physically and cognitively to accomplish these tasks can lead to temper tantrums. They feel overwhelmed with this frustration and strike out at anybody or anything. The prudent parent will not get involved in these "fits" but will let the child express his frustration and then comfort him or her and guide him or her to accomplish the tasks (Tamis-LeMonda & Bornstein, 1991).

The most important lessons that health professionals can teach during this time is allowing toddlers to explore within safe boundaries, vent their frustrations, guide and teach new tasks patiently while allowing the toddlers to take their time learning at their own pace. Parents need to realize that the young children are not being personal or bad when they get frustrated, but are overwhelmed at times.

Another major characteristic of toddlers is their egocentrism, that is, they believe that they are the center of their universe (Papalia, Olds, & Feldman,

2004). They are cognitively unable to see another point of view other than their own. Long discourses and logical explanations are lost on them. They are not capable of understanding the concepts of other's needs or feelings.

Play is a very important part of this time during which toddlers learn about the world and different roles. In addition, the role of play is a major milestone in the development of thought (Bornstein & O'Reilly, 1993; Užgiris & Raeff, 1995). Most of the play of the young child is parallel rather than interactive with other children. Because of their egocentrism and irreversible thinking, forcing toddlers to share their toys or loved objects makes them think that they are giving them away permanently—that the objects will be gone. That is due to Piaget's stage of irreversible thinking (Papalia et al., 2004). Recently, however, the newest theories suggest that Piaget may have underestimated the ability of early toddlers to understand permanence. Some children are capable of knowing that an object still exists, but the egocentrism may interfere with the sharing. Accordingly, when toddlers hurt or cut themselves, they cannot imagine that they will heal. The cut is there forever and may cause them great distress. They may scream and point at the cut for hours. Parents need to make the toddler "whole," that is, put a bandage on the cut. It is out of sight and out of mind and thus not stressful. These recent findings in Piagetian thinking point out that each child is unique and must be assessed and treated as an individual.

Young children are easily frustrated and are unable to articulate clearly what they want or able to perform some tasks that they want to do independently. Thus, the negative or "terrible twos" are normal manifestations of this time period. Parents who understand that these are normal, expected behaviors can guide and direct without the "war of wills" dominating this time. Findings are consistent with the proposal that in early development active resistance to parents often reflects children's motivation to control events, not poor parenting or strained parent–child relationships (Dix, Stewart, Gershoff, & Day, 2007). Health professionals can teach, reinforce, and reward these parents and create a home environment that is more thriving than distressing.

In summary, the child in early childhood is egocentric, incapable of reversible thinking, self-centered, and striving for limited independence while still wanting to be dependent and safe (Bornstein & Haynes, 1998; Garrett et al., 1994).

Middle Childhood

During this time, the child is capable of more independence and can tolerate more time away from parents and caretakers. In fact, going to school, visiting friends, going to camp, and having sleepovers are all necessary for this independence to flourish.

According to Erickson (Papalia et al., 2004), this time is dominated by the psychologic tasks of industry versus inferiority. This is the time when children begin to "work" at learning about the world and their place in it. The work of this time is school and social learning. Accomplishing tasks of reading and writing and getting along with peers and others gives children a sense of industry and mastery. Being unable—whether because of physical, psychological, or social problems—to accomplish these tasks may lead to a sense of failure and inferiority (Havighurst, 1972).

Piaget refers to this time as concrete thinking in which children can understand and master sensory memory, which is a type of holding tank for past experiences. Eventually, children of this age develop a working memory in which mental representations are prepared for and recalled. This enables the child to learn and recall the alphabet and numbers and experiences (Papalia et al., 2004). Social learning goes along with this type of cognitive development.

The most important support that parents can provide during this time is to grant the independence gradually for the child to experience the world and form the mental representations and recall them. Supporting children's experiences and work in school and social situations enables children to feel that they are capable. This success is subsequently built on throughout the years and leads to a competent, independent adult.

Primarily parents can provide a place where children can work on school work, ideally in their own room. In addition, they must have proper nutrition and exercise and enough sleep. They need periodic checkups and developmental assessments, as well as hearing and sight exams. Sensory deficits can be very detrimental to children's learning and socialization (Bugental & Goodnow, 1998).

Teachers, health professionals, and parents need to form cooperative relationships during these years so that school-age children understand and can be supported in the work of this critical time. Frequent communication among these groups is essential to a cohesive experience for the child of school age.

Adolescence

In most of human history, adolescence was not viewed as a continuation of childhood. After a child could go out and do some kind of work to support the family, that is what was expected. The prolonged incubation period of adolescence is a rather new notion, especially since the beginning of the

1900s. Of course, now children have several more years beyond school age, even beyond high school to prepare for independent life (Hauser, 1991).

According to Erickson (Papalia et al., 2004), the chief task of adolescence is to resolve the "identity crisis versus identity confusion." This task is achieved by modifying and synthesizing earlier identifications and organizing their abilities and interests, needs, and desires so that they can be expressed in a social context (Feldman & Elliott, 1990). The social context of adolescents is mainly associated with their peers during this time. Sometimes parents feel that peers are more important in their influence on their teenagers; however, it has been shown that parental and early experiences are still most influential. Thus, parents should not assume that they are not important to their children or that they do not listen. The common cultural idea of teenagers automatically being rebellious as expected may lead to more conflict, as teenagers then think that they have "permission" to act out.

Much of the conflict between parents and adolescents can be attributed to the adolescents striving for independence. They need to experience the world on their own terms, to try out their adult roles. Adolescents typically are starting to assume more permanent plans to lead separate lives from their parents such as college attendance, acquiring jobs, or seeking partners. If parents do not agree with these goals, they may exert a great deal of pressure on their offspring to conform to the parents' expectations; however, to be competent, the adolescent needs the space and experiences to make their own way even mistakes. Parents' knowledge of this stage of adolescence may truncate a great deal of conflict (Feldman & Elliott, 1990; Hauser & Bowlds, 1990).

POOR PARENTING EXAMPLES

If you want to be a good parent, be lucky enough to have good parents. That situation would be the ideal for all, but that is not always the case. It is a common occurrence for parents to find themselves acting just like their own parents. Many are taken aback by sounding like their parents in talking to their children. There are many indications cited in the literature (Hardy, Astone, Brooks-Gunn, Shapiro, & Miller, 1998). The learned parental role is a very compelling and persistent one. Learning and role theories remain major explanations for this phenomenon (Papoušek & Papoušek, 2002).

Discipline Versus Punishment

Although it is well known by health professions, it can be very difficult for them to understand that even abused children love their parents and may subsequently grow up to be abusers themselves. Breaking the chain of abuse is a major goal of child advocates. The key to changing unwanted learned parental behavior is learning and reinforcement.

One of the most controversial and recalcitrant parenting behaviors is spanking or other forms of physical punishment. Several research studies have shown that spanking is an inappropriate form of punishment that may have long-lasting negative effects on the child (Straus & Gelles, 1986). Research indicates that the majority of Americans have employed spanking as a discipline strategy at some point during their parenting history. Spanking is typically defined as striking the child on the buttocks or extremities with an open hand without inflicting physical injury. It is distinguished from physical abuse, which consists of beatings and other forms of extreme physical force that inflict bodily injury. Whereas spanking is a normative practice within the United States, physical abuse is not socially acceptable and is punishable by law. Although normative, spanking is used with varying frequency, depending on child attributes (e.g., age, gender, and temperament), parental characteristics (e.g., age, education, ethnicity, psychological well-being, and religious conservatism), and contextual factors (e.g., poverty and social support) (Korbin, Coulton, & Lindstrom-Ufuti, 2000; Rohner, Kean, & Cournoyer, 1991).

It is well documented that black parents employ spanking more frequently than European Americans, even after controlling for socioeconomic status (Smith & Brooks-Gunn, 1997). Blacks are also more likely than European Americans to use spanking as an appropriate display of discipline and parenting (Korbin et al., 2000; Mosby, Rawls, & Meehan, 1999).

Clearly, there is a greater need for more cultural research regarding these so-called normative parenting strategies. The empirical literature on spanking has been reviewed extensively. The most recent and comprehensive review, completed by Gershoff (2002), consists of a meta-analysis of 88 studies. Gershoff examined the relationship between corporal punishment and compliance of the child, moral internalization, aggression, criminal and antisocial behavior, quality of the parent–child relationship, mental health, and abuse. Spanking tended to be associated with immediate compliance of the child (i.e., desisting the behavior targeted by the punishment), which Gershoff (2002) considered to be the only positive outcome evident in her review. On the negative side, spanking was associated with decreased internalization of morals, diminished quality of parent–child relationships, poorer child and adult mental health, increased delinquency and antisocial behavior for children, and increased criminal and antisocial behavior for adults; spanking also was associated with an increased risk of being a victim of abuse or abusing one's own child or spouse. Reanalyses of studies have underscored the importance of how spanking is defined. Several studies in Gershoff's review included rather harsh punishment that would qualified as physical abuse (e.g., slapping in the face and hitting with an object). Reanalyses indicated the outcomes were more negative in those studies than in studies of less severe punishment (Baumrind et al., 2002).

Not all reviews reveal the same findings. Some found that very mild spanking used as a backup for mild disciplinary effects may not be detrimental and indeed can reduce noncompliance and fighting (Larzelere, 2000). It would be difficult to identify a consensus among researchers beyond a few key points. First, the deleterious effects of corporal punishment are likely to be a function of severity and frequency. Harsh punishment is associated with many untoward consequences, including increased morbidity and mortality for major adult forms of illness (e.g., heart disease, cancer, and lung disease) (Krug et al., 2002). Second, the effects of mild, occasional spanking (an oxymoron to some people) that is a backup to other disciplinary procedures such as time out from reinforcement or reasoning, that is physically noninjurious, that involves an open hand to hit the extremities or buttocks, and that inflicts temporary pain are not so clear (Baumrind et al., 2002). Again, there is no advocacy of corporal punishment in this latter view, but merely an acknowledgment that the research does not speak to the consequence of occasional spanking.

Goals of Parent Discipline

Presumably, the goals of disciplining children are to decrease some behaviors (e.g., tantrums, talking back, and disobedience), to develop others (e.g., problem solving, playing cooperatively, and completing homework), and to promote socialization more generally. It is not at all clear from studies that punishment is among the better strategies for accomplishing these behavior-change goals. For example, decreasing and eliminating inappropriate child behavior in the home can be achieved through positive reinforcement techniques, time outs, and explanations.

The use of spanking raises questions regarding the goals of discipline: whether any punishment is needed to attain them, whether punishment is needed, and whether hitting has any benefit over noncorporal punishment. Spanking seldom is the best method to discipline children, and it should be pointed out that the U.S. Surgeon General and the American Academy of Pediatrics have recommended against spanking and other corporal punishment.

The practice of physical punishment continues, however, and is seen by many parents as acceptable. The anecdotal experience of most parents is often stated as, "I was spanked as a child, and it didn't hurt me"; therefore, many parents continue this practice without investigating other disciplinary options.

A major source of confusion concerns the difference between discipline and punishment. Discipline is the setting of boundaries and limits for the child's behavior. Punishment is the consequences of breaking the rules or overstepping the boundaries. Methods of discipline and punishment need to be included in all parenting classes. Some parents fear that if spanking is eliminated altogether that they will be left with no means to discipline their children. This mistaken idea stems from a lack of knowledge or belief in other options, for example, restriction of privileges, depriving the child of a desired toy or event, and time outs, all accompanied with age-appropriate explanations.

GUIDELINES FOR DISCIPLINE

1. Parents show unconditional love. They do not withdraw love if a child misbehaves.
2. Discipline and explanations should be age appropriate.
3. Punishment fits the crime. Do not overreact or underreact to a child's breaking of the rules.
4. Children must know the rules and what is expected of them before they are presumed "guilty."
5. Children must know the consequences if the rules are broken.
6. There must be consistency of rules and expectations. There should not be confusion of "yes" today and "no" tomorrow.
7. Give children a framework of security to grow and grow away from family.
8. Avoid hitting, bullying, and not explaining what the child has done wrong. Truncating any disagreements by saying "do as I say, not as I do" or "because I said so."
9. Use restriction of privileges by setting limits on child's desired activities, such as television, video games, and play.
10. Use role modification and exploration of the problem. Try to see the child's view as well. Use compromise if warranted.
11. Give children choices and more control over their lives gradually as they mature such as giving chores, allowances, expecting them to cooperate within the family and help out for the mutual good.

Communication with Children

Parents who tell the child to do one thing or another that may or may not make sense to the child may answer the child's question of "why?" with the answer, "because I said so." Although this reply may truncate further explanations and complaints, ultimately, it is not satisfying or instructive for the child. All adults are bigger and more powerful than children, and therefore, there really is not any contest on who will win the argument or discussion; the ultimate goal is to teach the child to be self directed. A rational explanation, again age appropriate, will help the child see the need and logic of certain actions (Dawber & Kuczynski, 1999). Children speak to others as they are spoken to. In other words, if they are insulted, yelled at, or berated, they may often mimic this communication pattern to others, including their parents. The parents who see themselves as "bosses" may punish the child for disrespect without realizing that they, themselves, have modeled this disrespectful communication. The social rules of society that reward civility and politeness in conversation may be unattainable to children who have never been exposed to that behavior. Their aggressiveness in speaking may interfere with their relationships in school and create learning difficulties.

Cognitive development occurs over several age groups, and what a child can understand in language and teaching increases as the child grows. Some parents, whether well meaning or not, will often expect a child to understand a concept or command that is confusing for the child. An example of this might be that a toddler is punished for saying "no" frequently to a parental command when saying "no" and trying out his independence is a normal developmental milestone of the toddler. The parent, unaware of this developmental stage, may view the frequent negative responses from the child as "rebellion" that must be quelled. A health professional working with the family can explain the difference between normal and usual communication and willfulness, thus sparing the child and family from discord.

Increasing Responsibility and Accountability

With more knowledge of child development, parents can gradually increase what is expected of their children. This includes giving them more freedom, responsibility, and very importantly making them accountable for their mistakes and failures. Many loving parents will try to do more for the child such as delaying the responsibilities of household chores, school work, and so forth. In addition, they may try to shield their children from the consequences of not doing what is expected for their age group. When children do not do their homework or share in work at home, they need to know that there are punishments or deprivations that can follow. Some examples may be going to summer school for makeup work or failing a grade or paying for a broken object out of their allowances. Although it may be hard for parents to see their child in a difficult situation, it is imperative that children learn that actions have consequences.

Parents can overprotect their children by not allowing them to visit outside their homes or doing things on their own. These practices do not allow the child to develop his or her own sense of responsibility and direction.

Sadly, there are also parents who are neglectful and by default let the child do whatever he or she can do to get by. This neglect has dire consequences for the child who has no directions or limits. A child without boundaries feels insecure and unloved.

There are patterns that can be identified that are not conducive to loving, capable parenting. These patterns have been identified in the literature and can be summarized in the following chart:

1. Poor communication
2. Violence and child abuse
3. Neglect—children left to cope on their own
4. Poor parental role models
5. Scapegoating of one or more children
6. Chaotic environment in the home including no set times for meals, sleep, and other activities such as homework
7. Little understanding of children's needs and child development
8. Children not allowed to express ideas or show anger or disappointment
9. Social isolation of the family with little of no backup from community or extended family

LACK OF RESOURCES

As of this date, in the United States, over 40 million families lack adequate health insurance, which is needed to care for a growing family properly. It has been estimated that 1 dollar spent on health promotion in children will save 4 dollars in sick care. The tradition of the U.S. healthcare system has been to disregard prevention and pay for complications and sick care (Holden & Buck, 2002; Rowe, Pan, & Ayoub, 2005).

Often when children are showing symptoms of illness, the parents will resist seeking care because they cannot afford the upfront costs of seeing doctors and other health professionals and paying the price of the medications prescribed. Thus, a child's minor illness may progress to a more serious stage, resulting in very expensive in hospital care.

Many families, especially poor ones, have complicated lives and relationships. Often there are single parents struggling to raise children alone with poor paying jobs or welfare (Brooks-Gunn, Klebanov, & Smith, 2001). Working single parents without extended family support may not be able to take children to clinic visits or extracurricular activities or teacher conferences. This may set up an attitude of "negligent parent" among healthcare professionals frustrated with these families. Much of the mismatch of healthcare professionals and poor families stems from lack of education of the parents and the expectations of health professionals.

The goal of health professionals working with these families needs to be dedicated to helping them find appropriate resources to support their families and help their children develop optimally. Health professionals are not the only persons in families' lives that can contribute to the welfare of the child. School teachers, counselors, and those in criminal justice can all collaborate for the good of the child. One of the most effective means of assessment and monitoring of children's progress and well-being can be the school nurse. More and more communities are using nurses to interface with the school, parents, and other health professionals.

CONCLUSION

The ultimate goal of parenting is to support a child into becoming a healthy, independent, and capable adult. Creating a positive, safe, and nurturing environment for a child begins at conception and continues through adolescence.

There are many dimensions to the parenting of children that can influence greatly the success or failure of this journey to adulthood. Of paramount importance are the availability of adequate resources, knowledge of growth and development, and the persistence of parenting patterns that tend to be reinforced and practiced throughout several previous generations. Breaking the negative traditions that include physical punishment and irrational expectations takes motivation, teaching, and reinforcement. Health professionals working with these families can teach, role model, counsel, and support positive parenting strategies.

Keeping the ultimate goal in the forefront—that is, raising children to be independent—may help these families accept normative childhood behaviors rather than punish them. This chapter examined the issues of parenting in the context of child development and appropriate parenting behaviors. Examples of assessments, teaching methods, and scenarios were presented.

Scenarios are helpful in illustrating real-life situations that can teach various aspects of parenting. The following scenarios look at a negative and a positive outlook of prenatal nutritional teaching.

Case Study 22-1

Nutrition in Pregnancy—Sarah

Sarah, an 18-year-old high school dropout, presents at the public health clinic asking for a pregnancy test. She has missed her period for 3 months and suspects that she is pregnant by her boyfriend. Sarah is 5' 2" tall and weighs 210 pounds. She works at a fast-food restaurant and eats most of her meals at her place of employment. Often, she brings home food for the rest of her family, which consists of her mother and younger sister who is 9 years old. All the family members are greatly overweight for their height. In addition, Sarah smokes one to two packs of cigarettes per day, as does her boyfriend.

After the test confirms Sarah's pregnancy, the nurse counsels Sarah about the schedule of prenatal visits and other considerations of pregnancy. The nurse then centers on Sarah's weight and unhealthy diet and smoking. The nurse informs Sarah that she is damaging her health and that of her newborn with the excess weight and smoking and risks developing diabetes. The nurse does not include a dietitian in her counseling. Sarah points out that her family depends on her job and the food she brings home. Her mother is a domestic worker who has an inconsistent income. When her mother cooks, it is mainly fried meat or bologna and beans. Fresh vegetables are rarely bought or served.

Sarah is given an appointment for a follow-up visit with the dietitian and a doctor in 1 month. Sarah does not keep this appointment because of a conflict with her job.

She continues her lapses in prenatal care, sporadically seeing a nurse practitioner until she finally delivers a 4.8 pound baby 5 weeks prematurely. Sarah's weight has risen to 268 pounds. The baby is placed in NICU for 7 days with mild respiratory distress and poor nutritional status. Eventually, the baby goes home, and Sarah's mother watches her and bottle feeds her and begins table food at 3 months. Sarah continues her present employment and weighs 275 pounds.

Unfortunately, Sarah's example is all too common. Many young people in this fast-food culture are grossly overweight and have little taste or money for nutritious food. Adding smoking to an already compromised health status makes pregnancy even more deleterious for the baby.

Case Study 22–2

Nutrition in Pregnancy—Tasha

Tasha, a 19-year-old high school graduate works in a hotel as a housekeeper and sometimes kitchen worker. She is exposed to a lot of rich foods and desserts, and she and other workers are often able to eat the remains of catering meals and room service. Tasha eats on the run often picking up whatever is available, usually french fries or cookies and chips. She is 5' 4" and weighs 192 pounds. She lives with her boyfriend, Carlos, and neither one does much cooking. Take home of fast food is the norm. Sometimes they go out for pizza and beer. Tasha and her boyfriend both smoke.

Tasha misses her period and suspects that she is pregnant. She seeks out a visit and test at the local clinic, and the positive pregnancy test is confirmed. After the initial assessment, the nurse calls in a registered dietitian who is a regular member on the prenatal team. A complete 48-hour recall of food intake by Tasha was documented and evaluated. A pattern of deficient eating or poor choices was identified and discussed with the client.

Table 22-2 shows an example of a nutritional assessment.

Table 22-2 Nutritional Assessment

Nutritional Assessment

Please list all the foods and the amounts you have eaten in the last 2 days:

		Day 1	
Breakfast	Lunch	Supper	Snacks
_____	_____	_____	_____
_____	_____	_____	_____
_____	_____	_____	_____
_____	_____	_____	_____

		Day 2	
Breakfast	Lunch	Supper	Snacks
_____	_____	_____	_____
_____	_____	_____	_____
_____	_____	_____	_____
_____	_____	_____	_____

(*Continues*)

Case Study 22-2 (*Continued*)

Reviewing this list, is this a typical list of foods you eat on a regular basis?

What foods do you like?

What foods do you dislike?

How much money do you have to spend for food each week?

Do you have any financial help with buying food (e.g., food stamps and WIC)?

Who does the cooking in your household?

Who does the food shopping in your household?

Teaching Guide

In the last several years, the need for certain vitamins and nutrients has been established for this time period to enhance the health of the mother and baby. One example is folic acid. It was learned that adequate folic acid can avoid neural tube defects such as spina bifida and other spine anomalies. In addition, it is the total nutritional status of the mother throughout her life that can affect the mental status of the developing child's brain, especially in the area of intelligence and learning. A lack of protein has been often cited in this area.

Using the assessment guide, the health professional identified what was lacking in Tasha's diet and made suggestions about addressing these deficiencies. For example, high-quality proteins were lacking (as is often the case with low income clients because these are the most expensive of all foods). Tasha's protein intake consisted more of hamburgers, hot dogs, and sausages. The health professional suggested some meatless protein substitutions and how they can be combined to create complete proteins, that is, proteins with all of the essential amino acids. The meatless proteins are inexpensive and can be served by combining beans and rice or tortillas, or adding milk to meatless meals. Cheaper alternatives to orange juice, a main source of vitamin C and folic acid, such as canned or frozen juices can be substituted for soft drinks and fresh squeezed juices. Frozen and canned vegetables and fruits are often much less expensive than their fresh counterparts.

All of these alternatives were discussed with Tasha and her boyfriend. The dietitian suggested that because hotel food was available to them they could make smarter choices about what to eat such as salads, vegetables, and high-quality proteins. In addition, the need for dairy products was stressed for Tasha. They even explored the opportunity that Tasha could learn some cooking techniques from the hotel chefs and cooks. After the importance of good nutrition on their baby was stressed, both Tasha and Carlos were more committed to eating healthier. In addition, after the effects of smoking on the developing fetus were explained, both agreed to try to stop or cut back on their smoking.

Because Tasha was considered a low-income mother, she was immediately referred to WIC, and an immediate enrollment was arranged that same day. Many publications are available for health professionals that address the adequate nutrients needed in pregnancy. Most importantly, the clients must be given practical, easy-to-read brochures to reinforce the teaching.

Tasha was given easy to follow menus and recipes that she and Carlos used to plan and eat better meals. With the assistance of the WIC program, her own efforts to eat better, and the support of the healthcare team, Tasha's nutritional status improved significantly. Tasha stopped smoking and made the rest of her prenatal visits on time.

Tasha delivered a 7-pound baby girl at 39 weeks who was healthy and required no additional time in the hospital. The assessment of the baby showed normal development.

REFERENCES

Baumrind, D., Larzelere, R. E., & Cowan, P. A. (2002). Ordinary physical punishment: is it harmful? Comment on Gershoff (2002). *Psychological Bulletin 28*(4), 580–589.

Benasich, A. A., & Brooks-Gunn, J. (1996). Maternal attitudes and knowledge of child-rearing: associations with family and child outcomes. *Child Development, 67,* 1186–1205.

Bornstein, M. H., & O'Reilly, A. W. (Eds.). (1993). *The role of play in the development of thought.* San Francisco: Jossey-Bass.

Bornstein, M. H., & Haynes, O. M. (1998). Vocabulary competence in early childhood: measurement, latent construct, and predictive validity. *Child Development, 69,* 654–671.

Bornstein, M. H. (2002). Parenting infants. In M. H. Bornstein (Ed.), *Handbook of parenting, Vol. 1: Children and parenting* (2nd ed., pp. 3–43). Mahwah, NJ: Erlbaum.

Bornstein, M. H. (2006). Parenting science and practice. In W. Damon & R. M. Lerner (Series Eds.) & I. E. Sigel & K. A. Renninger (Vol. Eds.), *Handbook of child psychology, vol. 4: Child psychology and practice* (6th ed., pp. 893–949). New York: Wiley.

Brooks-Gunn, J., Klebanov, P., & Smith, J. (2001). Effects of combining public assistance and employment on mothers and their young children. *Women & Health, 32,* 179–210.

Bugental, D. B., & Goodnow, J. G. (1998). Socialization processes. In W. Damon (Series Ed.) & N. Eisenberg (Vol. Ed.), *Handbook of child psychology, vol 3: Social, emotional, and personality development* (pp. 389–462). New York: Wiley.

Chase-Lansdale, P. L., Wakschlage, L. S., & Brooks-Gunn, J. (1995). A psychological perspective on the development of caring in children and youth: the role of the family. *Journal of Adolescence, 18,* 515–556.

Dawber, T., & Kuczynski, L. (1999). The question of ownness: influence of relationship context on parental socialization strategies. *Journal of Social and Personal Relationships, 16,* 475–493.

Demick, J. (2002). Stages of parental development. In M. H. Bornstein (Ed.), *Handbook of parenting, vol. 3: Status and social conditions of parenting* (2nd ed., pp. 389–413). Mahwah, NJ: Erlbaum.

Dix, T., Stewart, A., Gershoff, E., & Day, H. (2007). Autonomy and children's reactions to being controlled: evidence that both compliance and defiance may be positive markers in early development. *Child Development, 78,* 1204–1221.

Edwards, C. P., & Liu, W. (2002). Parenting toddlers. In M. H. Bornstein (Ed.), *Handbook of parenting, vol. 1: Children and parenting* (2nd ed., pp. 45–71). Mahwah, NJ: Erlbaum.

Elster, A. B., McAnarney, E. R., & Lamb, M. E. (1983). Parental behavior of adolescent mothers. *Pediatrics, 71,* 494–503.

Emde, R. N. (2000). Next steps in emotional availability research. *Attachment and Human Development, 2,* 242–248.

Feldman, S., & Elliott, G. (Eds.). (1990). *At the threshold: the developing adolescent.* Cambridge, MA: Harvard University Press.

Garrett, P., Ferron, J., Ng'andu, N., Bryant, D., & Harbin, G. (1994). A structural model for the developmental status of young children. *Journal of Marriage and the Family, 56,* 147–163.

Gershoff, E. (2002). Corporal punishment by parents and associated child behaviors and experiences: a meta-analytic and theoretical review. *Psychological Bulletin, 128, 539–579.*

Hardy, J., Astone, N. M., Brooks-Gunn, J., Shapiro, S., & Miller, T. (1998). Like mother, like child: intergenerational patterns of age at first birth and associations with childhood and adolescent characteristics and adult outcome in the second generation. *Developmental Psychology, 34,* 1220–1232.

Hauser, S. T. (1991). *Adolescents and their families.* New York: Free Press.

Hauser, S. T.; & Bowlds, M. K. (1990). Stress, coping, and adaptation. In S. S. Feldman & G. R. Elliott (Eds.), *At the threshold: the developing adolescent* (pp. 388–413). Cambridge, MA: Harvard University Press.

Havighurst, R. J. (1972). *Developmental tasks and education* (3rd ed.). New York: David McKay.

Hockenberry, M., Wilson, D., Winkelstein, M., & Kline, N. (2003). *Nursing care of infants and children* (7th ed.). St. Louis: Mosby.

Holden, G. W., & Buck, M. J. (2002). Parental attitudes toward childrearing. In M. H. Bornstein (Ed.), *Handbook of parenting, vol. 3: Status and social conditions of parenting* (2nd ed., pp. 537–562). Mahwah, NJ: Erlbaum.

Korbin, J., Coulton, C., & Lindstrom-Ufuti, H. (2000). Neighborhood views and etiology of child maltreatment. *Child Abuse and Neglect, 24,* 1509–1527.

Krug, E. G., Mercy, J. A., Dahlberg, L. L., Zwi, A. B. (2002). The world report on violence and health. *Lancet, 360*(9339), 1083–1088.

Larzelere, R. (2000). Child outcomes of nonabusive and customary physical punishment by parents: an updated literature review. *Clinical Child & Family Psychology Review, 3*(4), 199–221.

Lowdermilk, D., & Perry, S. (2004). *Maternity and women's health care* (8th ed.). St. Louis: Mosby.

Mosby, L., Rawls, A., & Meehan, A. (1999). An examination of African-American child rearing narratives. *Journal of Comparative Family Studies, 30,* 489–521.

Papalia, D., Olds, S., & Feldman, R. (2004). *Human development* (9th ed.). New York: McGraw Hill.

Papoušek, H., & Papoušek, M. (2002). Intuitive parenting. In M. H. Bornstein (Ed.), *Handbook of parenting, vol. 2: Biology and ecology of parenting* (2nd ed., pp. 183–203). Mahwah, NJ: Erlbaum.

Potts, N., & Mandleco, B. (2007). *Pediatric nursing: caring for children and their families* (2nd ed.). Clifton Park, NY: Thomson Delmar Learning.

Rohner, R., Kean, K., & Cournoyer, D. (1991). Effects of corporal punishment, perceived caretaker warmth, and cultural beliefs on the psychological adjustment in St. Kitts, West Indies. *Journal of Marriage and Family, 53,* 681–693.

Rowe, M., Pan, B., & Ayoub, C. (2005). Predictors of maternal talk to children: a longitudinal study of low-income families. *Parenting: Science and Practice, 5,* 285–310.

Sirignano, S. W., & Lachman, M. E. (1985). Personality change during the transition to parenthood: the role of perceived infant temperament. *Child Development, 21,* 558–567.

Smith, J. R., & Brooks-Gunn, J. (1997). Correlates and consequences of harsh discipline for young children. *Archives of Pediatrics & Adolescent Medicine, 151*(8), 777–786.

Straus, M. A., & Gelles, R. J. (1986). Societal change and change in family violence from 1975 to 1985. *Journal of Marriage & Family, 48*(3), 465–479.

Tamis-LeMonda, C. S., & Bornstein, M. H. (1991). Individual variation, correspondence, stability, and change in mother and toddler play. *Infant Behavior and Development, 14,* 143–162.

Teti, D. M., & Candelaria, M. A. (2002). Parenting competence. In M. H. Bornstein (Ed.), *Handbook of parenting, vol. 4: Social conditions and applied parenting* (2nd ed., pp. 149–180). Mahwah, NJ: Erlbaum.

Užgiris, I. Č., & Raeff, C. (1995). Play in parent–child interactions. In M. H. Bornstein (Ed.), *Handbook of parenting, vol. 4: Applied and practical parenting* (pp. 353–376). Mahwah, NJ: Erlbaum.

Chapter 23

Asthma in Adults and Children

Susan J. Sommer, Julie Shurtleff, & Pamela Kelly

INTRODUCTION

Asthma is a chronic disease of the lungs that affects more than 20 million Americans, including 6.5 million children, and causes 4,000 to 5,000 asthma deaths per year (Akinbami, 2006). Asthma is a disease that is characterized by chronic inflammation of the airways in response to inhalation of irritants and allergens. The resulting edema and excess mucus in the airways produces reversible airway obstruction. This inflammation also causes bronchospasm and makes these muscles hypersensitive and hyperresponsive to a wide variety of "triggers," like irritants such as cigarette smoke, upper respiratory infections, exercise, and laughing.

Our growing understanding of asthma over the past 25 years has allowed for the development of very effective medications and methods of delivery to control the underlying chronic inflammation and the more acute symptoms that characterize the disease such as—wheezing, coughing, shortness of breath, and chest tightness; nevertheless, overall rates of asthma in the United States have doubled in the last 2 decades. Many families continue to suffer the heavy burden of asthma—disturbed sleep, limited activities, frequent emergency room visits or hospitalizations, and absences from school and work—often accepting these as inevitable consequences of asthma. Asthma continues to be a leading cause of hospital admissions for children. There are large and growing health disparities based on race, ethnicity, and socioeconomic status, with the highest prevalence and mortality rates among Puerto Ricans, followed by non-Hispanic blacks.

Beginning in 1991, the treatment of asthma has been defined by the *Guidelines for the Diagnosis and Management of Asthma* developed by the National Asthma Education and Prevention Program of the National Heart, Lung and Blood Institute (NHLBI), with an important update in 2007. These guidelines outline four major components in asthma management: measures of assessment and monitoring, control of factors contributing to asthma severity, pharmacologic therapy, and education for a partnership in asthma care. Asthma self-management is a cornerstone to effective asthma care. Along with our growing knowledge of asthma has come an increasingly central need to educate those affected by asthma so that they can become active partners in the daily management and monitoring of their disease. Effective self-management requires a thorough understanding of asthma, its pathophysiology, the different roles of controller and quick relief medications, the asthma action plan (AAP), recognition of early symptoms, the correct use of delivery devices, and control of environmental triggers. This chapter outlines the key topics that providers and educators working with people with asthma should address, as well as shares teaching approaches that have been demonstrated through research and clinical experience to produce reductions in hospitalizations and emergency room visits and improvements in quality of life.

OVERVIEW

Asthma self-management education requires reinforcement at *every* asthma-related encounter at *all* points of care by *all* members of the healthcare team—during the traditional office visit, on the telephone, in the emergency room, home, and community setting. Even those patients or parents who have been dealing with asthma for years may have forgotten or have misconceptions about their asthma management and control. Most importantly, the education should be interactive and tailored to the individual or audience (Liu & Feekery, 2001).

Beginning a visit or teaching session with open-ended questions gives the provider or educator excellent insight into the patient's level of asthma control and baseline knowledge about the disease. This also shows respect for the individual or families' experience: What are your concerns about you/your child's asthma? How has asthma affected each of your lives? What has worked for you and what hasn't? What does it mean to have asthma in your family or culture? What are your goals for your asthma treatment? As educators and healthcare providers, our aim is to empower patients and parents to become self-advocates and active partners in their asthma care. This exchange of information and ideas, with ample opportunities for questions and problem solving, sets the tone for this partnership.

Above all, asthma education cannot include *only* facts about asthma, but must also include skills training in asthma self-management—medication skills, self-monitoring techniques, management of exacerbations, and environmental controls—and promote self-efficacy and confidence (NHLBI, 1997, 2007; see Appendix 23-I).

What Is Asthma?

If you ask most patients this question, they will describe the coughing, wheezing, and shortness of breath that they feel when they have an asthma attack, in other words their asthma *symptoms*, and if you ask them what the cause of those symptoms are they will describe their *asthma triggers*: the cigarette smoke, an upper respiratory infection. These are important pieces of information for the asthma educator so that you can understand what kind of asthma control your patient has and be able to personalize your message to the patient's main concerns; nevertheless, very few patients remember hearing about the underlying airway inflammation that sets this entire process in motion, and often, they do not understand why they need anything other than their quick-relief medication to relieve their symptoms. In fact, in a cohort of 98 inner-city adults hospitalized for asthma, 53% believed they only had asthma at times when they were symptomatic, what the authors of this study called the "no symptoms, no asthma belief" (Halm, Mora, & Leventhal, 2006). The authors suggested asking patients this single question as a way to identify patients with this belief system, "Do you think you have asthma all of the time, or only when you are having symptoms?"

Show your patients graphics and models. You will continue to refer back to them throughout your teaching session. After a patient or parent has seen a picture or model showing the difference between a normal airway and "asthmatic airways," they are more able to have the conversation about how to control their asthma.

Why Do I Have to Take Medicine When I Feel Fine?

Referring back to your graphic of the airways, you can begin to discuss the difference between quick-relief bronchodilators that act on the smooth muscles and inhaled steroids and other controller medications that act on the airway inflammation. With this visual aid, the asthma educator can indicate the bronchoconstriction that is relieved by beta-2 agonists and the inflammation of the lining of the airways, which requires controller medication for those with symptoms of persistent asthma.

It has been well documented in the literature that controller medications, in particular inhaled steroids, which are considered first-line treatment for persistent asthma, are frequently not taken as prescribed. Various studies have shown that there remain many fears and misconceptions about this group of medications, with 23% to 34% of parents of children with persistent asthma reporting strong concerns or worries about these medications. These concerns were associated with poor adherence (Conn et al., 2005; Farber et al., 2003), as was the misunderstanding among adults of the preventative role of inhaled steroids (Boulet, 1998). More often than not, these concerns are not discussed with the healthcare provider (Boulet, 1998). A study on barriers to antiinflammatory medication use in children found that families that were poorer, less educated, and particularly black families had significantly more negative attitudes about these medications and less understanding about how they work (Yoos, Kitzman, & McMullen, 2003). Another commonly held belief is that inhaled steroids are "addictive" and will lose their effectiveness over time or require ever higher doses to be effective.

Identify and address any misconceptions or fears about asthma medications, in particular inhaled steroids, in order to increase adherence to these medications. The word "steroid" has many negative connotations in our society, such as the much publicized abuse of anabolic steroids by athletes and the perception that all medications with steroids have many side effects. Often the most publicized side effects, such as weight gain, loss of bone density, and stunted growth, relate to long-term treatment with oral steroids rather than the low to medium doses of inhaled steroids that most patients receive. There are several ways to address these concerns. Asthma educators should certainly share what is known about the safety profile of these medications. For example, new data show that children who chronically use inhaled steroids, although having some delayed growth in the first year of use, do, in fact, reach their normal adult height (Allen, 2006). According to the NHLBI guidelines, it is always recommended that the lowest dose to control asthma symptoms be used, thus arguing for routine asthma follow-up visits to monitor the response and allow for adjustment of controller medications. It is often helpful to compare the dose of an inhaled steroid with the amount of steroid in a "steroid burst," that is, a short course of oral steroids used to treat an acute exacerbation, which is often equal in dose to a year's worth of a moderate dose of inhaled steroid. It may be necessary to clarify the difference between anabolic steroids and the glucocorticoid steroids that are used in asthma.

The Asthma Action Plan

Develop an AAP with patients. Although each individual's asthma is different, in general, asthma control is achieved through a combination of measures that should include a written asthma AAP. Asthma self-management by the patient or parents, as well as the partnership between patients and clinicians, is central to the NHLBI guidelines. These guidelines recommend that clinicians provide an individualized AAP, ideally developed with the patient's or family's input, to all asthma patients. Using the traffic light symbol with green, yellow, and red zones, the AAP provides patients with a simple outline of their medications and when to use them. Reviewing the AAP with patients provides the asthma educator with the opportunity to cover many of the key points that patients need to know to be partners in their asthma management. For example, when discussing the Green Zone medications, the asthma educator can review the underlying inflammation that causes asthma and the role of controller medications. The Yellow Zone's emphasis on early signs and symptoms provides a perfect opportunity for the educator to help patients identify their own early warning signs and what measures to take, such as adjusting their medications, to prevent an exacerbation. The Red Zone indicates a need for immediate medical attention. A common error that patients make is to stay at home, despite increasing and ineffective use of beta-2 agonists (albuterol). The AAP can be tailored to indicate that if quick-relief medication is required more frequently than every 4 hours they should seek medical attention. The AAP also allows for patients to use their peak flow readings in addition to their symptoms to help guide them to the appropriate zone.

The AAP is an extremely helpful tool for asthma educators, school nurses, and other healthcare providers who interact with the patient around his or her asthma. The AAP provides a common understanding of the current medication regimen. The AAP is a working document and may change often based on such factors as changes in severity, exposure to environmental triggers, or patient preferences in dosing frequency or delivery device. For this reason, people with asthma also need regularly scheduled follow-up visits with their healthcare providers to reassess the AAP with frequency of visits generally every 3 to 6 months, depending on the severity, seasonal triggers, and asthma control of each patient. This frequency may increase to every month for those patients with poor asthma control or recently hospitalized or seen in the emergency room. This is a point often lost on patients and families with busy lives or other pressing problems.

Review asthma medication on an ongoing basis. Asking patients to bring their medications to each visit or to show them to you during a home visit allows you to review what medications the patient is taking and whether they are adhering to their current regimen. If the patient has been seen for an urgent care visit or by a different provider in the interim, they also may have been prescribed a different medication or a different dose, or the patient may have become confused by conflicting plans. This is also a time when the educator or provider can check refill dates as a way to gauge adherence.

Observe medication delivery technique at each encounter. Never assume that your patient, even someone who has been using the same device for years, is using it correctly. Depending on the actual technique used, the amount of medication that is actually reaching the airways may vary widely. By asking the patient to demonstrate his or her use of their inhaled medications at each encounter, one often uncovers errors in technique, such as failure to use a spacer or to take and hold a deep breath. Many patients, both children and adults, do not realize that spacers are now recommended for everyone who uses a non–breath-actuated metered dose inhaler (MDI).

Multiple studies have found errors in device technique among both adults and children, which improved with repeated educational sessions. In one sample of 42 mostly white children with good asthma control, aged 7 to 11 years old from middle- to upper-income households, 92% of the children had fair to poor MDI technique at pretest, whereas only 19% had incorrect technique after two instruction sessions, spaced no more than 4 weeks apart (Burkhart, Rayens, & Bowman, 2004). Among the most common mistakes identified in the study were (1) failure to hold their breath for at least 10 seconds after inhalation, (2) failure to shake the medication adequately, (3) not taking a deep enough breath, and (4) not using a spacer for those devices. In a separate study of 200 children, Kamps, Brand, and Roorda (2002) found that a single instruction session, typically done at the time the medication is first prescribed, is not adequate to ensure correct inhaler technique over time. Among patients who were newly referred to the asthma clinic where this study took place, 57% demonstrated correct technique of their inhaler device at the first visit, with 78.6% using their MDI with spacer correctly, and only 26.3% using their dry powder inhaler (DPI) correctly. Three subsequent instruction sessions by a pulmonologist or asthma nurse were needed for children or their parents to achieve 100% accuracy using MDI with spacer and 94.7% for a DPI. Among MDI users, incorrect preparation of the device, especially failing to shake the canister, was the most common error. For patients using DPIs, the most common mistake was failure to inhale forcefully and deeply. More instruction sessions were also necessary to achieve correct DPI use than for MDI with spacer. The authors of this study recommended that the inhalation technique should be checked at every follow-up visit.

What Is "Good Asthma Control"?

One of the most revealing conversations to have with patients and parents is the discussion of what we as clinicians and asthma educators mean by "asthma control." Patients and parents of children with asthma often accept impairment of activity as inevitable. Symptoms are controlled by limiting exercise and play or keeping a child home from school because of cold weather. Every parent of a child with asthma can identify with the loss of sleep that comes with the frequent nighttime coughing that occurs when asthma is poorly controlled. These same patients and families are often not aware that the goal of current asthma treatment is to eliminate or minimize such restrictions. Thus, people with asthma can live active lives, exercise, sleep through the night and attend school or work regularly.

The Rule of 2s is a simple way to remind patients and parents of what they should expect from their asthma management plan. If a person with asthma is symptomatic or using their quick-relief bronchodilator medication (1) more than two times a week during the day or (2) more than two times a month at night, or needing to refill the prescription for quick-relief medication more than two times a year, then his or her asthma is not well-controlled.

The Asthma Control Test

The Asthma Control Test (ACT), a quick and simple self-administered patient questionnaire, has been developed and validated to assess asthma control (Schatz et al., 2006). This questionnaire has been modified for children as well and can be used by the asthma educator as a screening tool at the beginning of an individual teaching session to identify patients with poor asthma control and to assess the efficacy of pharmacologic and environmental interventions. Another important goal of the ACT is to empower patients and parents to communicate with their healthcare provider if their current medications do not adequately control their asthma or if they begin to note a decline in their asthma control.

Help your patients identify their asthma triggers so that they can modify their environment and/or behavior to reduce exposure. Some triggers are universal and well known, such as secondhand smoke or strong cleaning products. Eighty percent of people with asthma also have an allergic component to their asthma. Often identifying these allergies is simple, for example, when an exposure produces an immediate allergic response to a specific trigger, such as exposure to a cat at a relative's house; however, at other times, the allergy is less obvious, especially when there is a perennial exposure to an allergen, such as dust mites or cockroaches. In these cases, it is often helpful to assist patients in requesting allergy testing.

There are specific allergy tests for many of the common allergens, such as dust mites, mouse and cockroach allergen, and various molds that may be present not only in the patient's home, but also in the schools and workplace. Together, the patient and asthma educator can review in detail the environments in which the patient spends time and identify known or potential triggers. There is further discussion in the section on Asthma Education in the Community of home environmental triggers and the unique role of the asthma home visitor to also help families mediate these often challenging environmental issues, especially in low-income, inner-city neighborhoods.

"His or her asthma came on all of a sudden. How do I know when he or she is getting sick?" When you review the history of an asthma exacerbation with the patient or family, there is often a history of several days or weeks of symptoms, usually coughing, especially at night, preceding the severe exacerbation that led them to seek emergency medical care. Accurate and timely symptom perception is another area that may be greatly improved through individualized and repetitive education with the patient or family. Usually patients and parents underestimate symptom severity, in particular coughing, which is often the first sign of declining asthma control and lung function (Butz et al., 2005).

Address the issue of tobacco and secondhand smoke. The issue of smoking deserves special attention, when discussing asthma triggers, as the health benefits for smoking cessation are so wide ranging for both smokers and those around them. Between 25% and 43% of all children are exposed to secondhand smoke. Among children with poorly controlled asthma, 51% had exposure to tobacco smoke (McGhan et al., 2006). Asthma educators have an excellent opportunity not only to educate about the dangers of smoking, but to also give information and referrals for help quitting (Winickoff et al., 2004).

Depending on the asthma educator's role, some or all of the brief intervention steps recommended in the 5As (U.S. Department of Health and Human Services, 2000) can be used to assist the educator in providing the important messages about cigarette smoking: (1) Ask about tobacco use at every visit. (2) Advise all tobacco users to quit. (3) Assess readiness to quit. (4) Assist tobacco users in quitting. (5) Arrange follow-up. Even brief interventions have been shown to increase quit rates. Offering tobacco treatment resources, such as quit lines, expert support and counseling, and assistance obtaining nicotine replacement products or other pharmacologic treatments, is within the realm of the asthma educator's role.

Tailor your teaching strategies to the individual. The asthma educator also needs to assess early on the recipients' learning style, primary language, and literacy level. Low literacy levels, as well as low health literacy (measured by reading comprehension of health-related materials), have been shown to result in poorer outcomes, such as more emergency room visits and hospitalizations, near-fatal asthma, inadequate MDI technique and ineffective self-management skills (DeWalt, Dilling, Rosenthal, & Pignone, 2007; Mancuso & Rincon, 2006; Williams, Baker, Honig, Lee, & Nowlan, 1998). For those patients with low literacy, for example, the health educator will want to adapt his or her teaching to include more verbal instruction, low-literacy reading materials, and other hands-on, interactive teaching strategies.

There are also an ever-increasing variety of modalities being studied to supplement one-on-one asthma education, including many interactive, computer-based programs that cross all health care and even community settings. These programs include touch-screen computer kiosks or tablet-style portable computers that guide the user through a series of questions and, based on their responses, produce recommendations to be shared with their provider based on the patient/parent's input and the current NHLBI asthma guidelines. These kiosks have been found to be easy-to-use by most users and can also be programmed for different languages and the option to hear the questions while reading along (Porter, Cai, Gribbons, Goldmann, & Kohane, 2004; Sockrider et al., 2006; Thompson, Lozano, & Christakis, 2007). Another study looked at a multimedia program in which children are guided through short, animated real-life vignettes on an exam room computer that can be viewed while the patient is waiting in the exam room to be seen for routine clinic visits. Each patient logs on with a password, and the program provides feedback to the learner and tracks their progress, reviewing material that was not understood in a previous session (Krishna, Balas, Francisco, & Konig, 2006). In particular, adolescents are a group that feel very comfortable on the Internet and may be better reached through a web-based tailored asthma program (Joseph, 2007).

ASTHMA EDUCATION IN THE COMMUNITY

The community setting offers many unique opportunities for asthma education. Foremost, the patients and families who most urgently need to be reached are often the same patients who, for complicated socioeconomic reasons, have poor access to and/or utilization of primary care. Thus, they may only be seen in the clinic or the emergency room during an asthma exacerbation, when there is little time for more thorough asthma education. Moving asthma education beyond the hospital or office setting into the communities and homes of our patients and their families provides them with easier access to the information that they need to avoid the emergency room in the future. Bringing asthma education to the community means not only holding asthma education sessions where our patients live and work, but also at times that are convenient and at venues that are familiar and accessible. Asthma education workshops may be held in day care centers, schools, shelters, community centers, libraries, housing developments, pharmacies, and religious organizations—wherever a group of adults, parents, or children affected by asthma can be assembled (Bryant-Stephens & Li, 2004; Kritikos, Armour, & Bosnic-Anticevich, 2007; Levy, Brugge, Peters, Clougherty, & Saddler, 2006). When working in low-income communities, sessions should be free, and child care should be offered. It is often helpful to offer some incentives to attend, such as a meal, a raffle for a HEPA vacuum cleaner or dust mite–proof bedding encasements, supermarket or pharmacy gift cards, and smaller giveaways, such as spacers, to create excitement about the event.

As with one-on-one sessions, group workshops function best when they are interactive. Although many people feel intimidated in the clinic or hospital setting, the community setting feels familiar and allows people to speak out and ask questions. Assuming that the group size permits, it is helpful to initially go around the room and ask attendees to introduce themselves and share how asthma affects them and their family. This gives the group leader information about the group; it also sets the tone for a discussion, rather than a lecture, in which participants can ask questions, support, and learn from each other. Depending on the cultural diversity of the group, a question about how asthma is treated in the participants' different cultures may start a lively discussion and also indicates to the group that their cultural perspectives and practices are respected and valued.

The impact of group members sharing successes and reinforcing educational messages was one aspect of a psychoeducational intervention designed by La Roche, Koinis-Mitchell, and Gualdron (2006) that was geared toward what was believed to be the more group- and relationship-oriented cultures of African American and Latino patients with asthma in this study. The intervention tested the belief that these groups would benefit from an educational approach that emphasized (1) participating in group sharing, (2) drawing on cultural beliefs and resources, (3) supporting collaborative asthma management within families, between families, and with their healthcare providers, and (4) placing the asthma symptoms within a socioeconomic context that takes into account the barriers and health disparities these populations often face. The treatment group had 50% fewer emergency department visits than the subjects that had the standard, psychoeducational group intervention and had almost double the impact of the control group that used routine medical care without any group educational sessions (La Roche et al., 2006).

Given the much higher rates of asthma among African American and Latino groups, hiring and training culturally and linguistically competent asthma educators has also been shown to increase success. A number of successful programs have trained lay health workers who live in the community to be asthma educators and outreach workers (Bryant-Stephens & Li, 2004; Primomo, Johnston, DiBiase, Nodolf, & Noren, 2006). These health workers, who also often have personal experience with asthma, have a more immediate rapport with clients and can break down many of the cultural barriers and distrust that healthcare professionals may encounter. For example, patients from cultures that defer to and want to please their healthcare provider may not be honest about what medications or home remedies they are actually using or what problems they or their children are having with asthma control.

The Home Visit

Educating families about home environmental triggers and how to reduce them has proven to be another critical component in improving asthma outcomes. Recently, a number of studies have looked at a multifaceted approach to home environmental interventions with home visitors helping families to identify, reduce, or eliminate the asthma triggers found in the home. Many of these programs have been shown to improve asthma control and quality of life, with reduced ER and unscheduled urgent care clinic visits, fewer missed school and work days, and increased symptom-free days (Krieger, Takaro, Song, & Weaver, 2005; Nicholas et al., 2005; Morgan et al., 2004).

The home visit offers many opportunities for individualized, comprehensive asthma education in an environment in which the patient feels most comfortable. Generally, the home visitor can also spend more time and provide more frequent visits than may be possible in the clinic setting. In addition, the visit allows the asthma educator to perform *with* the patient and family a home environmental assessment, thus identifying potential or known asthma triggers. Often many family members will be involved in the visit, thus broadening the reach of educational messages.

Typically, an initial home visit takes at least an hour and will include a review of "asthma basics," as well as a home environmental assessment. At this time, a variety of misunderstandings and problems may come to light, such as discrepancies between medications the patient is actually using and what is on the AAP, the lack of a spacer, or expired or discontinued medications that the patient is still using. As in the office visit, the home visit is another opportunity for the patient to demonstrate the correct use of the asthma devices and to review the green, yellow, and red zone treatments.

The home environmental assessment involves a room-by-room assessment for the presence of known, or likely, asthma triggers. This should be left for the latter part of the visit so that the home visitor and patient have established a relationship and there is a spirit of working together to improve the client's asthma. A nonjudgmental approach is essential to conducting an environmental assessment. First, recognize and praise the steps that the patient or parent has taken to manage his or her child's asthma, including opening their house to the visitor to do the environmental assessment. Families have different standards and abilities around housekeeping, and there may be barriers to having a clean, orderly house (such as depression, overcrowding, and lack of storage space) or substandard housing conditions (such as pests or mold). Generally, the home visitor pays special attention to the bedroom, as the patient with asthma spends so many hours there. Knowing the patient's specific asthma triggers (e.g., if he or she has tested positive for dust mite allergy) also helps the home visitor target those interventions that are going to help the most.

Many useful tools can be found on the Internet to aid the home visitor. The Environmental Protection Agency has many free educational materials and checklists on home environmental triggers (see Resources). The home visitor, whether a professional or a community outreach worker, is also an important link between the patient and the primary care provider or asthma specialist. The home visitor can convey information about patient symptoms and environmental barriers to asthma control, as well as help coordinate follow-up visits.

Integrated Pest Management

Cockroach and rodent infestations are endemic in many inner-city neighborhoods and given the allergenic nature of these pests, asthma educators, especially those visiting the homes, need to be well-versed in Integrated Pest Management. Unfortunately, many families use highly toxic, aerosolized and even illegal pesticides to control infestations in their homes. *Integrated pest management* is the term used to describe a method of pest control that minimizes pesticide use and applies common sense practices of denying pests: (1) entry to homes by filling in all holes or cracks; (2) food, by using tightly covered garbage cans, storing food in pest-proof containers, such as Tupperware, and cleaning up all food and dishes after meals; and (3) places to live and hide, such as clutter or cardboard boxes. Then, if needed, the least amount of the least toxic, nonaerosolized pesticides can be applied by a licensed pest control company, thus minimizing exposure of inhabitants to these dangerous chemicals.

Exercise

Our message to patients with asthma is this: "You can control your asthma so that you can be active and exercise." In fact, we want our patients to exercise to improve their lung function, avoid or reduce obesity, and gain the many other health benefits of exercise. For children, in particular, combining asthma education with exercise and other fun activities, such as asthma swim programs and asthma camps, can provide them with peer support, while learning self-monitoring skills and becoming more confident about playing and exercising like other children (Buckner et al., 2005). For those patients who, sadly, live in unsafe neighborhoods and cannot safely go outside to exercise or play, the asthma educator can be a resource in identifying affordable exercise opportunities in their communities.

Schools

For children, the school nurse is an essential partner in the education of the child and his or her parents around asthma and should always receive a copy of the AAP. There are many curricula, including the American Lung Association's *Open Airways for Schools* for school-age children (Clark et al.,

2004) and the Asthma and Allergy Foundation of America's *Power Breathing* course for adolescents, available that can be used in the school setting. The schools can also be a setting for parent education workshops about asthma.

THE AMBULATORY CARE SETTING

Within the ambulatory setting, particularly primary care, the ability to treat and manage a chronic and variable illness, such as asthma, can be a daunting task. This is particularly true with the present structure of health care that calls for large patient panels and increasing demands on both provider and nursing staff time. In a survey conducted with parents regarding the asthma education they received from their children's providers, it was found that the more complex issues involved in asthma self-management—such as establishing goals of treatment, chronic management of asthma, and learning to work in partnership with the healthcare provider—were less likely to be taught than the more concrete skills of using an MDI or managing an asthma attack (McMullen et al., 2007). Nevertheless, the patient/provider partnership is considered one of the essential elements in successful asthma management (NHLBI, 2007; Peterson-Sweeney et al., 2007). In order to foster this partnership, the healthcare provider and the larger ambulatory care team need to develop creative systems of asthma education that will meet patient and caregivers' needs.

As mentioned in the overview, the provider and other members of the asthma team must engage the patient in a conversation about his or her concerns, identifying with the patient short- and long-term goals of asthma treatment, for example, attending school or work regularly, taking dance lessons, or playing football. This provides the healthcare team with important information regarding how to motivate the patient around his or her asthma management. It also gives the provider an opportunity to explain the healthcare team's own goals and expectations of "good asthma control" and how these relate to the patient's own goals. By seeing a patient for regular asthma follow-up, the patient and provider can reassess periodically whether their goals are being met and what adjustments might need to take place. This also builds a strong relationship that fosters mutual understanding between the patient and provider (McMullen et al., 2007; Peterson-Sweeney, McMullen, Yoos, Kitzman, 2003).

The concept of regular follow-up care during times of stable asthma symptoms as well as times of illness is one of which both patients and even providers need to be reminded. In reality, the patient who is being seen for asthma is often at the clinic because of an exacerbation. Although far from ideal, the clinic staff can use this as an opportunity to engage the patient in a learning discussion, not a lecture, about his or her asthma. What were the triggers and early warning signs, and could this exacerbation have been avoided or treated earlier? Do the controller medications need adjusting, or are there issues of adherence that need to be addressed? Ideally, the patient should return in a couple of weeks for a more focused and lengthier follow-up visit. Emphasizing the importance of this visit and implementing reminder calls may help to encourage patients and families to attend this follow-up appointment. The provider and nursing staff should keep in mind, however, that a percentage of patients will not keep their follow-up appointments after this exacerbation is over. Thus, *each* ambulatory encounter, both scheduled and unscheduled, must include a review of the AAP, adjustments in medications, if indicated, and teaching on asthma self-care management.

Interventions

This section reviews a variety of steps that the ambulatory care team and other clinic staff can creatively use to maximize the impact of asthma education, given the realities of a busy ambulatory clinic:

1. Designate a clinical staff person, whether a nurse, health educator, nurse practitioner, or other trained staff, with dedicated time to provide asthma education and follow-up for patients who need education beyond the standard 15-minute office visit. This would include those who are newly diagnosed, have poor asthma control, need additional instruction on their devices or home self-management with an AAP, or have had a recent emergency room visit or hospitalization (Self, Chrisman, Mason, & Rumbak, 2005). Office practices may also want to encourage staff to prepare for the asthma educator certification examination. This certification process helps to develop a cadre of professionals with expertise and ensures teaching that is in line with current standards and promotes best practice in the clinic.

2. Create a multidisciplinary "asthma team" in your clinic, which should include clinicians and nurses who can focus on best practices and medical management (Cabana, Slish, Brown, & Clark, 2004; Walders et al., 2006). Involving social workers and case managers is important in order to aid families with issues such as substandard housing and lack of insurance or medication coverage that can have a negative impact on a family's ability to carry out effective self-care management. Other staff, such as

practice managers, may also be involved in looking at quality improvement measures and changes in administrative systems that may further develop asthma management within practices. This may also be helpful in addressing shortfalls in asthma management based on insurers' Health Care Effectiveness Data and Information Set measures, and health plan "report cards" that are increasingly connected to reimbursement. Such measures generally include a current AAP for all patients with asthma and the prescription of controller medications to all patients that meet criteria for persistent asthma, according to current NHLBI guidelines.

The asthma team may also be responsible for chart audits and ongoing clinical staff in-services, as studies continue to reveal that a significant number of providers do not adhere to current NHLBI guidelines (Halm et al., 2005) or underestimate asthma among their patients (Halterman et al., 2002). Asthma education programs for healthcare providers, particularly targeting providers serving low-income, urban families, have been successful at enhancing provider communication and counseling techniques used in teaching asthma self-management skills to patients and families (Brown, Bratton, Cabana, Kaciroti, & Clark, 2004).

3. Develop an asthma database or registry to facilitate reminders to patients to schedule routine asthma follow-up. This system can also be useful in the fall for reminders for flu vaccine administration, as well as identifying patients who tend to have exacerbations during particular allergy seasons or those who are at risk because of other medical or social reasons (Noble, Smith, & Windley, 2006). In this way, the clinic staff can more effectively focus on the needs of individuals within the providers' large patient panels.

4. Assure that families are familiar with the office triage system, after hours, and urgent care policies. For example, many practices are set up to accommodate urgent care visits and encourage patients and families to "check in" with the asthma or triage nurse at the outset of upper respiratory illnesses or exacerbations and before going to the emergency room, in case it would be more appropriate to come to the clinic. Provide patients with a list of important numbers in a format that they will keep at hand, such as a refrigerator magnet or as part of the AAP itself. Such systems extend the concept of partnership among the provider and patients.

5. Sponsor clinic and community asthma information events, and provide up-to-date lists of community programs, such as asthma camps, advocacy and home-visiting agencies, and exercise programs (Bentley et al., 2005).

For pediatric patients, communicating with school nurses, coaches, and after-school teachers after parental consent provides the child with a network of adults who are involved in other areas of the child's life and can be aware of early signs of an exacerbation, as well as support the child in following the AAP.

6. Display colorful posters illustrating normal and inflamed airways and educational materials geared to the ages, reading levels, and languages of your clinic's population in the clinic waiting and exam rooms. There are also many videos on asthma that can be running along with videos on other educational topics in the waiting room. These materials should be used as supplements, not substitutes, for the interactive, nonjudgmental discussion about asthma that must take place between the clinic staff and the patient. As always, adapt your teaching strategy to the individual's learning style. Alternative teaching tools such as an asthma kiosk or multimedia programs appeal to a wide range of patients and may be particularly appealing to adolescents and young adults.

7. Develop easy-to-use tools and checklists for documentation of both assessment of asthma control and asthma education at each visit. For those offices using an electronic medical record, online documentation, including an online AAP, allows providers, triage nurses, and asthma educators to coordinate care better and be sure that they are referring to the current AAP. Plans are easily edited online, and changes can be communicated more reliably back and forth between primary care providers and asthma specialists, especially if they work within the same institution or network.

8. Collaborate closely with an allergy or pulmonary specialist. NHLBI outlines criteria for early and timely referral to an asthma specialist. Some primary care practices have even arranged for a specialist to have designated clinic sessions within the primary care setting, thus increasing the accessibility of specialty care to patients and enhancing the coordination of asthma care between primary care providers and specialists.

EDUCATION IN THE IN-PATIENT SETTING

Asthma continues to be one of the major hospital admission diagnoses in children, accounting for more than $3 billion in direct costs for hospitalizations alone, not to mention the indirect costs of missed days of work and school (Banasiak & Meadows-Oliver, 2004). Major health disparities exist: For example, blacks are hospitalized for asthma at a rate more than three times that of whites (American Lung Association, 2006). As with missed school days or limitations of activity, many patients and their families, having experienced multiple hospitalizations in the past, accept hospitalizations as a fact of life with asthma. We now consider most asthma hospitalizations preventable; therefore, a hospitalization signals serious gaps in asthma care that both healthcare providers and patients/families need to share responsibility to prevent.

People are often more motivated to change their behavior after a stressful, negative event; thus, a hospitalization may be an opportune time to convey critical patient/family asthma education (Ebbinghaus & Bahrainwala, 2003; Osman & Calder, 2004). While recognizing that several members of the healthcare team will be providing asthma education during the course of the admission, generally, a nurse will be providing the majority of the formal asthma education. As in the clinic, the nurse should have a variety of materials and modalities at hand, including graphics of airways, videos, and brochures suitable for the populations being served. Before beginning to teach, however, the nurse's first step is to listen in a nonjudgmental way to the patient/family's understanding of what led to the admission. In this way, the nurse can begin to create an alliance with the patient and hopefully arrive at a common goal of preventing future hospitalizations. Reviewing not only the day of admission but also the days or even weeks before the admission will also help the nurse assess both baseline asthma control and early warning signs.

Nonadherence to medications and delay in seeking treatment are two of the most common and preventable reasons for admission. Even though the consequences of nonadherence are all too clear to the healthcare team, this connection may be far from obvious to the patient, who has little understanding of the role of the different medications. Nonadherence often involves stopping inhaled steroids on one's own. Identifying the underlying reason is critical to approaching this issue effectively. Although fears or misconceptions about these medications are the most common cause, the inability to pay for these much more expensive medications (or even co-pays) is another possibility that should be explored, as this would require a very different solution.

Halm et al. (2005) found that 73% of an inner-city adult cohort delayed treatment an average of 7.3 days before going to see their provider or to the emergency room. The reasons noted included a lack of a usual source of care, difficulty getting advice over the telephone or scheduling an urgent care visit, the patient's uncertainty that he or she was sick or belief that the exacerbation would resolve on its own; patient's fear of hospitalization; and a lack of written AAPs that detailed what to do when symptoms were worsening. They also found that delaying treatment is often accompanied by dangerous overuse of albuterol in the hours or days leading up to the hospitalization; therefore, taking the current episode as an example, the nurse can again show with airway graphics how the repeated dosing of albuterol was not treating the ever-worsening inflammation that resulted in the hospitalization. Patients benefit from clear messages regarding how frequently albuterol can be used at home and that early contact with a medical provider, whether the primary care provider or asthma specialist, will increase the likelihood that the exacerbation can be treated before it becomes severe. These instructions should also be detailed in a written AAP.

Teaching and preparing for discharge should be an ongoing process throughout the hospitalization. Providing education over several short—approximately 15- to 30-minute—sessions, rather than overwhelming the already stressed patient/family with too much information, has been found to work well (Osman et al., 2002). Some hospitals also offer group asthma education sessions on the inpatient units. These can be a time-effective way to convey "asthma basics" if there are several patients on the unit with asthma, as well as offer patients/families an opportunity to support and learn from each other. To increase attendance at these sessions, it is often helpful to provide healthy snacks and allow children to attend. Patients/parents should always be encouraged to follow up with any additional questions with their nurse or primary care provider after discharge.

No matter in which setting the education takes place or who provides the teaching, the same fundamental asthma topics should be covered. Before discharge, parents should have a basic understanding of asthma signs and symptoms, triggers, and ways to control and avoid them; medications and devices; and what to do in the event of an asthma attack (Cote, 2001; Sockrider et al., 2006). A written individualized AAP should be updated (or developed, if one does not already exist), reviewed carefully, and sent home with all patients (Sockrider et al., 2006). They should additionally be instructed to bring this plan to their follow-up visit with their primary care provider, as the plan may change as the patient's condition improves. Patients should also begin using whatever devices with which they will be discharged, including their albuterol MDI with spacer, while in house and be able to demonstrate correct technique, ideally on several occasions, before discharge.

It may be necessary to get social work or case managers involved during an admission to assist with issues related to insurance, transportation, or housing. Patients often present with lapsed insurance policies and have difficulty navigating the system to obtain new coverage. The nurse or social worker should clarify whether the patient or family will be able to afford the medications and the equipment that they are prescribed on discharge and if not make alternative arrangements to obtain them. Families should always be told to call the hospital or the primary care provider if they cannot obtain the medications for any reason.

The nurse should emphasize the importance of preventative care and regular medical monitoring and follow-up. It is also essential that every patient have a primary care provider identified on discharge. Although patients may feel better by the time they leave the hospital, the nurse should stress that it generally takes 6 to 8 weeks for the airways to return to baseline after a severe exacerbation; therefore, they need to finish all medications, such as oral steroids; continue to follow the AAP they are given; report any recurrence of symptoms promptly; and have close follow-up, perhaps initially every 2 weeks or monthly, with their primary care provider or asthma specialist. Follow-up appointments should ideally be scheduled before discharge.

As in the ambulatory setting, it is important to provide staff development on an ongoing basis. Depending on the size of the institution and the volume of asthma admissions, a designated clinician within the hospital, such as an asthma clinical nurse specialist, is very effective in providing regular in-services to both ambulatory and inpatient nurses and residents on NHLBI guidelines, hospital protocols (such as discharging all patients with an AAP), and quality improvement efforts.

SUMMARY

Asthma continues to be a disease with high morbidity and significant mortality, despite tremendous advances in medical management. National asthma management guidelines include asthma education at every asthma-related encounter as a key component in improving asthma outcomes. Asthma education must be tailored to the individual, promote a partnership between healthcare providers and their patients/families, include a written AAP, and teach asthma self-management skills with a focus on achieving "good asthma control." Additionally, asthma educators and healthcare providers must address environmental triggers, as well as the many other barriers to asthma control that some of our most vulnerable patients face. Hospitals, clinics, insurers, and community agencies face the urgent, yet exciting challenge of training staff and developing new systems to deliver the kind of quality asthma education that will allow people with asthma to live active, healthy lives.

Case Study 23–1

Home Visit

Johnny is a 10-year-old boy who has had asthma since 1 year of age. He has had one to two hospitalizations per year and three emergency room visits and four courses of prednisone in the past year. Johnny is the only one in the family with asthma and is obese.

The last time he was seen in the emergency room he was referred to the asthma nurse educator for a home visit. The asthma nurse spoke to the pediatrician, who said that mom expresses a lot of discomfort about using daily inhaled steroids because of the risk of side effects. She is not giving her son the inhaled corticosteroids.

Home Visit by Asthma Nurse Educator

Assessment

The asthma nurse educator begins with open-ended questions to mom and Johnny about how asthma has affected their lives in terms of quality of life and what goals they have around Johnny's asthma.

Mom is a single mother with a 12th-grade education. She feels very stressed by her full-time job and by Johnny's asthma. Johnny has missed 10 days of school, and mom has missed 10 days of work in the last 6 months. Johnny is using his albuterol inhaler four to five times per week during the day and six times a month at night. Johnny was recently seen by an allergy clinic and was found to be allergic to dust mites, tree and grass pollen, cats, dogs, and mice.

Mom finds herself often limiting Johnny's physical activities to avoid exacerbations. She states that she is always hypervigilant and aware that she may have to drop what she's doing at a moment's notice to rush Johnny to the hospital. Mom would love to not worry so much about Johnny and to let him play like other kids.

The nurse introduces the concept of asthma control. "We want Johnny to be able to run, play, attend school and sleep through the night like other children and we believe this is definitely achievable." Mom and the nurse agree on these mutual goals.

(Continues)

Case Study 23–1 (*Continued*)

Education

Despite that Johnny has had asthma for years, mom does not remember ever hearing an explanation of asthma pathophysiology or how his medicines work. The nurse showed mom and Johnny graphics and models of airways that are normal, mildly inflamed, and severely inflamed. The nurse also goes through Johnny's medications and explains the difference between quick-relief and controller medications, relating it back to the airway graphics.

Mom's fears about inhaled steroids are explored and addressed. Mom takes a lot of pride in her efforts to manage Johnny's asthma. The nurse explains the concept of "asthma control" in terms of Johnny's symptoms, frequency of need for quick-relief medications, and limitations on his quality of life.

The nurse explores the discrepancy between mom's desire for better asthma control, her clear efforts to take good care of Johnny and his asthma, and her reluctance to use inhaled steroids. Although mom is still not sure about side effects, mom agrees to start inhaled corticosteroids and schedule an appointment with Johnny's pediatrician in 2 weeks to review his AAP and asthma control.

AAP

Mom and child cannot put their hands on his AAP—they took their copy to the school nurse. Because Johnny does not have an AAP, the asthma educator assists mom and Johnny in drafting an AAP based on his most recent medications. The nurse also discusses routine asthma follow-up every 3 months, as Johnny has moderate persistent asthma and his AAP needs to be reviewed to see whether it is controlling his asthma and whether any medications need to be changed. She also reviews early signs of asthma exacerbations and the importance of communicating with his clinic, when Johnny regularly needs his quick relief medicine more than two times a week during the day, more than two times a month at night, or when his yellow zone measures are not working to resolve an asthma attack quickly.

Asthma Devices

The nurse asks mom to bring out Johnny's medications and devices. Johnny does not have a spacer, nor does he or mom know how to use one. The nurse has brought a spacer device and demonstrates how to use it. She has Johnny do repeat demonstrations, making corrections and adjustments until he has performed the steps correctly.

Home Environmental Assessment

Johnny lives in an apartment in an older building with carpeting, no pets (though several close relatives have cats), and no mice or cockroaches; mother smokes "outside." Johnny does not have dust mite–proof bedding encasements, despite his dust mite allergy; the couch is leather, thus reducing the dust mite exposure from that common source. Bedding encasements are provided to the family, and additional information is provided about cleaning and laundering recommendations. Because the landlord refuses to remove the carpeting, the mother is also provided with information about a HEPA (high-efficiency particulate air) vacuum cleaner.

Environmental Tobacco Smoke

Mom actually smokes in the hallway right outside their apartment. She sprays an air freshener, when she comes back inside. Mom was encouraged to sign a "smoke-free pledge" and smoke completely outside both the apartment building and her car. She is also advised to avoid air fresheners that can be an airway irritant and trigger asthma symptoms. The nurse explains the negative effects that even cigarette smoke on her clothes may have on her son's asthma and advises mom to stop smoking. Although mom was not ready to quit, she did agree to smoke outside the building. The nurse gives mom some literature on smoking cessation and suggests they talk about it again at the next visit.

Discussion

The asthma nurse educator has given mom the time to express her concerns and then establish mutual goals for Johnny's asthma. The home visit allows the nurse to both provide comprehensive asthma education, tailored to Johnny's and his mother's particular needs, and assess and address home environmental triggers.

Case Study 23–2

Ambulatory Care

Ms. Carter is a 33-year-old stay-at-home mother who brings her three children to you for primary care. Her children are 3 months, 4 years old, and 6 years old (Kyle). Her children's father works the night shift. Her 3 month old is still not sleeping through the night and is breastfeeding. Her 4 year old is adjusting to her new baby brother and has some notable regression since the birth of the baby. Her 6 year old has just begun kindergarten and is doing well except that he has had multiple upper respiratory illness symptoms since the start of the school year. This has led to increased urgent-care visits and increased albuterol use in the past month. Mom is anxious because October is fast approaching, and historically, October has been particularly difficult for Kyle's asthma. Mom is quite nervous about being at home with the three children at night, as her next door neighbor was burglarized 2 months ago. The family obtained a dog recently for protection. During the past few visits, you have increased the dosage of Kyle's nebulized Budesonide. Despite this, Kyle has been on two courses of steroids, and by the looks of his symptoms today, he may need another course. Mom has many questions about the safety of Budesonide at each visit, in response to which you have given her written handouts on the way out of the clinic. Mom mentions that Kyle's teacher says Kyle is increasingly active and fidgety at school. Mom also reports that he has become increasingly rambunctious, and his father feels that all of the "medications are making him hyper." You again tell her that this is the necessary treatment and that his behavior is likely in response to the new baby and will resolve with time. Mom also reports that Kyle has a "constant runny nose." You attribute this to the multiple upper respiratory illnesses since the start of school. You reassure her that this will get better in the spring. Mom says that she has not yet filled the prescription for Budesonide. You assume that she has lost the prescription and give her another one for the third time. Kyle is stable enough to leave, and you give his mother a paper to make a follow-up appointment and tell her again that she is not helping her son get better by keeping the dog in the house. Mom goes to the desk to make an appointment but leaves without making it since her 4 year old is having a temper tantrum.

Why is this patient not doing well?

Discussion

In this case, the provider has not truly addressed the mother's concerns. Foremost, mom is clearly overwhelmed and has many other factors influencing her ability to care for Kyle's asthma. The provider seems rushed and only addresses Kyle's acute symptoms, when, in fact, an in-depth discussion about the goals of the family and the barriers that they face in controlling Kyle's asthma is needed. Although removing the dog might be ideal, it may not be realistic given mom's safety concerns. Providing empathy for her situation and offering alternatives, such as keeping the dog out of Kyle's room and having Kyle wash his hands after contact, might be more useful. A referral to an allergist for skin testing could provide objective information about Kyle's allergies.

Mom comes to the clinic worried about Kyle's frequent asthma attacks and fears, based on experience, that it may get even worse in the month of October. What history might suggest that Kyle's asthma attacks are due to seasonal allergies rather than frequent upper respiratory infections? The provider fails to assess for allergies, which may be a significant component of Kyle's asthma.

Mom clearly states that she has questions about the safety of inhaled steroids and has not yet filled the prescription the provider gave her at the previous visit. The provider misses the opportunity to explore mom's concerns and explain the role of controller versus rescue medications. Giving mom positive feedback about her observations of Kyle's asthma patterns and developing a common goal of controlling his asthma better this fall would be one way to approach the conversation about controller medications. Because mom also feels that all of the albuterol is making Kyle "hyper," the goal of greatly decreasing the amount of albuterol Kyle needs by using a low dose of daily controller medication may be one that mom is interested in trying.

An assessment is also needed to identify any other reasons that Kyle is not receiving his controller medication. Are there insurance issues with which a social worker might be able to assist? Is there another family member, possibly the father, who has conflicting health beliefs about using daily medication? (If so, that individual should be encouraged to come to a follow-up visit.) Would mom find an inhaled steroid delivered via an MDI with spacer quicker and more convenient than Budesonide, which needs to be given via nebulizer? What other kinds of supports can be put in place for mom?

(Continues)

Case Study 23–2 (*Continued*)

The provider could also request to contact the school nurse/teacher to discuss concerns both about Kyle's "hyperactivity" and his asthma. Setting up a separate follow-up visit in the next few weeks for a more thorough discussion about Kyle's behavioral issues may again help mom to feel that this is a collaborative relationship and that her concerns have been heard.

Of course, all of these issues may be difficult for the individual provider to cover during a busy clinic session. This family would benefit from a referral to an asthma nurse educator in the clinic or a home visitor, who would be able to take more time to address mom's concerns and provide a thorough, interactive teaching session. This additional person could also provide close follow-up of Kyle's progress and adherence to medications. This approach would likely be more effective for both a busy new mom and a busy provider.

This case study highlights the importance of communication, a partnership between patient/parent and provider, and regular follow-up visits in comprehensive asthma care. Provision of dedicated asthma visits at regular intervals is essential for the management of a chronic disease such as asthma, with routine visits generally on a seasonal basis because of the variability of this illness. The individual provider as well as the entire clinic system needs to develop creative and coordinated strategies to handle this family's needs, as well as the challenges of the providers' daily schedule.

WEB RESOURCES

Environmental Protection Agency
www.epa.gov/iaq/asthma
www.epa.gov/asthma/publications.html

American Lung Association
www.lungusa.org

Asthma and Allergy Foundation of America
www.aafa.org

Allergy and Asthma Network, Mothers of Asthmatics
www.breatherville.org

National Heart, Lung and Blood Institute Asthma Guidelines, 2007
www.nhlbi.nih.gov/guidelines/asthma

APPENDIX 23-1

ASTHMA BASICS

Definition

- Chronic (recurrent) inflammatory disorder of the airways
- 3 Mechanisms
  - Muscles tightening around airways
  - Increased inflammation in airways
  - Increased mucus production
- Swelling in the lungs makes it difficult for the air to get through
- Inflammation that may also make the air passages more sensitive to things that may trigger asthma

Asthma "Triggers"

- Allergies (pollen, dust, mold, mildew, animal dander, cockroach/rodent debris, and certain foods)
- Irritants (smoke, pollution, household/workplace chemicals, and perfume)
- Exercise
- Upper respiratory infections
- Cold air/changes in weather
- Excitement (crying and hard laughing)

Early Warning Signs

- First signs of a cold
- Cough
- Shortness of breath
- Tight chest
- Wheezing
- Fatigue
- Restlessness

When to Call for Help

- When breathing does not improve within 10 to 20 minutes of using inhaler
- When too short of breath to walk, talk, or play
- When skin is pulling in between ribs or above collarbone on inhalation

Medications

- Long-term "controller" medications
  - For persistent asthmatics
  - Taken daily
  - Reduces inflammation/swelling
- Quick relief "rescue" medications—albuterol
  - Provides prompt treatment
  - Relaxes muscles around airways
  - Does not decrease swelling
  - May be used before exercise or every 4 to 6 hours, as needed
  - Should always be used with a "spacer"

Rule of 2s

If you regularly

- Wake up at night due to asthma more than 2 times a month
- Use a quick-relief inhaler (puffer) more than 2 times a week
- Refill your quick-relief inhaler prescription more than 2 times a year

then your asthma is not well controlled!

APPENDIX 23-2

INHALED STEROIDS: FREQUENTLY ASKED QUESTIONS

Q: What are inhaled steroids, and how do they work?

A: In order to understand how inhaled steroids work, we need to review what asthma is.

People with asthma have airways that are more sensitive than normal to irritants or other "triggers," such as dust, colds, or pollen. This extra sensitivity leads to inflammation (redness and swelling) of the lining of the tiny airways deep in the lungs. The inflammation in turn causes extra mucus production and tightening of airway muscles that wind around the bronchial tubes like laces. Both the swelling inside and the muscle tightening around the airways make it very difficult for air to pass through, resulting in the common asthma symptoms of wheeze, cough, shortness of breath, and chest tightness (see **Figure 23-1**).

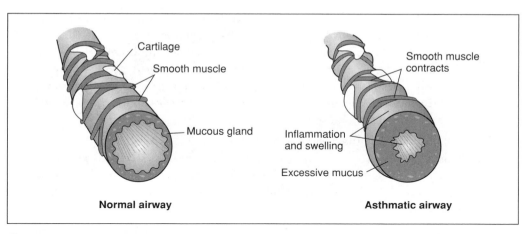

Figure 23-1

When you give your child albuterol by pump or nebulizer machine to relieve his or her symptoms, you are only treating the muscle tightening around the outside of the airway. These medicines, often called "quick-relief medications," do not help the inflammation on the inside of the airway that caused the muscles to tighten up in the first place.

That is where a group of medicines called corticosteroids comes in. These medicines work to reduce the swelling, both opening up the airway and making the airways less sensitive or "twitchy" when they come in contact with other triggers. These are often called "controller medications" and need to be taken every day in order to be effective.

Q: Are these the same as the steroids ("roids") that athletes and body-builders use to build up muscle?

A: No! Corticosteroids are a completely different kind of steroid from the anabolic steroids that some athletes misuse. Unfortunately, they're both called "steroids" for short. Corticosteroids do not build muscle nor do they have the dangerous side effects of anabolic steroids.

Q: Will inhaled steroids stunt my child's growth or cause him or her to gain weight? What are the side effects?

A: Many of the side effects that parents have heard about with long-term steroid use have to do with long-term use of the much higher doses of oral steroids, such as prednisone (Orapred), that are used for severe asthma attacks or occasionally for severe asthma, when even high doses of inhaled steroids do not work well enough. Studies of large numbers of children have found that even children who have been taking inhaled steroids for years reach their full, expected adult height, although possibly at a slightly slower pace during the first year of use. Likewise, weight gain is only a problem with long-term use of oral steroids.

In comparison, the dose your child receives using a steroid inhaler every day is a tiny dose, as it is going directly to the airways where it is needed to decrease inflammation. This is similar to using a steroid cream for eczema. In fact, one 5-day course of oral steroids is equal to over a year of inhaled steroids!

Inhaled steroids can occasionally cause "thrush," a minor fungal infection of the mouth, or hoarseness. The risk of these symptoms can be reduced by using a spacer and having your child either rinse his or her mouth out or brush his or her teeth after using the inhaled steroid.

Q: Are inhaled steroids addictive?

A: No. Like other chronic (long-term) illnesses—for example, high blood pressure—asthma generally needs to be treated with daily medication in order to prevent symptoms or worsening of the disease. This does not mean the medications are addictive, only that the medicine is needed to control the illness. On the other hand, we do worry about overuse of albuterol as a substitute for good asthma control, as this overuse can cause albuterol to stop working well.

Q: I do not feel comfortable giving my child inhaled steroids every day. My child is fine now. Can I stop them?

A: When your child's asthma is under control talk to your healthcare provider about adjusting the dose of your child's medications to the lowest dose that will control his or her asthma symptoms. You and your child's provider can figure out together what dose of inhaled steroid is going to keep your child healthy and active. Do not stop giving the daily controller (preventive) medications on your own! It is very possible that your child feels fine because of the inhaled steroids. If you stop them, the airway swelling will most likely return, and your child may end up in the emergency room with a bad asthma attack.

Meanwhile, the benefits of daily controller medications are tremendous. Your child will be able to run and play, attend school without a lot of sick days, and sleep through the night!

Developed by the Children's Hospital Boston Community Asthma Initiative, used with permission.

REFERENCES

Akinbami, L. (2006). *Asthma prevalence, health care use and mortality: United States, 2003–05.* Health E Stats, National Center for Health Statistics, Centers for Disease Control and Prevention. Retrieved September 9, 2007, from www.cdc.gov/nchs/products/pubs/pubd/hestats/ashtma03-05/asthma03-05.htm.

Allen, D. B. (2006). Effects of inhaled steroids on growth, bone metabolism, and adrenal function. *Advances in Pediatrics, 53,* 101–110.

American Lung Association. (2006). *Health disparities in lung disease 2006.* Retrieved June 21, 2007, from www.lungusa.org.

Banasiak, N., & Meadows-Oliver, M. (2004). Inpatient asthma clinical pathways for the pediatric patient: an integrative review of the literature. *Pediatric Nursing, 30*(6), 447–450.

Bentley, J. M., Ludlow, T., Meier, K., & Baydala, L. (2005). A community-based approach to pediatric asthma education. *Canadian Journal of Respiratory Therapy 41*(5), 24–29

Boulet, L. P. (1998). Perception of the role and potential side effects of inhaled corticosteroids among asthmatic patients. *Chest, 113,* 587–592.

Brown, R., Bratton, S. L., Cabana, M. D., Kaciroti, N., & Clark, N. M. (2004). Physician asthma education program improves outcomes for children of low-income families. *Chest, 126,* 369–374.

Bryant-Stephens, T., & Li, Y. (2004). Community asthma education program for parents of urban asthmatic children. *Journal of the National Medical Association, 94*(7), 954–960.

Buckner, E. B., Hawkins, A. M., Stover, L., Brakefield, J., Simmons, S., Foster, C., Payne, S., Newsome, J., & Dubois, G. (2005). Knowledge, resilience, and effectiveness of education in a young teen asthma camp. *Pediatric Nursing, 31*(3), 201–210.

Burkhart, P., Rayens, M. K., & Bowman, R. K. (2004). An evaluation of children's metered-dose inhaler technique for asthma medications. *Nursing Clinics of North America, 40,* 167–182.

Butz, A. M., Syron, L., Johnson, B., Spaulding, J., Walker, M., & Bollinger, M. E. (2005). Home-based asthma self-management education for inner-city children. *Public Health Nursing, 22*(3), 189–199.

Cabana, M. D., Slish, K. K., Brown, R., & Clark, N. M. (2004). Pediatrician attitudes and practice regarding collaborative asthma education. *Clinical Pediatrics, 43,* 269–274.

Clark, N. M., Brown, R., Joseph, C. L. M., Anderson, E. W., Liu, M., & Valerio, M. A. (2004). Effects of a comprehensive school-based asthma program on symptoms, parent management, grades, and absenteeism. *Chest, 125,* 1674–1679.

Conn, K. M., Halterman, J. S., Fisher, S. G., Yoos, H. L., Chin, N. P., & Szilagyi, P. G. (2005). Parental beliefs about medications and medication adherence among urban children with asthma. *Ambulatory Pediatrics, 5*(5), 306–310.

DeWalt, D. A., Dilling, M. H., Rosenthal, M. S., & Pignone, M. P. (2007). Low parental literacy is associated with worse asthma care measures in children. *Ambulatory Pediatrics, 7*(1), 25–31.

Ebbinghaus, S., & Bahrainwala, A. (2003). Asthma management by an inpatient asthma care team. *Pediatric Nursing, 29*(3), 177–183.

Farber, H. J., Capra, A. M., Finkelstein, J. A., Lozano, P., Quesenberry, C. P., Jensvold, N. G., Chi, F. W., & Lieu, T. A. (2003). Misunderstanding of asthma controller medications: association with nonadherence. *The Journal of Asthma, 40*(1), 17–25.

Halm, E. A., Wisnivesky, J. P., & Leventhal, H. (2005). Quality and access to care among a cohort of inner-city adults with asthma: who gets guideline concordant care? *Chest, 128*(4), 1943–1950.

Halm, E. A., Mora, P., & Leventhal, H. (2006). No symptoms, no asthma: The acute episodic disease belief is associated with poor self-management among inner-city adults with persistent asthma. *Chest, 129*(3), 573–580.

Halterman, J. S., Yoos, H. L., Kaczorowski, J. M., McConnochie, K., Holzhauer, R. J., Conn, K. M., Lauver, S., & Szilagy, P. G. (2002). Providers underestimate symptom severity among urban children with asthma. *Archives of Pediatric and Adolescent Medicine, 156,* 141–146.

Joseph, C. L. (2007). Asthma in adolescents research team: A web-based, tailored asthma management program for urban African-American high school students. *American Journal of Respiratory Critical Care Medicine, 175*(9), 888–895.

Kamps, A. W. A., Brand, P. L. P., & Roorda, R. J. (2002). Determinants of correct inhalation technique in children attending a hospital-based asthma clinic. *Acta Pediatrica, 91,* 159–163.

Krieger, J. W., Takaro, T. K., Song, L., & Weaver, M. (2005). The Seattle-King County healthy homes project: A randomized, controlled trial of a community health worker intervention to decrease exposure to indoor asthma triggers. *American Journal of Public Health, 95*(4), 652–659.

Krishna, S., Balas, E. A., Francisco, B. D., & Konig, P. (2006). Effective and sustainable multimedia education for children with asthma: A randomized controlled trial. *Children's Health Care, 35*(1), 75–90.

Kritikos, V., Armour, C. L., & Bosnic-Anticevich, S. Z. (2007). Interactive small-group asthma education in the community pharmacy setting: a pilot study. *Journal of Asthma, 44*(1), 57–64.

La Roche, M. J., Koinis-Mitchell, D., & Gualdron, L. (2006). A culturally competent asthma management intervention: A randomized controlled pilot study. *Annals of Allergy, Asthma and Immunology, 98,* 80–85.

Levy, J. I., Brugge, D., Peters, J., Clougherty, S., & Saddler, S. S. (2006). A community-based participatory research study of multifaceted in-home environmental interventions for pediatric asthmatics in public housing. *Social Science and Medicine, 63,* 2191–2203.

Liu, C., & Feekery, C. (2001). Can asthma education improve clinical outcomes? An evaluation of a pediatric asthma education program. *Journal of Asthma, 38*(3), 269–278.

Mancuso, C. A., & Rincon, M. (2006). Impact of health literacy on longitudinal asthma outcomes. *Journal of General Internal Medicine, 21*(8), 813–817.

McGhan, S. L., MacDonald, C., James, D. E., Naidu, P., Wong, E., Sharpe, H., Hessel, P. A., & Befus, A. D. (2006). Factors associated with poor asthma control in children aged 5 to 13 years. *Canadian Respiratory Journal, 13*(1), 23–29.

McMullen, A., Yoos, H. L., Anson, E., Kitzmann, H., Halterman, J. S., & Arcoleo, K. S. (2007). Asthma care of children in clinical practice: do parents report receiving appropriate education? *Pediatric Nursing, 33*(1), 37–44.

Morgan, W. J., Crain, E. F., Gruchalla, R. S., O'Connor, G. T., Kattan, M., Evans, R., Stout, J., Malindzak, G., Smartt, E., Plaut, M., Walter, M., Vaughn, B., & Mitchell, H. (2004). Results of a home-based environmental intervention among urban children with asthma. *New England Journal of Medicine, 351*(11), 1068–1680.

National Heart, Lung, and Blood Institute. (1997). *National Asthma Education and Prevention Program Expert Panel Report 2: guidelines for the diagnosis and management of asthma.* NIH Publication No. 97-4051. Bethesda, MD: U.S. Department of Health and Human Services; National Institutes of Health.

National Heart, Lung, and Blood Institute. (2007). *National Asthma Education and Prevention Program Expert Panel Report 3: guidelines for the diagnosis and management of asthma.* NIH Publication No. 08-4051 (prepublication copy). Bethesda, MD: U.S. Department of Health and Human Services; National Institutes of Health.

Nicholas, S. W., Hutchinson, V. E., Ortiz, B., Klihr-Beall, S., Jean-Louis, B., Shoemaker, K., Singleton, C., Kredell, J., Swaner, R., Vaughn, R. D., Northridge, M. E., Cushman, L. F., Polley, E. & Golembeski, C. (2005). Reducing childhood asthma through community-based service delivery—New York City, 2001–2004. *MMWR, 54*(1), 11–13.

Noble, M. J., Smith, J. R., & Windley, J. (2006). A controlled retrospective pilot study of an "at-risk asthma register" in primary care. *Primary Care Respiratory Journal, 15,* 116–124.

Osman, L. M., Calder, C., Godden, D. J., Friend, J. A. R., McKenzie, L., Legge, J. S., & Douglas, J. G. (2002). A randomized trial of self-management planning for adult patients admitted to hospital with acute asthma. *Thorax, 57,* 869–874.

Osman, L., & Calder, C. (2004). Implementing asthma education programmes in paediatric respiratory care: settings, timing, people and evaluation. *Paediatric Respiratory Reviews, 5*(2), 140–146.

Peterson-Sweeney, K., McMullen, A., Yoos, H. L., & Kitzmann, H. (2003). Parental perceptions of their child's asthma: management and medication use. *Journal of Pediatric Health Care, 17,* 118–125.

Peterson-Sweeney, K., McMullen, A., Yoos, H. L., Kitzmann, H., Halterman, J. S., Arcoleo, K. S., & Anson, E. (2007). Impact of asthma education received from health care providers on parental illness representation in childhood asthma. *Research in Nursing and Health, 30,* 203–212.

Porter, S. C., Cai, Z., Gribbons, W., Goldmann, D., & Kohane, I. S. (2004). The asthma kiosk: a patient-centered technology for collaborative decision support in the emergency department. *Journal of the American Medical Informatics Association, 11*(6), 458–467.

Primomo, J., Johnston, S., DiBiase, F., Nodolf, J., & Noren, L. (2006). Evaluation of a community-based outreach worker program for children with asthma. *Public Health Nursing, 23*(3), 234–241.

Schatz, M., Sorkness, C. A., Li, J. T., Marcus, P., Murray, J. J., Nathan, R. A., Kosinski, M., Pendergraft, T. B., & Jhingran, P. (2006). Asthma control test: reliability, validity, and responsiveness in patients not previously followed by asthma specialists. *Journal of Allergy and Clinical Immunology, 117*(3), 549–556.

Self, T., Chrisman, C. R., Mason, D. L., & Rumbak, M. J. (2005). Reducing emergency department visits and hospitalizations in African American and Hispanic patients with asthma: a 15-year review. *Journal of Asthma, 42,* 807–812.

Sockrider, M. M., Abramson, S., Brooks, E., Caviness, A. C., Pilney, S., Koerner, C., & Macias, C. G. (2006). Delivering tailored asthma family education in a pediatric emergency department setting: a pilot study. *Pediatrics, 117,* S135–S144.

Thompson, D. A., Lozano, P., & Christakis, D. A. (2007). Parent use of touchscreen computer kiosks for child health promotion in community settings. *Pediatrics, 119,* 427–434.

U.S. Department of Health and Human Services. (2000, November). *With understanding and improving health and objectives for improving health* (2nd ed.). 2 vols. *Healthy People 2010.* Washington, DC: U.S. Government Printing Office.

Walders, N., Kercsmar, C., Schluchter, M., Redline, S., Dirchner, H. L., Drotar, D. (2006). An interdisciplinary intervention for undertreated pediatric asthma. *Chest, 129,* 292–299.

Williams, M. V., Baker, D. W., Honig, E. G., Lee, T. M., & Nowlan, A. (1998). Inadequate literacy is a barrier to asthma knowledge and self-care. *Chest, 114,* 1008–1015.

Winickoff, J. P., Berkowitz, A. B., Brooks, K., Tanski, S. E., Geller, A., Thomson, C., Lando, H. A., Curry, S., Muramoto, M., Prokhorov, A. V., Best, D., Weitzman, M., & Robert, L. (2004). State-of-the-art interventions for office-based parental tobacco control. *Pediatrics, 115,* 750–760.

Yoos, H. L., Kitzman, H., & McMullen, A. (2003). Barriers to anti-inflammatory medication use in childhood asthma. *Ambulatory Pediatrics, 3(*4), 181–190.

Chapter 24

Diabetes in Adults and Children

Barbara B. Chase

INTRODUCTION

Diabetes mellitus type 1 and type 2 are both complex, multisystem diseases that require ongoing self-management by patients and families in collaboration with their healthcare providers. An understanding of the disease process, the necessary patient self-management skills, and the process of behavior change through personal empowerment are all imperative to the diabetes educator's success in working with patients. This chapter gives an overview of these essential topics, gives some concrete suggestions for teaching strategies, and uses case studies as examples. An extensive list of resources is offered for readers who desire more detailed information.

Diabetes is a disease that is characterized by hyperglycemia caused by insulin deficiency. In type 1 diabetes, autoimmune destruction of the pancreatic beta cells occurs relatively quickly and completely, leaving the patient, usually a child or adolescent, in need of exogenous insulin to survive. Treatment consists of multiple daily doses of insulin, as near physiologic as possible, adjusted to be in balance with the patient's physical activity and food intake. Type 1 diabetes occurs in only 0.5% of the population, and only 5% to 10% of the total number of patients with diabetes have type 1

(National Institute of Diabetes and Digestive and Kidney Diseases, 2007), but its early onset and lifelong course, along with the potential for acute and chronic consequences, profoundly affect the lives of individuals with this diagnosis.

Although type 2 diabetes is being seen with increasing frequency in overweight children, it is usually a disease of adults. Type 2 diabetes is characterized by insulin resistance, often related to elevated body mass index, which leads to excessive demand on the pancreas to produce insulin. Over time, beta-cell function decreases, and progressive hyperglycemia is the result. Characteristic of this disease is endothelial dysfunction, which causes insulin resistance as well as hypertension, hyperlipidemia, and beta-cell insufficiency. Treatment of type 2 diabetes starts with diet modifications to control and evenly distribute calories throughout the day and regular exercise to decrease insulin resistance and manage weight. If metabolic control is not achieved with these measures, various oral medications to reduce hepatic glucose output, improve insulin production, or increase insulin sensitivity are added to the treatment plan. If one or two oral medications are insufficient to produce control, insulin injections to replace endogenous insulin are added to the program.

In both type 1 and type 2 diabetes, vigorous management of blood pressure to 130/80 or less, control of lipids to low-density lipoprotein levels of 100 or less, and the addition of once-daily aspirin have been shown to decrease cardiovascular risk and should be considered as part of the overall treatment plan. Also, the patient's level of microalbuminuria must be measured, and if elevated, an angiotensin-converting enzyme inhibitor or angiotensin 2 receptor blocker should be added to the medication program for renal protection if the blood pressure is adequate to tolerate the medication's hypotensive effect. Care for all individuals with diabetes must include special attention to eye care in order to prevent, detect, and treat retinopathy; podiatric care to detect neuropathy and prevent infections and ulcers; and careful routine healthcare maintenance, including dental care and immunizations.

After steady increases in the past century, the incidence and prevalence of type 2 diabetes have skyrocketed worldwide in the past 20 years. As of 2005, 20.8 million Americans (7% of the U.S. population) had been estimated to have all types of diabetes, with 30% of those unaware of their diagnosis (National Institute of Diabetes and Digestive and Kidney Diseases, 2007). According to the American Diabetes Association (ADA), 18.3% or 8.6 million people over the age of 60 have been diagnosed with the disease

(Mensing, 2006). Both type 1 and type 2 diabetes carry the risk of acute complications brought on by hyperglycemia and hypoglycemia and of the chronic complications of microvascular disease (retinopathy, nephropathy, and neuropathy) and macrovascular disease (heart attack and stroke), making them a significant public health problem. Unfortunately, only about 10% of people diagnosed with diabetes have participated in formal diabetes education programs (Mensing, 2006).

The challenge for health professionals in working with patients with diabetes is not only to impart complicated information and multiple skills, but also to foster a climate of empowerment in which patients will come to understand that it is appropriate for them to be responsible for diabetes self-management on a day-to-day basis (Anderson & Funnell, 2005; Mensing, 2006; Funnell & Lasichak, 2004). As such, this chapter addresses not only the content areas for education and skills development but also discusses strategies for attitude and behavior change to optimize life with diabetes.

CONTENT AREAS OF PATIENT EDUCATION

The recent epidemic level of diabetes in the United States has prompted many healthcare organizations to develop formal diabetes education programs. The ADA requires that 10 content areas of diabetes education be covered in the diabetes self-management education (DSME) programs they consider for their Education Program Recognition (Funnell & Lasichak, 2004). In order to be reimbursed by Medicare, DSME programs, which cover up to 10 hours of education in the initial education year and 2 hours per year thereafter, must be ADA recognized; therefore, most DSME group or one-to-one programs are designed to meet this standard, with additions or customization of the program as needed.

Many healthcare professionals may become involved with the education of patients with diabetes, and some role groups such as registered nurses, registered dietitians, licensed social workers, psychologists, or exercise physiologists may be eligible to qualify for the Certified Diabetes Educator credential. This credential must be held by at least one member of any ADA-recognized DSME program.

Although the 10 ADA-recommended content areas that should be addressed with each patient, or in the case of young children, with responsible family members, they may be addressed in any order or in any creative format that is appropriate to the situation. As in any patient teaching situation, an assessment of the patient or family's readiness to learn, previous knowledge, learning style, developmental stage, barriers to learning, and time available are among the issues to be considered. The content areas are described later here.

Topic I: What Is Diabetes?

The contents of this section should start with a definition of diabetes mellitus as a disorder caused by lack of insulin, a hormone produced by the pancreas, a small organ behind the stomach. In type 1 diabetes, more common in children and young adults, no insulin can be produced, and insulin is always needed to sustain life, so exogenous insulin is always needed. In contrast, type 2 diabetes, more common in adults, often presents with a partial and gradual decrease in insulin production, allowing phased-in treatment with diet, exercise, oral medications and insulin. Diabetes is treatable, but not curable at this time. Risk factors for type 1 diabetes include heredity, formation of antibodies against one's own cells, and certain viral infections. Predisposing factors for type 2 diabetes include heredity, overweight, age, ethnicity, and stressors such as pregnancy, surgery, infections, and steroid medications.

The educator should explain to patients and families that when individuals eat the food is broken down into glucose, which then passes from the stomach and small intestine to the bloodstream, where it is distributed to the body's cells to be used inside the cells to create energy. Normally, when glucose enters the blood after a meal, the rise in blood glucose causes the pancreas to release insulin. This is important because insulin is needed for the glucose to enter the cells. Insulin acts as a key to open the cells for the glucose to enter. Because glucose is allowed into the cells, glucose in the blood stays in the normal range, from 70 to 100 mg/dL. When people have diabetes, a lack of insulin prevents the glucose from entering the cells, and thus, it remains in the blood stream, where it is referred to as high blood glucose, high blood sugar, or hyperglycemia. During the time that these patients' cells cannot get fuel (in the form of glucose) to come inside to produce energy, the kidneys try to eliminate the elevated sugar levels in the blood by producing extra urine. Eventually, this polyuria leads to dehydration, which causes increased thirst or polydipsia, and because the cells are starving for fuel, a sensation of increased hunger or polyphagia occurs. Unfortunately, at the same time, these people are losing calories in the urine, losing weight, and feeling fatigued.

All of these symptoms are the classic symptoms of diabetes. The diagnosis is usually made with a simple blood test showing the random blood glucose equal to or greater than 200 mg/dL with some of the above symptoms or the fasting blood glucose equal to or greater than 126 mg/dL on two separate occasions. A blood test patients have with regularity to measure the level of metabolic control is called the hemoglobin A1C. This test measures the amount of glucose red blood cells are exposed to over time and is usually elevated at the time diabetes is detected. The goal for patients with diabetes is to keep the hemoglobin A1C as close to normal as possible but no more than 7%.

The educator should introduce the concept of self-management early and frequently in the education process, emphasizing that this knowledge will be used on a daily basis to make choices and decisions that will affect both short- and long-term health. Brief explanations of treatment with the goals of balancing diet and exercise with basal and bolus insulin should be introduced if the patient has type 1 diabetes. If the patient has type 2 diabetes, the phased-in approach to treatment should be introduced, starting with balanced distribution of food throughout the day, with calorie, carbohydrate, or fat modifications if indicated, and adding planned daily exercise. Then as needed, add oral medications in a step fashion and/or insulin.

Topic II: How Can I Learn to Live with Diabetes?

This topic addresses the patient and family's psychosocial adjustment to living with a chronic disease. Patients need recognition that what they are going through is not easy. Points of discussion should concentrate on diabetes as a chronic illness, which will surely affect the person's lifestyle and self-perception. It is essential that patients recognize the personal meaning diabetes has for them and that they become aware of their feelings about having diabetes such as denial, anger, or depression, which are common and can become barriers to optimal self-care. The importance of developing coping skills to process these feelings is emphasized and, by definition, must be very individualized. Depression screening should be done, as depression is very common among patients with diabetes, and referral to and consultation with mental health providers are often indicated. Furthermore, educators must help individuals explore their support systems and assist them to create the kind of encouragement; assistance, care, and backup that they need to initially cope with a new diagnosis and later will need in an ongoing way to adapt to their new life demands (Mensing, 2006; Anderson & Funnell, 2005). Topics from this section should be brought into the discussion repeatedly as other topics are discussed, and family members or friends should be included in the conversation whenever possible. Often feelings about having a chronic disease surface long after the diagnosis is made; thus, the process of adaptation may be ongoing throughout the patient's life.

Topic III: What Do I Need to Know About Food?

Nutrition education must speak to the role of diet in diabetes self-management, a complicated and emotional topic. Family members must be included in this segment of the educational process if they are to become knowledgeable and supportive about the patient's nutrition goals. Patients and their families must be taught the reasons for meal planning in general and also specifically in relationship to the other components of their treatment plan such as medication and exercise. Emphasis must be placed on the importance of meal timing, portion size, and balancing fats, proteins, and carbohydrates each time patients eat. In order to accomplish this goal, patients must learn the fat, protein, and carbohydrate content of foods, as well as the classification of foods into groups, such as meat, dairy, grains/starchy vegetables, vegetables, fruits, and fats. Particular attention should be paid to how various types of foods affect blood sugar in general, with an emphasis placed on how individual patients can determine through home blood glucose testing, the specific effect particular foods or portions have on them personally. Meal planning skills like the plate method of measuring portions, the use of carbohydrate counting, especially if the patient requires insulin, and the importance of label reading should all be taught. Patients and families should also be taught skills and gain some proficiency in planned shopping, cooking at home, eating in restaurants, eating on social occasions, and using alcohol as it applies to them (Funnell & Lasichak, 2004). Referral to a registered dietitian to develop a specific, customized nutrition plan is optimal for all patients, as some need emphasis on weight reduction, whereas others need to learn carbohydrate counting or to pay special attention to lipid management or sodium restriction. These visits often need to be ongoing as patients and their families make changes and adjustments in their dietary habits. When working with patients and families, educators must explore and reflect with them on the psychologic significance food has for them. In doing this, patients will become more aware of their own emotional needs surrounding food, which can help them to make informed choices based on their personal goals.

Topic IV: What Do I Need to Know About Physical Activity and Exercise?

In this part of the education program, patients are encouraged to appreciate the beneficial role physical activity plays in lowering blood pressure and cholesterol, relieving tension and stress, improving cardiovascular function, as well as its effect on lowering blood sugar and burning calories. In discussing this topic, patients are encouraged to examine their preferences and choose a program that will best fit their personal needs while at the same time meet the targets of what has been medically recommended for them. Patients should include stretching, aerobic, and resistive training activity in their programs. The effect that exercise has on glucose metabolism and the precautions, self-monitoring, and self-treatment activities necessary to exercise safely are discussed in detail and include carrying identification and a carbohydrate source, choosing appropriate clothing and footwear, testing pre-exercise and postexercise blood glucose, adjusting food intake, monitoring of heart rate, perceived exertion, and fluid requirements, and adjusting oral medication timing and insulin dosing. Emphasis is placed on helping patients to choose a combination of physical activities that they can incorporate into their lifestyles over a lifetime. Although some physical activities may be related to sports or recreation, others may be modifications in daily transportation arrangements or household chore activities. Like dietary adaptations, physical lifestyle changes must be made by the patient using accurate information to make informed decisions and then employing the use of self-management strategies to achieve long-term change.

Topic V: How Are Oral Medications Used to Treat Diabetes?

This section of the education sequence for patients is not appropriate for patients with type 1 diabetes and can be brief if type 2 patients are not yet on medication. It should be more detailed when one or more oral medications are needed to achieve metabolic control. Patients should understand that oral medications are not insulin, but all act to lower blood glucose levels in several different ways. They should understand that the oral medications work together with their meal and exercise plans and that one, two, or sometimes three classes of medications are used together to manage blood glucose levels when the pancreas is still able to produce some insulin. Patients should be reminded that even with good blood glucose control, eventually the pancreas will not be able to produce insulin, and the patient will need to transition to insulin use.

Five classes of oral medication are commonly used, the first three with the most frequency:

Biguanides—for example, metformin (Glucophage)—is often started as a first oral drug, especially in overweight patients with mildly elevated glucose levels. This improves fasting glucose, inhibits the release of glucose from the liver and improves uptake of glucose in other parts of the body, and does not cause weight gain or hypoglycemia if used alone. It can cause gastrointestinal side effects that are lessened over time and when taken with a meal. It is available in the long-acting form and is not to be used if patient has liver, kidney, or heart failure or in those over 80 years old. Patients need to be counseled about lactic acidosis, use of contrast material and alcohol, and avoidance of over-the-counter cimetidine use.

Sulfonylureas—for example, glipizide (Glucotrol) or glimepiride (Amaryl)—are often used in combination with other oral medications. They improve premeal blood glucose levels, stimulate the pancreatic beta cells to increase production of insulin, and can cause weight gain and hypoglycemia; they are available in long-acting forms.

Thiazolidinediones (TZDs)—for example, rosiglitazone (Avandia) or pioglitazone (Actos)—are often used in combination with other oral medications. They reduce insulin resistance, inhibit the release of glucose from liver and improve uptake in other parts of the body, do not cause hypoglycemia when used alone, must not be used if patient has liver or heart disease, and may cause edema. Recent reports have suggested a possible relationship between rosiglitazone and increased cardiac events. Although the results are open to interpretation and the drug has not been removed from the market, it is being used with caution at this time.

Meglitinides—for example, repaglinide (Prandin) or nateglinide (Starlix)—are used alone or with other oral medications but not with alpha-glucosidase inhibitors. They improve postmeal blood sugar elevations, cause pancreatic beta cells to release insulin, should be taken only up to 30 minutes before meal because they are fast acting, and can cause hypoglycemia; thus, patients should not take them if the meal is omitted.

Alpha-glucosidase inhibitors—for example, acarbose (Precose) or miglitol (Glyset)—are used with other oral agents except the TZDs or with insulin, although not with the rapid-acting analogues. They blunt the rise in post meal blood sugars; slow carbohydrate absorption; do not cause hypoglycemia if taken alone. They should be taken with start of a meal and can cause bloating, gas, and diarrhea.

DPP-4 inhibitors are a relative new class of medication. Sitagliptin, marketed as Januvia, helps the body's own ability to manage glucose levels by increasing the active levels of hormones called incretins in the body by blocking an enzyme called DPP. It may be used with other oral diabetes medication; it improves fasting and postprandial glucose and does not cause hypoglycemia. This medication is taken once daily and has few side effects. In the United States, the popularity of this medication has been diminished by the high cost, which has been largely not covered by insurance plans.

Specific patient instructions about oral medication should include the drug's generic and trade names, usual doses, mode of action, how and when they should be taken, possible side effects, care and storage, and when to hold or call their provider for dosing advice (Funnell & Lasichak, 2004).

Topic VI: When Does a Patient Need Insulin?

Insulin is the subject that most patients least want to discuss. Many are fearful of the injections and have concerns about what starting insulin means about their health. The educator should begin by reviewing that insulin is a protein produced by the pancreas. It attaches itself to the body's cells, allowing glucose to go inside where it is changed into energy for that cell. Patients always need exogenous insulin injections if they have type 1 diabetes because they no longer produce any of their own insulin. Patients with type 2 diabetes need insulin when the beta cells of the pancreas no longer respond to oral medications and diabetes control can no longer be achieved with oral medications alone. The ultimate goal of insulin therapy in type 1 diabetes is to approximate the functioning of normal pancreas, and in type 2 diabetes, it is often used with oral medications to keep the blood glucose as close to normal as possible. With the recent development of nonpeaking basal insulin and rapid-acting analog insulin, along with the development of technology, which would allow continuous glucose monitors to communicate with insulin pumps, we are coming ever closer to achieving the goal of an artificial pancreas. Nevertheless, most patients will not have access to this level of technology in the near future and will need to learn to give themselves insulin injections.

To best manage their diabetes, patients who self-administer insulin must understand not only how to administer it but also what kind of insulin has been prescribed for them and how it works. They should know that exogenous insulin is made in the laboratory using recombinant DNA technology so that it is very pure. Most patients use U-100 insulin, which means that 1 cc (cubic centimeter) of insulin contains 100 units of insulin and comes in 10 cc bottles or 3 cc cartridges or pens. As long as the temperature is less than 86°F, the insulin bottle or pen being currently used can be kept about a month at room temperature, which is the best temperature for injection. Extra bottles or pens should be kept in the refrigerator but not frozen and should be carried on, not checked with luggage, when traveling. Patients should always check the label for the expiration date and the bottle or pen contents to make sure that it has not changed in color or appearance.

Patients should know that all insulin is classified by its onset and duration of action. Like the oral medications, they have both generic and trade names, and new products are being released with increasing frequency. The rapid-acting insulins are lispro (Humalog), aspart (Novolog), and glulisine (Apidra). They are given at meal times and act so quickly that some patients eat before giving their injection to make sure that the insulin does not start working before their meal begins to be absorbed and to be able to count the carbohydrates they have just ingested in order to calculate the appropriate number of units needed to cover the meal. These insulins' peak action is in about 1 hour and lasts 2 to 4 hours. Short-acting or regular insulin, with an onset in 30 to 60 minutes, peaks in 2 to 5 hours, and the duration is from 6 to 16 hours; it is used with decreasing frequency because the newer insulins more closely resemble the physiologic response of the pancreas to rising blood sugar. Intermediate-acting insulin, such as NPH, can take from 1 to over 2 hours to begin to act, peak several hours after that, and then continually diminish in strength ending at 22 to 24 hours. NPH is given alone or mixed with rapid or short-acting insulin once or twice a day. Long-acting insulin like Ultralente is no longer used in the United States now that non-peaking, long-acting basal insulins like glargine (Lantus) and detemir (Levemir) have become available. These newer insulins do not peak, and thus, they are used as background insulin, usually once but sometimes twice in 24 hours. Either bolus insulin, using a rapid-acting form or oral medications, is used with them to cover meal time blood sugar elevations. Another way to cover meal times is to give an insulin mixture containing 50% to 75% intermediate acting insulin and 25% to 50% rapid or short-acting insulin, which comes already mixed in the bottle in one of those proportions.

To administer insulin, patients will use either syringes or pen devices. After use, these items can be disposed of in a plastic or metal container with a screw cap and placed in the regular trash. When giving insulin, patients should know what their blood sugar is and what their meal exercise plans will be. They must be taught the importance of timing, hand washing, choice and preparation of injection site on abdomen, thigh, or upper arm, preparation of the correct dose of insulin, use of the specific device, and injection technique. The intensity of blood glucose testing and insulin administration varies depending on the type of diabetes the patient has, their lifestyle, personal goals, and preferences; however, the goal is always to replace the work of the pancreas by providing basal and sometimes bolus patterns which maintain target blood glucose levels.

Although not insulin, a new injectable medication exenatide, marketed as Byetta, has become available. It is given within the hour before the two largest meals of the day using a prefilled disposable pen. It is administered and stored the same as an insulin pen. Exenatide works by slowing the emptying of the stomach and therefore the processing of digestion and the elevation of postmeal blood glucose. Exenatide can be used with metformin, sulfonylureas, or TZDs to help manage postprandial blood glucose. If given with sulfonylureas, it can cause low blood glucose, necessitating a decrease in the sulfonylurea dose. Exenatide's major side effects are nausea, vomiting, and bloating, all of which decrease with the use of the medication. Because of nausea and decreased appetite, exenatide may lead to weight loss. Patients with renal failure or severe gastroparesis should not use exenatide.

Topic VII: Why Do I Have to Test My Own Blood Glucose?

Self-monitoring of blood glucose (SMBG) is an important tool that patients use to determine how meal timing, particular foods or portions, exercise, stress, and medication all affect the blood glucose; therefore, it is important that educators emphasize not only the technical procedure, but also the meaning of results and the benefits of regular testing. Many monitors are available to patients and should be chosen based on their usability, cost, and preferred features like memory, computer download ability, or need for coding. The process of SMBG should be taught early in the education sequence and includes hand washing, the use of lancet devices, the rotation and use of lateral fingers, coding and quality testing the monitor, trouble shooting and the use of toll-free numbers, the use of monitor memory, and manual recording of results or downloading the monitor memory to better recognize trends.

Patients should understand that glucose levels change throughout the day and night. The frequency and timing of SMBG depend on the intensity of treatment with insulin or oral medications, degree of exercise, timing of meals, congruity of SMBG with A1C testing, and personal tolerance for testing. Some patients test up to eight times a day, checking fasting and premeal and postmeal results, as well as pre-exercise and postexercise and bedtime readings. Others check but once a day, sometimes checking a fasting glucose, but on other days, they may choose one of the other times to test. Patients should set individual goals for testing frequency and SMBG results with their healthcare team based on their treatment plan; however, for many patients, fasting and premeal finger stick results should be in the 90- to 130-mg/dL range, and 2-hour postmeal results should be less than 180 mg/dL (Funnell & Lasichak, 2004). When results are outside of these ranges, patients should reflect on what variables might have been responsible, such as skipping a meal, eating too much at one time, or eating too much of a certain food; increased or decreased exercise; omitting medicines or taking the wrong dose; illness or stress; or monitor error.

SMBG gives patients information that allows them to make informed decisions about their own care. They can confirm or rule out hypoglycemia as a cause for symptoms, determine when a bedtime snack might be needed to prevent nocturnal hypoglycemia, or determine the effects of exercise or food on blood glucose. Teaching about SMBG is an opportunity to reinforce the concept of self-empowerment with patients (Anderson & Funnell, 2005). When patients learn to look for patterns in their blood glucose results, they learn to use the results to problem solve by making adjustments in their diet and exercise and working with their healthcare team to make adjustments in their medications.

Topic VIII: What Do They Mean When They Say "Acute Complications?"

Educating patients about acute complications means helping them to understand how to prevent, recognize, and treat high and low blood glucose levels and how to manage sick days. Before discussing this topic, patients should have a working knowledge of basic diabetes pathophysiology, the treatment with medications, and the effects of diet, exercise, and stress on blood glucose. They should also have an appreciation for the role of SMBG. Most patients benefit from a review of these topics to remind them that balancing the factors that raise and lower blood glucose must now be consciously managed by them because their bodies have lost the ability to do so automatically.

Hypoglycemia, which is sometimes referred to as an insulin reaction, is defined as a blood glucose level less than 70 mg/dL. If patients have had significantly elevated blood glucose readings for a long time, they may feel the symptoms of hypoglycemia when blood glucose levels are actually much higher than this. Low blood glucose occurs when there is an excess of the forces that lower blood sugar such as too much exogenous insulin, sulfonylurea medication, or exercise or too few calories because of too little food. Hypoglycemia can be avoided by paying attention to the timing of medications, exercise, and meals and using SMBG to detect patterns. Patients may experience sudden sweating, weakness, hunger, anxiety, trembling, fast heart-beat, irritability and inability to think clearly, headache, drowsiness, numbness or tingling around lips, confusion, and if severe, even seizures, coma, and death. If the episode happens at night, patients may wake because of nightmares or sweating, or they may awaken in the morning with a headache. At the other end of the spectrum, some patients can have extremely low blood glucose levels with none of the usual symptoms or no symptoms at all. This phenomenon is called hypoglycemia unawareness; it can be very dangerous and must be managed with care. Patients with hypoglycemia unawareness often have very subtle minisymptoms; thus, educators must work with these patients to help them avoid potential low blood glucose events, as well as to learn to recognize their unique signs of low blood glucose.

Patients should check their blood glucose as soon as they think that they are having a hypoglycemic reaction, and if the results are low, they should treat hypoglycemia promptly with a carbohydrate source such as sugar, juice, or glucose tablets or paste. Patients who use insulin or sulfonylureas must always carry a carbohydrate source and should wear and carry identification alerting others to their diabetic status. If patients have symptoms that could be hypoglycemia but they are not able to use their monitor for any reason, they should treat the hypoglycemia first, and test the blood sugar as soon as it is possible to do so. At 10 to 15 minutes after treatment, patients should recheck their blood glucose levels to make sure that they are back in a safe range, and if not, they need to repeat the treatment or have a snack. After the event has been treated, patients should always reflect on why hypoglycemia occurred in order to avoid recurrences. If patients have repeated hypoglycemia, they should communicate with their diabetes management team to work on making changes in their treatment plan. All patients with diabetes should carry or wear identification noting their medical problems, but patients with frequent or unrecognized hypoglycemia should be educated that they are at particularly increased risk (Funnell & Lasichak, 2004).

Hyperglycemia is defined as a fasting or premeal glucose more than 130 mg/dL, a postmeal reading more than 180 mg/dL, or a hemoglobin A1C more than 7. It is caused by too little blood glucose lowering factors such as insulin, oral medications, or exercise or an excess of things that raise blood glucose such as too many calories, increased weight, infection, or stress. Mild hyperglycemia may not give any symptoms, but will show up in SMBG testing, which is one reason why it is important to test on a regular basis. Higher levels of blood glucose will cause increased urination, thirst, fatigue, and blurred vision and, if severe, may cause dehydration, lethargy, confusion, coma, and even stroke.

Patients with type 1 diabetes should know that they are at particular risk when hyperglycemic because their complete lack of insulin forces the breakdown of body fat and protein, which produces acidic waste products called ketones. These ketones can build up in the blood and cause a condition called ketoacidosis, which is a serious chemical imbalance and can, if untreated, lead to death; therefore, patients with type 1 diabetes should test their blood or urine for ketones frequently when they have a blood glucose reading more than 300 mg/dL or when they are feeling sick. If patients with type 1 diabetes have ketones that do not go away when they increase their intake of sugar-free liquids, they should call their healthcare team or go to an emergency department for treatment. Even if unable to test, patients with symptoms of ketoacidosis should go to the nearest emergency department. Symptoms of ketoacidosis include all of the symptoms of hyperglycemia plus fruity breath, fast, deep breathing, anorexia, nausea, vomiting, abdominal pain, and mental changes, including coma.

The treatment of hyperglycemia depends on the degree and the cause of the elevated blood glucose. Every patient with diabetes has occasional high readings, and this is to be expected; however, patients should always reflect on possible reasons for the increased readings such as dietary indiscretions, omitted or expired medication doses, or symptoms of an infection; however, if blood glucose readings remain above target or are over 300 mg/dL or patients are experiencing symptoms of hyperglycemia, dehydration, or ketosis, they must contact their healthcare team to work together to modify their plan of care.

Everyone gets minor illnesses like colds and stomach upsets, and people with diabetes are no exception; therefore, all patients with diabetes should know what to do when they have a sick day. If they suspect they have a fever, they should check their temperature and report any reading more than 101°F to their health team. They should check their blood glucose readings as often as every 4 hours, and in type 1 diabetes, ketones should be tested as well. Patients should know that if they are able they should eat normally, and if not, they should eat carbohydrates or drink high carbohydrate liquids. Any patient with blood glucose readings that are more than 300 mg/dL who cannot tolerate liquids or who has positive ketone results should contact his or her healthcare team (Funnell & Lasichak, 2004).

Topic IX: How Can I Prevent Chronic Complications?

Although many patients know little about diabetes when they are first diagnosed, many know at least some of the complications and fear them. Patients who have misinformation and preconceptions about the complications of diabetes often bring feelings of hopelessness and helplessness to their experience of having diabetes. These patients have difficulty engaging in self-care, feeling that complications are inevitable no matter what they do. It is especially important to emphasize the recent improvements in chronic complication reduction with patients who may have seen the long-term effects of diabetes in older family members for whom the current information regarding the positive effects of tight management were not available. Patients must have up-to-date information in order to recognize the importance of prevention, recognition, and early treatment for chronic complications related to diabetes. As well, the principles of information-based decision making and empowerment must always be emphasized when working with these patients.

Patients with diabetes should understand that diabetes can affect both the large and small blood vessels of the circulatory system and can damage the nervous system. Large blood vessel damage most often occurs in the heart and lower extremities. It is caused by arteriosclerosis, which is a buildup of fats and plaque in the inside wall of an artery. This causes the passage for blood flow to become narrowed and creates the risk that a piece of the plaque will break loose. If circulation is interrupted by either of these factors, the tissue downstream suffers from decreased oxygen supply and can be damaged or die. When this happens in the heart, it can cause a heart attack. When it happens in the brain, it can cause a stroke, and when it happens in the legs and feet, it can cause both severe pain with walking as well as skin ulcers and slow healing, both of which can lead to infections and amputations. Because heart disease is a major cause of death for patients with diabetes, they must understand the reasons for decreasing their risk factors even if they have no symptoms of heart disease at the present time; therefore, controlling blood glucose, lipids, and blood pressure, not smoking, exercising regularly, and maintaining normal weight are all important ways to reduce the risk of heart disease. Many patients are also advised to take low dose aspirin as a way to reduce the risk of heart attack.

Small blood vessel disease takes place in the kidneys and the eyes. In the kidney, nephropathy occurs when the small blood vessels that function to filter waste products from the blood become less effective and waste products build up in the blood. Early on in this process there are no symptoms, however; thus, it is necessary to test blood and urine regularly to detect the early signs of kidney dysfunction. The best way to avoid kidney damage is to keep the blood glucose and blood pressure in normal range and if indicated to take one of the two classes of medications that have been shown to delay the progression if nephropathy, angiotensin-converting enzyme inhibitors or if they are contraindicated, angiotensin 2 receptor blockers, as directed by the patient's healthcare team. In the event that kidney failure progresses to a severe degree, patients have the options of dialysis or kidney transplant.

Retinopathy is also a small vessel disease affecting the retina of the eye, which is at the back of the eye and acts like the film in a camera to capture images sent through the lens. Retinopathy occurs when the blood vessels in the retina develop defects and leak blood into the eye. Over time, the retina heals, but scars or abnormal vessel growth may result, causing progressively decreased vision. If scar tissue pulls on the retina, it can cause a sudden loss of vision because of a detachment of the retina, which is an eye emergency requiring immediate care in the emergency room. Prevention of retinopathy has been demonstrated (DCCT Research Group, 1993) by the management of blood glucose to normal or near-normal levels and of blood pressure maintenance at normal levels. The importance of regular dilated eye examinations cannot be overemphasized, as no symptoms are present in early retinopathy and early treatment can stop or delay the progression of eye damage and preserve vision. The treatment for retinopathy is laser therapy of the retina, which can slow or prevent development of abnormal blood vessels. Patients with diabetes also have a higher incidence of cataracts, caused by accumulated glucose in the lens. The treatment for cataracts is removal of the lens and replacement with a prosthesis, which produces excellent results.

Diabetes may also damage the nervous system causing neuropathy. If the sensory nerves are affected, patients experience increased or decreased sensation, tingling, pain, or burning, usually in the legs and feet but also sometimes in the hands. Sometimes extremity pain becomes a management problem, or sensation is so impaired that patients cannot feel when they injure themselves. Together with decreased circulation of the lower extremities, which can slow healing and lead to infections, neuropathy is a major contributor to patients needing amputations. When motor nerves are damaged, patients have muscle weakness, and when autonomic nerves are damaged, body functions that are normally controlled without conscious thought are affected. Autonomic nerve damage can lead to the discomfort of delayed emptying of the stomach, constipation, diarrhea, dizziness when standing because of low blood pressure, urinary incontinence or retention, and sexual dysfunction. Although treatments are available to manage pain, such as medications and transcutaneous nerve stimulation, neuropathy is a difficult problem to manage. Intensive treatment of blood glucose has been linked to a 60% risk reduction for neuropathy (DCCT Research Group, 1993; UK Prospective Diabetes Study Group, 1998).

Patients with diabetes need to know that recent advances in diabetes research have shown that maintenance of near normal blood glucose levels, aggressive management of blood pressure to 130/80 or less, control of lipids, especially reduction of the low-density lipoprotein cholesterol to less than 100, treatment of microalbuminuria with angiotensin-converting enzyme inhibitors, and the use of low dose aspirin can all contribute to decreased long-term complications of diabetes. The reduction of other cardiovascular risk factors such as smoking, excessive weight, or lack of exercise is also important. To achieve these goals, patients should see their care team regularly to evaluate their blood pressure, lipids, HbA1C, urine microalbumin, and eyes and to receive foot and dental care and routine immunizations.

Topic X: Is It Really Possible to Change a Person's Habits?

The topic of behavior change must be introduced early in the education process and must consistently be reinforced throughout the educational program to be effective. All patients with diabetes should come to terms with what diabetes means for them, as discussed in Topic II. For some patients, this process will be long, ongoing, and often painful. They should understand that because they have a chronic disease they need more regular consultations with their health team to monitor their control and to update and maintain preventative care. Most patients need to make at least some changes in their diet and exercise habits and must learn to monitor their home blood glucose. Many must learn to take medications, including insulin. Patients should be asked early on in the education process to examine their own readiness for change. Do they see diabetes as a serious threat to their health? Do they believe that making changes will benefit them? Do they think that changing some of their habits will be impossible or too big a sacrifice? Do they have more pressing or immediate physical, social, or psychological needs or priorities? Although education is necessary for patients to make informed decisions, until patients are ready to make some movement toward change, no amount of diabetes education will lead to change and optimal self-management. After readiness for change is evident, learning and implementing strategies that support change can help patients to modify their habits (Mensing, 2006; Anderson & Funnell, 2005).

One key strategy that empowers patients to make successful change is to make a plan. First, patients should be asked to try to define the problem. What is the biggest concern or the most difficult part of having diabetes? What are their feelings surrounding this problem? What are their long-term goals? What are the benefits and barriers to reaching them? What short-term, concrete steps can they take toward reaching one of their goals? What are they ready to do? What could a short term goal be? Although one patient may be ready to start testing their blood glucose regularly but not be ready to start exercising, the opposite might be true for another person. How can they get support? What will they do? (It should be specific and measurable.) When will it start? How will they measure success? After a trial, they should evaluate how their plan worked. What went right and what went wrong? What will they do next time? What did they learn? After change has occurred, patients need time and support to make this new behavior a habit, and after new habits are formed, they should be used as building blocks to strengthen patients' confidence in their ability to change (Mensing, 2006). Achieving change is an ongoing process; thus, even after the information giving phase of diabetes education is completed, patients often benefit from ongoing support in the form of educator visits, support groups, or peer counseling.

Healthcare workers sometimes become frustrated with "noncompliant" patients who appear to not follow medical advice or do what is best for them. It should be remembered that optimal diabetes self-management demands more learning, change, and adaptation than most individuals can comfortably accommodate. Diabetes educators should consider that coaching others to change is an art. It requires reflection, insight, patience, trust, and respect on the part of both the patient and the healthcare worker. In keeping an open mind when working on the acquisition of diabetes self-management skills, both patients and educators will become more creative in their artistry.

TEACHING STRATEGIES

Whether it is a quick visit for a respiratory infection or a phone contact to titrate insulin, every healthcare encounter with a patient with diabetes has the potential to become a teachable moment and should be captured. Learning to do a quick assessment if the patient is not known to the educator, focusing on the salient points of diabetes self-management relevant to the situation, eliciting post instruction feedback, and adjusting instructions based on need and patient understanding are all techniques that are used in the office to make sure diabetes care is woven into primary care. The unfortunate reality is that far too many patients have only had diabetes education in this haphazard way. Although many patients are emotionally well adjusted, financially secure, adapt well to change, possess high levels of health literacy, and are able to access complicated information independently, many more do not share all of these qualities; therefore, the model for diabetes education should be a comprehensive, interactive, and individualized program for each patient that begins with a complete patient assessment as soon after diagnosis as possible. How old is the patient and at what developmental stage? How long has he or she had diabetes? Does he or she have complications? What level of education has he or she had in school? At what level does he or she function? What instruction has he or she had regarding his diabetes? What does he or she already know? What misconceptions does he or she have? What is his or her support system? What has been his or her previous family, work, school, or community experience regarding diabetes? What have his or her daily lifestyle and habits been like? What are his or her health and cultural beliefs? What is his or her economic and insurance status? What issues have caused problems? What does he or she want? These and many other factors affect an individual's response to learning new information and adapting to change, making it important for the educator to have insight into the patient point of view. A comprehensive assessment gives the diabetes educator information to determine the model of instruction that will best suit the patient's learning needs. An excellent discussion of and more detailed and specific information regarding patient assessments can be found in Chapter 25 of *The Art and Science of Diabetes Self-Management Education* (Mensing, 2006).

Group DSME is a popular method of both information giving and coaching. Because this method of education can be designed to fit the needs of a specific group of individuals, meetings can be scheduled for evenings or weekends and can consist of multiple short sessions or be designed as two half-day retreats. Group work has the benefit of sharing information with more patients at one time while simultaneously encouraging an exchange of ideas and experiences among the participants. These peer interactions can be powerful forces in stimulating readiness for change, movement toward a plan for change, or support and acknowledgment for changes already accomplished. Moreover, bonds may form between members that provide emotional and problem-solving support during as well as long after the group sessions are completed. Often, the DSME group reconvenes for a few hours every year thereafter to refresh and update both the educational and the social aspects of their work.

Typically, before group DSME begins, patients have a one-to-one visit with an educator to assess their needs and appropriateness for group work. At a later date, the group convenes for several sessions, and the diabetes educator uses the 10 topics discussed previously here as curriculum for the program. Although some groups have a separate didactic session using PowerPoint slides or flip charts and a separate discussion period, other educators prefer to weave the curriculum into interactive activities such as games or story telling. An example of an interactive exercise is Conversation Mapping (Healthy Interactions Inc., 2007), where the educator guides the DSME participants in conversations prompted by the images presented on a large tabletop display similar to a board game. In addition to providing prompts for the ten recommended topics for education, the conversation map makes it seem more natural for patients to share their own experiences as they follow the map. Adaptations can be made to accommodate different age groups or number of patients.

Another creative method to engage patients in conversation about diabetes is the "Magic Eight" questions developed by Arthur Kleinman (in Mensing, 2006).

1. What do you call the problem?
2. What do you think has caused the problem?
3. Why do you think it started when it did?
4. What do you think the sickness does? How does it work?
5. How severe is the sickness? Will it have a short or a long course?
6. What kind of treatment do you think you (or the person) should receive? What are the most important results you hope will be achieved from this treatment?
7. What are the chief problems the sickness has caused?
8. What do you fear most about the sickness?

This method of engaging patients in conversation regarding diabetes is especially helpful with groups who may have different cultural and health beliefs or who may feel overwhelmed by the complexity of information before them.

The same curriculum covering the 10 content areas can be offered to individuals who are not right for group work because of preference or other physical, mental, or emotional factors. Visits with the educator can be scheduled in any way a practice can accommodate them. As with the group sessions described previously here, family and friends are encouraged to participate in the educational sessions. For some of the same reasons that they are not well suited for group work, these patients may be more difficult to engage in their own self-care; however, the one-to-one patient–educator relationship, the ability to individualize completely teaching methods and pace, and the increased number of hours devoted to one patient should be used to offset these barriers.

Support from family, friends, peers, and the healthcare team can be crucial to patients who are making the transition from knowledge acquisition to self-management skills. For this reason, some programs offer ongoing support groups for patients struggling to implement what they have learned into their daily lives. Support groups can offer patients a place to examine and process feelings of frustration and failure, regroup and reprioritize their plans, grow and adapt to life with a chronic disease, and celebrate and share their successes. Above all, they encourage peer support in the community and reinforce that patients are not alone in their journey.

SUMMARY

Types 1 and 2 diabetes mellitus are both complex, multisystem diseases that require ongoing self-management by patients and families in collaboration with their healthcare providers. In order to work with patients and families successfully, diabetes educators must possess an understanding of the disease process, knowledge of the required patient self-management skills, and an appreciation of the process of behavior change through personal empowerment. This chapter gives the diabetes educator basic tools to teach patients what they need to know to live well with diabetes. Sections address the pathophysiology of diabetes and explain the usual treatments with diet, exercise, and oral and injected medications. They discuss the significance of SMBG and the importance of the patient's psychological adjustment. Topics teach the prevention, recognition, and treatment of acute and chronic complications and explore the concept of habit change as patients become empowered by knowledge. Examples of comprehensive teaching strategies using DSME curriculum are given.

Case Study 24–1

B.D. is a 69-year-old woman referred for diabetes teaching to the nurse by her primary care doctor. She was not certain whether she had diabetes. She had an elevated A1C of 7.3% for at least 2 years, with random serum glucose levels varying from under 100 mg/dL to occasionally over 200 mg/dL. She had a complicated medical history, including hypertension, hyperlipidemia, history of atrial flutter, renal artery stenosis, gout, osteoarthritis, hypothyroidism, and cataracts; she was on 12 medications. She had no known family history of diabetes. She was overweight with a body mass index of 32 and had seen a dietitian years ago for weight loss. She was physically

(Continues)

Case Study 24–1 (*Continued*)

inactive; her walking was limited because of arthritis in her knees. As a retired educator, she lived alone but had friends, family, and nieces involved in her life.

A review of her eating habits showed she had a high-carbohydrate diet:

> Breakfast: cream of wheat, tea, fruit, and toast or English muffin
> Lunch: grilled cheese or tuna sandwich and orange juice and water
> Supper: meat or fish with vegetable, potato, or pasta
> Desserts: cookies at lunch or supper
> Snacks: occasional crackers at bedtime and candy

She was not testing her blood sugar. An office exam included a finger stick blood sugar of 175 mg/dL at 2 hours after her lunch. Her weight was 205 pounds, and her height was 5' 7".

The nurse's evaluation was that this is an intelligent woman with a complicated medical history. Her history of random sugars of 200 mg/dL or more with A1Cs in the 7.3% confirmed that she had diabetes, about which she had little knowledge. The main goal of the first session therefore was to educate the patient to the basics of diabetes care.

Of the 10 recommended education content areas, those addressed on this visit were

- *Diabetes disease process:* definition of type 2 diabetes, risk factors, symptoms, natural history of the disease, and treatment.
- *Nutrition:* emphasis on weight reduction through lower fat and portion control, influence of carbohydrates on blood sugar, and dietitian appointment scheduled.
- *Physical activity:* increase as tolerated and try both walking and swimming.
- *Medications:* those used in type 2 diabetes briefly reviewed.
- *Blood glucose self-monitoring and using results:* taught how to use monitor and obtain equipment for use, instructed to test before and 2 hours after meals and record.
- *Chronic complications and goals of control to reduce CV risk factors:* "the ABCs," or A1C, blood pressure, cholesterol.
- *Goal setting and problem solving:* introduce concepts of self-management using up-to-date information and personal goals, responsibility, and empowerment.
- Psychosocial adjustment: coping with the confirmation of her diagnosis.

The nurse's evaluation of the patient's response to teaching was that the patient was highly motivated and very engaged in the teaching session. She deferred group class because of knee pain when sitting for long periods and preferred going to one-to-one teaching. She agreed to phone contact and return appointment in a few weeks. The patient accepted written information to reinforce the materials discussed in visit today and covering additional information if patient desires to go further.

On the return appointment, the patient had been testing home blood glucose readings and found that she was having postprandial sugar excursions in the 200s. This informed her of the importance of modifying diet to prevent these rises. She had attempted more physical activity and found that swimming was far preferable to walking, and in fact helped her knees to feel better. She was swimming 5 days per week. After seeing the dietitian, modifying her diet, increasing her exercise, and continuing her blood glucose monitoring, her postprandial sugars dropped to goal levels of under 180 mg/dL, and her A1C dropped to 6.7%. Her weight decreased 7 pounds to 198 pounds. Patient had read the teaching materials given to her at the last visit and had appropriate questions seeking more details.

Discussion

This was a patient who was unaware of her diagnosis until she had her first contact with the nurse educator. Unfortunately, she had had the diagnosis for some time before she became aware. Nevertheless, when informed about the facts, she openly accepted her diagnosis and responsibility for home management. She was able to understand materials taught in the one-to-one setting, motivated enough to read the materials given for home use, kept her appointment with the dietitian, and made some dietary adjustments based on that visit. In addition, the patient was able to circumvent a barrier to exercise by finding a way to swim five times per week. This level of engagement, understanding, and readiness for change enabled this patient to reach her goal A1C after one education visit. Nevertheless, some patients have a very positive first response to the diagnosis only to later fall into depression or denial; therefore, it would be important for the educator to continue to see this patient on a regular basis to complete the curriculum and possibly refer her to a support or peer group.

Barbara B. Chase and Katherine Hurxthal

Case Study 24–2

This case involves a common and less than ideal patient teaching situation in which the nurse is asked to teach a patient who was urgently overbooked into the schedule for the reason of "very poorly controlled diabetes, needing to start insulin immediately." It was the first visit for B.D., a 62-year-old black man referred to the office for diabetes management. He had a history of type 2 diabetes for 3 years and had been on oral medications, glipizide and metformin, with very poor control. His hemoglobin A1C was 10.3%. He had been recently seen in the emergency room with a rash, probably caused by lisinopril. The lisinopril was discontinued, but he had elevated blood sugars in the 400s. Thus, he was referred to this practice. Other medical problems included hypertension, hyperlipidemia, coronary artery disease, and status post–coronary artery bypass graft surgery. B.D. had a large knowledge deficit regarding his diabetes, as previously documented by his endocrinologist, and would need ongoing teaching with the nurse and dietitian. At the time of the first visit, however, he had marked hyperglycemic symptoms and needed to get on insulin immediately. He did not follow any particular diet plan, did not test his blood glucose, and worked two jobs, one of which was physically active and the other sedentary. He admitted that although it was his intention to take his medications as advised, he rarely got all of the doses in because of competing priorities like work and falling asleep before taking them. He lived alone and had a full kitchen but did little cooking for himself.

In this classic example of "survival teaching," of the 10 content areas, only a few were addressed because of time constraints.

- *Diabetes disease process:* brief review of the fact that type 2 diabetes often requires the use of insulin because of the natural history of the disease.
- *Nutrition:* importance of avoiding obviously high carbohydrate fluids and eating at regular mealtimes; dietitian appointment scheduled.
- *Medications:* very simple description of Lantus; administration with pen, basics of timing, dosing, site selection, care of pen, disposal of needles.
- *Monitoring:* use of meter. Patient does not have his meter with him or her and does not recall brand; therefore, new meter and equipment given. Medical assistant to review meter use with patient after visit. Test if possible before meals and at bedtime, at least twice a day; record and bring results and monitor to office visits.

- *Acute complications and goals of control:* hypoglycemia and preprandial glucose goals.
- *Goal setting and problem solving:* advancing Lantus every 3 to 4 days based on fasting blood sugar.

This is the nurse's evaluation of patient response to teaching: This less than ideal scenario for patient education is not uncommon; the basics are taught with the understanding that ongoing review and education are mandatory. The patient was attentive and cooperative but somewhat passive during the visit. Because of the limited time and the large amount of information exchange that were needed, it was not possible to individualize instruction as much as would be desired in one-to-one DSME. Social and personal information was obtained from the chart, rather than the patient, and no attempt was made to engage the patient in reflection regarding his feelings about diabetes his understanding about self-care and his personal goals. Also, no attempt was made to determine whether the patient has a support system or the potential to develop one. The patient was at least able to demonstrate that he could test blood glucose and give insulin after instruction. Directions regarding dose and advancing dose were written out for the patient, thus reinforcing verbal instructions. The plan was that B.D. was to follow up with his physician and the nurse on the telephone during the upcoming days and to return to the nurse in a week.

Unfortunately, after calling the office the day after the visit for insulin titration review, the patient missed his follow-up appointment with the nurse and the dietitian. When the nurse called to follow up, the patient apologized, saying that he had to work. Based on his history of blood glucose results, his insulin was titrated that day by phone, and an appointment was set up for him on his next day off. The nurse made sure that the secretary would call the day before to remind him of his upcoming appointment.

Discussion

This patient needs a complete assessment at the next visit. Although it is possible to teach technical skills and facts in isolation, it is never optimal and can lead to misunderstandings, confusion, and frustration for both the patient and the healthcare team. After more is understood about B.D.'s situation, his readiness to change, and his support system, it will be possible to work with him to develop

(Continues)

Case Study 24–2 (*Continued*)

personal goals and devise a plan for success. Given his history of long-term poor diabetes control, lack of knowledge, and limited resources, it would be important to reach out to him and accommodate his needs for appointment times, frequency of visits, and intensity of DSME work. Support group or peer coaching may be ways to engage this patient in the self-care that he desperately needs to begin in order to prevent complications.

Case Study 24–3

G.S. was a 15-year-old male admitted to a pediatric inpatient unit after 3 days of nausea, vomiting, and lethargy. He was found to have a blood glucose level in the mid-600s and was ketotic. His parents reported that G.S. had been entirely well until 2 weeks before admission when he had come down with an upper respiratory infection that caused a cough and nasal congestion. He had been taking over-the-counter cold medicines that caused him to have a dry mouth and increased thirst. The medicine and the cold also made him very tired. They noticed that he was urinating frequently but attributed that to the increased fluid intake. They also noted that he seemed to have lost a few pounds, but attributed that to the respiratory illness and the fact that G.S. might be having another growth spurt, as he had done the year before when he had gained height. To their surprise, G.S. and his parents were told that he has type 1 diabetes and would need insulin.

After hydration and insulin, G.S.'s blood glucose levels came down into the 130–180 mg/dL range. The next day G.S. reported that he felt like himself again and wanted to go home. The attending physician explained that before going home, G.S. and his family would have to learn how to give insulin and how to manage his diet. He arranged for the diabetes nurse educator and the dietitian to meet with G.S. and his family. The nurse educator spent over 2 hours with the family. She covered all 10 content areas of education recommended by the ADA. She instructed, demonstrated, and required repeat demonstrations for both blood glucose monitoring with a meter and subcutaneous insulin administration using a pen device. G.S. was to give basal insulin once a day and sliding scale rapid acting insulin with meals.

The dietitian worked with the family for over an hour. She reviewed carbohydrates, portions, timing, and the need to balance food groups. She introduced the concept of carbohydrate counting and gave G.S. and his family a book to look up how many grams of carbohydrate there are in various foods. Because G.S. and his family lived about an hour from the hospital, his care would be taken over by a physician in his community; therefore, after these education sessions, G.S. was discharged with prescriptions, some written information on diabetes, and instructions to make an appointment with his local doctor within 10 days.

When they arrived at home, G.S.'s mother made an appointment with the local physician. Unfortunately, there were no appointments for over a month. G.S. did very well for the rest of the week, as it was school vacation. He tested his finger stick blood glucose every morning, recorded it, took sliding scale if needed, and ate the breakfast his mother had prepared for him. He did the same before lunch and dinner and tested again before bedtime. His blood glucose readings were all less than 200 mg/dL, and he had not had any low readings or hypoglycemia symptoms; however, as soon as he returned to school, he began to encounter difficulty. First, he had never eaten breakfast in the past and soon started skipping it again. He did not want to test his blood glucose or give insulin at school, and thus, he ate lunch without knowing what his blood glucose was and without administering any insulin. At supper time, his readings were sometimes high, and thus, he gave sliding scale but then did not eat much to "make up" for the high readings and help bring down the blood glucose results. After several readings in the 300s before supper, he became erratic about testing, not wanting to know bad news. His parents had informed the school administration about his new diagnosis, and he had met with the nurse; however, this made him feel awkward. Furthermore, he was encouraged by her not to do any sports till his diabetes was stable, which made him really angry. By the end of his second week back at school, G.S. was no longer checking his blood glucose because he did not know how to interpret the results and did not want to check at school, and he was no longer taking sliding scale insulin. He was, however, taking his bedtime insulin and writing down made-up results in his record book to assure his parents that everything was okay. On the Saturday before his appointment with his doctor, he checked his fasting blood glucose, and it was 375 mg/dL. He gave his sliding scale, ate some toast, and decided to go for a run to get back in shape. He became hypoglycemic while exercising and fortunately was noticed by a neighbor who called the police. He was taken to the local urgent care, where his blood glucose was 27 mg/dL.

(Continues)

Case Study 24-3 (*Continued*)

Discussion

Although this patient and his family were given information while he was hospitalized, there was insufficient time to do an initial assessment of their learning needs. Also, at the time that they were educated, they had known about the diagnosis for less than 48 hours and had not had sufficient time to process this or the enormous amount of information they were given in just a few hours before discharge. Furthermore, follow-up care was not coordinated by the hospital team, and no phone follow-up was offered, resulting in a long delay before care was resumed and leaving the patient and his family with no medical support system in the interim.

Supporting teens as they learn diabetes self-management can be a daunting task given the patient's need for independence and flexibility; however, in this case, a better understanding of the patient's daily schedule, activities, habits, and feelings regarding blood glucose testing, insulin administration, and carbohydrate counting could have produced a plan that would afford G.S. better control. When frequent visits are not possible, phone follow-up is invaluable to newly diagnosed patients as they adjust to the idea of having diabetes and grapple with the new challenges that arise every day.

Case Study 24-4

T.P. was 10 years old when she was diagnosed with type 1 diabetes. She had had the "flu" for several weeks and was losing weight, feeling tired, and thirsty all of the time. She had even wet the bed once in the middle of the night. When her doctor saw her in the office, he immediately suspected diabetes and confirmed it with a finger stick showing her blood glucose to be 500 mg/dL. Her hemoglobin A1C was 11. T.P. did not really understand what the doctor was telling her mother, but in recalling that day, she could tell by the look on her mother's face that it was not good. T.P. went to the emergency room with her mother, and her father joined them there. She had to have an intravenous line, which hurt and frightened her, but her parents were with her; after it was in, it was not so bad. At the end of the day, her blood glucose had come down to near-normal levels, and she felt much better.

It was then that she learned that she would have to have injections every day. She now can recall feeling confused and upset.

T.P. went home from the emergency room that evening but went back to her doctor's office the next day and joined a "program." In the program, children and their parents met with a diabetes educator and then attended classes with the nurse and dietitian several times a week for 2 weeks and then came back once a month for as long as they needed to do so. In the program, T.P. and her parents learned about diabetes. The nurse and the dietitian covered all of the content areas recommended by the ADA by using slides, pictures, games, food, glucose monitors, and insulin pens and pumps. They talked with other people who also had diabetes, and T.P. learned about a special program in the summer just for children. After 2 weeks, T.P. went back to school, but she and her mother went to the program meeting once a month for most of a year. The program worked with the school nurse to make sure everyone knew what to do. The nurse tested her blood glucose and gave her insulin. Although T.P. did not like the sticks, she did like the attention, and she liked the school nurse.

Eventually, T.P. learned to test her own blood glucose and did it four to six times a day. She also learned to give her own insulin injections, long acting at night and rapid acting before meals, using a pen device. Sometimes T.P. had low blood glucose symptoms after gym class or when she did not eat all of her lunch. She recognized the symptoms of hypoglycemia, however, and quickly treated them with a glucose source. Once a month, she and her mother had a phone visit with the program to discuss the trends of her blood glucose results. From these consultations, she began to understand how food, exercise, and insulin work together and how to manage her blood glucose.

T.P. started college this year and is living in a dormitory. She hopes to become a nurse. She tests her blood glucose multiple times a day, and at this time, she is using an insulin pump. Her hemoglobin A1C is 6.2.

Discussion

This case is close to ideal. The diagnosing physician was aware of the DSME program affiliated with his practice and did not hesitate to refer the patient and her family early in their process of adaptation to a new illness. The family had the resources to attend many sessions so that they were able to benefit from the group support, as well as become comfortable with the information made available to them. T.P. adjusted to her diagnosis and became an active participant in her own care, resulting in excellent metabolic control of her diabetes.

RESOURCES

Jo-Ann Barrett

American Diabetes Association. (2003). *Exchange lists for meal planning.* Alexandria, VA: Author.

American Diabetes Association. (2004). *Medical management of type 1 diabetes* (4th ed.). Alexandria, VA: Author.

American Diabetes Association. (2008). Clinical practice recommendations 2008. *Diabetes Care, 31*(Suppl. 1).

Anderson, B., & Funnell, M. (2005). *The art of empowerment: Stories and strategies for diabetes educators* (2nd ed.). Alexandria, VA: American Diabetes Association.

Anderson, B., & Rubin, R. (2002). *Practical psychology for diabetes clinicians* (2nd ed.). Alexandria, VA: American Diabetes Association.

Armstrong, D. G., & Lavery, L. A. (Eds.). (2006). *Clinical care of the diabetic foot.* Alexandria, VA: American Diabetes Association.

Beaser, R. S. (2003). *Joslin's diabetes deskbook.* Boston: Joslin Diabetes Center.

Childs, B., Cypress, M., & Spollett, G. (Eds.). (2005). *Complete nurse's guide to diabetes care.* Alexandria, VA: American Diabetes Association.

Franz, M. J., & Bantle, J. P. (2003). *American Diabetes Association guide to medical nutrition therapy for diabetes.* Alexandria, VA: American Diabetes Association.

Healthy Interactions Inc. (2007). *Conversation maps.* Retrieved January 27, 2008, from http://www.healthyi.com.

Johnson, P. D. (2003). *Teenagers with type 1 diabetes: a curriculum for adolescents and families.* Alexandria, VA: American Diabetes Association.

Jovanovic, L. (2008). *Medical management of pregnancy complicated by diabetes* (3rd ed.). Alexandria, VA: American Diabetes Association.

Kahn, C. R. (Ed.). (2004). *Joslin's diabetes mellitus* (14th ed.). New York: Lippincott, Williams and Wilkins.

Kaufman, F. R. (2005). *Diabesity: The obesity-diabetes epidemic that threatens America—and what we must do to stop it.* Westminster, MD: Bantam Dell.

Klingensmith, G. (2003). *Intensive diabetes management* (3rd ed.). Alexandria, VA: American Diabetes Association.

Lebovitz, H. (2004). *Therapy for diabetes mellitus and related disorders.* Alexandria, VA: American Diabetes Association.

Mensing, C. (Ed.). (2006). *The art and science of diabetes self-management education.* Chicago: American Association of Diabetes Educators.

Pastors, J. G. (Ed.). (2003). *Diabetes nutrition Q&A for health professionals.* Alexandria, VA: American Diabetes Association.

Ross, T. A., Boucher, J. L., & O'Connell, B. S. (Eds.). (2005). *Guide to diabetes medical nutrition therapy and education.* Chicago: American Dietetic Association.

Ruderman, N., Devlin, J., Schneider, S. (Eds.). (2002). *Handbook of Exercise in Diabetes.* Alexandria, VA: American Diabetes Association.

Scheiner, G. (2004). *Think like a pancreas.* New York: Marlowe.

Thomas, A. M. (2005). *Guide to gestational diabetes mellitus.* Chicago: American Dietetic Association.

Warshaw, H. S., & Kulkarni, K. (2004). *ADA complete guide to carb counting.* Alexandria, VA: American Diabetes Association.

Zimmerman, B. (2004). *Medical management of type 2 diabetes* (5th ed.). Alexandria, VA: American Diabetes Association.

REFERENCES

Anderson, B., & Funnell, M. (Eds.). (2005). *The art of empowerment: stories and strategies for diabetes educato*rs (2nd ed.). Alexandria, VA: American Diabetes Association.

DCCT Research Group. (1993). The effect of intensive treatment of diabetes on the development and progression of long term complications in insulin-dependent diabetes mellitus. *New England Journal of Medicine, 329,* 977–986.

Funnell, M., & Lasichak, A. J. (Eds.). (2004). *Life with diabetes* (3rd ed.). Alexandria, VA: American Diabetes Association.

Healthy Interactions Inc. (2007). *Conversation maps.* Retrieved January 27, 2008, from http://www.healthyi.com/.

Mensing, C. (Ed.). (2006). *The art and science of diabetes self-management education.* Chicago: American Association of Diabetes Educators.

National Institute of Diabetes and Digestive and Kidney Diseases. (2007). *Diabetes in America* (2nd ed.). Bethesda, MD: National Institutes of Health.

UK Prospective Diabetes Study Group. (1998). Intensive blood glucose control with sulfonylureas or insulin compared with conventional treatment and risk of complications in patients with type 2 diabetes (KUPDS 33). *The Lancet, 352,* 837–853.

Chapter 25

Teaching Patients with Cardiovascular Disease

Terry Mahan Buttaro

INTRODUCTION

Improving communication between patients and healthcare providers is a major recommendation from *Healthy People 2010* and the Institute of Medicine (2001). An integral component of communication in healthcare is education. Teaching people about their health and encouraging them to ask questions aid in promoting wellness and empowerment. What is teaching really, however? Historically, in health care, teaching meant telling the patient what to do or not do, but effective communication between patients and healthcare providers is really a partnership, a shared experience. Understanding this concept and appreciating the benefit of the teaching/learning process in our patient encounters will help our patients to develop the knowledge and motivation necessary for their healthcare needs.

Cardiovascular (CV) disease is the leading cause of death in this country for both men and women (American Heart Association [AHA], 2007a). Motivating our patients and ourselves to learn about risk factors for heart disease, lifestyle changes, and prevention and treatment strategies is of paramount importance to decrease the morbidity and mortality associated with this multifaceted disorder. This chapter is intended to highlight important concepts in controlling the risk factors associated with CV disease and suggests teaching techniques that will encourage patients to take charge of their health and well-being.

Most often associated with heart attacks and strokes, CV encompasses a broad range of diseases and disorders. The heart and/or blood vessels can be affected, and the cause can be either congenital or acquired. Hypertension, atherosclerosis, coronary artery disease (CAD), valvular heart disease, dys- rhythmias, heart failure, and peripheral vascular disease are the more com- mon disorders associated with CV disease.

Almost 80 million people in the United States have CV disease (AHA, 2007a); 72,000,000 have been diagnosed with hypertension, and almost 16 million have known CAD. Half of those with CAD have had a myocardial infarction, and the other half have angina (AHA, 2007a).

The prevalence of CV disease is partly related to inactivity (Carnethon, Gulati, & Greenland, 2005). Ethnicity, heredity, race, gender, and age are risk factors that cannot be changed, but physical inactivity, obesity, smoking, hypertension, dyslipidemia, and type 2 diabetes mellitus are modifiable risk factors that can significantly decrease the risk for CAD and sudden cardiac death (AHA, 2007b).

The challenge for healthcare providers is to identify each patient's risk factors for CV disease and then to teach the patient appropriately about the disease, the potential risks, and appropriate interventions. The primary imperative is to promote patient understanding and empower the patient to make lifestyle changes that will decrease morbidity and mortality. CV disease is insidious and starts early in life, long before patients are symptomatic. Thus, promoting a healthy lifestyle for all our patients, young and old, is a healthcare provider imperative.

PATIENT TEACHING AND CARDIOVASCULAR DISEASE

The rationale for patient teaching is to enhance patient understanding of dis- ease processes, as well as the recommended treatments, but if teaching is to be effective, the methods used must first capture the patient's attention (Katz, 1997). Interesting the patient in the information is vital, but it is equally important to determine the patient's primary language and his or her health literacy (i.e., the ability to process, understand, and attain information) (Hage, 2008). Other concepts to consider are to focus the teaching on what the patient needs to know now and keeping the teaching straightforward and understandable (Falvo, 2004; Katz, 1997).

The information when communicated appropriately helps patients real- ize that lifestyle changes and the suggested medications and interventions can help avoid disease progression (Falvo, 2004). An additional goal of patient education is to motivate patients to take charge of their health. This partnership of patient and healthcare provider is essential in the prevention and treatment of all diseases and disorders.

To reduce the risks of CV disease, primary and secondary prevention treatment strategies are targeted at all modifiable risk factors: smoking, obesity, physical inactivity, hyperglycemia, hypertension, and dyslipidemia. Smoking and hypertension are often considered the most important modifiable risk factors, but patient risk factor profiles do differ. Discussing with the patient their individual CV risk profile (i.e., Framingham Risk Score) can help motivate the patient to make lifestyle changes that will decrease his or her cardiovascular risk (AHA, 2002).

SMOKING CESSATION

Cigarette smoking is clearly associated with CV disease and is a significant cause of heart attacks and strokes (AHA, 2007c,d). According to the AHA, most smokers want to discontinue smoking; in the past 40 years, 40% of smokers have been able to stop. Because most people do want to stop smoking, it is important to encourage smoking cessation at all encounters. The transtheoretical model of change theory suggests that asking patients whether they have considered trying to stop smoking and then providing information about the benefit of stopping can help those in the precontemplation stage of change consider the risks of continued smoking (DiClemente et al., 1991). According to DiClemente et al., the awareness of these risks helps patients move from the precontemplation stage to the contemplation stage of smoking cessation and then onto the determination stage where the patient states, "I know I need to stop" (**Table 25-1**). This is the crucial moment for healthcare providers. By assisting the patient in developing a plan to stop smoking, the patient is empowered to take action and stop smoking. Continued support enables the patient to sustain the change and prevent relapse.

Table 25-1 The Processes of Behavioral Change

Precontemplation
Contemplation
Determination
Action
Maintenance
Relapse

Change is difficult, and patients can become discouraged and relapse. Thus, it is essential that healthcare providers understand the importance of encouragement and understanding. Harassing patients to stop smoking, lose weight, or comply with treatment recommendations is never helpful. Instead, it is crucial to listen to the patient, acknowledge how difficult change is, and offer the patient supportive resources (Falvo, 2004). Regularly scheduled visits with the primary care provider allow the provider to ask the patient what would be helpful for the patient when he or she next tries to stop smoking. Continued support and counseling techniques encourage the patient to make a plan to stop smoking and consider substitute behaviors for smoking.

According to Jorenby (2001), self-help information for smoking cessation has not been proven to be effective, but counseling combined with nicotine replacement (e.g., gum, patches, nasal sprays, or inhalers) and bupropion, an antidepressant, can be helpful. Varenicline (Chantix) is a newer pharmacologic agent designed to help patients stop smoking that was efficacious in phase 3 trials (Jorenby et al., 2006; Tonstad et al., 2006). Varenicline is not a nicotine replacement, but works by blocking cravings for nicotine. It cannot be used in combination with the other stop-smoking agents; a support telephone program is available for patients using this product.

OBESITY

Despite a growing awareness of the dangers associated with obesity, the number of overweight Americans is steadily increasing. The 2003–2004 National Health and Nutrition Examination Survey (NHANES) revealed that 32.9% of Americans aged 20 to 74 are overweight (Centers for Disease Control [CDC], 2007a). This is double the number of overweight Americans identified in the first NHANES survey conducted between 1976 and 1980 (CDC, 2007a). Unfortunately, this trend is affecting Americans of all ages as the number of overweight children more than doubled between the first and second NHANES survey (CDC, 2007a). The causes of this epidemic are multifactorial, although calorie consumption in excess of energy expenditure is the prime reason for this epidemic (CDC, 2007a). When teaching patients about weight control, it is important to consider factors that impact weight control: patient age, culture, socioeconomic status, genetics, metabolism, behavior, stress, environment, and amount of physical activity (CDC, 2007a; Siegel, 2007).

The National Institutes of Health defines obesity as a body mass index (BMI) greater than or equal to 30 kg/m². Ideal BMI for adults ranges from 18.5 to 24.9. A BMI greater than ideal is associated with dyslipidemia, hyperglycemia, and hypertension and increases the risk of CAD. Even a small decrease in weight can decrease CV risk, and thus, encouraging patients to start with an initial 5-pound weight loss, with a weight loss goal of 10 to 20 pounds will be beneficial.

Recommendations for weight loss are innumerable, and fad diets abound; however, helping patients develop a sensible eating and exercise plan is far more valuable for developing a healthy lifestyle. Healthcare providers can be very instrumental in promoting weight loss by encouraging patients to make small lifestyle dietary changes that help promote weight loss and improve glucose control. Motivation is crucial, but it is essential that the healthcare provider realize the frustration and difficulty many patients have with weight control. Partnering with the patient to encourage behavioral change is an integral component of weight management (Gordon, Fergus, Koo, & Takeuchi, 2007). Promoting a social network or "buddy system" for patients to support them while trying to lose weight can also be beneficial as a support system at home and at work can be helpful especially if others in the network are also trying to change their eating habits.

A 24-hour dietary review helps the patient and provider understand how calories are consumed. Encouraging the patient to record "each mouthful" is also useful so that patients can then understand that the "mouthful" of ice cream or candy, although seemingly inconsequential, contributes to weight gain. The dietary review allows the provider the opportunity to discuss with the patient small changes that can be helpful (e.g., encouraging the patient to eat a piece of fruit during the day rather than drinking juice and stressing the importance of portion control with examples of appropriate servings). Although a weight loss diet may be indicated for obese patients, strategies that allow a patient to lose 0.5 to 1 pound per month or 10% of body weight in 6 months may be more successful in the long run (**Table 25-2**).

The Dietary Approaches to Stop Hypertension (DASH) diet is often recommended for patients with CV disease, primarily because it is beneficial for patients with hypertension (Appel et al., 2006); however, it is a sensible diet plan that emphasizes portion control while encouraging fruits, vegetables, fiber, and lower amounts of fat and cholesterol. The basic DASH diet is a 2,000-calorie per day diet that will help many patients lose weight, but the dietary plan can be modified to 1,800 calories per day or less.

Table 25-2 Lifestyle Changes to Help Promote Weight Loss

1. Eliminate juice drinks and sugared soft drinks.
2. Avoid alcohol. Substitute "lite" beer for regular beer.
3. Eat small amounts several times a day.
4. Monitor size of portions carefully (3 ounces of meat at dinner, equivalent in size to a deck of cards). Order the smallest serving size (ice cream, drinks, and food) when eating away from home.
5. Avoid cream, whipped cream, ice cream, whole milk, caramel, and other sugar syrups when ordering iced coffees.
6. Weigh and record your weight daily.
7. Avoid fried foods and foods with trans-fats. Steam, stir-fry, bake, and broil!
8. Use canola, corn, olive, soybean, or sunflower oil. Avoid lard, coconut, palm, and partially hydrogenated vegetable oil.
9. Limit yourself to one "sweet" (two small cookies, low-fat yogurt, or a serving of unsweetened canned fruit) per day (for most people, this should be after dinner), but avoid concentrated sweets (doughnuts, pie, and cake).
10. Substitute fish or chicken for meat.

For some patients, the DASH diet may seem too complicated or stringent. For most of us, it is easier to make lifestyle changes one step at a time. By decreasing caloric intake by just 100 calories, almost 1 pound of weight can be lost in a month.

PHYSICAL INACTIVITY

A lack of exercise impacts weight control and is associated with hypertension, hyperglycemia, dementia, dyslipidemia, CAD, and strokes in both men and women. Studies suggest that exercise helps increase high-density lipoprotein (HDL) cholesterol while decreasing triglycerides, total and low-density lipoprotein (LDL) cholesterol, atherosclerosis, and improving endothelial function (Bowles, Woodman, & Laughlin, 2000; Petersen & Pedersen, 2005).

The AHA recommendations for primary CV disease prevention include a minimum of 30 minutes of moderate intensity exercise each day (AHA, 2007b). This type of exercise is considered endurance or aerobic exercise, but resistance exercise to improve muscle strength is also important.

For all patients, the best exercise is the one they like and will do on a regular basis. For many patients, walking briskly is a reasonable way to exercise, and walking for 10 minutes three or more times each day may be as effective as daily exercising for 30 minutes to an hour (Jakicic, Wing, Butler, & Robertson, 1995). Taking 10,000 steps a day has also been recommended as a goal for cardiovascular fitness, although currently, there are no studies to support this recommendation that seems to be primarily media based; however, using a pedometer to encourage walking as a means to cardiovascular health seems reasonable. A review by Tudor-Locke and Bassett (2004) revealed that active adults did take 10,000 steps per day. Unfortunately, older adults might not be able to manage that many steps, and children would likely need even more steps a day to prevent obesity.

Other appropriate aerobic exercise activities include swimming, dancing, bicycling, and cross-country skiing. The goal for maximum intensity exercise is to increase the heart rate to a target rate for 20 minutes. The target heart rate, which should not be exceeded during exercise, is calculated by subtracting the patient's age from 220. For patients beginning an exercise program, moderate intensity exercise is recommended. For these patients, the heart rate goal during exercise is 50% to 70% of the maximum target heart rate (Peterson, 2007; Pollock et al., 1998).

Calisthenics and weight lifting are forms of resistance training. Building muscular strength for all muscle groups is beneficial, although for this type of exercise, some patients (e.g., older people or patients with diabetic retinopathy) will need medical clearance to prevent injury. A physical therapist consultation may also be beneficial to help patients learn proper resistance techniques.

In today's world, regular physical activity is impacted by many factors: time, work, weather, and family commitments. Patients often know they need to exercise, but barriers abound. Exercise is more doable for most of us if we have a partner to exercise with, and thus, encouraging families or friends to exercise together can inspire patients to motivate others.

Motivational interviewing has been suggested as one method that may be beneficial in helping patients develop their own exercise plan (Perry & Bennett, 2006). Motivational interviewing is based on the transtheoretical model of change (Table 25-1) and encourages the patient to discuss the benefit of exercise. The healthcare provider listens and acknowledges the patient's explanation of the barriers to exercise and then facilitates the discussion by encouraging the patient to consider a feasible daily exercise plan.

Most patients can begin a moderate intensity exercise program and not require exercise stress testing. Patients with obesity, a history of heart disease (including genetic heart disease), diabetes, a sedentary lifestyle, or increased CV disease risk factors (e.g., age, family history, smoking, hypertension, and hyperlipidemia) should talk with their healthcare provider before starting a vigorous exercise program. An exercise stress test may be indicated for these individuals before an exercise program is started. Patients need to understand that any chest, neck, or jaw discomfort; left arm pain; lightheadedness or fainting; or a cold sweat during exercise means that the patient should stop exercising immediately and call the healthcare provider or 911.

CARDIAC REHABILITATION

Patients with a history of CV disease or a history of a myocardial infarction, heart failure, percutaneous coronary artery angioplasty or stenting, or coronary artery bypass surgery are candidates for a cardiac rehabilitation exercise program. Cardiac rehabilitation is an individually designed program of secondary prevention to improve patients' quality of life, decrease cardiovascular risk factors, and enhance function (AHA, 2007d). Patients are medically supervised during exercise, and adjustments are made to medications and the exercise regimen as needed. In addition, patients receive educational information about their cardiac disorder, medications, physical limitations, and continued risk factors (AHA, 2007c). Psychosocial support, vocational counseling, and risk reduction strategies are emphasized. By engaging patients in healthy behaviors and explaining how smoking, high blood pressure, medications, and other factors impact the heart, cardiac rehabilitation encourages patients to take control of their health and reduces morbidity and mortality (AHA, 2007b,c,d).

HYPERGLYCEMIA

About 14.6 million people in the United States have been diagnosed with diabetes, and another 6.2 million people have diabetes but have not yet been diagnosed (CDC, 2007b). Many others have impaired fasting blood sugars or glucose tolerance, which increases their risk for diabetes. The importance of controlling blood sugar cannot be understated if the macrovascular and microvascular complications that cause arteriosclerosis, atherosclerosis, neuropathies, and nephropathies are to be avoided. Understanding the importance of normal blood sugar levels, nutritional and medication therapy, and lifestyle changes is fundamental for these patients and their families if CV disease is to be averted.

Cardiovascular risk reduction for patients with hyperglycemia is comprehensive. Blood pressure control; reduction of triglycerides, LDLs; and total cholesterol; and smoking cessation, weight control, and daily exercise are as important as glucose control.

The patient and collaborative health team (i.e., healthcare provider, physician specialist, diabetes educator, and nutritionist) partnership can help promote normoglycemia by helping the patient actively take charge of his or her blood sugar control. A low-calorie, low-fat, high-complex carbohydrate diet and an appropriate exercise regimen are recommended; however, the goal is to help the patient develop healthy eating habits based not only on carbohydrate counting, but also on the patient's culture, food likes and dislikes, and lifestyle. Exercise recommendations are similar to those previously described, although hypoglycemia is a potential risk especially in patients with type 1 diabetes. A snack before exercise is often recommended. Recognizing the signs and symptoms of hyperglycemia and hypoglycemia and having an understanding of treatments are also very important.

Diabetes care is best accomplished by empowering the patient/family with knowledge and self-management skills. Often, however, psychosocial issues are an impediment to learning and self-management. This is true with all diseases and disorders, but can be particularly true with patients who have diabetes. These concerns are frequently evident when a patient is first diagnosed, but are really ongoing.

HYPERTENSION

Worldwide, hypertension is the major risk factor for mortality related to CV disease (Chobanian et al., 2003). Lowering systolic blood pressure to less than 120 and diastolic blood pressure less than 80 can reduce the risk of stroke, heart attacks, and heart and kidney failure, especially if other CV disease risk factors are also reduced. Lifestyle changes that can help decrease blood pressure include decreasing alcohol consumption, weight loss, aerobic exercise, and the DASH diet. Many patients will also need a combination of antihypertensive medications from different classes to control blood pressure adequately, although continued exercise and weight loss can sometimes negate the need for life-long pharmacologic therapy.

Because high blood pressure is an asymptomatic disorder and really an abstract concept for many patients, it is especially important to explore the patient's thoughts about hypertension. Some cultures have home remedies to treat hypertension (e.g., garlic, vinegar, certain foods, and herbal preparation), and some patients do not want to take any medications. Others cannot really afford the costs of three or more medications for blood pressure control. Exploring these issues in a caring, respectful manner is critical. It is important to respect people's cultural beliefs, but also helpful to talk with them about other ways to treat high blood pressure, plus discuss and show or draw pictures that illustrate how increased blood pressure can cause a heart attack, stroke, or kidney failure. Patients should know what the target blood pressure is and be encouraged to check (and record) their blood pressure at home or at the local drug store or senior center.

Despite lifestyle changes, some patients will require medications to control blood pressure. Many patients will require three or more medications from different pharmacologic classes. Explaining this initially is particularly important so that patients can understand that each medication works in a different way to lower blood pressure and decrease the risks of cardiovascular and renal disease. When a medication is added, it is helpful to discuss the potential side effects with the patient and include simple written instructions to reinforce when and how the medication is taken as well as information concerning the need to call the healthcare provider if the medicine causes any untoward effects.

DYSLIPIDEMIA

Lipid disorders are prevalent in the United States and are a concerning risk factor for CV disease. This disorder can be genetic or associated with diet. The current National Cholesterol Education Program's Adult Treatment Panel III Guidelines recommend a total cholesterol level of less than 200 mg/dl and a LDL level less than 100 mg/dl (Grundy et al., 2004). For patients with high risk factors or known CV disease, the optimal LDL is less then 70 mg/dl (Grundy et al., 2004). Triglycerides, an element of lipoprotein, are a risk factor for CV disease when greater than normal (150 mg/dl), whereas HDL, usually considered cardioprotective (especially when higher than 60 mg/dl), is an additional CV risk factor if less than 40 mg/dl. Many patients actually have a mixed dyslipidemia consisting of a low HDL and high LDLs and triglycerides. Mixed dyslipidemia is often associated with a disorder commonly known as the metabolic syndrome, a consternation of CV risk factors that also includes hypertension, hyperinsulinemia, and central obesity.

Lifestyle changes include weight loss, exercise, and dietary therapy. These are very important in the control of dyslipidemia and impact the other associated CV risk factors (e.g., obesity, hypertension, and hyperglycemia). Exercise, especially if aerobic, will increase HDLs and decrease total cholesterol, LDLs, and triglycerides. Recommended dietary changes include limiting saturated fats to less than 7% and total fats to 25% to 30% of each day's calories. Monounsaturated fats from olive oils and nuts (1.5 ounces of walnuts, almonds, pecans, or pistachios each day) are best: saturated fats (meat and dairy products and palm and coconut oils) and transfatty acids should be avoided. The recommended amount of total daily cholesterol is less than 200 mg.

Cultural practices are incorporated into dietary planning by collaborating with the patient and family, and it is helpful to realize that it may be easier for the patient to make one change at a time. In general, changes in diet that are helpful for controlling cholesterol include increasing dietary fiber by eating 1.5 cups of oatmeal and five servings (0.5 cup) of fruits (apples, berries, oranges, and prunes) or vegetables (carrots and sweet potatoes) daily. Substituting chicken, fish, nuts, or 4 ounces of tofu or beans for meat is beneficial, and these are good sources of protein. Soy milk is a good substitute for milk, but skim milk is also acceptable.

For some patients, medications are indicated, but it is important that patients understand that the need for medication therapy in the treatment of dyslipidemia, hypertension, or hyperglycemia does not necessarily reflect patient failure. Sometimes lifestyle changes are just not enough. The HMG-CoA reductase inhibitors, commonly known as the statins, are most often prescribed medications for dyslipidemia. The statins are effective for increasing HDL cholesterol and lowering total cholesterol, LDLs, and triglycerides. Many patients are concerned about this class of drugs because of the reports of liver failure and muscle breakdown, although these adverse effects are uncommon. Gemfibrozil, a fibric acid, increases HDL and decreases triglycerides, but is not as efficacious in decreasing LDLs and can also cause liver toxicity. Niacin (nicotinic acid) is also appropriate for treating dyslipidemia, but the gastrointestinal disturbances, flushing, and dry, itchy skin are more challenging for many patients. For patients who cannot take these medications, the bile acid sequestrants and cholesterol absorption inhibitors may have fewer side effects. When lifestyle changes and single drug therapy do not lower cholesterol levels to the desired goals, combination therapy can be used.

ASPIRIN AND CV DISEASE

Many people take an aspirin each day, as studies suggest its efficacy for those with known CV disease (AHA, 1997); however, there are risks associated with aspirin use (e.g., gastrointestinal bleeding and hemorrhagic stroke), and thus, it is important that each patient discuss the risks and benefits with his or her healthcare provider.

TEACHING TECHNIQUES

Perhaps, the most essential aspect of patient teaching is the relationship between the patient and the healthcare provider. The relationship itself is affected by the patient's previous encounters with you as well as previous experiences the patient may have had with other healthcare providers. The goal is to have each encounter be a positive experience for the patient so that the patient feels better and is empowered to make changes. It is the patient–provider relationship combined with the patient's empowerment that helps promote the collaborative bond necessary for patient understanding and education.

The patient needs to feel that the provider is focused on the patient. Sensing that the provider cares about the patient's well-being and values the patient's participation in healthcare planning is integral. Whether meeting the patient in the hospital or office, the provider should greet the patient and patient's family and introduce himself or herself. A firm handshake, if culturally appropriate, helps impart trust and respect. It is also important that the provider avoid prejudice so that the patient will feel respected both as a person and for his or her beliefs (Buttaro & Trybulski, 2008).

A quiet setting free from interruptions and distractions helps center the dialogue and creates the educational environment. Sitting at eye level across from the patient facilitates eye contact and enhances the interaction while allowing the healthcare provider to monitor the patient's reactions conscientiously (Buttaro & Trybulski, 2008). Listening attentively to any concerns or questions helps prevent misunderstandings and allows for clarifications. Although electronic medical records are valuable for accessing and recording patient information, it is very important that the healthcare provider focus on the patient so that the computer is not viewed as a barrier to the patient/provider relationship.

Patient education also needs to be centered on the patient and family's needs rather than on what the provider thinks the patient (or family) needs to know (Scott & Thompson, 2003). Because healthcare issues can impact all aspects of a patient's and family's life, it is preferable to ask about patient concerns first in an encounter and be certain to address these concerns. After the patient's issues are addressed, the encounter can be centered on the patient's educational needs. In CV disease, patients really need to know that often the disease is multifactorial (i.e., many patients with CV disease will have hypertension, dyslipidemia, and other risk factors). Knowing all of the risk factors is helpful for patients. It is also useful that the patient understand what the goal blood pressure or LDL or blood sugar should be. For some patients, writing this information and documenting their progress for them can be beneficial in promoting their understanding.

Other important considerations in patient education that are particularly important in the treatment of CV disease include the patient's motivation to change, cultural beliefs, and their cognitive and economic status. Cultural understanding helps prevent misunderstandings and medication errors in addition to strengthening the trust between the patient and provider. Awareness of the patient's cognitive abilities and health literacy aids the provider in appropriately helping the patient understand the physiologic changes and treatments.

The complexity of CV disease requires careful explanation, as well as written information that the patient can understand. According to Hoffmann and Worrall (2004), the instructions should be simple and written at the lowest possible reading level in the patient's language. The information should be accurate, pertinent, and culturally appropriate (Hoffmann & Worrall, 2004). Some educational materials are general and explain their disease or dietary recommendations (e.g., a low cholesterol diet) in terms the patient can understand. Often, however, patients need specific information that is printed clearly (or typed) explaining when it is important to call the doctor. For example, for a patient diagnosed with heart failure, the healthcare provider might write this:

1. Weigh yourself every day and write it down.
2. If you gain more than 2 pounds in 2 days, take one furosemide tablet (this is the fluid pill).
3. If you need to take more than two fluid pills in 1 week, call the office and let us know. We may want to see you and do a blood test.
4. Call the office or go to the emergency room if you have shortness of breath or any chest discomfort.

Some patients will benefit from group learning and others will find support groups helpful. Educational resources on the Internet can be useful for some patients if they have Internet access.

SUMMARY

Every healthcare provider has a theory or philosophy about patient care. Sometimes during an encounter with a patient we remember why we chose health care as a profession, but it is easy in the stress of every day life and responsibilities to forget. To care for our patients effectively and to teach them about their health, it is critical that we appreciate each patient as an individual with different needs and learning styles. It is not possible or reasonable to teach each patient everything that they need to know in one encounter; however, after any educational patient encounter, it is helpful to have the patient restate relevant instructions as well as information about signs and symptoms that the patient should report to the doctor or healthcare provider.

The difference between success and failure in health education as documented in the following case studies may be a need for more in-depth assessment, compromise, and follow-up. It would be important to ensure that

Mrs. M. understood the seriousness of her condition, and to work with her to try to find ways to fit medications and required lifestyle changes into her daily life, as was done for Mrs. N. Even small changes may foster a better outcome.

Case Study 25-1

Mrs. M is a 42-year-old married, self-employed female. She does not smoke but has a history of hypertension controlled with hydrochlorothiazide and lisinopril. She often does not keep her appointments because her business demands so much of her time. On a recent visit, she complains of bilateral leg discomfort while walking and some dyspnea on exertion. An exercise stress test is ordered, but the results are not conclusive. Her blood tests, however, revealed an elevated fasting blood sugar and a hemoglobin A1C indicating type 2 diabetes mellitus. Her lipid profile is also abnormal, but she refuses treatment for both the high blood sugar and mixed dyslipidemia because she just does not want to take any more medicines. She also refuses to test her blood sugars at home stating, "I don't want to stick my fingers everyday." She is given a diabetic, low-fat, low-cholesterol diet and an appointment to see her doctor in follow-up. She misses her next two appointments. Several months after her last office visit, she complains of chest discomfort while out with her family. She is immediately brought to the local emergency room but dies of a massive heart attack.

Case Study 25-2

Mrs. N is a married, 75-year-old female who has always been in good health. Recently, her blood pressure has been elevated, and she was started on hydrochlorothiazide. She returns for a follow-up blood pressure check, but her blood pressure is even higher: 178/106. Lisinopril, 10 milligrams a day, is added, but her blood pressure remains elevated, sometimes as high as 200/96, despite weekly visits to the doctor's office and the addition of more medications to control her blood pressure. At each visit, she becomes more distraught about this change in her health, yet all diagnostic tests are negative. She develops shortness of breath and is admitted to the hospital and started on furosemide, a diuretic. An echocardiogram reveals diastolic heart failure, but the cardiologist believes that the heart failure is caused by the uncontrolled high blood pressure. While in the hospital, her blood pressure is better: 140–150/50–60. She is discharged from the hospital on furosemide, 80 mg daily; lisinopril, 40 mg daily; Cardizem, 240 mg daily; and metoprolol, 50 mg twice a day; however, at her follow-up office visit, her blood pressure is again elevated, and she complains that her breathing is heavy. Mrs. N is asked whether she is taking her medications, and she says, "Not all of them. They make me tired and I don't feel like myself."

The healthcare provider sits down with the patient and asks whether the patient knows what medicine is making her tired and learns what medicines the patient is taking. The healthcare provider explains with a picture how the high blood pressure is affecting Mrs. N's heart. She also tells the patient that there are many blood pressure medicines available, and by working together, she is sure that Mrs. N can feel better and have well-controlled blood pressure. Mrs. N agrees to keep a diary and return weekly. Within a few weeks, Mrs. N's blood pressure is controlled at 120–130/70–80, and she feels better. She has continued to do well over the past year and has had no evidence of heart failure.

WEB RESOURCES

American Association of Diabetic Educators
www.aadenet.org

American Diabetes Association
www.diabetes.org

American Heart Association
http://www.americanheart.org/downloadable/heart/
1166712318459HS_StatsInsideText.pdf.
AHA: www.americanheart.org

American Stroke Association
www.StrokeAssociation.org/Power

Black Women's Health Imperative
www.Blackwomenshealth.org

Centers for Disease Control and Prevention
www.cdc.gov/

Framingham Risk Calculator
http://circ.ahajournals.org/cgi/reprint/106/25/3143 [p 3230]

America on the Move: 100 Ways to Cut 100 Calories
www.americaonthemove.org

National Heart, Lung, and Blood Institute
Health Behavior Change: A Guide for Practitioners
www.nhlbi.gov/health/index.htm.

The DASH Diet
www.nhlbi.nih.gov/health/public/heart/hbp/dash/new_dash.pdf

Smoking Cessation Strategies for the 21st Century
http://circ.ahajournals.org/cgi/content/full/104/11/e51

Way2Quit
http://www.quit.com

REFERENCES

American Heart Association. (1997). Aspirin as a therapeutic agent in cardiovascular disease: a statement for healthcare professionals from the American Heart Association. *Circulation, 96,* 2751–2753.

American Heart Association. (2007a). Heart disease and stroke statistics: 2007 update. Dallas, TX. Retrieved June 14, 2007, from http://www.americanheart.org/downloadable/heart/1166712318459HS_StatsInsideText.pdf.

American Heart Association. (2007b). Primary prevention in the adult. Retrieved July 5, 2007, from http://www.americanheart.org/presenter.jhtml?identifier=4704.

American Heart Association. (2007c). Cigarette smoking and cardiovascular disease: AHA scientific position. Retrieved July 5, 2007, http://www.americanheart.org/presenter.jhtml?identifier=4545.

American Heart Association. (2007d). Smoking cessation. Retrieved June 14, 2007, from http://www.americanheart.org/presenter.jhtml?identifier=4731.

American Heart Association. (2007e). Cardiac rehabilitation. Retrieved July 8, 2007, from http://www.americanheart.org/presenter.jhtml?identifier=4490.

Appel, L. J., Brands, M. W., Daniels, S. R., Karanja, N., Elmer, P. J., & Sacks, F. M. (2006). Dietary approaches to prevent and treat hypertension: a scientific statement from the American Heart Association. *Hypertension, 47,* 296.

Bowles, D., Woodman, C., & Laughlin, M. (2000). Coronary smooth muscle and endothelial adaptations to exercise training. *Exercise and Sport Sciences Reviews, 28*(2), 57–62.

Buttaro, T. M., & Trybulski, J. (2008). The provider–patient relationship. In T. M. Buttaro, J. Trybulski, P. P. Bailey, & J. Sandberg-Cook (Eds.), *Primary care: a collaborative practice* (3rd ed.). St. Louis: Mosby.

Carnethon, M. R., Gulati, M., & Greenland, P. (2005). Prevalence and cardiovascular disease correlates of low cardiorespiratory fitness in adolescents and adults. *JAMA, 294,* 2981–2988.

Centers for Disease Control and Prevention. (2007a). Department of Health and Human Services. Overweight and obesity. Retrieved June 29, 2007, from http://www.cdc.gov/nccdphp/dnpa/obesity/index.htm.

Centers for Disease Control and Prevention. (2007b). National diabetes fact sheet. Retrieved July 10, 2007, from http://www.cdc.gov/diabetes/pubs/estimates05.htm#prev.

Chobanian, A. V., Bakris, G. L., Black, H. R., Cushman, W. C., Green, L. A., Izzo, J. L. Jr., Jones, D. W., Materson, B. J., Oparil, S., Wright, J. T. Jr., Roccella, E. J., et al. (2003). The seventh report of the Joint National Committee on Prevention, Detection, Evaluation, and Treatment of High Blood Pressure. *JAMA, 289,* 2560–2571.

DiClemente, C. C., Prochaska, J. O., Fairhurst, S. K., Velicer, W. F., Vekasquz, M. M., & Rossi, J. S. (1991). The process of smoking cessation: an analysis of precontemplation, contemplation, and preparation stages of change. *Journal of Consulting and Clinical Psychology, 59*(20), 295–304.

Falvo, D. R. (2004). *Effective patient education: a guide to increased compliance* (3rd ed.). Sudbury, MA: Jones and Bartlett.

Gordon, D., Fergus, P., Koo, J., & Takeuchi, R. K. (2007). Lifestyle assessment. In T. M. Buttaro, J. Trybulski, P. P. Bailey, & J. Sandberg-Cook (Eds.), *Primary care: a collaborative practice* (3rd ed.). St. Louis: Mosby.

Grundy, S. M., Cleeman, J. I., Bairey Merz, C. N., Brewer, H. B. Jr., Hunninghake, D. B., Pasternak, R. C., Smith, S. C. Jr., & Stone, N. J. (2004). Implications of recent clinical trials for National Education Program Adult Treatment Guidelines III. *Circulation, 110,* 227–239. Retrieved July 26, 2007, from http://www.nhlbi.nih.gov/guidelines/cholesterol/atp3upd04.pdf.

Hage, B. (2008). Health literacy. In T. M. Buttaro, J. Trybulski, P. P. Bailey, & J. Sandberg-Cook. (Eds.), *Primary care: a collaborative practice* (3rd ed.). St. Louis: Mosby.

Hoffmann, T., & Worrall, L. (2004). Designing effective written health education materials: considerations for health professional. *Disability and Rehabilitation, 26*(19), 1166–1173.

Institute of Medicine. (2001). *Crossing the quality chasm: a new health system for the 21st century.* Washington, DC: National Academies Press.

Jakicic, J. M., Wing, R. R., Butler, B. A., & Robertson, R. J. (1995). Prescribing exercise in multiple short bouts versus one continuous bout: effects on adherence, cardiorespiratory fitness, and weight loss in overweight women. *International Journal of Obesity, 19,* 893–901.

Jorenby, D. E. (2001). Smoking cessation strategies for the 21st century. *Circulation, 104,* e51.

Jorenby, D. E., Taylor, H., Rigotti, N. A., Azoulay, S., Watsky, E. J., Williams, K. E. Billing, C. B., Gong, J., Reeves, K. E. (2006). Efficacy of varenicline, an alpha-4 beta-2 nicotinic acetylcholine receptor partial agonist, vs. placebo or sustained-release bupropion for smoking cessation: a randomized controlled trial. *JAMA, 296,* 56–63.

Katz, J. R. (1997). Providing effective patient teaching. *American Journal of Nursing, 97*(5), 33–36.

Perry, C. K., & Bennett, J. A. (2006). Heart disease prevention in women: Promoting exercise. *Journal of the American Academy of Nurse Practitioners, 18*(12), 568–573.

Petersen, M., & Pedersen, B. (2005). The anti-inflammatory effect of exercise. *Journal of Applied Physiology, 98,* 1154–1162.

Peterson, J. A. (2007). Get moving! Physical activity counseling in primary care. *Journal of the American Academy of Nurse Practitioners, 19*(7), 349–357.

Pollock, M., Gaesser, G., Butcher, J., Despres, J., Dishman, R., Franklin, B. A., Garber, C. E. (1998). The recommended quantity and quality of exercise for developing cardiorespiratory and muscular fitness, and flexibility in healthy adults. *Medicine & Science in Sport & Exercise, 30*(6), 975–991.

Scott J. T., & Thompson, D. R. (2003). Assessing the information needs of post-myocardial infarction patients: a systematic review. *Patient Education and Counseling, 50*(2), 167–177.

Siegel, J. H. (2007). Obesity. In T. M. Buttaro, J. Trybulski, P. P. Bailey, & J. Sandberg-Cook (Eds.), *Primary care: a collaborative practice* (3rd ed.). St. Louis: Mosby.

Tonstad, S., Tennesen, P., Hajek, P., Williams, K. E., Billing, C., & Reeves, K. R. (2006). Effect of maintenance therapy with varenicline on smoking cessation: a randomized controlled trial. *JAMA, 296,* 64–71.

Tudor-Locke, C., & Bassett, D. R. (2004). How many steps/day are enough? Preliminary pedometer indices for public health. *Sports Medicine, 34*(1), 1–8.

U.S. Department of Health and Human Services. (2000, November). *Healthy people 2010: understanding and improving health* (2nd ed.). Washington, DC: U.S. Government Printing Office.

Chapter 26

Education for Patients and Families After Stroke: A Multifaceted Approach

Anne Marie Dupre & Lynn Foord

INTRODUCTION

Stroke is a major cause of disability in the United States, resulting in both temporary and permanent loss of function. The extent of disability varies from patient to patient and is dependent on the extent and location of the lesion, age, and any pre-existing chronic illnesses (Gordon et al., 2004; Vanetzian, 1997). For many stroke survivors, admission to a rehabilitative facility, outpatient care, and/or home care may be necessary to resume their premorbid level of functional mobility and psychosocial functioning. Physical rehabilitation often consists of neuromuscular re-education, retraining in functional mobility, and training in activities of daily living (ADLs). For many patients, speech therapy and retraining for cognition and perception may be necessary should deficits in these areas interfere with or delay a patient's recovery (Galaneau, 1993). Education is an essential part of any patient's rehabilitation throughout the continuum of care from the acute episode through discharge. Various forms of educational methods have been used in the care of patients with strokes, including written material, structured educational programs, individual education, and counseling.

In this chapter, we explore these many facets of instruction that are provided to patients and their families after a stroke. Instruction must be both written and verbal; instruction must address both knowledge and skills. Furthermore, the instruction must be directed toward both patients and families, and the instruction must be timed for when the patient and the family are ready to learn. Supportive education and coping skills must also be provided in the form of counseling, sometimes extending long after the patient has been discharged. The purpose of this chapter is to explore these many facets of instruction and how they can affect the successful outcome for stroke survivors and their families.

Written educational material is the most common medium addressed by the research and was the focus of most of the studies analyzed for this chapter. The advantages of written information are that it is consistent, reusable, and portable; it can be delivered in a flexible schedule, and it is amenable to a self paced learning style (Hoffman & McKenna, 2006). Despite these benefits, several studies have indicated that few patients, 26% (Hanger, Walker, Paterson, McBride, & Sainsbury, 1998) and 12% (Wellwood, Dennis, & Warlow, 1994), could recall receiving any written information. Studies of the effectiveness of written information as a stand-alone intervention for stroke patients and their caregivers reported inconclusive results (Hoffman & McKenna, 2006; Nolan, Nolan, & Booth, 2001). One obvious limitation of written educational material is that it can be effective only when it can be read and understood. Impaired reading ability may be found in patients who have suffered a stroke and have residual deficits such as aphasia, impaired cognition, and/or visual and perceptual impairments. Hoffman (2006) completed a study analyzing the reading ability of patients who had suffered a stroke and their caregivers. Based on their findings, they proposed recommendations for improving the written information for stroke education. Hoffman's findings indicated that (1) written information should be written at the lowest reading level possible (52% of the patients could not read beyond an eighth-grade level); (2) materials need to cover all stroke related topics and should be tailored to meet the individual needs of the patients and caregivers; and (3) written information should be paired with and reinforce verbal education. (See also Chapters 5 and 14 for more information about patient instruction.)

Successful physical rehabilitation requires motor learning. For motor learning to occur, the learner must construct both declarative memories, measured by verbal recall, and procedural memories, measured by the ability to perform a skillful movement. When skills such as dressing, bathing, transfers, bed mobility, and ambulation are practiced in therapy, the information or skills are stored as procedural memories, and the patient demonstrates learning by performing the skills independently. Learning that requires the patient to be consciously aware when processing the information, such as medication schedules or medication side effects, is stored as declarative memories. Research has indicated that the likelihood that someone will repeat a behavior learned, whether it is procedural or declarative, increases when there is positive reinforcement, when the learner rates the activity with moderate degree of difficulty (Vanetzian, 1997), and when the patient is motivated to solve a recognized problem (Mold, McKevitt, & Wolfe, 2003; Wachters-Kaufmann et al., 2005).

Ted's case demonstrates how declarative and procedural memories are used to promote learning successfully during his rehabilitation after a stroke.

Case Study 26-1

Ted is a 36-year-old male who suffered a right frontal parietal arteriovenous malformation (AVM) bleed while surfing on vacation in Oregon. He was medically stabilized and transferred to a rehabilitation facility for 3 weeks. He then received outpatient therapy with a focus on left lower extremity stability and functional mobility training.

Ted's rehabilitation is complicated by a complete left ACL tear that occurred 3 years ago without repair, hypertension, and a continued history of smoking (one pack a day). Ted is single, lives alone, has a supportive girlfriend, and works as a nurse at a local skilled nursing facility.

Ted's educational background as a nurse provided him with some declarative knowledge of stroke rehabilitation and associated risk factors. For example, Ted was able to explain when and how he used his ACL brace, indicating both declarative and procedural knowledge regarding his decision not to repair his ACL tear.

Given Ted's excellent background knowledge, the focus of his education after the stroke was on how to manage the effects of a stroke superimposed on a complete ACL tear. His rehabilitation team discussed why aggressive stability/mobility training would be critical to his return to work and his active lifestyle of surfing, fishing, diving, and hiking. He nodded and agreed to the goals that were mutually determined. Ted came to most appointments and worked hard; however, he continued to smoke, and he was not doing very much at home except watching television. Despite having developed mutually agreed-on goals with his rehabilitation team, Ted's lack of follow through indicated that effective learning had not occurred; therefore, a new approach was used to show Ted that even at this early stage of recovery his goals of hiking and walking on the beach were reasonable goals to attain. The new approach tapped into his procedural memory by having him walk on the treadmill at an incline to simulate hiking and having him walk on a large piece of soft foam without his shoes to simulate walking on the beach. Although Ted did experience lower-extremity instability and shortness of breath during these activities, the intent of these instructional activities was to help Ted problem solve what was required for him to get better while providing him with an activity that he would deem as moderately difficult. With a lot of positive reinforcement as he faced these challenges, Ted learned that his goals were achievable, and the rehabilitation team soon observed changes in his behavior.

In this example, Ted had to feel procedurally what it took to meet his goals and learn how to problem solve in order to achieve them. After the initial demonstration, every therapy session concluded with him "hiking" on the treadmill and "walking the beach" on the foam. Gradually, his speed and endurance for each activity increased. By the end of 10 weeks, Ted had made an appointment to talk with his physician regarding help to quit smoking, and he went on his first short hike with his girlfriend.

Ted was lucky. He had received immediate attention after his stroke, which limited the effects on his mobility to residual weakness, and he had no cognitive and/or perceptual deficits. Ted was young, and he had a valuable knowledge base to help him problem solve and make the appropriate changes in his behavior after the right educational approach was applied. Providing Ted with only written information or giving him another lecture would not have worked. Ted needed to experience that even though his goals were difficult to obtain they were achievable.

Steve's rehabilitation after his stroke was not as successful, even though the same principle of addressing both declarative and procedural learning was applied.

Case Study 26-2

> Steve is a 54-year-old male s/p right CVA with left hemiparesis. Impairments included left neglect and poor insight into his deficits. Past medical history includes alcohol abuse and smoking. He is divorced and lives alone. He has no children and he works as a cable repairman.

During Steve's rehabilitation, he demonstrated excellent motor recovery, similar to Ted, but his functional recovery was limited. While Ted's recovery was compromised because of a total ACL tear, Steve was limited by poor insight and left neglect. Because of his inattention, Steve would experience multiple falls while ambulating, requiring physical assistance from his therapist to prevent falling to the ground. As the time for Steve's discharge approached, the rehabilitation team recommended a supervised setting, and Steve became angry and very defensive. He would deny ever experiencing any loss of balance, making statements like "I've never fallen," "this would never happen at home," or "I will be just fine once I am home."

After many frustrating therapy sessions and family meetings, the physical therapist proposed a new teaching approach to help Steve experience his loss of balance. Now, during each treatment, when Steve experienced a loss of balance, the therapist would delay her assistance, allowing Steve to feel his lack of postural adjustment and hopefully recognize that he was about to fall. Despite weeks of such training and discussions with his rehabilitation team, Steve still insisted on going home alone. In this case, neither declarative nor procedural learning had occurred, despite the multiple attempts by all of the disciplines involved in Steve's rehabilitation. If Steve were to be successful at home, he would require insight into his limitations.

In Steve's case, there were significant differences between his expectations about his recovery and the expectations held by the health professionals who worked with him about his functional mobility and level of independence that he would be able to achieve. The health professional sees Steve as he is post stroke, with all of his accumulated deficits. Meanwhile, Steve sees himself only as he was before the stroke. Steve's perception is especially common among patients who have experienced frontal lobe damage and demonstrate poor insight into their disability as is occurring with Steve.

When the expectations held by the healthcare providers are significantly different from those held by the patient, it becomes quite difficult to develop meaningful goals for the patient and his or her family. The difficulty in Steve's case as in others like it relates to the patient's learning readiness. It may be that Steve is not ready to learn new skills and make changes in his life at this time. After a stroke, barriers to patient's readiness to learn can be temporary or permanent. The most common barriers include depression, a lack of insight or denial of functional limitations, perceptual deficits such as left neglect, anxiety, cognitive impairment, and aphasia; however, one of the problems in today's healthcare system is that teaching occurs at the convenience of the insurance companies and hospitals, which may not coincide with the patient's readiness to learn. If Steve could be given more time to practice in the hospital or at home with trained family members, it is possible that there could be sufficient healing and learning to improve his functional outcome.

Steve's case demonstrates how after a stroke patients may not only lose mobility because of a hemiparesis, but they may also experience cognitive and perceptual deficits that can affect the length of their rehabilitation and their ultimate functional outcome (Galaneau, 1993; Zinn et al., 2004). In a systematic review (Palmer & Glass, 2003) to determine the predictors of disability after stroke, social support was found to be among the most robust and consistent predictors of poststroke functional recovery. It has also been reported that the availability of caregivers is associated with improved mobility (Palmer & Glass, 2003) and improved ADLs (Anderson et al., 2002) because of the emotional support coming from the caregiver.

It has been shown that a network of family support (Palmer & Glass, 2003) and sufficient family income (Kendall & Terry, 1996) lower the risk of long-term placement for many patients. In many instances, in order for patients who have survived a stroke to be discharged home, a supportive family is usually indicated (Mold, McKevitt, & Wolfe, 2003; Palmer & Glass, 2003; Visser-Meily et al., 2005).

Family support is not only about providing encouragement to maximize recovery of muscle strength, range of motion (ROM), or functional mobility; for many patients going home, it is also about changing pre-established family roles and responsibilities to provide the necessary physical and emotional support needed for the patient's successful return to the home setting. Family members may find it difficult to change their roles and identity, especially if the patient is aphasic or has cognitive deficits that require the caregiver to adjust their communication. Changing the dynamics within the family may be a very difficult process for both the patient and the caregivers. For example, if prior to the stroke the patient was primarily responsible for transportation, finances, and home maintenance, these roles and responsibilities might now have to be transferred to the caregiver, leaving the patient feeling powerless and the caregiver overwhelmed. The challenge is to create an environment that balances care with assistance, while encouraging the stroke survivor to regain independence.

Robert's case is an example of a successful discharge to home where teaching was provided to the patient and a supportive network of family and friends acted as caregivers.

Case Study 26-3

Robert is an 81-year-old male with a resolving left cerebrovascular accident (CVA), expressive aphasia, dysphasia, left neglect, and right hemiparesis. His past medical history is significant for hypertension, coronary artery disease

(CAD), myocardial infarction, and coronary artery bypass graft (CABG) x3. It is 2.5 months after insult, and Robert has shown little motor return in his right arm and leg. Because of difficulty swallowing, he continues to require tube feedings. He is nonambulatory and requires assistance for all mobility and ADL skills.

Robert has a supportive wife who is also 81 years old and is fragile; she cannot provide any physical assistance for Robert. Before his stroke, Robert took care of their finances and was responsible for all driving, shopping, yard work, home repairs, vacuuming, and laundry. Robert has a strong network of friends, siblings, children, and grandchildren who live locally.

Robert's family and friends insisted on a home discharge, despite his limited recovery and the significant level of care that he would require at home. It was their insistence and their dedication to come in everyday and learn how to assist Robert and support him and his wife that made this discharge a success. This family considered the care of Robert and his wife as their responsibility. They met with nursing to learn about medications and feedings, with nutrition to talk about diet, and with physical and occupational therapy to learn about the equipment and physical assistance that would be required.

Although all families go through a similar preparation before discharge, what made this potentially difficult discharge a success was the ability of everyone involved to organize themselves to assume their new role in the care of their father, grandfather, or friend. They found friends to make meals, involved the children in the physical care of their father, and paid for help when the family could not contribute. More important than the physical care that was provided was their emotional support for Robert. They had a way of making Robert feel important and in control at a time when he had lost all of his independence and control. A poignant example of their support was their involvement in the one thing Robert loved the most, the Boston Red Sox. For most games throughout the season, someone would come by and spend time with him in watching the game. This activity allowed Robert and his family to see him as he was before the stroke—a big Red Sox fan. This small activity empowered Robert because it was not about his stroke or lack of independence but about sharing his love for the game with his friends and family, just as he had done before his stroke.

A key element in the success of this case was that the family involvement was initiated before Robert's discharge home. This gave the family time to understand and prepare for their level of commitment and their new roles and responsibilities while still relying on the rehabilitation staff to care for their father. Another key element that was perhaps more important than the family's acceptance of their new role was Robert's acceptance of his disability. His acceptance of his new role allowed him to focus on what was important to him: spending time with his family and friends and, of course, watching the Red Sox. After Robert had accepted his disability and his family saw him being happy again, their feelings of sadness, grief, fear, and anger at their father's disability began to dwindle, and it became easier for them to assume their new roles and responsibilities.

Robert's case would have turned out differently if he had been depressed and/or if his family had not been able to accept their parent's disability. Ruth's case demonstrates an example of this where the discharge home did not go well.

Case Study 26-4

> Ruth is a 79-year-old female who suffered a left CVA with impairments, including aphasia, right neglect, thalamic mutism, and right hemiparesis. Her past medical history is significant for hypertension, chronic obstructive pulmonary disease, and severe osteoarthritis of both knees. In addition, Ruth is extremely hard of hearing.
>
> It has been 4 months since the insult, and Ruth has demonstrated minimal motor return and functional mobility, and she continues to be nonambulatory secondary to the severe osteoarthritis in both knees. Before the stroke, Ruth lived in the independent living section of an assisted-living facility. She has a supportive daughter and son who work full time and live locally.

Ruth's therapy and prognosis were very similar to Robert's, and she worked with the same rehabilitation team. Although Ruth demonstrated little functional return, her family insisted on taking her home. The family expected that their mom would walk and insisted that walking should be a focus of therapy. The rehabilitation team had many discussions with the family about why ambulation was too painful for Ruth given her limited knee range of motion and pain from the severe osteoarthritis. The team tried to explain that walking would be even more difficult for Ruth now given her decreased strength and endurance because of the stroke. In response, the family would just acknowledge that their mom always had pain and persisted that "we just have to work through it." Thus, the therapist decided to invite the family to therapy to see their mom's limitations, pain, and struggles. The family came to several therapy sessions, and despite what they saw and the verbal explanations offered by the rehabilitation team, the family chose to ignore the team's recommendation and instead spent their time encouraging their mom to stand despite her pain, cries, and closed eyes. In this case, despite multiple attempts, the family could still not accept their mom's disability.

In Ruth's case, like Steve's, the expectations of the family were different from the expectations of healthcare providers. To the rehabilitation team, it is as if the family is seeing their mom without the deficits from her stroke. For Ruth's family, a successful outcome in rehabilitation was defined as walking; when this was not achieved, they saw their mom's therapy as a failure.

Even though her rehabilitation outcome was not what they had expected, Ruth's family did take their mom home with numerous home care services; however, after about 2 months, when the home care services started to dwindle, Ruth started to show a decline, and she was readmitted to the hospital. It is not unusual during the early stages of discharge when all services are in place for the family to feel a somewhat false sense of support. Within several months of returning home from the hospital, social support networks tend to diminish, leaving the family and the patient isolated at a time when support is most critical to a positive outcome following the stroke (Kendall et al., 2007). This sense of isolation may compound the overwhelming nature of the situation, leading to psychological difficulties and potentially catastrophic outcomes (Watson & Quinn, 1998). Research has suggested that it takes 1 or 2 years after stroke recovery for psychological and social outcomes to stabilize while many supportive services are cut back after several months (Kendall et al., 2007).

This sense of feeling overwhelmed and isolated may also occur for Robert's family, despite the success of his discharge. Although Robert's social network was large, it was really one daughter who took charge to organize both the physical and the emotional components of her parents' care. This is an overwhelming responsibility for one person, and it was likely that she would sooner or later require some counseling. Ideally, the goal would be for Robert to take on more of the responsibility of his care gradually, perhaps communicating and coordinating part of his care and needs. A gradual shift of responsibilities in this direction would decrease his daughter's stress and increase his own level of independence and power in the family.

There are few studies on the effects of education and counseling for patients and families after discharge. In one controlled study (Evans, Matlock, Bishop, Stranahan, & Pederson, 1988), families receiving counseling and education demonstrated less deterioration of problem solving and communication compared with controls. Counseling also appeared to support the benefits of education and resulted in better patient adjustment at 1 year (Hoffman & McKenna, 2006; Palmer & Glass, 2003). Visser-Meily et al. (2005) in a systematic review showed that up to 3 years after a stroke, counseling increased confidence and knowledge about patient care and provided active coping strategies that most likely led to positive outcomes.

The amount of time that patients spend in both inpatient and outpatient rehabilitation has become shorter and shorter, which means that families are being asked to do more and more with less help than before. This increased burden may cause families to feel overwhelmed, disempowered, and depressed (Palmer & Glass, 2003). More research is needed to learn about the impact on patient care and family function of shorter stays in rehabilitation along with decreases in community services.

In the meantime, it is important for healthcare providers to consider the many facets of education that can improve their patient's recovery and support the family. Although rehabilitation time is limited, we must be prepared to offer verbal and written instructions that address both declarative and procedural learning. We must be attentive to the readiness of both patients and their supportive family members to learn new skills, new roles, and new responsibilities. We may need to creatively structure our time with patients to provide the instruction they need at the time they are best able to absorb it and implement it. Finally, we must continue to advocate for access to counseling for patients and families when it can help to improve their ability to cope successfully with the effects of the stroke.

Clinicians have many skills that we can provide to our patients, and when we include the many facets of patient and family education as part of our care, we can significantly increase the patient's ultimate return to his or her highest possible level of independence as well as the family's ability to support their loved one along the way.

REFERENCES

Anderson, H., Erikson, K., Brown, A., Schultz-Larsen, K., & Forchhammer, B. (2002). Follow-up services for stroke survivors after hospital discharge: a randomized control study. *Clinical Rehabilitation, 16,* 593–603.

Evans, R. L., Matlock, A., Bishop, D. S., Stranahan, A., & Pederson, C. (1988). Family intervention after stroke: does counseling or education help? *Stroke, 19,* 1243–1249.

Galaneau, L. (1993). An interdisciplinary approach to mobility and safety education for caregivers and stroke patients. *Rehabilitation Nursing, 18*(6), 395–399.

Gordon, N., Gulanick, M., Costa, F., Fletcher, G., Franklin, B., Roth, E., & Shepard, T. (2004). Physical activity and exercise recommendations for stroke survivors: an American Heart Association scientific statement from the Council on Clinical

Cardiology, Subcommittee on Exercise, Cardiac Rehabilitation, and Prevention; the Council on Cardiovascular Nursing; the Council on Nutrition, Physical Activity, and Metabolism; and the Stroke Council. *Stroke Journal of the American Heart Association, 35,* 1230–1240.

Hanger, H., Walker, C., Paterson, L., McBride, S., & Sainsbury, R. (1998).What do patients and their carers want to know about stroke? A two-year follow-up study. *Clinical Rehabilitation, 12,* 45–52.

Hoffman, T., & McKenna, K. (2006). Analysis of stroke patients' and carers' reading ability and the content and design of written materials: recommendations for improving written stroke information. *Patient Education and Counseling, 60,* 286–293.

Kendall, E., & Terry, D. (1996). Psychosocial adjustment following closed head injury: a model for predicting outcome. *Neuropsychological Rehabilitation, 6,* 16–23.

Kendall, E., Catalano, T., Kuipers, P., Posner, N., Buys, N., & Charker, J. (2007). Recovery following stroke: the role of self-management education. *Social Science and Medicine, 64,* 735–746.

Mold, F., McKevitt, C., & Wolfe, C. (2003). A review and commentary of the social factors which influence stroke care: issues of inequality in qualitative literature. *Health and Social Care in the Community, 11,* 405–414.

Nolan, J., Nolan, M., & Booth, A. (2001). Developing the nurse's role in patient education: rehabilitation as a case example. *International Journal of Nursing Studies, 38,* 163–173.

Palmer, S., & Glass, T. (2003). Family function in stroke recovery: a review. *Rehabilitation Psychology, 48,* 255–265.

Vanetzian, E. (1997). Learning readiness for patient teaching in stroke rehabilitation. *Journal of Advanced Nursing, 26,* 589–594.

Visser-Meily, A., Heugten, C., Post, M., Schepers, V., & Lindeman, E. (2005). Intervention studies for caregivers of stroke patients: a critical review. *Patient Education and Counseling, 56,* 257–267.

Wachters-Kaufmann, C., Schuling, J., The, H., & Meyboom-de-Jong, B. (2005). Actual desired information provision after a stroke. *Patient Education and Counseling, 56,* 211–217.

Watson, L. D., & Quinn, D. (1998). Stages of stroke. *British Journal of Nursing, 7,* 631–640.

Wellwood, I., Dennis, M., & Warlow, C. (1994). Perceptions and knowledge of stroke among surviving patients with stroke and their carers. *Age Ageing, 23,* 293–298.

Zinn, S., Dudley, T., Bosworth, H., Hoenig, H., Duncan, P., & Horner, R. (2004). The effect of poststroke cognitive impairment on the rehabilitation process and functional outcome. *Archives of Physical Medicine Rehabilitation, 85,* 1084–1090.

Chapter 27

The Cancer Patient: Adult and Child

Susan DeCristofaro, Judith I. Balboni, & Martha Young

INTRODUCTION

In spite of the increase in early detection and advancements in treatment, cancer is still a life-altering experience that is now recognized as a chronic illness. For the adult and pediatric patient, the trajectory of treatment can vary from days to weeks and/or from months to years. Technical information highways enhance patient learning, and the quest for information ensures a patient's right to informed consent. In the new millennium, standard treatments include surgery, radiation, and chemotherapy; however, various other fields of research, including the Human Genome Project, HIV research, angiogenesis inhibitors, immunotherapy, monoclonal antibodies, brachytherapy, vaccines, and sentinel node biopsies, bring new discoveries that are changing the once terminal prognosis of days past.

Inherent in the role of the healthcare provider is patient and family education. Materials available through the National Cancer Institute, the American Cancer Society, the Cancer Patient Education Network (CPEN), and the Lance Armstrong Foundation are only a few of the resources available to support this essential education.

This chapter offers practical guidance for the healthcare provider who is currently in or transitioning to an education role in oncology. Also discussed are the importance and development of a learning resource center for adults and a program using dramatic art to educate both adults and children, as well as a prevention model for teaching smoking cessation to young adults in the community.

THE ROLE OF CANCER PATIENT EDUCATOR

Entering the field of patient education is not foreign to healthcare providers. Providers seek to educate patients and to support and help patients care for themselves. They inform patients and families about disease and chronic illness, a variety of medical tests and procedures, and the types and complexities of treatment. Instruction on what to expect, what to look for, what to report, and when to seek further medical attention is essential. The nurse who educates about cancer, treatment regimens, and follow-up will have an effect on how patients carry out their activities of daily living, as well as the psychosocial impact the illness has on the patient and family.

There are many facets of patient education in cancer care. They encompass knowledge of the disease process, chemotherapy protocols, medications, clinical trials, side-effect management, and supportive care. The role of the educator includes a tremendous amount of psychosocial understanding and interaction with patients and families. The healthcare provider helps the patient to understand the cancer diagnosis, its treatment, and possible outcomes. The provider will witness a profound impact on the coping mechanisms of the patient, loved ones, and caregivers.

Healthcare providers who have excelled in another specialty can bring their clinical skills and experience to the transition to oncology (Saca-Hazboun, 2007). Transitioning to oncology requires mentoring and attention to technical, physical, and psychological skills (Saca-Hazboun, 2007). Working with a preceptor or having a mentor relationship with an experienced provider in the field fosters the transition into the new role.

Transitioning from a field where one is accomplished can sometimes bring anxiety about being discovered as less than expert in the new role. This process, also known as imposter phenomenon (Clance & Imes, 1978), was first described as a feeling of phoniness typically experienced by women who are high achievers. Today, this term refers to the "normal temporary experience that occurs when a professional transitions from a position with a high level of competency to a new one" (Saca-Hazboun, 2007).

Several other resources are available to nurses transitioning to the field of cancer care or education that are extremely valuable. In addition to orientation and professional development courses offered by an employer, continuing education courses offered by professional oncology organizations can help to establish a foundation of knowledge. One organization is the Oncology Nurses Society (ONS), which offers courses such as Radiation Oncology and Chemotherapy and Biotherapy. There are resources at the ONS website that cover a wide spectrum of subjects to further the nurse's oncology knowledge.

The CPEN provides cancer patient educators with additional resources and support. CPEN promotes best practice models and patient education resources to colleagues. CPEN provides a source of support for networking and sharing with other healthcare professionals and adult and pediatric patient educators. Additional materials for patient education instruction are the National Cancer Institute's *Trainer's Guide for Cancer Education* and the ONS's *Advocacy in Health Care: Teaching Patients, Caregivers, and Professionals.*

It is essential to be aware of the multitude of patient education resources available to patients and families in order to assist them with obtaining the information that they need to manage a cancer diagnosis. The provider will need to explore the wide variety of resources available on cancer information websites, in professional journals, books, pamphlets, and magazines, as well as to stay abreast of state and regional cancer support groups and disease-centered organizations. It is essential to stay informed, join professional list-serve groups, and subscribe to newsletters produced by various cancer-related groups. These efforts can help keep the nurse current and in step with the daily issues and concerns faced by oncology patients and their families.

EDUCATING THE PEDIATRIC CANCER PATIENT

Chemotherapy, radiation, stem cell transplant, hair loss, isolation, and fatigue are, too say the least, atypical experience for most children and adolescents. With missed opportunities on the baseball team and absences from school, the healthcare team works diligently to create supportive programs and normative childhood experiences. Education is a common aspect of childhood. For many, it starts in preschool and continues for the next 14 to 18 years. How do healthcare providers translate the natural ability of children to learn new concepts with the foreign experiences of diagnosis and treatment? This is often the goal of child life specialists, nurses, and other healthcare providers working with the pediatric oncology population.

A family resource center can provide an environment to foster learning. Information can be centralized with easy access to computers and comfortable places to read. A resource center can provide a place for patients and their family members to find support and empowerment through information. A wide variety of classes can be offered, both to educate parents and to provide opportunities for exploring integrative therapies such as yoga, art, or music. A cooking class, for example, can provide patients and their siblings the opportunity to create healthy snacks for themselves, enjoying the process at a time when there can be many struggles related to eating. Parents have the opportunity to talk with a nutritionist, to look through brochures and cookbooks, and to use other parents as a resource helping them to realize that they are not alone while coping with their child's food issues.

If the creation of a family resource center for your pediatric population is not a reality, there are many other ways that you can create a learning environment in your healthcare facility: create mobile resource carts, hold classes in conference rooms, advertise programs on fliers in exam rooms or on plasma screens in waiting areas, design creative displays within the institute, or make toolkits of information to bring to patients. Whether staffing a resource room or a mobile education program, the following text will highlight the unique skill set needed to educate pediatric cancer patients and their family members effectively.

PLAY AS AN EDUCATIONAL TOOL

Play has a crucial role in the development of children from birth through adolescence. Play may foster both fine and gross motor development as well as promote intellectual development by encouraging problem solving, perspective taking, language development, exploration, logic, and memory (Isenberg & Quisenberry, 2002). Children approximately 7 to 12 years old, for instance, may enjoy games based on rules, as it helps develop logical thought. Play also creates opportunities for children to develop socially and often leads to the development of compromising skills, resources for coping with disagreements, and the opportunity to explore social roles. When children begin elementary school, previous experiences with other children have hopefully provided them with the social skills needed to engage in cooperative play (Thompson & Standford, 1981). Finally, play is a crucial tool for the child in navigating emotional development. Through activities alone and with others, children are able to express themselves, practice how to manage feelings, and may learn to care and empathize with others.

Play is not only essential for children at home and in school; it is also crucial for children in medical settings. Healthcare play has benefits in addition to fostering normative development. Play may help children express their fears and anxieties, reveal misconceptions about medical care, provide the child with a sense of mastery and control over their environment, and promote communication with others in an atmosphere that can be isolating (Gaynard et al., 1998). Play is a resource that when tapped by educators can act as a springboard for learning. Many of the fundamental qualities coincide with what we hope are the benefits of patient education: exploration, interaction, creativity, and understanding. With complex medical procedures and concepts to explain, play is pivotal. We can help children translate life experiences, even complicated ones like cranial radiation, through play.

Some medical play may be nondirected, or child led; let children experiment with safe medical equipment such as stethoscopes, blood pressure cuffs, bandages, and medical tape. As they practice cleaning an injection site or pretending to put on EMLA cream, they are making meaning of their medical experiences. Educators can also create opportunities to teach through directed medical play. As children experiment, introduce sequential steps of a procedure or suggest methods of coping such as deep breathing. Allowing children to play the role of the doctor or nurse may help them to comprehend better a procedure, lessen anxiety, and further empower the child. Such complex theories, treatments, and procedures can be taught through play before children have the language to comprehend them.

Just as a preschool classroom has an area for experimental play, so should your pediatric resource center. Substitute the child-sized kitchen appliances for child-sized exam tables and dolls with central lines or prosthetic limbs. Instead of a dollhouse, provide a hospital or clinic with plastic medical equipment. There are countless ways to provide opportunities for medical play. Patients might make a collage with medical equipment, or use plastic syringes for water play or painting.

Using play as a method of implementing education to the pediatric cancer patient is an invaluable tool. It is essential that all healthcare providers working with this population gain awareness of the power of play to maximize both teaching and learning.

CHILD DEVELOPMENT

Rapid physical, social, emotional, and cognitive development occurs during childhood. When familiarizing pediatric patients with the healthcare experiences that they may encounter, educators must have a keen knowledge of normative child development to provide accurate and appropriate explanations, images, medical equipment, or models.

Having a port-a-catheter placed, for instance, is often one of the first surgeries for pediatric oncology patients. Regardless of the patient's age, healthcare providers should spend time explaining the sequence, nature, and reason for the procedure. The type and amount of information shared when educating patients about a port-a-catheter placement, however, will vary depending on age and stage of development. Educators working with a 4-year-old patient would likely spend more time emphasizing what the port looks like, so that when it is under the skin, the typically imaginative preschooler has a realistic understanding of its appearance and use. Educators working with an adolescent patient might focus on explaining what their chest might look like after surgery, perhaps using pictures of other adolescent patients: where it will be placed, its small size, and what the scar might look like. For this population, acknowledgment of appearance concerns is critical at a time when acceptance from peers and body image are typical worries.

With cognitive development in mind, language use is another facet that should be given careful consideration. Terms used by adults in the medical field do not always translate to patients, especially children. Such misconceptions can cause great anxiety. It is important for an educator to be aware of literal interpretations of the terms such as "dressing change" or "draw labs." Confusion can be avoided by taking the time to explain, "Next they will take off your bandage and put on a new one" or "take a small amount of your blood for testing."

The treatment of cancer includes many complex procedures that may be very difficult to explain in child friendly terms. When educating pediatric patients and family members, explain the purpose for the procedure and how long it might take; describe the procedure step by step and plan and rehearse coping strategies. When simplifying complex medical language, remember to use simple language that includes sensory information, how things might feel, smell, or sound (Gaynard et al., 1998). Describing Betadine as brown and explaining that EMLA cream might feel cold are important sensory experiences to review when educating pediatric oncology patients about lumbar punctures, for example. Injecting lidocaine, one step in many lumbar punctures, might be translated, as "this medicine might feel warm when it goes in. It will make the area on your back numb so that nothing hurts."

It is essential for educators to be aware of and to consider the various stages of growth and development when planning teaching opportunities in order to minimize fear and anxiety and to maximize coping. This will not only make the experience better for the patient and family but also for the person delivering the care.

FAMILY-CENTERED CARE

Family-centered care is an innovative approach to the planning, delivery, and evaluation of health care that is grounded in mutually beneficial partnerships among healthcare patients, families, and providers (The Institute for Family-Centered Care, 2007). When a child, adolescent, or adult is diagnosed with cancer, the entire family is involved. Educators need to assure that resources are available for everyone: children, teens, siblings, parents, grandparents, boyfriends, aunts, and others.

Parents in particular have a unique role as caregivers. They frequently carry a great deal of responsibility in making treatment choices for their child. Parents often want to gather as much information as possible in making those decisions. Patient education materials need to reflect these needs. Teaching classes, facilitating search requests for information, and providing materials on support for caregivers can help ease this burden. Of additional benefit is connecting families with one another, either informally in a resource center, or formally through support groups at the hospital, online, or over the telephone.

Educators should also play a role in providing the siblings of pediatric oncology patients with the resources they need. Using medical play to teach about new treatments and procedures will not only empower the sibling but may also clear up misconceptions about their brother or sister's medical experiences. Many resources are also available, such as books written from the point of view of siblings, summer camp opportunities, and support organizations such as SuperSibs (www.supersibs.org).

Not only must an educator recognize the needs of different members of a family—an educator must recognize the needs of different families. Materials must be accessible in a variety of languages and education levels. If not available, work with your interpreter services department to create new materials. Providing equal access to information is critical. Families that, unfortunately, are used to struggling to locate resources will find it comforting to find information easily as a patient.

CREATING A PATIENT FAMILY INTERACTIVE RESOURCE CENTER

The creation of a learning resource place such as a kiosk, small room, or a more established large center should provide easy access to reliable and state-of-the-art oncology-related information. Many resource centers have brochures, medical reference texts, computers for Internet searches, books,

DVDs, and videotapes for loan. Planning for a learning resource center depends on the needs of the institution or community office practice, the patients served, funding, designated space, and staff. Direct administration may arise from the nursing education department or, if in a larger institution, the patient family education department. Day-to-day operations are most often supervised and staffed by a registered nurse, a strong administrative staff, and trained volunteers. In the pediatric oncology setting, a child life specialist can offer leadership and expertise.

The location of the learning center depends on the services that will be provided, as well as the mission of the institution or practice. In a large hospital or clinic, the center is frequently within the lobby or near public access. An ideal space will lend itself to multiple venues including support groups, classes, and quiet reading or meditation space and uses background music to promote a peaceful milieu.

When faced with limited staffing resources, consider graduate or undergraduate student interns to supplement work demands. Volunteers can also be an excellent resource to staff; however, they may require supervision. There are many talents and skills a volunteer can bring to the learning resource center. Volunteers will need training usually provided by a nurse and other members of the oncology health team. Creating a DVD of a live taped formal training will allow additional volunteers to be oriented at different points of the year. A plan for competency testing and continuing education offers further best practice. Having the novice volunteer shadow experienced volunteers is helpful in the outpatient and especially the inpatient setting.

Budget and Funding

In planning for a center, two distinct budgets should be considered. Start-up costs include staff, books, computers, and resource materials, followed by costs to keep operations current. To be prudent, one should start with a small operation with room to grow, rather than have the center run out of funds. Working with development personnel is critical in the planning for necessary funding to begin and for ongoing operations of the center to continue. Staff can promote programs, hang fliers, and create displays, but having families share a book they found helpful or pictures of their Make a Wish trip is the best advertisement available. Constructing a welcoming, comfortable, and fun environment in the resource center creates a space where learning is shared on a daily basis. Staff is available to facilitate these conversations and provide knowledge and access to resources.

Staffing a resource center that is accessible to all means dialoging with interdisciplinary staff to provide optimal support of the patient and collaborating with outside organizations, both on a national and local level. Although there is much to be considered, in the author's experience the most critical task is creating a supportive environment. If your family resource center contains only books and computers, the only people that will use the information are information seekers. What about parents that are not sure how to help their child in school but are too shy to ask? What about the sister that wants to meet other siblings but is not sure whether there is a place for her?

Scope of Services

An effective resource center should provide the means for patient empowerment through education, access to information, opportunities to develop mutually supportive relationships with other patients and their families, and outreach to clients of the larger community. A cancer diagnosis generates the need for information. Regardless of the patient's age, collaborating patient learning needs with the healthcare team is needed throughout treatment. The resource center cannot work in a "silo." A reference room and/or lending library should provide patients and families with a comfortable place to learn about their illness, explore treatment options, and become familiar with supportive resources. A private consult room within the center will provide the space necessary for one-on-one teaching, consultation, meditation, DVD, or video reviewing and effective emotional support.

A center should provide information covering a broad spectrum of oncology-related resources:

- Books catalogued by diagnosis and/or brochures by subject
- DVDs, audiovisual materials, and computers
- Educational classes (i.e., introduction to treatment, blood counts, advanced directives)
- Recommended updated websites in a handout and bookmarked on the computer
- Foreign language materials
- Reference medical texts
- CDs for listening and relaxation

Suggestions for sections or divisions of information include the following:

- Cancer prevention
- Caregiver support
- Chemotherapy fact sheets

- Clinical trials
- Diet and nutrition
- Disease-specific information, general cancer, and specific types
- Employment and financial issues
- Explaining cancer to children
- Genetics
- Hospice corner and bereavement for both children and adults
- Inspirational and spiritual concerns
- Integrated therapies
- Palliative care
- Stress management and survivorship
- Symptom management

Tracking patron visits and detailing how many people visit the learning space can be helpful to capture data on visitors who use the resource center. Electronic counters are available to record patrons if volunteers or staff cannot attend to the center.

Circulation Services

One of the most important decisions will be to determine whether any or all of the learning center materials will be available for circulation. A policy and procedure manual can be developed to specify who may borrow and which items may circulate. Establish whether the loan library is for patients or open to the community. A regional center with patients traveling long distances might offer lending privileges over many weeks and a mail return system. A library management system should allow bar code scanning of materials, which is useful in high-volume learning resource centers. Whether or not you are working in a dedicated cancer hospital or in a general hospital within a unit specific to hematology oncology patients, creating a learning resource space is possible.

Criteria for the Selection of Materials

Based on set materials selection criteria, patrons should be made aware that not all materials are appropriate. The ability to access print or computerized information does not imply approval, recommendation, or endorsement of the host facility. This is to release the learning center from liability and to encourage patients to ask the nurse or healthcare provider any specific patient-related questions. A process for reviewing challenged materials should be established.

This is an example of a disclaimer:

> The resource center staff members do not monitor and have no control over the information accessed through the Internet. The Internet offers access to many valuable sources of information; however, not all sources on the Internet provide current, accurate, or complete information. We encourage you to be a critical information consumer by evaluating the information you receive from the Internet rigorously. You may ask a staff person for specific Internet sites that deal with evaluation.

The following criteria may be used to evaluate reference materials:

- Medical accuracy
- Credibility
- Sponsorship/authorship
- Content
- Audience
- Disclosure

Internet Use and Warning Signs

Online information can be misleading, making it difficult to know what online information to trust. The Pew Internet Project's "On Line Health Search 2006" report found that 80% of American users, or about 113 million adults, have searched for health information online. The U.S. Federal Trade Commission has developed a list of the following claims that bring suspicion:

- Claims of scientific breakthrough
- Claims that a product can cure a range of illnesses, including cancer
- Case histories of people who have had amazing results but with no scientific basis
- Claims of a "money-back" guarantee

Consumers may use general-purpose engines rather than medical sites or portals to find information. It is therefore prudent to use criteria to evaluate websites before listing suggestions for patients and families:

- Any good health-related website should make known the party responsible for the site information. Many health sites post information collected from other websites—original sources should be clearly labeled. Websites should have a policy on how they link to other sites. Unless you are actively reviewing all websites, aim for conservative sites for patients to use. Several websites are listed at the end of this chapter, but the letters at the end of the URL address offer a clue about who runs a site.

- ○ .edu is an education system
- ○ .org is nonprofit
- ○ .com is usually run by commercial for profit or private source
- ○ .gov denotes a federal government sponsored site

- For medical information, professional and scientific qualification is needed. Websites that do not list the company name, physical address, phone number, or contact information are usually not credible.
- Information should be continuously reviewed and updated. Even if the information remains unchanged, site owners should ensure timely valid reviews.
- Avoid chat rooms. Chat room discussions are frequently not supervised.
- Know how the site pays for its existence. Sites that sell products or are sponsored by a drug company will need an established policy on the ethical concerns that surround those issues.

Code of Ethics

The code of ethics describes the values and responsibilities of the staff of the center, providing the highest level of service to patrons regardless of race, color, creed, and so forth. The American Library Association, the American Nurses Association, and the Medical Library Association have examples of ethical standards a learning center may adopt.

Choosing Items for Collection

With the large amount of consumer resources available, it can be difficult to choose the most authoritative titles. Here are some suggestions:

- Materials can be obtained at no cost from the National Cancer Institute, the American Cancer Society, the Leukemia and Lymphoma Society, the Lance Armstrong Association, and numerous other nonprofit associations.
- The date of publication is important, especially if the resource discusses treatment. Nothing treatment related over 5 years old is recommended.
- Look for reviews from other respected organizations. Reviews from *Library Journal* and Doody's are excellent resources.

- CAPAIS, a consumer and health information section of the Medical Library Association, provides a website on how to set up and operationalize a consumer health library.

When reviewing patient education materials, consider low literacy and plain language:

- Content should be limited to essential information.
- Literacy or plain language suggests a reading level at sixth grade or lower.
- Graphics should promote white space, bullets, and larger font size.
- The material should encourage the reader to interact and should be stimulating.
- The material should be culturally appropriate and presented in a positive manner.

Leading Patrons to Your Center

To help guide visitors to the resource center, there should be mention of the location of the center listed at all entrances, stairwells, and elevators and eye-catching signage. If you have a pediatric room, a banner or flag helps to bring parent awareness. A glass door opens visibility, as do lights, music, window displays, and an LCD screen promoting class events, trivia questions, and support group listings. An 800 number assists those traveling from outside the local neighborhood. A link to the main institute call center will help assist patients in navigating the hospital or ambulatory care center.

Creating welcoming events compels people to enter the center. Book talks with the author present, and light refreshments add a hub of activity and a welcoming milieu. Interfacing with clinicians for luncheon get-togethers or small department staff meetings in the center encourages clinician buy-in. A patient orientation class will grab the attention of patients, families, and different departments. Offering a weekly orientation class as well as by appointment classes brings high visibility and immediate patient family satisfaction.

Program Evaluation

Program evaluation is a necessary process that helps to determine how the program meets its goals. When planning a resource center, consider how program services will be evaluated. Potential costs can be added to the operating budget and issues regarding statistics, and staff responsibilities can be identified for future consideration. A patient survey form might be developed as a postage-paid mailer. Suggestion survey questions might include the following:

- Was this your first visit?
- What resources did you use?
- How would you rate the helpfulness of the staff?
- Do you feel your interactions were handled confidentially?
- Please list the topics of information you received.
- Would you recommend the resource room to other people?
- Are you a patient, friend of a patient, patient from another institution, spouse, or another family member?
- Please indicate classes and education topics of interest.
- Would you like your name on our mailing list?
- Other comments

Members of CPEN have shared lessons learned in the process of developing and managing a cancer learning resource center that can be helpful advice and pearls of wisdom (**Table 27-1**).

Table 27-1 Shared Lessons from CPEN Members

Staff and Volunteers

- Your staff, whether paid or volunteer, is the public face of your center. Select staff with good people skills who are motivated to provide excellent customer service.
- Interview and screen all students and volunteers. Provide guidance, supervision, a well organized interdepartmental training, and competency testing. Volunteers mean well and try hard, but quality of service varies from day to day and volunteer to volunteer.
- Do not underestimate the number of staff/volunteers you may need.
- Older volunteers or volunteers who have retired may be more likely to need extended periods of time off to travel, visit family, care for family, and so forth. Remain flexible and require notice of time off well in advance.

Work Ethics

- Think outside the box. Be flexible. Take risks, and run with your ideas.
- Make the work atmosphere a fun and enjoyable place to be.
- Provide periodic forums for discussion, track inquiries by search request forms, and survey or interview patients, families, and staff looking for gaps in materials or services.

Collaborative Partnerships and Marketing

- Consider a professional librarian as a consultant.
- Listen, network, and collaborate with the healthcare team of patient and all disease centers.
- Partner with key external agencies (i.e., American Cancer Society, Leukemia and Lymphoma Society, State Public Health Department, and local and area schools).

Table 27-1 Shared Lessons from CPEN Members (*Continued*)

- Talk about what your center does all the time and everywhere you go!
- Bring small groups of clinicians into your space. Orient new staff to specific resources for their patients.
- Use cancer survivors (patients and family council members) as advocates in evaluating new programs, services, and materials.
- "Never eat lunch alone." Make friends with staff from all disciplines who will help you spread the word about your services.
- Invite disease-specific groups or cancer site-specific visiting physician work groups to tour the center, to recommend disease-specific reference materials, and to participate in disease-specific book or materials review.
- Offer free take away "gift" items with information about your center on them: bookmarkers, key rings, pens, and special education pamphlets.

General and Physical Space

- Background music can be very soothing.
- Keep an updated web list for distribution.
- Make sure that your center is wheelchair accessible. Add a doorbell if necessary.
- Someone should be in the center at all times the center is open. Do not leave valuable and personal items unattended.
- A picture says a thousand words. Have photographs, illustrated anatomy books, models, and displays to teach and reinforce education messages.
- Take time to review other institution's websites. Utilize the CPEN listserv for questions. Network with other institutions for development of policies and procedures.
- Keep materials current within 5 years of copyright date.
- Do not worry about starting out and needing to have everything in the beginning. You can always add to your collection as you go along.
- Use the NCI free booklet: *Criteria and Guidelines for Establishing Comprehensive Cancer Patient Education Services.*
- Visit other consumer health libraries/resource centers. Share ideas and accomplishments.
- Videotapes may not be a worthwhile investment as they rarely get updated, but many individuals prefer them to books.
- Offer a disability section including samples of accessible aids (i.e., the machine from the Talking Book Library).
- Although printed material takes up a lot of space, patrons usually prefer printed publications or brochures. A slat wall is the best product for pamphlets.
- Printers, copiers, and telephones are a must. A fax is helpful as well.
- In purchasing books, talk with pharmaceutical representatives about obtaining an unrestricted educational grant. Use funds to buy books for the disease symptom management issues for which their company promotes the research.
- Ask the medical director of individual centers (gastrointestinal, brain, lung, gynecology, etc.) to recommend the best textbook in the field for your "reference" section. Then ask them to help buy it—they usually do!

A comprehensive patient resource center exists at the Dana-Farber Cancer Institute in Boston, Massachusetts. The Eleanor and Maxwell Blum Patient and Family Resource Center provides information and resources for varied learning needs and serves 17,000 patron visits a year. The mission statement fosters easy access to multimedia information, interactive nurse-led education programs, multicultural materials, and varied readability levels and promotes opportunity for private consultation when needed.

Case Study 27-1

The Eleanor and Maxwell Blum Resource Center

In 1996, the Dana-Farber Cancer Institute in Boston, Massachusetts recognized the need for a patient family resource center. An interdisciplinary committee was formed and met over a 12-month period. Members of a physician-led committee included staff from nursing, social work, development, the medical library, the communications department, the volunteer director, and a patient. The result of this process is the Eleanor and Maxwell Blum Resource Center and its satellites. These facilities provide the means for patient empowerment through education, access to information, opportunities to develop mutually supportive relationships with other patients and their families, and outreach to the larger community. The resource center program continues to foster the belief that patients and their healthcare providers are partners, actively participating together in information sharing and decision making.

At Dana Farber, a phlebotomy space was converted to establish a visible space as a resource center in the main lobby. The budget for establishing the resource center at the Dana-Farber Cancer Institute with books, materials and first-year furniture, computers, and furnishings was $60,000. The floor plan was a low-budget item where shelves and bookcases, Macintosh computers, and comfortable seating were incorporated to accommodate the space. The pastoral care department donated a peaceful, colored glass-paneled door that had been on an inpatient unit. This brought attention and high visibility to the new construction and quickly encouraged foot traffic. Susan Decristofaro, MS, RN, an oncology nurse, was appointed the leadership role and oversaw the daily operations of the center and the curriculum for training volunteers. The center has a full-time child life specialist, along with support from a host of student interns and trained volunteers.

The mission statement of the resource center bridges four institutions: Dana-Farber Cancer Institute, along with the combined efforts of Massachusetts General Hospital, Brigham and Women's Hospital, and Children's Hospital Boston. The center is committed to providing the highest level of care to cancer patients and their families through a combination of excellent treatment, education, and cutting-edge cancer research.

In the Blum Pediatric Resource Center, patients are drawn to the resource room by the sound of guitar lessons during music therapy, the smells of apple crisp during cooking class, or the need for a quiet space and the peaceful breathing of yoga. In addition, the center offers the Creative Arts Program with its own art studio and uses art, dance/movement, drama, music, humor, writing, and poetry as an integral part of patient education. The private consult area serves well for music lessons. During these experiences, patients and family members meet, and the real work of information sharing and support begins.

THE USE OF ART TO PROMOTE EDUCATION

Research suggests that creative arts have healing effects on the mind and body. Studies show that engagement in the creative process positively affects physiological functioning and can relieve pain and suffering. The creative arts program, housed within the patient and family education department at Dana-Farber Cancer Institute, was founded in 1997. Both adult and pediatric patients participating in the creative arts program experience the healing nature of the arts through painting, drama, dance, humor, writing, and poetry. Although creative art has been thought of in relation to children and young adult, it is appropriate for all ages (Sternberg, 1997).

The Adventures of Cell Zappers, written at Dana-Farber Cancer Institute, is a simple, light-hearted play that explains chemotherapy, surgery, and radiation treatments to adult and pediatric oncology patients and their families. Live interactive heroes and villains transform overwhelming, difficult-to-understand medical information into comprehensible learning in a nonthreatening way. The theatre troupe included multidisciplinary institute staff and local university students all volunteering as actors, portraying personalities such as Wally White Blood Cell, Adrian Adriamycin, Captain Chemo, and Lt. Ray Radiation. Responses from both adult and pediatric patients and families found this drama offered a satisfactory method for learning more about cancer, its treatment, and heightened awareness of the physical, emotional, and spiritual self.

The play *SunSense* is used as part of an educational curriculum designed to promote sun-safe behaviors among third grade students in Boston Public Elementary Schools. Set in a classroom, characters learn about their friend Billy's weekend at the beach and subsequent severe sunburn. After a trip to the hospital, Billy becomes an expert on the sun, why protecting his skin is important, and ways to be safe in the sun. Using diagrams, song and comedy, he returns to tell his classmates all about what he has learned. The value of *SunSense* as an educational tool is demonstrated by the children who watch in full attention and are able to answer questions accurately about sun safety. The program elicited an overwhelmingly positive response as students enjoyed learning. The authors continue to explore the use of dramatic art as a creative and interactive teaching method. Used in tandem with traditional treatment, drama can ease the burden of cancer patients and empower oncology nurses, among others, with additional educational resources.

Both *The Adventures of Cell Zappers* and *SunSense* were written in an attempt to improve learning. Experience has demonstrated that nurse educator and child life specialist should continue to collaborate and find teaching opportunities that stimulate learning in the affective domain to facilitate understanding and ease associated emotions (Hurtig & Stewin, 1990; Sawatzky, 1998).

Drama facilitates the use of emotion to develop empathy with characters, mood, situations, and content (O'Hara, 1984). Drama may offer experiential learning by involving audience participation and identifying with imaginary character roles and situations (O'Neil, Lambert, Linnell, & Warr-Wood, 1976). Drama builds on the existing knowledge patients, families, and/or elementary school children may have of cancer and enriches their knowledge of the subject.

Fundamental to the value of any dramatic production is the process of reflection. This can take place in discussion with questions and answers during or after the drama, in written evaluation or in achieved insights shared with others after further thinking (O'Neil, Lambert, Linnell, & Warr-Wood, 1976). Because education about the life-threatening aspect of cancer, treatment, and its prevention is complicated, one must be sensitive that not all persons are comfortable with gaining cancer information. Knowledge is a powerful resource for adults and children living with cancer and for persons of all ages learning how to prevent cancer. Ground rules for both *Cell Zappers* and *Sunsense* require language to be nonthreatening, nonoffensive, and at a literacy level that met both adult and child's understanding. Drama also requires the play be sensitive to language, scenery, effects, props, and music.

Introducing drama in patient education requires strategic planning. Adding drama to the creative arts program at Dana-Farber Cancer Institute required a necessary shift in staff attitude as the writing of both plays was explored. The aim of using drama was (1) to help the learner connect with sensitive and complex medical terminology related to cancer, (2) to improve understanding of how cancer occurs at a cellular level, (3) to explain chemotherapy, surgery, and radiation treatments and their side effects, and (4) to help alleviate anxiety and fear associated with cancer in an effort to teach principles of cancer prevention.

Choosing an adolescent young adult as the main characters in both plays was a deliberate attempt to attract both adults and children. The fantasy aspect of both plays opened possibilities for learning that are unavailable in real life. How the players co-create and organize themselves in the imaginative endeavor provides a wealth of information about the vulnerability of a patient in *The Adventures of Cell Zappers* undergoing treatment and in *Sunsense* of how a serious sunburn and a trip to the emergency room changes everything for a student and his friends.

The use of drama as an experiential method in teaching patients and the lay public has proved to be beneficial. Active involvement in artistic expression involves all five senses and improves learning (Curtis, 1999). Both dramas inspired viewers to reflect on how they felt while watching each play and how they might cope and, in effect, change behaviors given a real situation. Comments on both adult and pediatric evaluation tools reflected improved understanding.

Using dramatic art as an education method, combined with traditional written and verbal education, provided additional resources for teaching. Educators need to use as many of the arts as possible to address different learning styles. Learning and healing need to be considered in terms of the whole brain: left and right hemispheres (Curtis, 1999). These plays, *The Adventures of Cell Zappers* and *Sunsense*, serve as examples for options to consider. Cancer education, although a challenging life issue, can be embraced using the stage.

CANCER PREVENTION EDUCATION: TOBACCO CESSATION

Educating patients, families, and the community about cancer prevention is an important aspect of the work of cancer patient educators. Although there are multiple initiatives in cancer prevention education, this section concentrates on the prevention of cancers associated with tobacco. This includes a review of the current cessation treatment guidelines, implementation of an outpatient tobacco cessation program, and a community outreach initiative in a specific cultural group.

Smoking is the number one cause of preventable death in the United States (Centers for Disease Control and Prevention, 1993). According to the 2004 Surgeon General's Report, smoking causes acute myeloid leukemia and cancer of the bladder, pharynx, oral cavity, esophagus, larynx, lung, kidney, pancreas, cervix, and stomach (U.S. Department of Health and Human Services [DHHS], 2004). Other diseases causally related to smoking include coronary artery and cardiovascular diseases, abdominal aortic aneurysm, pneumonia, some reproductive effects, and sudden infant death syndrome (DHHS, 2004).

GUIDELINES

In 2008, updated U.S. Public Health Guidelines were established to assist clinicians and tobacco treatment specialists in treating tobacco use and to provide information about cessation practices. The following are a few of the key recommendations according to the guidelines.

- Tobacco dependence is a chronic condition that requires repeated interventions and multiple attempts to quit.
- Clinicians and health care delivery systems need to consistently identify and document tobacco use status and treat every tobacco user seen.
- Clinicians should encourage every patient willing to make a quit attempt to use the counseling treatments and medications recommended in the guidelines.
- Brief tobacco dependence treatment is effective and should be offered to every patient who uses tobacco.
- Individual, group, and telephone counseling are effective. Practical counseling (problem solving/skills training) and social support delivered as part of treatment are two components of counseling that are especially effective.
- Clinicians should use motivational treatments to increase future quit attempts for tobacco users who are currently unwilling to quit.
- In treating tobacco dependence, counseling and medication are effective when used by themselves. However the combination of counseling and medication are more effective than either used alone.

The established guidelines suggest that providers approach patients with the five As: ask, advise, assess, assist, and arrange. These words represent a specific action for the healthcare provider to address.

- *Ask* the patient if they use tobacco. This action will identify users.
- *Advise* the patient. Urge the patient to quit.
- *Assess* the willingness of the patient to quit.
- *Assist* the patient in quitting.
- *Arrange* for follow-up contact for the patient.

For patients who are unwilling to quit, the goal of the guidelines is to enhance motivation to quit with the five Rs: relevance, risks, rewards, roadblocks, and repetition.

- *Relevance:* Encourage the patient to state why quitting is personally relevant.
- *Risks:* Ask the patient to identify potential consequences of tobacco use.
- *Rewards:* Ask the patient to identify benefits of quitting.
- *Roadblocks:* Ask the patient to identify barriers to quitting.
- *Repetition:* For the unmotivated patient, motivational intervention should be repeated with each visit to the clinic.

For the patient who has recently quit, guidance and assistance with relapse prevention need to be provided.

Another recommendation from the clinical practice guidelines focused on the area of pharmacotherapies. Because numerous effective treatments are now available, it is recommended that they be used in all patients attempting to quit smoking, with the exception of those who present medical contraindications to treatment or specific populations for which there is insufficient evidence of effectiveness (DHHS, 2000).

There are seven first-line medications which can reliably increase long-term smoking abstinence rates. The medications include five nicotine products: gum, patch, inhaler, lozenge, and nasal spray, and two non-nicotine medications, bupropion SR and varenicline (DHHS, 2000). The guidelines also recommend that clinicians consider the use of certain combinations of medications that have been identified as effective.

COMPONENTS OF AN OUTPATIENT TOBACCO CESSATION PROGRAM

The tobacco cessation course used at Dana-Farber Cancer Institute in Boston is a structured, multicomponent, 8-week course. A multicomponent program is made of interrelated phases: preparation, quitting, and relapse prevention, with some methods and principles useful in more than one phase (Abrams et al., 2003). The course content is adapted from the Massachusetts General Hospital Quit Smoking Service and the University of Massachusetts Medical School: Tobacco Treatment Specialist training program models (2006). The class instruction and counseling time are 1 hour per week in either individual or group settings to facilitate the needs of the individual. The weekly lesson plan reviews the goals and objectives and what topics or activities will be addressed and highlights an inspirational quote each week for motivation.

The course is available to patients, family members, institution staff, or the general public. Participants enter the program either by clinician or self-referral. Scheduled meeting times of the course are varied and flexible. Course fees consist of a counseling fee and written materials; however, any pharmacologic treatment is an additional cost.

Entry components of the program include an intake form that reviews smoking and social and medical histories. A measure of the level of nicotine dependence is done with the Fagerstrom Tolerance Questionnaire (Fagerstrom, 1978) and the Heaviness of Smoking Index (Heatherton et al., 1989). A contract for the course outlining expectations is provided. Both the participant and the counselor sign the contract, agreeing to abide by the language. Participants wishing to have nicotine replacement therapy (NRT) provided by the counselor need to have their primary care provider sign a NRT permission form. Participants who prefer not to purchase NRT through the program may purchase their own over-the-counter NRT at a pharmacy. In addition to over-the-counter NRT products, there are other first- and second-line tobacco cessation treatment regimens available, which would require a prescription by the participant's healthcare provider.

Each class has a separate focus. The program starts with exercises to start the participant on the journey of stopping tobacco use. The process includes a review of the Stages of Change (Prochaska & DiClemente, 1983), which consist of precontemplation, contemplation, preparation, action, and maintenance. The stages help the participant identify with certain behaviors associated with change. Also included in this cycle is relapse, which can interrupt the process of change at any particular stage. The review of the importance/confidence scale helps to establish motivation to change and builds awareness about the readiness to become tobacco free. The Decisional Balance Scale (Velicer, DiClemente, Prochaska, & Brandenburg, 1985) helps to identify and assess factors that are for and against smoking and for and against quitting—the expected behavior change. These exercises help to determine readiness to change.

The next key component of the program is building the foundation, understanding the smoking pattern, and learning stress management. Included in this work is a good-bye letter, which is written by the participant to their cigarettes or other form of tobacco. The process of writing and journaling can be very cathartic for participants. The written expression can be a source of reinforcement for continued abstinence during times of craving and potential relapse.

Understanding nicotine addiction, potential triggers, barriers to quitting, and potential solutions can be an intense awakening for some tobacco users. Understanding smoking patterns and potential problems can assist with preventing or changing situations in order to maintain a smoke-free life. Setting a quit date is a very powerful development during the course: The smoker has reviewed his or her smoking patterns, has worked toward controlling his or her environment, and now is setting up the date to be free from tobacco.

Continued support and the power of positive thinking can be very empowering. Repeating affirmations can assist in changing a smoker's thought process to identify as a nonsmoker. After time, participants need to concentrate less or spend less time thinking about not smoking, and eventually, their new thought process identifies them as a nonsmoker.

Another component of the course work is rating withdrawal symptoms on a scale and revisiting the tool each week to rate the symptoms. This process helps the participant identify which symptom may be a problem area and how to address it. Frequently, it can be a tool for reinforcing behavior, as the participant can often see marked improvement and lessening of withdrawal symptoms associated with tobacco cessation.

Important instruction is also included about body awareness. Work is focused on eating patterns, the food pyramid, and exercise. With heightened taste buds and a slower metabolism, some individuals can gain some weight during the tobacco cessation process. Learning how to plan their diet and to incorporate exercise into their daily routine can be beneficial to the participants and prevent some unwelcome additional body fat.

Toward the completion of the program, a significant amount of time is spent on holding resistance, sticking with the program, and concentrating on relapse prevention. At times, obstacles may appear and challenge the quest to become a nontobacco user. During these times, it is beneficial for the individual to review their reasons for quitting and to reread their words of goodbye to tobacco, thus empowering them to remain tobacco free. Referrals to support groups, telephone quit lines, referral services, and quit tobacco websites can be very helpful in the first stages of quitting and in ongoing cessation.

Case Study 27-2

Bringing the Tobacco Cessation Program to Youth and Young Adults in the Asian Community

Asian Americans are one of the fastest growing ethnic groups in the United States. In addition to the numerous countries of origin, multiple languages, and associated dialects, there are also varying levels of acculturation in the United

States (Matthews-Juarez & Weinberg, 2006). An understanding of the relationship between acculturation and smoking in this population is an important step toward developing more pertinent prevention and cessation programs (Ma et al., 2004).

According to a 1999 compilation of myths and facts related to Asian American Health in Massachusetts, many believe that the prevalence of smoking is low among Asian Americans, whereas the facts reported Asian Americans in Massachusetts had a higher rate of smoking at 26.9% as compared with 22.5% in the general population (CEO Services, 1999). In addition, a 2000 National Youth Tobacco Survey reported the largest increase in smoking rates among any ethnic group was found in Asian American youth from 7th to 12th grade. They had the lowest teen smoking rates in middle school and the second highest by senior year (Asian Pacific Partners for Empowerment and Leadership, 2002). Because of the level of smoking and tobacco use in this population and the need for cessation programs in this community, a pilot initiative was established.

Community Outreach Pilot Program

As a community outreach initiative, the tobacco treatment program was brought to a service agency in the Asian community in Boston. The goals of this initiative were to expand the program into the community, identify the current and future needs of this community in relation to tobacco use and cessation, and to evaluate the current smoking cessation program for use with a specific cultural group.

Getting Started

A relationship was established with a service agency that mentors Asian youth and adolescents to young adults. This program offers education, youth development programs, and prevention and intervention services. In addition, youth leadership and social and recreational activities are supported.

In fostering the new relationship, much ground work needed to be done to accomplish the desired outcome. This work included a community assessment, which included meetings with the community agency leaders regarding the need for a program in their community. Planning meetings were also held with the smoking cessation program's tobacco team to review feasibility and to develop an action plan. One-to-one interviews were conducted with mentors in the medical field and the Asian community to review cultural beliefs in this population.

After the proposal for the program was in place, the funding for the program was secured from the community benefits program. The funding provided for program costs, including instructor salary, transportation, education materials, and NRT.

The Group

The cessation group started with eight participants, seven male and one female, ranging in age from 18 to 26 years. All were English speaking and were either born in the United States or have lived in the United States for an extended period of time. All group members started smoking in their early teen years and had smoked for several years. The importance scale of quitting tobacco was varied, the majority with midrange levels to the highest on the scale. Reporting of the participants' confidence levels was mainly in the midrange, and support rating was the lowest of the three factors. For many, this was the first attempt at quitting smoking.

All were given the course materials, a three-ring binder notebook with the class lessons and worksheets, and a collection of tobacco cessation booklets, pamphlets, and leaflets. The regular smoking cessation curriculum was used for this group, and some key observations were made.

Lessons Learned: Sharing

In the group setting, sharing among the group was very difficult and at some times absent, depending on the subject matter. In this culture, family is the center of the social structure. Privacy is very important to Asian Americans; therefore, family matters are not willingly discussed outside of the family with strangers (Matthews-Juarez & Weinberg, 2006). In order to facilitate learning about each individual and to compensate for the lack of information from group sharing, private meeting time was scheduled, one half hour before and after each weekly meeting time, in order to have one-to-one conferencing time. This change in procedure greatly enhanced the process and enabled the facilitator of the group to learn more about the individual participant. Telephone contact and e-mail correspondence were two other methods of communication available for all. In order to compensate for the lack of shared feelings, especially those related to stress, the facilitator described scenarios and potential sources of stress to the participants. Recognition of the signs of stress, increased awareness about how stress can manifest itself, and ways to handle stress were important lessons to share. Although there was a lack of verbal sharing, there was evidence of nonverbal communication by shaking and nodding of the head and glancing of the eyes. These actions assisted the group to be engaged. Follow-up communication with the individuals confirmed this.

Lessons Learned: Writing

As mentioned earlier in the components of the cessation program, writing the good-bye letter, a form of creative expression, can be a very cathartic and powerful piece of the tobacco cessation process. At first some participants may be resistant to the idea and activity, but they usually take part in the process. In this setting, there was unanimous disapproval of the exercise and unwillingness to participate. The class was encouraged to be creative and to write a letter, a poem, or a short note or make a song, rap, or anything that would convey how they felt about ending the relationship with their cigarettes. It was stressed that is was something that would not need to be shared with others if they chose not to. Not one participant wrote a note. It was later learned that writing, especially long passages, is difficult for these youth and young adults. The agency leaders report that these individuals often do not go to college because of the college entrance essay writing requirements and the lack of confidence. Classes to support writing efforts are held at the agency, but there is still some resistance.

Lessons Learned: Support

Another observation involved support and the group's perceptions about it. Many of the intake forms indicated low levels of support rated on the scale.

Many of the participants felt that their peers would not support them in their attempts to quit smoking. Several reported they would have a very difficult time asking their peers for assistance in their cessation attempts. To ask someone to refrain from smoking or to change a shared behavior, in order to help them avoid triggers to smoking, was something they could not see themselves doing. The group also reported that they did not feel that they could be a catalyst for change by encouraging others in their own community to quit, if they themselves quit smoking. In follow-up communication with agency leaders, much work is done surrounding having a voice and being proactive for others. The difference is how it is presented. Generally, ideas and communication will come forth if the question is asked on behalf of others and not themselves. Conformity is important to Asian American families, and there is an expectation that the family member will adhere to societal and family norms, thus not bringing shame to the family (Matthews-Juarez & Weinberg, 2006). The group reported that family members and being perceived as a "thug," not the health effects of tobacco, discourage youth against smoking. Because of this experience, many participants reported their family members did not know about their smoking and thus were not supported in quitting. The group was given information on websites for quit-smoking information and support. In addition, a toll-free smoker's quit-line number was also made available to the group for support.

Lessons Learned: Education

The benefits of quitting tobacco and the subsequent positive changes and improvement in health are reviewed as part of the course curriculum. In discussion with the group, it became clear to the author, evidenced by the number of health related questions, that there is a need for more information and health education for this population. Additional instruction time was spent discussing the body and how the body functions.

Lessons Learned: NRT Dosing

A study that reviewed ethnic differences in nicotine metabolism reported nicotine clearance and cigarette intake were lower in Chinese Americans when compared with whites and Latinos, which may explain lower lung cancer rates in Chinese Americans. In line with this report, the results of this study might have implications for dosing NRT in Chinese Americans (Benowitz, Perez-Stable, Herrera, & Jacob, 2002), which the tobacco program medical director was consulted about. Taking into consideration the reported low cigarette intake of some of the participants, a lower dose of nicotine was recommended. The lowered dose was insufficient for the participants, partially related to incorrect cigarette counts. Half of the class participants reported less cigarette intake than they actually consumed. When dose recommendations were based on actual cigarette counts, the participants were able to tolerate the regular dosing. The results of this study will be taken into consideration in the future as needed.

Lessons Learned: Cultural Differences

Bringing the tobacco cessation program to the Asian American community was a new endeavor for the author. At the beginning, there was a concern related to being a non-Asian and whether that fact would have an effect on the class. Class discussions were very open, and cultural differences were discussed freely during the class. The class participants spoke very freely and proudly of their culture, beliefs, and practices. At the end of the program, it appeared that being different added to the class, sharing and learning new aspects of each other's lives. The agency leaders also felt that the course taught by a non-Asian had a great impact, as it was not "traditional" in its presentation.

The Results and Follow-Up

The classes started with eight participants. There was one member who quit the program after 2 weeks because of a conflict with a new job opportunity. Seven members completed the 8-week course. Four participants quit smoking, and three did not. Everyone in the class except one made at least one quit attempt.

A follow-up and reunion class was held 5 months after the start of the program. The seven participants met and exchanged stories and experiences. One participant remained a nonsmoker, and the other three who had quit relapsed. The cause of the relapse was attributed to stress and social triggers. Three participants, who never quit, continued to smoke. It was reported, however, that all had a reduction in the number and amount of cigarettes consumed.

Next Steps for the Future

Continuing the tobacco cessation program in the Asian community would be beneficial. Program changes implemented in this pilot initiative will remain in the future. Restructuring the curriculum to include more education and guest speakers on different topics and creating a support group network after the initial 8-week course are recommended to assist the new nonsmokers with relapse prevention. Another future goal is to build partnerships with other community organizations to expand the program. It will be kept in mind that the level of acculturation needs to be taken into account and the curriculum and language structured accordingly. It is also a recommendation to develop a new curriculum targeting youth and teens. This would include education about tobacco prevention and the health effects related to tobacco use.

Summary

Educating about the prevention of cancers and other diseases is a very important aspect of a cancer patient educator's role. Tobacco cessation can save lives and improve the general health of so many Americans. It is important that these efforts assist all Americans and that every effort is made to reach the underserved communities.

CONCLUSION

This chapter presents the key concepts in educating patients and families. The healthcare provider involved in education needs to know how best to ensure comprehension of the patient's diagnosis, treatment, and experience based on specific attributes such as age or spoken language of the patient and their family. Pediatric cancer patients may need more participatory learning, like playing with medical supplies, to understand what an adult acquires through words. Using the various methods of teaching patients about cancer also includes establishing a base of knowledge not only with the adult or pediatric patient but to include family and other caregivers, which offers the ideal patient outcome.

Introducing and explaining cancer diagnoses, treatments, and prevention to patients and families are essential to a cancer patient educator's role. The nurse, child life specialist, and other healthcare providers benefit from a closer look at patient and family education through the many methods available for teaching, including electronic and literary resources, play, art, equal access to information, prevention, and reaching out to the community. By staying current with new medical, psychological, and support knowledge, educators can effectively provide patients and families with the tools that they need to understand and manage their cancer experience.

RESOURCES

Gates, R. A., & Fin, R. M. (2007). *Oncology nursing secrets* (3rd ed.). Retrieved from www.cancerpatienteducation.org.

Oncology Nurses Society. (2004). *Manual for radiation oncology nursing practice and education.* Pittsburg, PA.

Oncology Nurses Society. (2005). *Chemotherapy and biotherapy guidelines and recommendations for practice* (2nd ed.). Pittsburg, PA.

Oncology Nurses Society. (2005). *Core curriculum for oncology nursing* (4th ed.). Pittsburg, PA.

Oncology Nurses Society. (2005). *Study guide for the core curriculum for oncology nursing.* Pittsburg, PA.

Shelton, B. K., Ziegfeld, C. R., & Olsen, M. M. (2004). *Manual of cancer nursing.* Sidney Kimmel Comprehensive Cancer Center at Johns Hopkins. Philadelphia: Lippincott, Williams, & Wilkins.

The Child Life Council. (2007). *Child life council activity recipe book.* Rockville, MD.

WEB RESOURCES

American Library Association: Code of Ethics
www.ala/oif.statementpols/codeofethics/codeethics.htm.

American Nurses Association
www.nursingworld.org/ethics/code/protected_nwcoe303.htm

Cancer Patient Education Network
www.cancerpatienteducation.org

Child Life Council
www.childlife.org

Medical Library Association
www.mlanet.org/about/ethics.html
www.caphis.mlanet.org/resources/index.html

Potential Vendors for Library Supplies

Highsmith: www.highsmith.com

Vernon Library Supplies: www.vernonlib.com

Demco: www.demco.com

The Library Store: www.thelibarystore.com

Library Management Systems

LibraryWorld: www.libraryworld.net/home.html

Athena Library Automations System:
www.sagebrush.corp.com/tech/athena.com

Resourcemate: www.resourcemate.com

Softlink: www.softlinkamerica.com

REFERENCES

Abrams, D. B., Niaura, R., Brown, R. A., Emmons, K. M., Goldstein, M. G., & Monti, P. M. (2003). *The tobacco dependence treatment handbook: a guide to best practices.* New York: Guilford.

Asian Pacific Partners for Empowerment and Leadership. (2002). Making tobacco relevant for Asian American and Pacific Islander communities. *APPEAL, Fall,* 1–14.

Benowitz, N. L., Perez-Stable, E. J., Herrera, B., & Jacob, P. III. (2002). Slower metabolism and reduced intake of nicotine from cigarette smoking in Chinese-Americans. *Journal of the National Cancer Institute, 94*(2), 108–115.

Cancer Patient Education Network. Retrieved May 20, 2007, from http://www.cancerpatienteducation.org/.

Centers for Disease Control and Prevention. (1993). Cigarette smoking: attributable mortality and years of potential life lost, United States, 1990. *Morbidity and*

Mortality Weekly Report, 42(33):645–649. Retrieved November 20, 2007, from http://www.cdc.gov/mmwr/preview/mmwrhtml/00021441.htm.

CEO Services. (1999). *Asian American health: myth and facts; Massachusetts: tobacco use and other substances.* Newton, MA: CEO Services. Retrieved May 16, 2007, from www.culturalcompetence2.com/articles/asianamericanmythandfacts.doc.

Clance, P. R., & Imes, S. (1978). The imposter phenomenon in high achieving women: dynamics and therapeutic intervention. *Psychotherapy Theory, Research and Practice, 15*(3), 1–8.

Curtis, A. M. (1999). Communicating with bereaved children: a drama therapy approach, *Illness, Crisis & Loss, 7*(2), 410–413.

Fagerstrom, K. (1978). Measuring degree of physical dependence to tobacco smoking with reference to individuation of treatment. *Addictive Behaviors, 3,* 235–241.

Gaynard, L., Wolfer, J., Goldberger, J., Thompson, R., Redburn L., & Laidley, L. (1998). *Psychosocial care of children in hospitals: a clinical practice manual from the ACCH child life research project.* Rockville, MA: Child Life Council.

Heatherton, T., Kozlowski, L., Frecker, R., Rickert, W., & Robinson, J. (1989). Measuring the heaviness of smoking: using self-reported time to the first cigarette of the day and number of cigarettes smoked per day. *British Journal of Addiction, 84*(7), 791–799.

Hurtig, W., & Stewin, L. (1990). The effect of death education and experience on nursing students' attitude towards death. *Journal of Advanced Nursing, 15,* 29–34.

The Institute for Family-Centered Care. (2007). Retrieved on April 30, 2007, from http://www.familycenteredcare.org.

Isenberg, J. P., & Quisenberry, N. (2002). Play: essential for all children. *ACEI Position Paper, Fall,* 33–39.

Ma, G. X., Tan, Y., Toubbeh, J. I., Su, X., Shive, S. E., & Lan, Y. (2004). Acculturation and smoking behaviors in Asian-American populations. *Health Education Research: Theory & Practice, 19*(6), 615–625.

Massachusetts General Hospital. MGH Quit Smoking Service, Boston, MA.

Matthews-Juarez, P., & Weinberg, A. (2006). *Cultural competence in cancer care: a health care professional's passport.* Houston, TX: Baylor College of Medicine, Intercultural Cancer Council.

O'Hara, M. (1984). Drama in education: a curriculum dilemma. *Theory into Practice, XXIII*(4), 315–320.

O'Neil, C., Lambert, A., Linnell, R., & Warr-Wood, J. (1976). *Drama guidelines. Drama structures: a practical handbook for teachers.* London: Heinemann.

Prochaska, J. O., & DiClemente, C. C. (1983). Stages and processes of self-change of smoking: toward an integrative model of change. *Journal of Consulting and Clinical Psychology, 51*(3), 390–395.

Saca-Hazboun, H. (2007). Building on a strong foundation: educating RNs from other specialties for oncology care. *ONS Connect, October,* 10–14.

Sawatzky, J. E. (1998). Nurse perceptions of changes impacting nursing practice. *Concern, 27*(5), 19–21.

Sternberg, P. (1997). Drama therapy presentation. NADT conference workshop. New York.

Thompson, R., & Standford, G. (1981). *Child life in hospitals: theory and practice.* Springfield, IL: Charles C Thomas.

University of Massachusetts Medical School. (2006). *Massachusetts tobacco treatment specialist training manual.* Worcester, MA: Division of Preventive and Behavioral Medicine Center for Tobacco Prevention and Control.

U.S. Department of Health and Human Services. (2000). *Treating tobacco use and dependence: clinical practice guideline.* Rockville, MD: DHHS.

U.S. Department of Health and Human Services. (2004). The health consequences of smoking: a report of the Surgeon General. U.S. Department of Health and Human Services, Centers for Disease Control and Prevention, National Center for Chronic Disease Prevention and Health Promotion, Office on Smoking and Health. Retrieved November 20, 2007, from http://www.cdc.gov/tobacco/data_statistics/sgr/sgr_2004/index.htm.

Velicer, W. F., DiClemente, C. C., Prochaska, J. O., & Brandenburg, N. (1985). A decisional balance measure for assessing and predicting smoking status. *Journal of Personality and Social Psychology, 48,* 1279–1289.

Chapter 28

Education for Arthritis, Joint Injury, and Replacement

Clare E. Safran-Norton

INTRODUCTION

Osteoarthritis (OA), formally known as "degenerative joint disease," is the most common form of arthritis experienced in the general population. It occurs throughout the lifespan as part of the normal aging process. OA can be found throughout the spine, especially in cervical and lumbar spine joints, as well as in the hands, hips, and knee joints. Typically, people in middle and older age groups experience OA more than those in younger age groups.

OA is often referred to as simply generic "arthritis" among the general population. It can be confused with rheumatoid arthritis, joint effusion, bursitis, cartilaginous microfractures, bone spurs, or meniscal tears. A more accurate definition of OA is a "non-inflammatory disorder of movable joints characterized by deterioration of articular cartilage" (Fagerson, 1998, p. 40). Typically, these degenerative changes of the cartilage are seen on radiographs and coincide with patient symptomatology such as joint pain, swelling, pain with changes in the weather, and pain with weight-bearing activities, that is, ambulation and stair climbing.

EPIDEMIOLOGY

The degenerative disease process of OA is slow, occurs over a long period of time, worsens with age, and can be correlated with gender. OA is more common in later years of life; that is, one third of people aged 65 years and older have positive radiograph findings for knee OA (Klipper, 2001), unless it is associated with trauma. Studies report that OA affects 12.1% of adults aged 25 to 74 years, which is an estimate of 20.7 million (1990 population estimates) U.S. adults (Lawrence et al., 1998). Other studies report the incidence rates of symptomatic OA as being greatest for knee OA (240 per 100,000 person-years) and least for hip OA (88 per 100,000 person-years) (Oliveria et al., 1995).

Relative to gender and OA, men are more likely to have OA if found before the age of 50, whereas after 50 years of age, there is a higher prevalence of OA in women than men (Buckwalter, Saltzman, & Brown, 2004). For women, the incidence for radiograph findings is highest for OA of the knee (4%) per year (Felson et al., 1995). Women also tend to have a higher risk for knee OA and hip OA (not hand) when compared with men (Srikanth et al., 2005). These gender differences between men and women appear to level off at around age 80 (Buckwalter et al., 2004).

This high prevalence of OA among women and men, the effects of OA on weight-bearing joints, and the association of these degenerative changes to limitation in functional mobility (Arthritis Foundation) have made OA an important public health issue. The degeneration of joint cartilage that occurs with OA leads to significant joint pain and loss of motion, which can lead to the inability to function independently and safely without pain. When joint pain and limitation in daily functional mobility inhibits a person's ability to carry out normal activities of daily living (ADLs) and instrumental activities of daily living (IADLs), surgical joint replacement is considered.

Two of the more common surgical joint arthroplasties are the total hip arthroplasty (THA) and the total knee arthroplasty (TKA). Estimates report about 400,000 hip and knee arthroplasties being surgically performed at a cost of $10 billion U.S. dollars (Lavernia et al., 1995) in healthcare expenditure annually. Relative to hospitalization, cost, and surgical interventions, OA accounts for 55% of all arthritis-related hospitalizations (Lethbridge-Cejku, Helmick, & Popovic, 2003) with knee and hip joint replacement procedures accounting for about 35% of total arthritis-related procedures during hospitalization (Gabriel et al., 1997).

Although there are not much data published on the association of OA and race, it has been reported that blacks and persons with low income tend to have lower rates of total knee replacement but higher complications and mortality than whites (Mahomed et al., 2002). Studies (Katz et al., 2004; Losina et al., 2004a, 2004b) have reported a positive association between high-volume hospitals and high-volume surgeons to good outcomes for patients undergoing TKA. These studies have also reported individuals with low income and minorities as more likely to have joint replacements performed in low-volume hospitals by low-volume surgeons. This lower rate of surgical intervention among blacks may be related to socioeconomic status, preconceived beliefs about surgery, medical interventions, and fear related to the surgery. These beliefs, demographics, and socioeconomic status are associated with low rates of total joint replacements for blacks. When considering health education and interventions for this group of patients, the healthcare provider needs to recognize the need for extra patient education, support services, and postoperative follow-up in order to improve their ability for a good outcome.

In addition to age, gender, socioeconomic status, and race, obesity is another important health issue that has an impact on OA. Obesity is defined as a person being more than 20% over their ideal weight, as a co-morbidity, which speeds up and exacerbates the degenerative process of OA in weight-bearing joints. A person with obesity has decreased space between joint surfaces, increased joint pressure within weight-bearing joints, and more degenerative wearing on the cartilaginous surfaces of the joints as the excessive weight of their body compresses the joint surfaces more than a person with an average body mass index. Because of this increased weight, people with obesity compromise their candidacy for joint replacement.

Persons with excessive weight also place high demands on their body organs for basic functioning. The impact of the extra strain on the organs in addition to the ability to tolerate anesthesia and a surgical procedure further compromises surgical candidacy for a patient with obesity. A new joint replacement has a margin of how much weight it can tolerate; therefore, obesity also decreases the life expectancy of a joint replacement and the ability for it to function successfully over time. Clearly, obesity is a significant co-morbidity for OA that affects the disease process as well as one's candidacy for a joint replacement. Here, healthcare providers may be asked to counsel and set up a weight reduction, nutrition, and exercise program for a patient in order to become a candidate for a joint replacement surgery.

Diagnosis of Hip Osteoarthritis

The American College of Rheumatology has created a diagnostic algorithm for hip OA. The diagnostic classification scheme for hip OA includes the following:

1. Hip pain
2. At least two of the following three features: erythrocyte sedimentation rate < 20 mm/hr, radiographic femoral or acetabular osteophytes, and radiographic joint space narrowing (superior, axial, and/or medial) (Altman et al., 1991)

This diagnostic algorithm for accurately diagnosing OA has very good validity with 89% sensitivity and 91% specificity. This classification algorithm is well published in the literature and is regularly used among clinicians.

Clinical Presentation

Common clinical features of OA include (Fagerson, 1998)

- Painful joint area with movement, pain with weight-bearing activities
- Increased pain with low barometric pressure (e.g., rain)
- Painful joint with rest
- Night pain in later stages of disease
- Referred pain
- Muscle spasm
- Progressive loss of range of motion (movement)
- Joint stiffness at rest, moderate joint effusion (edema)
- Thickened joints
- Joint crepitus (sometimes audible)
- Gait deviations (limping with ambulation)
- Functional limitations (e.g., stairs and transfers)

Specific to the hip joint, a patient may experience the following:

- Pain in the hip joint with ambulation
- Loss of hip range of motion
- Hip joint contracture (most frequently in adduction, flexion, and external rotation)

- Occasional deformity as a result of incongruity of the femoral head and acetabulum
- Antalgic (painful) gait
- Trendelenburg gait (weakness of the gluteus medius muscle)
- Leg length discrepancy from subchondral collapse

Radiographically, one can expect to see (Fagerson, 1998)

- Loss of joint space
- Subchondral cysts
- Osteophytes
- Bone collapse
- Loose bodies
- Possible bone/joint deformity

Specific to the knee joint, one might see:

- Signs and symptoms of pain, and swelling
- Loss of range of motion
- Decreases in functional mobility
- Muscle length restrictions and limitations in gait

Radiographic joint space narrowing superior, axial, and/or medial are common.

Medical Interventions for OA

General recommendations (Hochberg et al., 1995) for intervention for a patient with OA may include

- Medications
- Exercises (e.g., pain-free weight-bearing and non–weight-bearing exercises)
- Weight-reduction program and education
- Lower-extremity braces or walking aids (e.g., crutch, cane, or walker, as indicated)
- Surgery
- Medications for OA may include the following:
  - Acetaminophen

    ○ Nonsteroidal anti-inflammatory drugs (NSAIDs) or COX-2 inhibitors
    ○ Capsaicin
    ○ Tramadol
    ○ Narcotic pain relievers (oxycodone, oxymorphone, or morphine)
    ○ Glucosamine

The use, dose, precautions, and contraindications of all medications should always be addressed and reviewed with each patient for each medication. Although there have not been specific studies correlating death to the use of NSAIDs in OA, there is a more recent concern of gastrointestinal bleeds related to the usage of NSAIDS as a potential cause of death for patients with OA (Sacks, Helmick, & Langmaid, 2004).

Exercises for patients with OA should encompass four concepts:

1. Encourage pain-free movement, high repetitions, low loads.
2. Challenge the patient's muscles to the extent that the muscles become fatigued and strengthened, but do not elicit injury nor pain.
3. Preserve joint integrity by use of assistive devices and patient education.
4. Preserve and improve functional status (i.e., walking programs and transfer training).

When prescribing exercises for a patient with OA, the exercises may or may not include resistance (e.g., weights, theraband, and resisted bicycling). The exercises should be performed in varied positions (e.g., gravity assisted, gravity resisted, or gravity minimized) and may sometimes be done in a pool using principles of aquatic therapy (e.g., buoyancy assisted or water resisted) to reduce the load on the joints while encouraging pain-free movement and muscle strength.

The most common surgical interventions for a patient with OA include THA and TKA. Basic elements of patient education and interventions are suggested in this text. Because many interventions are patient and surgeon specific, a list of resources for the most current and comprehensive surgical techniques and procedures, physical and occupational therapy programs, medications, and general interventions associated with postoperative care is suggested in the back of the chapter.

In addition to medical management using medications, surgical interventions, and therapeutic exercise, some modifiable and nonmodifiable risk factors have recently been identified and associated with OA and should be included in patient education (Felson, 2004; Felson & Zhang, 1998; Felson et al., 1995; Jordan et al., 2007; Rossignol et al., 2005).

Modifiable risk factors for men and women include the following:

- Excess body mass (especially knee OA)
- Obesity
- Injuries sustained from sports, work, or trauma
- Occupational hazards such as heavy lifting, extreme knee flexion, and repetitive motions
- Manual or physical labor that requires excessive mechanical stressors on the tissues
- Muscle imbalances (muscles that are too tight with opposing muscles that are too weak)

For men, some occupational hazards may include the following:

- Construction work
- Farm work
- Professional athletics or industry jobs that require heavy or repetitive lifting or sustaining positions of extreme joint flexion

For women, some occupational hazards may include

- Sewing
- Factory assembly lines
- Cleaning
- Waitressing
- Farming
- Retail

Nonmodifiable risk factors associated with OA are those predisposing factors that a person cannot control or change. These nonmodifiable risk factors include the following:

- Body composition
- Joint and extremity malalignment
- Gender (most often female)
- Age (increases with age and levels around age 80)

- Race (some Asian populations have lower risk of OA and blacks may be predisposed to worse outcomes) (Hawker, 2006)
- Genetic predisposition for OA
- Body type associated with increase risk of developing OA such as joint malalignment

A recent report (Felson, 2004; Felson & Zhang, 1998) indicated that about 20% to 35% of knee OA and about 50% of hip and hand OA may be genetically determined. According to the Centers for Disease Control, other possible risk factors of OA include the following: estrogen deficiency (ERT may reduce risk of knee/hip OA), osteoporosis (inversely related to OA), use of vitamins C, E, and D (equivocal reports), and C-reactive protein (increased risk with higher levels). All of these risks (modifiable and nonmodifiable) should be considered and addressed as a part of patient education.

Teaching Techniques for Health Education for Patients with Joint Replacements

Much of the literature on patient outcomes status after surgical intervention for a joint replacement is correlated with preoperative status. Although a healthcare provider has limited ability to improve some preoperative impairments, some patient education, exercises, and functional ability can be addressed and improved prior to surgery. Here, preoperative patient education includes explanation of medical procedure, functional training with assistive devices (i.e., walker, crutches, and cane), ambulation and weight-bearing status, transfers (i.e., bed mobility and toilet transfers), stair climbing, transfers in and out of bed, seat heights for THA, and joint precautions for THA. Exercises include strengthening the lower-extremity muscles and optimizing range of motion if a restriction is related to a shortened muscle that can be stretched.

THA

Patient education for hip precautions after a THA is mostly based on the surgical approach. There are three types of surgical approaches for performing a THA:

1. Posterior lateral
2. Anterior lateral
3. Lateral

The preference for the surgical approach is typically dependent on the surgeon, their training, their personal preference, and good outcomes. The

Table 28-1 THA Precautions

Surgical Approach	Hip Precautions
Posterior lateral	No hip flexion beyond 90 degrees in combination with internal rotation; hip flexion allowed with external rotation and MD permission; no hip adduction, no internal rotation
Anterior lateral	No hip extension, no adduction, no internal rotation
Lateral	No adduction

following THA precautions are typically associated with each type of surgical procedure, although surgical preferences should be noted and applied for each patient appropriately (**Table 28-1**).

Today, some surgeons are performing minimally invasive TKA instead of these more traditional open surgical replacements. These newer techniques are less invasive and are typically chosen to preserve loss of blood, increase healing time, and limit scarring of tissues; however, current literature demonstrates some higher incidence of dislocation and wearing of the joint surfaces if not placed in ideal alignment. The literature reports better outcomes with higher volume surgeons, experienced surgeons, and careful selection criteria for patient population. It appears that there are good outcomes with this less invasive procedure when there is an experienced surgeon and the ability to create a good prosthetic alignment with a smaller incision (Cioppa-Mosca et al., 2006; Hawker, 2006).

Additional patient education (Peak, 2005) includes the following:

- Avoid pillows under knee to prevent hip flexion contracture
- Use abduction pillow when lying supine (on your back)
- Comply with restricted weight-bearing status
- Gait training with assistive device
- Use adaptive equipment as indicated
  - Long-handled reacher, shoe horn, sponge, and stocking aide
- Sit on elevated toilet seat, car seat, and chair at home
- Use raised bathtub seat and bathtub safety bars as indicated
- Comply with therapeutic exercises as prescribed

Research Outcomes for Patient's Status Post THA

Recent research on successful outcomes (March et al., 1999) for patient's status post THA demonstrates positive effects for therapy intervention (Sashika, Matsuba, & Watanabe, 1996) and surgical procedures for improvement with functional mobility. A 6-week home exercise program (e.g., range of motion exercises, eccentric hip abduction exercises, and isometric exercises) was effective in long-term follow-up for patients with THA (Sashika et al., 1996). A study by Mahomed et al. (2002) reported that preoperative status was the main determinant of postoperative status, but greater education and more positive expectations were also significant predictors of better postoperative pain and functional status.

TKA

There are generally two types of total knee arthroplasties to consider:

1. The standard TKA
2. The minimally invasive TKA

Patient education following TKA includes the following:

- Avoid pillows under knee to prevent hip flexion contracture
- Comply with daily range of motion exercises
- Comply with pain and edema control reduction techniques such as ice, quadriceps exercises, and range of motion exercises
- Comply with restricted weight-bearing status
- Have gait training with assistive device
- Use adaptive equipment as indicated
  - Long-handled reacher, shoe horn, sponge, and stocking aide
- Use raised bathtub seat and bathtub safety bars as indicated
- Comply with therapeutic exercises as prescribed

In addition to these intervention suggestions, it is recommended that activities such as swimming, cycling, and power walking be chosen to maintain low joint loads after a total knee replacement. These types of activities do not require high joint compression or high joint loads as do skiing, jogging, and hiking. Extended repetitive activities will shorten the life expectancy of a new joint. In short, minimization of wear and tear is the main factor in preservation of joint replacements and improving long-term outcomes in patients with TKA (Kuster, 2002).

Research Outcomes for Patient's Status Post TKA

To date, there are no long-term (10 years or more) follow-up studies on the newer technique (e.g., minimally invasive TKA), but there are good long-term outcomes on the standard TKA. Physicians may agree or disagree on which approach has better outcomes. In a recent study by Bonutti et al. (2004), the authors noted that there may be a discrepancy in what a doctor determines to be a good outcome versus a patient's idea of a good outcome. For example, patients appear to be interested and concerned with pain and time to recover, whereas doctors are most concerned with functional outcomes. Bonutti et al. suggest that their clinical investigation of patient's status after minimally invasive TKA reduced hospital stays, decreased postoperative pain, decreased the need for rehabilitation, and increased patients' ability to return to functional status more quickly. Being able to compare and contrast the positive and negative outcomes for total knee replacements is important to include in patient education and health promotion.

The National Institutes of Health published a consensus statement in 2003 on the outcomes of total knee replacement. Here, a panel of experts representing the fields of orthopedics, rheumatology, internal medicine, nursing, physical therapy, rehabilitation, biostatistics, epidemiology, health-related services research, and a patient status after TKA concluded that the research supports the long-term (20 years or more) outcomes for TKA. The article reported patients to have substantial improvement in pain, functional status, and overall quality of life. There was a consensus that perioperative interventions improved outcomes of TKA, some of which included systemic antibiotic prophylaxis, aggressive postoperative pain management, perioperative risk assessment and management of medical conditions, and preoperative education. Contraindications for TKA included persistent infection, poor bone quality, significantly restricted use of quadriceps muscle, poor skin condition, and poor vascular supply. Factors associated with hospital high volume were associated with better outcomes, and factors associated with the surgeon's case volume, technique, and type of prosthesis also had better outcomes for TKA; therefore, NIH supported current research findings and promoted the use of TKA when indicated.

Research Outcomes Questionnaire for the Healthcare Provider

Relative to functional outcomes, it is important for the healthcare provider to determine a good outcome for a patient after medical intervention. Although many institutions require preadmission and postadmission surveys, there are good outcome measures established in the literature that may be used as good indicators for outcomes for patients with OA. Two more common outcome measures used in medicine are the SF-36 and the WOMAC (Western Ontario and McMaster Universities Osteoarthritis Index).

The SF-36 is a scale used to report on ability to function. March et al. (1999) demonstrated significant improvement in health-related quality of life after joint replacements in most scales of the SF-36 scores, especially in the areas of physical function, role, and body pain. In their study, patients' status after hip arthroplasty improved as well as or better than population normals on all scales, whereas those patients' status after knee arthroplasty improved their scores on the SF-36, but physical function and body pain scales were worse than the population norm; therefore, the patients who underwent a total hip replacement had higher levels of satisfaction with their level of function and pain than those patients who underwent a TKA.

Another study by similar authors (Bachmeier et al., 2001) compared the usefulness of two outcome measures for patients with OA who had undergone THA and TKA: the WOMAC and the Medical Outcomes Study SF-36 Health Survey (MOS SF-36). Here, Bachmeier et al. demonstrated significant and meaningful changes in outcomes after both types of lower-extremity joint replacements. Recommendations of the authors were to use the WOMAC for short-term outcomes (less than 6 months) and the MOS SF-36 for outcomes greater than 6 months' duration. Overall, their results had similar findings to the previous study where the outcomes on the patients with THA were better than the outcomes for patients' status after knee THA.

Relative to health education, it is important to be able to explain to patients and their families that there have been good studies published describing successful recovery of function and decreased pain for patients who have undergone these surgeries. Also, waiting too late for a total joint replacement can actually have a negative effect on future outcomes. A study by Fortin et al. (1999) considered functional outcomes in matched patient populations in Canada (socialized medicine) and the United States. Here, patients in both geographical sites were comparable in age, gender, time to surgery, and proportion of hip and knee joint replacement surgeries; however, the patients in Canada had a lower level of functional status before their surgery and more pain than their U.S. counterparts. Assessments performed after surgery revealed lower scores for those patients who had lower preoperative physical function and more pain than those with higher preoperative function; therefore, the researchers concluded that surgery performed later in the natural progression of the disease process of OA and functional decline may result in worse postoperative functional status.

The following section lists some examples and ideas for application of this material to real patient cases. There are two successful outcomes: one status after THA and the other status after TKA. A brief discussion with rationale for decisions and support toward an optimal outcome is included.

Case Study 28–1

Mary is a 78-year-old female status post right THA 2 days ago secondary to hip OA. This is the patient's first THA surgery. She is currently in an inpatient hospital rehabilitation center for a 1-week stay to include physical therapy, occupational therapy, nursing, and social services. The patient is a widow, residing alone in an elevated apartment senior housing structure, and she has no family nearby. She has one daughter who resides in Texas with three high school-aged children; the daughter is unable to come to visit until the weekend. The patient will be in the rehabilitation unit until she is independent and safe with all THA precautions, bed mobility, transfers (e.g., sit to stand, car transfers, and bathtub and toilet transfers), walking, stair negotiation, and most ADLs (e.g., dressing, bathing, toileting, taking medications, and eating). She can be discharged home with a home care service to provide further management of her medical issues, medications, progression of functional status, walking, and IADLs (e.g., meal preparation, grocery shopping, and household cleaning).

Successful Outcome

Success in this case relies on good patient education for Mary, which includes medical management (monitoring medications) and the ability to understand and carry out total hip replacement precautions. Mary should also be instructed in how to function safely within her own home environment and how to engage safely in ADLs and IADLs. Mary lives alone and does not have family support nearby; therefore, it was critically important to allow her to be transferred to a medical facility that could take care of her until she is ready to be discharged home safely. Although an inpatient rehabilitation stay is more expensive than care at home, it is recommended in this situation because Mary resides alone, does not have family nearby, and is not at a safe level at day 2 after surgery to return home safely.

There are many various types of facilities that would allow a patient postoperative from hip surgery to have a rehabilitation stay in order to allow them to be safe enough to go home with ongoing support and medical services. This type of temporary institutional care is recommended to allow the patient to have intensive rehabilitation, which will allow the patient an optimal outcome in a short period of time. The extent to which a patient qualifies for a medical or rehabilitation facility largely depends on his or her medical needs and their insurance coverage. It is likely that Mary has either Medicare or Medicaid; she may also have an additional type of supplemental insurance coverage that would pay for a brief period of rehabilitation prior to her discharge to home.

Case Study 28–2

Ralph is an 84-year-old man who recently underwent bilateral total knee arthroplasties 3 days ago. He was discharged home over the weekend with a walker, with orders for partial weight bearing for bilateral lower extremities. The home healthcare physical therapist evaluated him the next day to perform his agency admission and evaluate further need for services. The physical therapist recommended that nursing evaluate him for wound care, medication management, and home healthcare supervision. Further recommendations were for an occupational therapy evaluation for bathing, dressing and toileting. The physical therapist will treat him 5 days per week for functional training, ambulation, range of motion, and exercises.

Successful Outcome

In Ralph's case, a successful outcome is dependent on the education regarding pain management and edema control, as well as restoration of early motion in both knees to assure a return to functional mobility. Because the patient has had both knees operated on at the same time, he will need intensive therapy, pain management, and a good understanding of early motion in order to have an optimal outcome.

Ralph is likely to have a successful outcome because he has home care services that evaluated and recommended services the day after he left the hospital. The physical therapist was an integral part of a team and recognized the need for the other disciplines to be involved with the patient's overall care plan. The physical therapist made appropriate and speedy referrals that addressed the needs of the patient in an efficient matter and assured a cost-effective use of services. It is likely that Ralph healed quickly and experienced a rapid restoration of movement and function with a successful overall outcome.

Unsuccessful Outcome

Research has demonstrated that being minority status and low income and having a joint replacement performed at a low-volume institution or by a low-volume surgeon may predispose patients to a less successful outcome. In these cases, education directed toward addressing patient expectations and follow-up care may improve the patient's ability achieve a good outcome.

In addition to patient education, some primary concerns for a healthcare provider in the education of a patient status post THA will include proper management of medications and effective instruction regarding hip replacement precautions. With regard to medications, the patient will typically be given an anticoagulant medication upon discharge for a short time. During this time frame, the patient will need to have blood drawn to monitor his or her levels of Coumadin. This is typically carried out by a home health nurse who is in regular contact with the patient's primary care physician.

The second significant educational concern for patients, healthcare providers, and surgeons is the understanding and demonstration of hip replacement precautions. This is dependent on the surgical approach that is performed and the patient's ability to understand and carry out hip precautions. If the patient is noncompliant with THA precautions, he or she is susceptible to hip dislocation. Hip dislocations can occur early if the precautions are not followed; they can also occur later in time if the tissues and hardware are compromised from noncompliance.

CONCLUSIONS

In summary, OA is a common type of arthritis with a high prevalence and incidence among middle-aged and older adults of both genders. To date, there are many supporting research studies validating a diagnostic algorithm to detect OA, studies to demonstrate the success of surgical and therapeutic interventions, and the ongoing need for patient education to minimize risk factors and maximize medical interventions. There is much that can be taught to patients preoperatively, postoperatively, and in the spirit of health promotion and wellness. The following sections provide further support in these endeavors to teach and promote optimal health care for all.

RESOURCES

American College of Rheumatology Diagnostic Criteria for OA: Altman, R., et al. (1991). The American College of Rheumatology criteria for the classification and reporting of osteoarthritis of the hip. *Arthritis and Rheumatology, 34,* 505–514.

eOrthopod: A Patient's Guide to Osteoarthritis of the Hip
www.eorthopod.com/public/patient_education/6501/osteoarthritis_
of_the_hip.html

Arthritis.com: Arthritis and your joints:
www.arthritis.com

Arthritis Foundation
http://ww2.arthritis.org/conditions/diseasecenter/OA/oa_epidemiology.asp

American College of Rheumatology: Guidelines
for Medical Management of Osteoarthritis
www.rheumatology.org/publications/guidelines/oa-hip/oa-hip.asp

Centers for Disease Control
www.cdc.org

Arthritis Practitioner: How to Detect and Treat OA Hip Pain
www.arthritispractitioner.com/article/6355

Joint Replacement Institute at St. Vincent Medical Center, Los Angeles, CA
Information for Prospective Patients, Postoperative Course: Hip
www.jri-docs.com/JRI_Prospective_Post_Hip.html

Patient UK: Osteoarthritis
www.patient.co.uk/showdoc/23068795/

Brigham and Women's Hospital: Occupational Therapy Standards of Care:
Total Hip Replacement
www.brighamandwomens.org

REFERENCES

Altman, R., Alarcon, G., Appelrouth, D., Bloch, D., Borenstein, D., & Brandt, K. (1991). The American College of Rheumatology criteria for the classification and reporting of osteoarthritis of the hip. *Arthritis and Rheumatology, 34,* 505–514.

Bachmeier, C. J. M., March, L. M., Cross, M. J., Lapsley, H. M., Tribe, K. L., Courtenay, B. G., & Brooks, P. M. (2001). A comparison of outcomes in osteoarthritis patients undergoing total hip and knee replacement surgery. *Osteoarthritis and Cartilage, 9*(2), 137–146.

Bonutti, P. M., Mont, M. A., McMahon, M., Ragland, P. S., & Kester, M. (2004). Minimally invasive total knee arthroplasty. *American Journal of Bone and Joint Surgery, 86-A*(2), 26–32.

Buckwalter, J. A., Saltzman, C., & Brown, T. (2004). The impact of osteoarthritis. *Clinical Orthopaedics Related Research, 427S,* S6–S15.

Cioppa-Mosca, J., Cahill, J. B., Cavanaugh, J. T., Corradi-Scalise, D., Rudnick, H., & Wolff, A. L. (2006). *Postsurgical rehabilitation guidelines for the orthopaedic clinician.* New York: Hospital for Special Surgery, Department of Rehabilitation, Mosby-Elsevier.

Fagerson, T. L. (1998). *The hip handbook.* Boston: Butterworth-Heinemann.

Felson, D. T. (2004). Risk factors for osteoarthritis. *Clinical Orthopaedics Related Research, 427S,* S16–S21.

Felson D. T., Naimark, A., Anderson, J., Kazis, L., Castelli, W., & Meenan, R. F. (1987). The prevalence of knee osteoarthritis in the elderly: the Framingham osteoarthritis study. *Arthritis & Rheumatism, 30*(8), 914–918.

Felson, D. T., & Zhang Y. (1998). An update on the epidemiology of knee and hip osteoarthritis with a view to prevention. *Arthritis & Rheumatism, 41*(8), 1343–1355.

Felson, D. T., Zhang, Y., Hannan, M. T., Naimark, A., Weissman, B. N., Aliabadi, P., & Levy, D. (1995). The incidence and natural history of knee osteoarthritis in the elderly: the Framingham osteoarthritis study. *Arthritis & Rheumatism, 38*(10), 1500–1505.

Fortin, P. R., Clarke, A. E., Joseph, L., Liang, M. H., Tanzer, M., Ferland, D., Phillips, C., Partridge, A. J., Belisle, P., Fossel, A. H., Mahomed, N., Sledge, C. B., & Katz, J. N. (1999). Outcomes of total hip and knee replacements: Preoperative functional status predicts outcomes at six months after surgery. *Arthritis & Rheumatism, 42*(8), 1722–1728.

Gabriel, S. E., Crowson, C. S., Campion, M. E., & O'Fallon, W. M. (1997). Direct medical costs unique to people with arthritis. *Journal of Rheumatology, 24*(4), 719–725.

Hawker, G. A. (2006). Who, when and why total joint replacement surgery? The patient's perspective. *Current Opinions in Rheumatology, 18*(5), 526–530.

Hochberg, M. C., Roy, D., Altman, K. D., Brandt, B. M., Clark, P. A., & Dieppe, M. R. (1995). Guidelines for the medical management of osteoarthritis. *Arthritis & Rheumatism, 38*(11), 1535–1540.

Jordan, J. M., Helmick, C. G., Renner, J. B., Luta, G., Dragomir, A. D., Woodard, J., Fang, F., Schwartz, T. A., Abbate, L. M., Callahan, L. F., Kalsbeek, W. D., & Hochberg, M. C. (2007). Prevalence of knee symptoms and radiographic and symptomatic knee osteoarthritis in African Americans and Caucasians: the Johnston County osteoarthritis project. *Journal of Rheumatology, 34*(1), 172–180.

Katz, J. N., Barrett, J., Mahomed, N. N., Baron, J. A., Wright, R. J., & Losina, E. (2004). Association between hospital and surgeon procedure volume and the outcomes of total knee replacement. *Journal of Bone & Joint Surgery American Volume, 86,* 1909–1916.

Klipper, J. H. (2001). *Primer on Rheumatic Diseases* (12th ed.). Atlanta, GA: Arthritis Foundation.

Kuster, M. S. (2002). Exercise recommendations after total joint replacement: a review of the current literature and proposal of scientifically based guidelines. *Sports Medicine, 32*(7), 433–445.

Lavernia, C. J., Drakeford, M. K., Tsao, A. K., Gittelsohn, A., Krackow, K. A., & Hungerford, D. S. (1995). Revision and primary hip and knee arthroplasty: a cost analysis. *Clinical Orthopaedics and Related Research, 2*(311), 136–141.

Lawrence, R. C., Helmick, C. G., Arnett, F. C., Deyo, R. A., Felson, D. T., Giannini, E. H., Heyse, S. P., Hirsch, R., Hochberg, M. C., Hunder, G. G., Liang, M. H., Pillemer, S. R., Steen, V. D., & Wolfe, F. (1998). Estimates of the prevalence of arthritis and selected musculoskeletal disorders in the United States. *Arthritis and Rheumatism, 41*(5), 778–799.

Lethbridge-Cejku, M., Helmick, C. G., & Popovic, J. R. (2003). Hospitalizations for arthritis and other rheumatic conditions: data from the 1976 National Hospital Discharge Survey. *Medical Care, 41*(12), 1367–1373.

Losina, E., Barrett J., Baron J. A., Levy, M., Phillips, C. B., & Katz, J. N. (2004a). Utilization of low-volume hospitals for total hip replacement. *Arthritis and Rheumatism, 15,* 836–842.

Losina, E., Barrett J., Mahomed, N. N., Baron, J. A., & Katz, J. N. (2004b). Early failures of total hip replacement: effect of surgeon volume. *Arthritis and Rheumatism, 50,* 1338–1343.

Mahomed, N. N., Liang, M. H., Cook, E. F., Daltroy, L. H., Fortin, P. R., Fossel, A. H., & Katz, J. N. (2002). The importance of patient expectations in predicting functional outcomes after total joint arthroplasty. *Journal of Rheumatology, 29,* 1273–1279.

March, L. M., Cross, M. J., Lapsley, H., Brnabic, A. J. M., Tribe, K. L., Bachmeier, C. J. M., Courtenay, B. G., & Brooks, P. M. (1999). Outcomes after hip or knee replacement surgery for OA: a prospective cohort study comparing patients' quality of life before and after surgery with age-related population norms. *Medical Journal of Australia, 171,* 235–238.

National Institutes of Health. (2003, December 8–10). *National Institutes of Health Consensus Statement.* NIH Consensus Development Conference on Total Knee Replacement. Retrieved from http://consensus.nih.gov/2003/2003TotalKnee Replacement117html.htm.

Oliveria, S. A., Felson, D. T., Reed, J. I., Cirillo, P. A., & Walker, A. M. (1995). Incidence of symptomatic hand, hip, and knee osteoarthritis among patients in a health maintenance organization. *Arthritis and Rheumatism, 38*(8), 1134–1141.

Peak, E. L. (2005). The role of patient restriction in reducing the prevalence of early dislocation following total hip arthroplasty. *Journal of Bone and Joint Surgery, 87-A*(2), 247–253.

Rossignol, M., Leclerc, A., Allaert, F. A., Rozenberg, S., Valat, J. P., Avouac, B., Coste, P., Litvak, E., & Hilliquin, P. (2005). Primary osteoarthritis of hip, knee and hand in relation to occupational exposure. *Occupational and Environmental Medicine, 62,*772–777.

Sacks, J. J., Helmick C. G., & Langmaid, G. (2004). Deaths from arthritis and other rheumatic conditions, United States, 1979–1998. *Journal of Rheumatology, 31,* 1823–1828.

Sashika, H., Matsuba, Y., & Watanabe, Y. (1996). Home program of physical therapy: effect on disabilities of patients with total hip arthroplasty. *Archives of Physical Medicine and Rehabilitation, 77*(3), 273–277.

Srikanth, V. K., Fryer, J. L., Zhai, G., Winzenberg, T. M., Hosmer, D., & Jones, G. (2005). A meta-analysis of sex difference prevalence, incidence and severity of osteoarthritis. *Osteoarthritis Cartilage, 13,* 769–781.

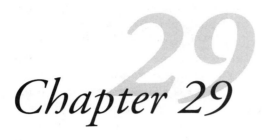

Chapter 29

Progressive Neurological Disorders

Nancy Lowenstein

INTRODUCTION

This chapter focuses on health promotion programs for two progressive neurological disorders for which there has been evidence to support health education and health promotion activities. These neurological conditions are multiple sclerosis and Parkinson's disease.

Multiple sclerosis is an autoimmune disease of the central nervous system in which the body attacks the myelin sheath that surrounds the nerves leaving scar tissue, known as sclerosis. This in turn disrupts the conduction of impulses over the affected nerve and produces a variety of symptoms. There are four categorizations of multiple sclerosis, as described by the National Multiple Sclerosis Society: relapsing remitting, secondary progressive, primary progressive, and progressive relapsing. The common thread for all of them is the gradual loss of both motor and some cognitive function; however, the extent and speed of progression are different for each individual with the disease. The most frequent symptoms are fatigue, walking, balance and coordination difficulties, bowel and bladder issues, visual issues, pain, spasticity, sexual dysfunction, and emotional problems, such as depression (www.nmss.org). Many of these symptoms are "silent" symptoms—that is, they are not visible to others. Often these symptoms, such as fatigue, cognitive or bladder issues, may be an individual's only symptoms; thus, with a lack of motor symptoms, the individual "looks good" or "healthy" to those who do not know that they have multiple sclerosis. This can lead to misunderstandings with family members, coworkers, and friends.

Parkinson's disease is a chronic and progressive movement disorder (www.pdf.org). It is caused by the death of the dopamine producing cells in the substantia nigra in the cerebral cortex. Dopamine is a neurotransmitter that influences movement and coordination. As dopamine diminishes, several symptoms develop. The most common are difficulty initiating movement, tremors (most notably in the hands, arms, legs, jaw, and face), rigidity and stiffness in the trunk and limbs, bradykinesia (slowed movement), impaired balance and coordination, and speech difficulties. Classically, individuals with Parkinson's disease have a "masked face" appearance, stooped posture, and a festinating gait (www.pdf.org).

Both multiple sclerosis and Parkinson's disease impact those close to the individual with the condition: families, coworkers, and friends. It is in this context that the individual can benefit from education regarding his or her disease. It is important that individuals learn how to communicate to others, to feel empowered, and to be able to advocate for themselves. Additionally, health education can assist the individual to manage new symptoms as they appear, deal with the unpredictability of the disease, and learn how to communicate his or her needs to others. Busting myths, providing up-to-date and accurate information, and providing resources for disease management are all important aspects of a good health promotion program.

HEALTH EDUCATION FOR MULTIPLE SCLEROSIS AND PARKINSON'S DISEASE

Literature on health and wellness programs for individuals with multiple sclerosis is growing and has a notable cross-cultural factor. Studies done in the United Kingdom, Australia, and the United States (Ennis, Thain, Bogglid, Baker, & Young, 2006; Nolte Elsworth, Sinclair, & Osborne, 2007) have focused on two primary areas in multiple sclerosis health management: fatigue management and health behaviors/lifestyle change. Frequently, these studies focus on the development of knowledge and skills, building self-efficacy, and individualized problem solving. Commonalities in these studies include offering a community-based series of classes for 6 to 8 weeks and teaching health management behaviors, including exercise, goal setting, and social support.

Additionally, Stuifbergen, Becker, Blozis, Timmerman, and Kullberg (2003) explored the effectiveness of a lifestyle change program that included "lifestyle adjustment; exercise and physical activity for fun, endurance, and strength; eating healthy; stress management; intimacy and sexuality; and women's health issues" (p. 470). They found that those women who participated in the study "succeeded in improving self-efficacy, health behaviors, and selected aspects of QOL (pain, mental health)" (p. 474). Ennis et al. (2006) completed a study of individuals with multiple sclerosis who had completed an 8-week multidisciplinary health promotion program "aimed at increasing knowledge, skills and confidence" (p. 783). They showed significant changes in health-promoting behaviors. Their group intervention was divided into segments that addressed "exercise and physical activity, lifestyle adjustment/ fatigue management, stress management, nutritional awareness, responsible health practices" (p. 786). Both studies used the Health Promoting Lifestyle Profile II as their outcome measure. This measure has six subscales related to health and well-being and asks participants to rate themselves on physical activity, spiritual growth, health responsibility, interpersonal relationships, nutrition, and stress management.

Another area of health promotion for individuals with multiple sclerosis is that of fatigue management. Fatigue is a primary and often debilitating symptom of multiple sclerosis and is one of the most common reasons, along with cognitive deficits, that individuals with multiple sclerosis stop working (www.nmss.org). Medications have inconsistent results in relieving fatigue, and in this author's experience, the energy management strategies that are often taught to clients require lifestyle change, changes in self-perception, and sometimes adjustment in family dynamics.

Unlike a general health promotion program, the fatigue management programs are specifically targeted toward one symptom: fatigue. In these programs, energy conservation techniques are taught to participants as a way of managing their fatigue. Marcia Finlayson (2005) describes these skills as "learn[ing] to evaluate their energy expenditures for daily activities, determine ways of modifying these activities, evaluate their rest-activity ratios, use their bodies to perform tasks efficiently, plan ahead to manage their fatigue and examine their use of adaptive equipment and community resources" (p. 267). In several studies by Finlayson (2005); Matuska, Mathiowetz, and Finlayson (2007); and Holberg and Finlayson (2007), the effects of a 6-week course to learn energy-conservation strategies found that those participants who did implement these strategies reported that they were effective in reducing fatigue and improving their daily performance.

There is much less literature specifically on self-management programs for individuals with Parkinson's disease. There is a body of evidence that looks at the effectiveness of different rehabilitation techniques, most notably two meta-analytic reviews for physical therapy and occupational therapy treatment (de Goede, Keus, Kwakkel, & Wagenaar, 2001; Murphy & Tickle-Degnen, 2001). Two studies that specifically looked at providing health education for individuals with Parkinson's disease are older (1994 and 1987). The study by Montgomery, Lieberman, Singh, and Fries (1994) provided a health education program by mail, individualized recommendations about diet, exercise, medication issues. The treatment group demonstrated significant improvement in performing activities of daily living when on and off their medications, and on the self-efficacy outcome measures, they had significantly more confidence in their ability to control their symptoms and disease issues. The study by Gauthier, Dalziel, and Gauthier (1987) involved a 5-week, 10-session occupational therapy group using mobility activities, rest, socialization, dexterity and functional activities, and education. Results at 6 months and 1 year showed fewer signs of bradykinesia and akathisia. Additionally, the treatment group reported greater psychological well-being. More recently, Ellis et al. (2005) completed a study of group physical therapy programs in two countries. The group programs consisted of 12 sessions, twice a week for 1.5 hours each. Each group consisted of "cardiovascular warm-up activities (5 min), stretching exercises (15 min), strengthening exercises in a functional context (15 min), functional training (15 min), gait training with auditory cueing (15 min), balance training and recreational games (15 min), and relaxation exercises (10 min)" (p. 628). Results of this study support gains in functional status and quality of life in relationship to mobility, but not in global quality of life. The lack of research supporting the use of wellness intervention for individuals with Parkinson's disease should not discourage health professionals from developing health promotion and wellness programs for individuals with Parkinson's disease, as there is a good body of evidence to support self-management for individuals with chronic disease.

TEACHING TECHNIQUES FOR HEALTH EDUCATION AND HEALTH PROMOTION FOR INDIVIDUALS WITH PROGRESSIVE NEUROLOGICAL DISEASE

Individuals with chronic diseases come to health promotion and health education groups at a variety of stages in the disease process. Some people may be newly diagnosed, wanting to learn as much as they can in order to be proactive. Others may have been functioning fairly well for a long period and are now experiencing changes that require them to examine their condition more closely, whereas still others may be fairly far along in their disease process and are looking for ways to continue to cope with the changes that are occurring to their mind and body. Additionally, no two individuals will experience their disease in the same way. For those with multiple sclerosis, some may experience more physical problems or more silent symptoms or more emotional issues. For those with Parkinson's disease, some may experience more tremor, more balance or ambulatory issues, or more cognitive issues. For these reasons, there is no single teaching method, but instead, many different techniques and strategies are used. Here are described some teaching strategies that have been found to be useful in leading health and wellness groups for individuals with multiple sclerosis and Parkinson's disease.

Leadership

Although lay leadership can be effective (as in support groups), having a group leader who has a background in the medical, allied health, or social work field provides the group with someone trained in running a group, knowledge of the condition, and experience working with individuals with the condition. These professionals can ensure that the materials being taught and discussed in the groups are based on valid and reliable information. It is also important for the leader to be very familiar with the condition(s) of the group participants. The leader must know the most recent medications and treatments, the disease course, common symptoms, and recent evidence.

Additionally, a co-leader who is an individual with the condition can provide a balance to the group leadership. This individual can talk from a lived experience of the disease, whereas the professional leader ensures the validity of the information. Additionally, members are open to hearing information from someone who has the same condition as them.

Workbook and Homework

A workbook is useful in providing key points, homework, and resources for each week's session. If exercises are involved, the workbook can have photos and descriptions of the exercises so that participants can do them on their own. The workbook can be formatted in many different ways, but the text should be written at a reading level for all participants (including those who may have cognitive or literacy issues). Additionally, with some disorders, especially multiple sclerosis, visual issues may be common, and the font size should be no smaller than 14 points (National Multiple Sclerosis Society requirements). A workbook can also include homework to be completed between sessions. Active engagement in the learning process is needed in order to make effective health behavior changes. This can be accomplished by asking participants to reflect on or practice each week's lesson and return to the next class with their homework completed. Sometimes the homework may relate to the class that is coming up, and thus, participants can prepare in advance. For instance, if the following week's session is focused on examining the home, the participant might be given a worksheet that asks him or her to look at how his or her home is set up, how many stairs, how often does he or she take the stairs and for what, and so forth. When students come to class, they have this information readily available for discussion and analysis.

Teaching Techniques

Many teaching techniques are appropriate for this population. Active learning techniques involve engaging the learners in a learning activity, as opposed to being lectured to. Techniques such as brainstorming, repetition, accountability, goal setting, and practice of newly learned skills are all good techniques. The use of tools such as video clips, flip charts, overheads, or PowerPoint slides in small numbers may also be used.

Brainstorming is a useful technique for exploring a variety of solutions to a specific problem or to a general issue. For instance, when brainstorming solutions to a task such as cooking, there may be specific problems for individuals in the group, as well as general problems that many people in the group share. Another advantage of brainstorming is that group members can see a variety of ways to address a problem or issue, as well as understand that many issues are common to all the group members.

Repetition allows for issues to be revisited several times throughout the 6- to 8-week group or in setting a weekly routine for the group. An example of a routine for a 2-hour group may be as follows:

15 minutes to review questions from previous weeks or for introductions

0.5 hour for exercise

0.5 hour for topic discussion

0.5 hour for goal setting

15 minutes to review homework and answer any questions

This timeline would be repeated each week with the same exercise routine repeated each week, a new or revisited discussion topic, and review of weekly goals.

Accountability and goal setting are related topics. Being accountable for doing homework and attending and participating in the group are all norms that can be set up during the initial group meeting. By inviting participants to be active in the group and in their learning, participants are more likely to invest in the learning process.

Goal setting requires participants to create goals that can be realistically met. Failure to achieve a goal is often because it was set unrealistically. Even our New Year's resolutions are often unrealistic. How many times have you set a New Year's resolution that you were going to start exercising, lose weight, stop biting your nails, stop smoking, and so forth? A few weeks into the new year, however, you most likely reverted to old behaviors and habits. The problem with these goals is that they are too vague and do not require any accountability. Goals should have a timeline and a specific and measurable outcome. By restating the goal so that it is more specific and also telling someone else your goal, the chance of achieving it is enhanced. For example, instead of setting a goal to start exercising, have the group member look at their history of exercising. When was the last time they did any? What type do they like? Have they ever exercised? Next, have the group member take that information, set a goal, such as "I will exercise two times this week, on Monday and Wednesday, for 15 minutes each time." This type of goal has a better chance of being met because there are specific days, a length of time, and a number of times. Now it feels less daunting to achieve this goal than the previous vague goal of "start to exercise." In a group, sharing goals is a good way for participants to be accountable for their goals and for helping each other become realistic in their goal setting.

Practicing new skills within the group is also a good technique. In this way, the group leader can ensure that the participants are performing the skill correctly and, if not, make corrections before bad habits are started. When working with individuals with Parkinson's disease, practicing a skill is essential, as you want "over learning" to occur so that the individual does not need to "think" about how to do the task.

SUMMARY

Individuals with chronic progressive neurological diseases have unique issues when it comes to educational programs. They face the uncertain nature of their disease course, medication management, family issues, and the progressive nature of the disease.

There is more evidence that supports health promotion education for individuals with multiple sclerosis than for those with Parkinson's disease;

however, there is a growing body of evidence that supports rehabilitation (physical therapy, occupational therapy, and speech therapy) for individuals with Parkinson's disease, and these principles can be incorporated into health promotion programs and groups.

Teaching techniques for these adult learners should include a variety of active learning techniques, practice, homework, and workbooks. Additionally, an effective group leader has knowledge of the condition and can manage the group process.

Case Study 29–1

Mrs. P is a 48-year-old female who has had multiple sclerosis for 10 years. She is married and has two teenage children. Mrs. P works full time as a paralegal in a busy, but small, law office. She has worked for the same employer for over 14 years, and she has disclosed her illness to her employer. Mrs. P signed up for a 6-week fatigue management course sponsored by the National Multiple Sclerosis Society. Mrs. P had to get permission from her employer to attend the course, as it met for 2 hours during the workday. Her job is high stress, and she has thought about reducing to part-time but feels that her family needs the money. There were 10 individuals in the first group. The course was set up to discuss, practice, or teach a new energy-conservation technique each week. There was weekly homework, a workbook, and several guest experts, including a neurologist, exercise physiologist, and physical therapist. The group was led by an occupational therapist. Mrs. P broke down in tears during the first meeting of the group, noting that she does not do anything for herself. She is exhausted by the time she gets home from work, yet still wants to manage dinner and other household chores and is very stressed. Much of her identity was tied up in being a wife and mother. The group was very supportive of each member and encouraged each other to try techniques learned, share their successes and barriers, and create a safe environment for sharing. Mrs. P attended all classes, did all of the homework, and was an active participant. She began to see the importance of making time for herself, and as the group progressed, she met with a personal trainer and began a regular exercise program. By the end of the program, Mrs. P had started to ask her family for help in household chores and began to think about reducing her hours at work. She had incorporated many of the energy-conservation strategies that she had learned into her life and had embraced a lifestyle change. At the final group meeting, Mrs. P proudly showed off her new manicure—the first one she had had in years!

Discussion

Mrs. P came to the group with a sense of desperation about her life and disease. She clearly had little sense of self-efficacy or control over her disease and had little communication with her family about her needs. She also had very little contact with other individuals with multiple sclerosis. For Mrs. P, the group was the first opportunity for her to learn that there were methods to manage her fatigue, to talk to others in similar circumstances and with similar issues, and to start to make lifestyle changes. The group provided her with tools to make changes, ways to identify her needs, and then communicate these to her family. She was able to move successfully from a feeling of hopelessness to one of empowerment.

Case Study 29–2

Ms. B was a 28-year-old woman who had been diagnosed with multiple sclerosis. She lived with a partner, worked part-time, and was taking a college-level class as a prerequisite for applying to graduate school, although she was not sure that she could complete the program. Ms. B enjoyed outdoor activities, such as hiking and biking, drove a stick-shift car, but used a cane for walking, as she had weakness in her left leg. She also had fatigue that impacted her energy levels and limited her ability to socialize and pursue leisure and vocational occupations. She attended a 6-week wellness program for individuals with multiple sclerosis. The group format consisted of a half-hour discussion, half-hour exercises, half-hour discussion, and half-hour goal setting. Two group leaders, one a healthcare professional, and the co-leader, an individual with multiple sclerosis facilitated group discussions. Discussion topics included fatigue, stress management, leisure, depression, cognitive issues, how to talk to your neurologist, and weekly goal setting. From the first group, Ms. B was an active participant in the group discussions. She learned to set realistic goals, which mostly revolved around time management in order to include

(Continues)

Case Study 29–2 (*Continued*)

an exercise routine and time for her school studies. By the end of the course, Ms. B had started a regular exercise routine and had bought a two-person kayak so that she could continue to enjoy her leisure pursuits in the outdoors. Several months later, Ms. B contacted the instructors to let them know that she had decided to give up her manual transmission car and buy one with an automatic transmission. She also decided to enroll in graduate school full-time.

Discussion

Ms. B was young when diagnosed with multiple sclerosis and had had very few physical symptoms for many years. She was motivated by the course to become empowered and make life decisions, not based on how her condition *may* change in the future, but on what she wanted to enjoy now. By learning techniques and getting the support of others with multiple sclerosis, she was able to explore the activities that were important to her (leisure, vocation, and transportation), learn techniques to manage symptoms, and make decisions based on her priorities, not on her disease. The course taught her lifestyle changes and ways to manage the uncertainties of her disease and provided a supportive environment with those who understood her condition to safely explore change.

Case Study 29–3

Mr. S is a 67-year-old man with Parkinson's disease. He lives alone in a third-floor walk-up apartment in an urban area. He is retired from his job as a professor and is divorced with adult children. He participated in a 6-week self-management program for individuals with Parkinson's disease as part of a study to explore the efficacy of a self-management program. The group met weekly for 2 hours following a set format consisting of mobility and speech exercises, ambulation training, skill practice, and discussion. Topics addressed throughout the program were all issues related to functioning with Parkinson's disease, such as using the telephone (soft voice, slurred speech), transferring out of chairs, bed mobility, handwriting and computer use (micrographia and tremor), dressing (movement limitation), and more. Mr. S was also visited weekly by an occupational therapist in his home while he was participating in the study. Mr. S's symptoms were well controlled by medications, with little variation when medications were at their peak (on/off times). He attended all of the group sessions and did the exercises and participated in the discussions; however, he also joked quite a lot during each session and was known as the group humorist. He consistently denied any problems associated with his condition, and during the brainstorming discussions, he frequently made comments that were not supportive of conditions of other group members. He did not practice the exercises outside of the group meetings, nor did he try any of the techniques discussed during the sessions. One of Mr. S's hobbies was using an exacto knife to cut out magazine pictures and make collages. These were quite beautiful pieces. Mr. S had a slight tremor and hand weakness but was not interested in learning any techniques to address this. He identified a few issues around meal preparation, but was not interested in addressing these during either the group or this home visit, noting he "would figure it out when he had to." Although he arrived to the group on time and made it to all of the sessions, he continually noted that he did not "have any of these problems."

Discussion

Mr. S's Parkinson's disease had not significantly impacted on his daily life, and although he knew his condition could worsen, Mr. S was comfortable with his functional level and did not see the necessity of changing his habits before it became necessary. Despite the emphasis during the self-management group that it was important to learn new habits before they were needed and that repetition was important in learning a new skill, Mr. S did not see a connection to his own life and condition. It is possible that when his condition begins to change that Mr. S will remember the techniques that were taught during the course and begin to use them.

REFERENCES

de Goede, C. J., Keus, S. H., Kwakkel, G., & Wagenaar, R. C. (2001). The effects of physical therapy in Parkinson's disease: a research synthesis. *Archives of Physical Medicine and Rehabilitation, 82,* 509–515.

Ellis, T., de Goede, C. J., Feldman, R. G., Wolters, E. C., Kwakkel, G., & Wagenaar, R. C. (2005). Efficacy of a physical therapy program in patients with Parkinson's disease: a randomized controlled trial. *Archives of Physical Medicine and Rehabilitation, 86,* 626–632.

Ennis, M., Thain, J., Bogglid, M., Baker, G. A., & Young, C. A. (2006). A randomized controlled trial of a health promotion education programme for people with multiple sclerosis. *Clinical Rehabilitation, 20,* 783–792.

Finlayson, M. (2005). Pilot study of an energy conservation education program delivered by telephone conference call to people with multiple sclerosis. *Neurorehabilitation, 20,* 267–277.

Gauthier, L., Dalziel, S., & Gauthier, S. (1987). Group occupational therapy improves functional status, decreases symptoms of clients with Parkinson's. *American Journal of Occupational Therapy, 41,* 360–365.

Holberg, C., & Finlayson, M. (2007). Factors influencing the use of energy conservation strategies by persons with multiple sclerosis. *American Journal of Occupational Therapy, 61,* 96–107.

Matuska, K., Mathiowetz, V., & Finlayson, M. (2007). Use and perceived effectiveness of energy conservation strategies for managing multiple sclerosis fatigue. *American Journal of Occupational Therapy, 61,* 62–69.

Montgomery, E. B., Lieberman, A., Singh, G., & Fries, J. F. (1994). Health education and promotion may improve ADL status and self-efficacy in clients with Parkinson's disease. *American Journal of Medicine, 97,* 429–435.

Murphy, S., & Tickle-Degnen, L. (2001). The effectiveness of occupational therapy-related treatments for persons with Parkinson's diseases: a meta-analytic review. *American Journal of Occupational Therapy, 55,* 385–392.

Nolte, S., Elsworth, G. F., Sinclair, A. J., & Osborne, R. H. (2007). The extent and breadth of benefits from participating in chronic disease self-management course: a national patient-reported outcomes survey. *Patient Education and Counseling, 65,* 351–360.

Stuifbergen, A. K., Becker, H., Blozis, S., Timmerman, G., & Kullberg, V. (2003). A randomized clinical trial of a wellness intervention for women with multiple sclerosis. *Archives of Physical Medicine & Rehabilitation, 84,* 467–476.

Chapter 30

Mental Health

Florence Keane

> *A great teacher turns learning into an exciting adventure.*
> —*Author unknown*

INTRODUCTION

Historically, mental health has been approached from a negative perspective and was only thought of as an illness. Over the years, the movements in health have seen a shift from any stigma or negative attitudes or phrases, such as mental illnesses, and have replaced them with more positive phrases. Thus, mental illness became mental health. The World Health Organization (WHO, 2007) offers the following definition: Mental health is a state of well-being in which the individual realizes his or her own abilities, can cope with the normal stresses of life, can work productively and fruitfully, and is able to make a contribution to the community; however, there is no clear cut definition for mental illness or mental health. Mental illness or health, for that matter, is influenced by cultural, family, and individual values. Take hallucinations, seeing things or hearing voices that are not seen or heard by others around, and delusions, false beliefs—this experience is highly valued in some cultures, and the one who is hallucinating or is delusional is revered. In other cultures, the experience is regarded as insanity and should be avoided and not mentioned at all.

A simple definition of mental illness could be a feeling or way of thinking by someone, or rather by the family, friends, and people around, that there is something that is not right. A sense of disharmony exists. It is this lack of understanding about what is happening that brings about the stereotyping and the stigma that is often associated with mental illness. Mental illness may be explained at the physical level as a malfunction in the brain, the personal level as a lack of self-care, and the societal level as the inability to interact well with others. Genetics too may play a role in mental illness; some mental illnesses run in families. The cultural factors of aging, immigration stress, racism, the belief that one's race is better than others, marginalization, sexism, and inadequate access to health care are all influences for the development of physical and mental disorders. Persons who emotionally are unable to cope with these prejudices, hostility toward them for being different, may develop the strange manifestations that we call mental illness.

Mental health is the attempt to restore harmony to the person, family, and friends. The person while on the road to improvement in mental health realizes that he or she has the ability to learn and the ability to feel, express, and manage his or her positive aspects and or emotions. Mental health is the result of positive coping to the emotions. Persons are able to form and maintain good relationships with others; they are able to cope and manage change and uncertainty successfully. Mental disorders are real health conditions just as cardiovascular or renal disease and mental health is fundamental to overall health.

BACKGROUND OF THE PROBLEM

The prevalence of mental health problems is much greater than one would imagine. Mental health problems are very common, and it is believed that one in every four persons, who has accessed the healthcare system, has had at least one incident of mental, neurological, or behavioral disorder (WHO, 2007). In the correctional system, one in every two youth who is incarcerated may have a serious mental health problem, according to the President's New Freedom Commission on Mental Health (2003). There are many more who are less likely to receive any kind of treatment. After the events of September 11, 2001, the nation's concern for safety has caused many added stressors to everyday life. The stresses of life, nowadays, have caused many persons to develop mental health problems. Today, mental illness counts for 15% of all illness in developed countries. Depression is second only to ischemic heart disease in terms of burden to society (National Institute of Mental Health

[NIMH], 2006). Bipolar disease, significant mood swings, is the most expensive mental healthcare problem, for both patients with the disease and their health insurance plan. In one study, the average lifetime cost per case ranged from $11,720 for persons with a single manic episode, elevated mood, and unusual thought pattern to $624,785 for persons with nonresponsive or chronic episodes (National Alliance for the Mentally Ill, 2000b).

CULTURE AND MENTAL HEALTH

Culture plays an important role in mental illness. Culture is the shared beliefs, values, and practices that guide persons in patterned ways of thinking and acting (Leininger, 2002). It is through cultural norms that persons decide what is normal or abnormal. Within each culture, there are world views that influence how the culture understands health and illness. If someone acts outside of the norms of their culture, they are considered as ill. This belief applies to mental illness when defining those who are mentally ill; however, one must be aware that the same behaviors that are acceptable in one culture may be regarded as mental illness in another culture. As previously mentioned, someone who has hallucinations may be regarded as having a gift of vision from God in one culture and psychotic by another culture. Mental illness is defined by behaviors; therefore, it is important to understand the behavior in order to be able to plan an appropriate, culturally sensitive intervention. Because the population of the United States is becoming more ethnically diverse, healthcare practitioners need to develop what is called cultural competence by learning about different cultures.

MENTAL DISORDERS

Mental health problems are increasing throughout the world. Mental health problems manifest themselves in the form of mental illness, as well as distress from abuse, violence, displacement, exploitation, and poverty. Some of the manifestations of mental disorders may be distressing only to the person, including disorders such as anxiety. In this instance, the disorder may present itself in such a way that the person spends a lot of time feeling miserable and worrying for no known reason. The disorder may also present itself in a way that may be upsetting to family and friends when the person withdraws from relationship, isolates himself or herself as occurs in depression, becomes manipulative, and has emotional outbursts against loved ones and others. Other behaviors of mental disorder affect society at large when the person displays acts of violence, substance abuse, and dependence. **Table 30-1** comprises a list of some mental disorders taken

Table 30-1 Partial Listing of Disorders

Mental Disorders	Neurobehavioral Brain Disorders	Disinhibition Syndrome
Anxiety disorders	Cognitive impairment disorders	Suicide
Eating disorders	Neuropsychiatric problems	Domestic violence
Mood disorders		Sexual violence
Schizophrenic disorders		Community violence
Substance-related disorders		
Personality disorders		
Spectrum disorders		

from the *Diagnostic and Statistical Manual of Mental Disorders* IV-TR (American Psychiatric Association [APA], 2000).

SOME THEORIES OF MENTAL ILLNESS

There are many theories of mental illness, and any theory could be of help to the practitioner in understanding mental health. Using a theory will allow the practitioner to have a more scientific base for providing care. One theory is the intrapersonal theory, which focuses on the feelings, thoughts, behaviors, and experiences of persons. Intrapersonal theorists believe that one's personality is shaped by events that happen very early in life. Sigmund Freud (1935) developed the first intrapersonal theory. He identified three components of personality: the id, ego (unconscious), and the superego (conscience); each play a role in a person's behavior. This theory is still very popular and is widely used today. Freud's theory is important in understanding how persons cope when dealing with issues such as anxiety and it provides an understanding of how persons use defense mechanisms to cope.

In the late 19th century, the focus shifted away from the individual to interpersonal relationships and events in the social context. Social-interpersonal theory was born. Harry Sullivan (1953) believed that persons should be studied within the context of relationships. Social interpersonal theories emphasize the developing influence of family and society. They believe that mental health problems are interpersonal problems. Sullivan believed that even the most seriously ill could be reached through human relationship of psychotherapy. Abraham Maslow (1963) viewed personality as self-actualizing. Persons were at peak when they fulfilled all of their potential. Before fulfillment could be attained persons had to meet certain needs, starting with basic physiological needs. The social-interpersonal theory allows one to see human behavior from a different viewpoint. The theory explains behavior within a social context and allows the reader to think about the influence of culture and society.

Behavioral theories focus on the person's actions, rather than on their thoughts and feelings. Behaviorists believe that all behavior is learned and therefore can be tailored to achieve the desired end through reward and punishment. Behaviorists believe that undesirable behaviors are learned and that they continue when reinforced. They believe that undesirable behaviors can be replaced with desirable ones (Skinner, 1953). The behaviorist theorists like the social-interpersonal theorists also looked at the personality. Skinner was not concerned with the way persons behaved as much as why they behaved the way they did and what was reinforcing the behavior. The emphasis was not on the past but the present. This is important to predict the trend in the undesirable behavior and to control the behavior. Behavior theories are important theories in client education, especially with mental health. Mental health providers can help persons understand more clearly what is to be gained or lost by behaving in a certain manner through using behavior theories.

Case Study 30-1

Alice, a 26-year-old female, was admitted to the facility on numerous occasions. Her admitting diagnoses are Axis I schizophrenia undifferentiated type, substance abuse disorder, Axis II borderline personality disorder, Axis III pseudo-seizures, and deep vein thrombosis—a blood clot in a deep vein in the leg.

It has been 1 year since her last admission. During this time, there have been several changes in the facility. There are many new staff nurses and mental health technicians; even the unit psychiatrist is new to the facility. Among the many changes, one that is particular displeasing to Alice is the fact that the hospital has now adopted a no-smoking policy.

Alice has been plotting a way to leave the hospital so that she can smoke. She contacted a friend on the outside, and he requested that she be allowed a home visit for a few hours one weekend, but that plan is stymied because he is restricted from leaving home himself, a consequence of drug charges.

Alice does not give up; she decides to play another card. She fakes a seizure. The new mental health technician, who was caring for her, panics when Alice falls to the floor and starts shaking. The mental health technician runs to call the new nurse, who also starts to panic and calls a code. The members of the code team arrive, and they are all in a state of panic as everyone tries unsuccessfully to start an intravenous line on Alice. The staff nurse calls 911. The emergency medical technicians arrive, and Alice is transferred to the local medical hospital, where she is admitted for 1 week while they do a workup for seizure on her. She returns to the facility after 1 week boasting to the other ladies about the wonderful treatment that she received at the hospital. Alice recounted how many cigarettes a day she was able to smoke, in this case five, and she offered to teach the other ladies how to fake a seizure. She faked a seizure every other week since this admission. The staff has called 911 every time, and she has been sent to the hospital each time. Her medical diagnosis from the hospital after each admission was pseudoseizure.

Case Study 30-2

Maureen is a 26-year-old female. This is her first admission to the facility.

Her diagnoses are Axis I schizophrenia undifferentiated type, Axis II borderline personality disorder, Axis III none.

On the first day of her admission, Maureen decided that the facility was too restricted for her; therefore, she decided to fake a seizure hoping the staff would transfer her to a medical hospital. She fell to the floor and started shaking. Of course, the staff panic and called a code. It was early in the day on a weekday, and thus, everyone was still at the facility. The psychiatrist ordered Ativan, a sedative, and the emergency medical technicians arrived and transported her to the hospital. She was sent back to the facility 5 days later with a medical diagnosis of pseudoseizures. Her mother visited the next day, and she told the staff that Maureen had demonstrated attention seeking and manipulative behaviors all of her life and that is why she had her committed to the facility. The mother swore that no harm would come to Maureen, and she begged the staff not to send Maureen to the hospital if she faked another seizure. Two days later Maureen again threw herself on the floor and started to shake. The staff again called a code. On this occasion, it was a weekend night, and the nurse practitioner who was on duty was familiar with the case. All attempts to arouse Maureen were unsuccessful, and thus, the nurse practitioner said, "Maureen I know you are faking this seizure, I will not be sending you to the hospital, so whenever you are ready to go to your room you may do so." Maureen did not respond; she continued to lie on the floor shaking. Again the nurse practitioner spoke. This time she said to the staff, "I believe Maureen wants to sleep on the floor tonight so go get her blanket from her room and let her sleep here." Within 5 minutes Maureen arose, went to her room and went to sleep without a word. The next week Maureen again tried to fake a seizure while the same nurse practitioner was on duty. After responding to the code, the nurse practitioner found Maureen lying on the floor shaking her body all over. The nurse practitioner told her to get up off the floor and go to her room, as that was the only place she would be sent to. Maureen got up spat at the nurse practitioner before going to her room. The nurse practitioner documented the incident, and it was reported to the psychiatrist the next day. As a result, Maureen lost all privileges for 2 weeks. She was confined to the unit and was not allowed to participate in any programs or activities. After about a month of going through the same routine, with Maureen faking seizures and the nurse practitioners refusing to treat her, Maureen gave up her undesirable behavior. Three months later, the nurse practitioner was on the unit visiting another person when Maureen came up to her and said, "I want to apologize for my previous bad behavior. I now have two jobs here. I have saved some money, and I will be going home in 6 weeks."

ANALYSIS OF CASE STUDIES 30-1 AND 30-2

In the previous examples, the Axis I diagnoses are those that are considered mental illnesses and can be treated by therapy and medications. The Axis II diagnoses are personality disorders; medication is not effective in treating these disorders, but some therapies such as behavior therapy and cognitive therapy have been proven to have some effect. The Axis III diagnoses are medical conditions (APA, 2000).

Looking back at the cases of Alice and Maureen, both persons were about equal in age, and they both had the same diagnoses. For many years, they had employed this manipulative, controlling, attention-seeking behavior in order to get what they want. In the first case, the staff fell right into Alice's trap. Alice won the first round, and she continued to play the same card throughout her admission. The staff was not wrong in calling 911. Even the emergency medical technicians were fooled by Alice's behavior. When Alice arrived at the hospital, she had even more shaking episodes. The emergency room nurse's notes documented that Alice had a witnessed seizure for 20 minutes. The attending physicians were concerned about treating a medical problem, and thus, they kept her at the hospital and ran every possible test known to rule out seizures. On each subsequent visit, the physicians were so afraid that this was a true case of seizure; not wanting to miss anything and be sued later, they again treated her for seizures each time. This all continued to reinforce the unwanted behavior. There was no desire for Alice to stop this undesirable behavior.

Maureen, on the other hand, did not get any reinforcement of her undesirable behavior. She soon became aware that as long as she continued to behave undesirably she was losing more than she was gaining. This quickly motivated her to want to change her behavior. When Maureen started to change her behavior, she was rewarded for changing. The reinforcement of the positive behavior encouraged her to continue being positive and do good things rather than to continue being controlling and manipulative. Her self-esteem and self-worth were also improved, and she no longer felt the need to seek attention by faking seizures.

Cognitive theorists believe that it is our ability to think and learn that makes us human. Our cognitive functions allow us to rationalize, make good judgment, interpret the world we live in, and learn new skills. Jean Piaget (1972) believed that the more one is exposed to things in the world around us the more intelligent one becomes. Beck and Freeman's (1990) theory was that it was not important what people did—what was important was how people viewed themselves and the world. Cognitive distortion occurs when people view themselves as being inadequate and have a negative misinterpretation of current events and a negative view of the future. The distortion may present as selective abstraction or focusing on certain information while ignoring contradictory information. Another distortion is overgeneralization, where information from one event is attached to numerous situations. Magnification occurs when insignificant events are aggrandized. Some persons also are caught up with superstitious thinking where they believe that events will be influenced by some mysterious force. Dichotomous thinking occurs when a person believes that everything is all or none. Everything must be all good or all bad. Cognitive theory is important because it assists with assessment and interventions. Analysis of the person's cognitive distortion can allow the practitioner to individualize the person's plan of care.

Neurobiological concepts place emphasis on the medical model. These concepts emphasize the fact that behaviors and emotional problems are illnesses like all others. Assessment is based on presenting symptoms. All illnesses are a result of toxins, lesions, or neurotransmitters, the chemicals used to relay transmission between cells. Social, economic, and medical advances such as new screening and testing instruments, new diagnostic tools, new medications, improvement in nutrition, and the control of infectious diseases have caused reduction in the incidence of disability for mental illness, or the incidence would be much higher than it is today. Some mental disorders such as schizophrenia are believed to have a genetic disposition. Some persons are believed to have a predisposition to mental illness, but they never become mentally ill (Paris, 1999). New medications such as the selective serotonin reuptake inhibitors provide new hope to many with mental illnesses. Researchers in many parts of the world are trying to determine the cause of mental illness as well as to design therapies that can treat persons more effectively. Do persons become mentally ill because of some genetic defect, or is it the stressors of the environment? This is the question that many researchers are asking today. It might be more practical to conclude that mental disorders are the result of the interaction between genes and the environment.

Nursing Theories

Many nurses have contributed to the practice of psychiatric mental health nursing, but Hildegarde Peplau is remembered more than any other for her work with psychiatric mental health nursing. Peplau (1952) was considered the mother of psychiatric mental health nursing. She was influenced by the work of Sullivan and his learning theory. She laid the foundation for psychiatric nursing in her textbook *Interpersonal Relations in Nursing* (1952). Peplau was the first nurse to identify psychiatric nursing as general nursing and as a specialty area. She was interested in the process by which nurses helped persons live more productive lives by making positive changes in their health and well-being. She wrote about the interpersonal process that makes health possible, and she encouraged nurses to listen carefully to patients so that they could develop therapeutic relationships through empathy. Peplau identified three stages of the nurse–patient relationship. The first stage is the introductory stage, where the person and the nurse begin to know each other. Next is the working stage; here the nurse applies his or her intervention to help the person toward wellness. The last stage is the termination stage, when the person is approaching wellness and there must be an end to the relationship as the person regains independence.

Gender differences do exist; the male brain is 10% larger than the female brain. The corpus callosum, which connects both hemispheres of the brain, is larger in the female (APA, 2000). There are also hormonal differences; women have more serotonin (5HT), the neurotransmitter that inhibits aggressive behavior, and men have higher levels of testosterone, making them more prone to be aggressive behaviors. Society also has different expectations for males and females. Currently, science has no clear-cut answer as to why there are differences in the disposition to certain mental disorders with males and females (APA, 2000) (**Table 30-2**).

Table 30-2 Mental Disorders and Their Predispositions

Female	Male	Both
Anxiety disorder	Learning disorders, attention deficit, autistic, Asperger's, hyperactivity	Bipolar disorder
Schizoaffective, borderline, histrionic	Antisocial, schizoid, obsessive-compulsive, narcissistic, personality	Oppositional defiant disorder
Depression, dysthymia	Schizophrenia	Avoidant personality
Eating disorder	Substance abuse disorder	
Alzheimer's disease	Vascular dementia	
	Tourette	

RISK FACTORS FOR MENTAL ILLNESS

The challenge for healthcare providers arises when screening for mental disorders. Providers must be able to recognize mental illness/disorders and implement the appropriate, evidenced-based treatment that is individualized and appropriate for the person. Many persons who present with somatic complaints have an underlying mental disturbance. Psychiatric illnesses are expected to contribute 11% to 15% of the world's diseases in the next century (American Nurses Association, 2000). As the population ages, many persons will be afflicted with Alzheimer's disease and other dementia and will decline in cognitive function. The stress of migration has accounted for many new immigrants receiving inappropriate diagnoses of various mental disorders.

The limited budgets of state hospitals and political actions have resulted in deinstitutionalization; the mentally ill were no longer placed in institutions. The Community Mental Health Law was enacted in 1963. This was a very important time in the history of mental health treatment. The media brought to light the inadequacy of care in the mental institutions. A large number of persons from public mental institutes were discharged to the community. These mentally ill persons very often ended up homeless, with reduced mental benefits because the medical coverage for mental care is 50% of the coverage for medical care (National Alliance for the Mentally Ill, 2000a). They often committed petty crimes, acts of violence, and many ended up incarcerated. Community health services could not keep up with the demand, and at the same time, there were many service men returning from the war that needed mental care.

That era also brought the discovery of psychiatric drugs, however, and new social reforms such as Social Security Disability, Medicaid, Medicare, Social Security Income, and Food Stamps were introduced. Anyone can be afflicted with a mental disorder. Practitioners at all levels should be aware of some of the signs and mental illness so that appropriate referrals can be made.

MENTAL ILLNESS PREVENTION AND MENTAL HEALTH PROMOTION

With new advances in technology and research, the hope is that researchers will be able to develop means to identify those who will be at risk for developing mental illness. Nurses and other healthcare providers who interact with the public play an important part in screening and identifying those at risk. Advances in communication through the Internet and other telehealth systems and advertising by drug companies on television and the radio are all making it possible for millions of people to get information and find help. There are many support groups and community agencies at the national and state levels through which information is disseminated. Providers can help destigmatize mental illness by forming alliances with agencies such as the NAMI. In the acute-care setting, the care of persons are coordinated by a team composed of nurses, social workers, occupational and activity therapists, psychiatrists, medical doctors, psychologists, pharmacists, and other workers.

Community mental health needs are different than those of the hospital. Support in the community may be provided in many traditional and nontraditional sites and manner. The community resource practitioner needs access to many resources to meet the need of persons with mental health issues. Persons in the community need assistance with their mental health, in addition to help with family and support systems. Most importantly, they need a place to live, and they will need financial and medical and mental treatment. Support is needed at the primary, secondary and tertiary levels. Depending on the age of the person, primary support may be provided through some type of day care center or school. The secondary level support may be at a crisis center, a shelter, some type of treatment center, nursing home, or hospice. Tertiary prevention is usually provided in a rehabilitation program or a community mental health center.

In order to screen for mental illness one must be able to conduct a culturally, appropriate mental status assessment. The type of mental status assessment may vary, depending on the circumstances of the client, but attempts should be made to complete the assessment at a later date. The mental status examination is similar to the physical examination on the medical side. Practitioners need to be aware that some medical disorders such as thyroid disorder, HIV, epilepsy, Huntington's disease, and many infections may mimic mental disorders.

When conducting a mental status examination, the practitioner should first collect personal information then start by assessing the ABCs:

- *Appearance and affect.* Is the person dressed appropriately? What about his or her level of hygiene? Are the pupils dilated or constricted? Describe his or her facial expression. Is the affect appropriate to the mood?
- *Behavior and speech.* Is there excessive or peculiar body movement, such as repetitive gestures? How would you describe the balance and gait? What about the eye contact (remember culture here)? Is the speech

rapid, slow, or normal? Is person talking in a loud, disturbing or cluttered manner?

- *Cognition and thought process.* What is the level of consciousness, alertness, and orientation? How is the memory (recent or remote)? Fund of knowledge, attention, abstract thinking, insight, and judgment? Are the thoughts disorganized? Is there flight of ideas? Do you recognize delusions, hallucinations, obsessions, or suicidal ideation?

The mental status examination is only one aspect of the assessment. Practitioners need to also perform a psychosocial assessment and a physical examination to plan culturally appropriate interventions. An extensive interview and history taking should follow using culturally appropriate rating scales to verify the data.

INTERVENTIONS

After a diagnosis has been formulated, using criteria from the *Diagnostic and Statistical Manual of Mental Disorders* IV-TR (APA, 2000), a plan of care should be implemented. The practitioner should use a theoretical framework along with critical thinking to support their judgment. Interventions should be evidenced based. Before practitioners formulate a plan of care, outcomes should be identified so that there can be effective evaluation of the plan of care.

The plan may involve some basic interventions such as counseling, self-care activities, health teaching, psychological interventions, and milieu therapy or more advanced interventions such as psychotherapy, pharmacotherapy, or referrals. Of course, the type of intervention will depend on the psychiatric diagnosis. Some more common diagnoses are anxiety disorders, mood disorders, personality disorders, and schizophrenic disorders.

Anxiety Disorders

Peplau (1968) identified anxiety as one of the most important concepts in psychiatric mental health nursing. Anxiety may be classified as mild, moderate, severe, or panic anxiety. Anxiety can be described as a feeling of apprehension or uneasiness resulting from a real or perceived threat. Some interventions for anxiety are

1. Remain with the person during anxiety attack.
2. Help the person identify their anxiety.

3. Encourage person to talk about feelings.
4. Explore coping mechanisms that worked in the past.
5. Provide outlet for working off anxiety such as exercising (punching bag).
6. Offer high-calorie fluids.
7. Offer medication as appropriate (antianxiety medications).

Mood Disorders

Depression is the fourth leading cause of disability in the United States (WHO, 2001). The incidence of depression greatly increases among people with a medical disorder. Some physical symptoms of depression are headache, fatigue, disturbed sleep, dizziness, chest pain and vague body pains, gastrointestinal complaints, and sexual dysfunctions. Depression represents a change in previous functions. Depression often strikes people who are dealing with a death in the family or a serious illness. They cannot get over the grief at their loss. Persons with depression usually present with at least five of the following disorders: depressed mood, anhedonia, poor appetite, insomnia, increased or decreased activity, and anergia, feelings of helplessness, hopelessness, low self-esteem, and recurrent thoughts of death or suicide (APA, 2003). Untreated depression may lead to suicide. Treatment for children is very often delayed because of ignorance on the part of the practitioner (Monsen & Thomas, 2006). Some interventions for depression are

1. Help person find alternate explanations to problems.
2. Help person to identify distortions and negative self-appraisal.
3. Encourage activities to raise self-esteem, coping skills.
4. Encourage exercise.
5. Encourage support groups.
6. Provide referrals.
7. Offer medications as appropriate (antidepressants).

Personality Disorders

Does the pattern of behavior differ from the expected behavior of the person's culture? Does it usually start in adolescence or early adulthood? Is it stable over time and lead to distress or impairment (APA, 2000)? According to the *Diagnostic and Statistical Manual of Mental Disorders* IV-TR, all personality disorders have four characteristics in common: (1) inflexible and maladaptive response to stress, (2) inability to work and love, (3) frequent interpersonal conflicts, and (4) an inability to maintain personal boundaries. Some interventions for personality disorders are

1. Discuss concerns about behavior with person.
2. Determine appropriate behavior expectations.
3. Establish consequences for chosen actions.
4. Set limits and refrain from arguing, bargaining.
5. Provide physical outlets for anger.
6. Encourage person to self-reward for successful outcomes.
7. Medications have not been proven effective with this population.

Schizophrenia

A devastating brain disease affects a person's thinking, language, emotions, social behavior, and ability to perceive reality accurately. Schizophrenia is described as a psychotic disorder. Psychosis refers to delusions, hallucinations, illusions, disorganized speech and thought, and/or disorganized, catatonic behavior (APA, 2000).

The symptoms of schizophrenia may be classified as positive and negative symptoms. Examples of positive symptoms are hallucinations, delusions, bizarre behavior, and paranoia; they are the symptoms that we are first aware of. Many practitioners believe that the negative symptoms such as anhedonia, apathy, lack of motivation, and poor thought process are more destructive than the positive symptoms because they make persons inert and unmotivated (Beng-Choon, Black, & Anderson, 2004). Persons with schizophrenia usually have a difficult time achieving optimal health. They are usually socially isolated. They do not have adequate information to health education and treatment programs, and the medications keep them sedated and with low levels of functioning (Beebe, 2007). Some treatments for schizophrenia are

1. Provide structure, support, and psychotherapy, including family therapy.
2. Offer medications as appropriate (psychotropic drugs/medications).
3. Protect client and others from harm.
4. Offer counseling and social skill training.
5. Set limits (milieu management and counseling).

Psychiatric Emergencies

Practitioners must be aware of crisis situations. The three basic types of crisis are (1) maturational, (2) situational, and (3) adventitious. Persons with preexisting mental health illnesses are prone to crisis. Crisis may lead to suicide, taking one's own life. In 2001, suicide was the leading cause of death (NIMH, 2006). Suicide is the third leading cause of death among 14 to 25 year olds (APA, 2006). There are many tools to help healthcare providers assess for suicidal potential. A popular scale is SAD PERSONS, developed by Patterson et al. (1983). The important skills for the provider include

1. Assessing for risk factors, including history of suicide, hopelessness, and helplessness and a plan of action.
2. Determine whether the age, gender, and previous suicide attempts put the person at higher risk.
3. Establish whether social support is lacking.
4. Determine whether there is a loss of rational thinking.
5. Look for a sudden switch in mood from sad to happy.

Some interventions for suicide prevention include

1. Provide activities that offer support, information, and education.
2. Provide counseling.
3. Provide safety through milieu therapy with suicide precautions.
4. Provide treatment for suicide in secondary settings.
5. Provide support and interventions to family and friends.
6. Offer antidepressants at adequate doses.

FAMILY TEACHING

The family has the task of recognizing that their loved one is mentally ill. Parents may have a difficult time accepting that their child has a mental disorder. Some mental disorders, such as cognitive disorders, psychotic disorders, mood disorders, and substance-related disorders, first diagnosed in infancy, childhood, or adolescence are identical to the disorders of adulthood. In addition, there are certain disorders that appear during the early developmental years and are identified according to the child's inability to perform. For those parents, it is essential that they recognize normal behavior patterns characteristic of the developmental milestone of the child. Disorders such as mental retardation, deficits in intellectual functioning, and autistic disorders, withdrawal of the child into self, are irreversible and can be managed at home, but caregivers need special teaching to deal with their loved ones. Other disorders such as self-mutilation, impaired social interaction, and disruptive disorder behaviors are more manageable with proper teaching.

It is the responsibility of the healthcare practitioners to teach family members how to care for their loved ones at home. They should realize that it might even be more beneficial to manage these clients in the home setting where they can receive individualized attention. Emphasis should be placed on situations that are life threatening. Safety and security of persons are the first priority. The family caregiver needs to be extremely patient. They should offer positive reinforcement to encourage repetition of positive actions and behaviors. It is important to anticipate the needs of the child until he or she is ready to start communicating. Some children are capable of learning just by developing habitual patterns. Many maladaptive behaviors can be averted if the cause of the behaviors is determined. Teach family caregivers that some behaviors, such as self-mutilating behavior, are usually caused by increasing anxiety, and thus, there must be a feeling of trust in order for the cause of the anxiety to be determined. Family caregivers should stay with the child during such time until a feeling of security has developed and the anxiety can be decreased.

At the other end of the spectrum are those persons, usually older persons, with disorders of delirium, dementia, and amnestic disorders. Here too, healthcare providers need to share successful interventions with caregivers, as they will be the ones caring for the persons when they are discharged home. Caregivers need to be taught that disorientation may lead to safety issues. Furniture needs to be rearranged to accommodate the person's disabilities; items that are used frequently should be within easy reach, and potentially harmful items such as cigarette lighters, matches, and sharp objects should be removed. Persons who have a tendency to wander should have an area where they can wander safely. Caregivers should be taught to use restraints very cautiously, or not at all, as restraining persons might result in increased agitation. Caregivers should stay calm when caring for these persons as their anxiety might be transferred to the persons cared for. Family caregivers must maintain a low level of stimuli at all times to help in decreasing anxiety. They should reorient the client as appropriate and have familiar objects around such as pictures of loved ones and have clocks and calendars in view to help with reality orientation.

Family members need to realize that alcoholism is a family illness. Persons with diagnoses of substance-related disorders such as alcoholism and drug abuse need family involvement to be successful in beating their habits. Programs should be geared toward family and support groups. The family will be the ones to identify the ineffective coping behaviors. Very often family members enjoy the role that they play while the person is disabled, and they do not want to relinquish this role. Family members should be taught to initiate and plan for lifestyle changes. They need to be taught to take action to change the destructive behaviors and alter the enabling behaviors that contribute to the person's addiction.

The person and the family need to be taught about their medications. Persons are noncompliant with medication because they do not like the side effects that they may experience. Persons and family members should be taught how to take their medication, that some drug–drug or drug–food interactions may occur, and that possible side effects of medications may occur. Most psychotropic medications may cause dizziness and or drowsiness. Teach persons and family not to drive or operate dangerous machines while taking medications. Medications should not be stopped abruptly but should be tapered down. Even though the person may believe that the symptoms have subsided, they should continue taking the medicine as some medications will not be effective until a period of four weeks. Alcohol and other central nervous system depressants should not be consumed while taking medications. Sunscreen and protective clothing should be used when going outdoors, as the skin will become more sensitive to sunburn with psychotropic medications. To prevent a sudden drop in blood pressure, persons should rise slowing when going from a sitting or lying to a standing position.

Finally, much has been written about caregivers' burden. It is the responsibility of the healthcare provider to assess that the caregiver is able to anticipate the person's needs and provide the appropriate care. Caregivers should be given appropriate information. The teaching does not have to be formal, but there should at least be an exchange of information to assist them with the responsibility they have been given. Caregivers need to be aware that they should not try to do it all themselves. They should know when they need assistance and where to find the help that they need. They should be encouraged to express their feelings, especially those of anger and resentment. Caregivers should be encouraged to attend support groups so that they can share their stories and learn from others who might have the same situation. They might learn new ways of coping and receive support from each other, which will help to relieve the burden of caregiving.

Case Study 30-3

Jerry, age 19 years, was a sophomore in college when his problems first started, or so he stated. He was always attracted to other young men, but he was unable to discuss this with anyone in the family. Jerry was an identical twin, and his twin brother Joe was "perfect." Joe always did better in school; Joe was the valedictorian of the graduating class, and he was the athletic one of the two brothers. The parents were always raving and praising Joe, whereas Jerry was considered the family clown. Jerry secretly started to hate his brother; he wanted to be the opposite of Joe, and thus, he succumbed to his feminine side and started a clandestine relationship with his college roommate.

The stress of going away to college, the secret life he was living, and trying to bid for his parents' attention became too much for Jerry. His anxiety became so intense that he started to do poorly in school and was placed on probation. He became extremely depressed. He went to see the school psychologist and was given a prescription for Xanax 2.5 mg for 7 days and was referred to a psychiatrist. When the prescription ran out, Jerry did not make an appointment to see the psychiatrist; instead, he got some illegal Xanax, and 1 week later he stopped going to all of his classes. He became very dependent on the Xanax bars he was buying illegally. His roommate became unenamored with him, as he had a change in personality. He became very irritable and easily argumentative and no longer wanted to leave the apartment.

One day after returning from the store he realized that he was locked out of the apartment. The roommate found that some of his belongings were missing, and he became afraid so he had the locks changed. Jerry became very angry; he broke the locks, forced himself into the apartment, and beat up the roommate. He was subsequently arrested and expelled from school.

The parents were devastated when they heard the news, but they realized that they were also at fault. They arranged for him to go to rehabilitation on the advice of their nurse practitioner and for the entire family to start counseling. He was diagnosed with substance abuse and depressive disorder NOS (not otherwise specified). Jerry went to rehabilitation for 6 months; the family stayed involved. After 6 months of cognitive therapy, there was a marked improvement in his disposition. He continued the cognitive therapy along with his antidepressant medications, and on his discharge, he enrolled in the community college near home so that they all could continue the family therapy.

Case Study 30-4

Pete was an only child. He lived in a nice neighborhood with his parents who were both professionals. His mother was a nurse, and she worked days at the local hospital; however, she also moonlighted at a nearby hospital 3 nights per week. His father was a police officer, and he worked varied shifts. Both parents were too busy with their own careers to pay much attention to their child. Pete had everything that an 18-year-old boy would want, but he was not happy. When he graduated from high school, the neighbors took him to the graduation ceremony along with their daughter Mindy. He felt alone in the world except for Mindy.

Pete was in love with Mindy. They had been going together since they were 13.

The counselor at Pete's school recommended that he and the entire family be evaluated by a psychologist or psychiatrist. Pete's mother made an appointment, and both she and Pete went for one visit. The psychologist suggested that the entire family start therapy, and he scheduled an appointment for the entire family to be evaluated. The father refused to go to therapy. "There is nothing wrong with Pete. He is just a teenager, and we have a good family life," he replied. The counselor was not able to persuade the parents of the seriousness of the situation. The parents never followed through, and after two missed appointments, the psychiatrist gave up. It was approaching the Christmas holidays, and Pete was on the phone talking to Mindy, as he tried to make plans for the holidays with her. Mindy had been acting strange for the past couple of months. Pete suspected that she wanted to break off the relationship, and he was determined that he would win her back. After talking on the phone for approximately 2 hours, Mindy was not budging. She told Pete that she thought he was still a baby and not man enough for her. Pete told Mindy to hold on. He went into his parent's bedroom (they were both working that night). He got his father's gun and shot himself in the head. He died 3 hours later after an unsuccessful attempt to resuscitate him at the local hospital.

ANALYSIS OF CASE STUDIES 30-3 AND 30-4

Both Pete and Jeff were very depressed, and their parents were oblivious to the situation. In Jeff's case, he was fortunate that he was away at school, and he sought help at the onset of his depression. He did not follow through with the original treatment plan, but when his situation got worse, he was able to get the help he needed. His family was there for him, and with the support of his family and his nurse practitioner, he was able to get treatment for his depression. Jeff and his family listened to the nurse practitioner as she described the signs and symptoms of depression. They were willing to try the family therapy and cognitive therapy, and medication was successful for Jeff. Pete, on the other hand, was isolated. Both parents were in the home, but they were unaware of their son's depression. They never had a chance to help Pete because his depression was so far gone, and now he was losing the one person he thought loved him. The family did not take the advice of the school counselor. The father remained in denial. The parents were not willing to try family therapy on the advice of the counselor or the psychiatrist. Parents need to be aware of the signs and symptoms of mental illness; they need to pay attention to their children, and they need to intervene before it is too late. It is important that they seek help and follow the advice and treatment plan as prescribed by healthcare professionals. Depression is a serious illness, and untreated depression can lead to suicide, as in the case of Pete. Young adolescent men are at high risk for suicide. Healthcare practitioners must teach families and caregivers to be attentive to their children and to watch for the signs and symptoms of depression with their loved ones, as they will be the first ones to recognize the abnormal behaviors.

Table 30-3 Key Terms

Anxiety	Ego	Prejudice
Bipolar	Grief	Psychosis
Crisis	Hallucinations	Psychotropic drugs
Culture	Id	Psychotherapy
Cultural competence	Loss	Racism
Deinstitutionalization	Mania	Schizophrenia
Dementia	Mental health	Stigma
Delusions	Mental illness	Suicide
Depression	Neurotransmitters	Superego
Diversity	Personality disorders	

SUMMARY

Entire text books have been written on the subject of mental illness/health by several different disciplines. This chapter has attempted to provide basic information on some of the major mental illnesses/disorders, different theories of mental illness, and the treatment for some of the major mental health problems today. Theories on mental health, along with the influence of culture, were introduced to provide a better understanding of mental illnesses/disorders in today's world. If people believe that mental illness is *not* a disease then they will not seek treatment. On the other hand, if people believe that mental illness *is* a disease then they will engage in health-promoting behaviors such as nutrition and exercise to avoid the disease. Mental illness may not be preventable, but we can certainly take steps toward promoting better mental health just as we promote health with other medical conditions (**Table 30-3**).

RESOURCES

The needs of the society today are different than in the 1950s when a great deal of emphasis was placed on mental illness. In those days, many families were ashamed of their mentally ill relatives, and thus, they kept them locked away in their homes. Very often they received no treatment at all. With new advances in science and medicine, the public at large has begun to gain more insight and be more educated about mental illnesses. Mentally ill persons are no longer locked away in their homes but are placed in institutions. When institutionalization became a problem, as is now the case, the mentally ill are discharged into the community. The problem that now exists and persists is due to the fact that many mentally ill persons are not aware of and/or are incapable of using the community resources that are available. Federal and state laws have mandated that resources be available for the mentally ill. The mentally ill are protected under the U.S. Code: Title 42, Chapter 114, Protection and Advocacy for Mentally Ill Individuals. Effective 2000, the Department of Children and Family protects the mentally ill. Some nationally available resources in the United States are as follows:

American Association for Geriatric Psychiatry
7910 Woodmont Avenue, Suite 1050
Bethesda, MD 20814-3004
www.aagpgpa.org

American Psychological Association
750 First Street, NE
Washington, DC 20002-4242
800-374-2721 (toll-free)
www.apa.org

Depression and Bipolar Support Alliance
730 N. Franklin St., Suite 501
Chicago, IL 60610-7224
800-826-3652
www.dballiance.org

National Alliance for the Mentally Ill
Colonial Place Three
2107 Wilson Boulevard, Suite 300
Arlington, VA 22201-3042
800-950-6264
www.nami.org

National Institute of Mental Health
6001 Executive Blvd., Room 8184, MSC 9663
Bethesda, MD 20892-9663
301-443-4513
866-415-8051 (TTY)
www.nimh.nih.gov

National Mental Health Association
2000 N. Beauregard St., 6th Floor
Alexandria, VA 22311
800-969-6642
www.nmha.org

REFERENCES

American Nurses Association. (2000). *Statement in the scope and standards of psychiatric-mental health clinical nursing practice.* Washington, DC: Author.

American Psychiatric Association. (2000). *Diagnostic and statistical manual of mental disorders (DSM-IV-TR)* (4th ed., text rev). Washington, DC: Author.

American Psychiatric Association. (2003). Practice guideline for the assessment and treatment of patients with suicidal behaviors. *American Journal of Psychiatry, 160*(11), 1–60.

Beck, A., & Freeman, A. (1990). *Cognitive therapy of personality disorders.* New York: Guilford.

Beebe, L. (2007). What can we learn from pilot studies? *Perspectives in psychiatric care, 43*(4), 213–218.

Beng-Choon, H., Black, D. W., & Anderson, N. C. (2004). Schizophrenia and other psychotic disorders. In R. E. Hales & S. C. Yudofsky (Eds.), *Essentials of clinical psychiatry* (2nd ed., p. 200). Washington, DC: American Psychiatric Publishing.

Freud, S. (1935). *A general introduction to psychoanalysis.* New York: Simon & Schuster.

Leininger, M. (2002). Culture care assessments for congruent competent practices. In M. Leininger & M. McFarland (Eds.), *Transcultural nursing: concepts, theories, research and practice* (3rd ed., pp. 117–144).

Maslow, A. (1963). *Toward a psychology of being.* Princeton, NJ: Van Nostrand.

Monson, R., & Thomas, D. (2006). Children's mental health. *Journal of Pediatric Nursing, 21*(6), 443–444.

National Alliance for the Mentally Ill. (2000a). *History and mission of NAMI.* Retrieved July 11, 2007, from www.nami.org/history.htm.

National Alliance for the Mentally Ill. (2000b). *Communities, bipolar disorder.* Retrieved July 11, 2007, from www.nami.org/templates.cfm.

National Institute of Mental Health. (2006). *The numbers count: mental disorders in America.* Retrieved from www.nimh.nih.gov/publicat/numbers.cfm.

Paris, J. (1999). *Nature and nurture in psychiatry.* Washington, DC: American Psychiatric Press.

Patterson, W., Dohn, H., Bird, G., & Patterson, G. (1983). Evaluation of suicidal patients: the SAD PERSONS scale. *Psychosomatics, 214*(4), 343–345.

Peplau, H. (1952). *Interpersonal relationships in nursing.* New York: G. P. Putnam.

Peplau, H. (1968). *Basic principles of patient counseling.* Washington, DC: Publication Cientifica.

Peplau, H. (1999). Psychotherapeutic strategies, 1968. *Perspectives in Psychiatric Care, 25*(3), 14–19.

Piaget, J. (1972). *The psychology of the child.* New York: Basic Books.

President's New Freedom Commission on Mental Health. (2003). Retrieved July 11, 2007, from www.mentalhealthcommission.gov.

Skinner, B. F. (1953). *Science and human behavior*. New York: Macmillan.

Sullivan, H. (1953). *The interpersonal theory of psychiatry*. New York: W.W. Norton.

World Health Organization. (2007). *Mental health*. Retrieved July 11, 2007, from www.who.int/mentalhealth/en/.

Chapter 31

Reproductive Issues for Men and Women

Flora Carter Flood

INTRODUCTION

As health professionals consider the plethora of complex and multidimensional phenomena and idealism bombarding individuals in our communities near and far, it is evident that there is still an urgent need for comprehensive sex education at all levels. Since the beginning of time, men and women have sought to be in control of their own reproductive destiny. The term sexuality is a complex, multidimensional phenomena that incorporates biological, psychological, interpersonal, and behavioral dimensions. In recent years, much debate has occurred over how much and when should information concerning these phenomena be provided. It is important to recognize that a wide range of normal sexual functioning exists, and ultimately, each individual and his or her partner defines sexuality within the context of factors such as gender, age, personal attitudes, and religious and cultural values (Sexuality and Reproductive Issues, n.d.). Comprehensive sex education that provides balanced and accurate information is essential to equip men and women with the necessary skill to achieve healthy sexuality throughout their lives (Lindberg, Santelli, & Singh, 2006). The goal of sex education is to help young people develop knowledge, autonomy, and the skills needed to make the transition to adulthood in good sexual health (Forrest & Kanabus, n.d.; American Conference on Population Development, 1999).

Although comprehensive sex education is broadly supported by U.S. health professionals, it is being increasingly replaced by abstinence only education. In 1999, 23% of secondary school sex education teachers taught abstinence as the only way to prevent pregnancy and sexually transmitted diseases (STDs); only 2% had done so in 1988. In 1999, one quarter of secondary education teachers said they were prohibited from teaching about contraception. Not only has the major expansion been in abstinence only programs, but restriction of other information was required. Federally funded abstinence education programs are required by law to teach that sexual activity outside of the context of marriage is likely to have harmful psychological and physical effects and that a mutually monogamous relationship in the context of marriage is the expected standard of human sexual activity. Discussion of the benefits of contraception is prohibited in these programs (Lindberg et al., 2006).

Good reproductive health should include freedom from risk of sexual diseases, the right to regulate one's own fertility with full knowledge of contraceptive choices, and the ability to control sexuality without being discriminated against because of age, marital status, income, or similar consideration. Unplanned and unwanted pregnancies pose major reproductive health problems to both women and men throughout the world (Maja, 2007).

REPRODUCTIVE HEALTH AND SEX EDUCATION

Reproductive health has been defined as a state of complete physical, mental, and social well-being and not merely the absence of disease or infirmity in all matters relating to the reproductive system and to its functions and processes. This implies that people are able to have a satisfying and safe sex life and that they have the capability to reproduce and the freedom to decide if, when, and how often to do so. It also includes sexual health, the purpose of which is the enhancement of life and personal relationships, and not merely counseling and care related to reproduction and STDs (UNFPA, 2000).

Puberty is the period of time when children begin to mature biologically, psychologically, socially, and cognitively. From the time we are born, our bodies are constantly going through changes. Puberty leads to adolescence, and each individual has his or her own time line. As you get nearer to puberty, the brain and pituitary gland release hormones that regulate the reproductive organs of both males and females. These hormones stimulate the ovaries of girls to produce other hormones called estrogen and progesterone and the testes of boys to produce testosterone. One of the first signs that puberty has begun is hair growth. Boys and girls begin to grow hair under their arms and in the pubic area. As puberty progresses, the hair becomes thicker, darker, and heavier. Boys will begin to grow hair on their faces. For girls, puberty can begin between the ages of 9 to 14 years. For boys, it will be around the age of 10 to 17 years. Reproductive years for women are customarily defined as ages 15 to 45 years. Reproductive health is a lifetime concern for both women and men from infancy to old age (Coolnurse.com, n.d.).

Young children and adolescents often learn about sexual matters and reproduction by observing adult behavior and from peers and older siblings. Unfortunately, such information may be limited and often erroneous. Recent research suggest that a variety of media sources and strategies that include mass media communication, computer-assisted instruction, and the Internet can be used effectively for increasing knowledge and changing attitudes on sexual health issue and for promoting responsible sexual behaviors among young people. Media interventions seem to be more effective to achieve these goals when complemented with interpersonal strategies.

School-based sex education can be an effective way of enhancing knowledge, attitudes, and behavior toward sexuality for young people (Delgado & Austin, 2007). Much research has been conducted about what works and what should be included in such programs. Most effective programs included the following elements:

- Emphasis on reducing specific risky behaviors
- Theories that explain what influences people's sexual choices and behavior
- Reinforcement of messages about sexual behavior and risk reduction
- Accurate information about contraception and birth control, risks associated with sexual activity, and methods of avoiding or deferring intercourse
- How to deal with peer and other social pressures on young people; opportunities to practice communication, negotiation, and assertion skills
- Opportunity to engage young peoples and help them to personalize the information.
- Strategies appropriate to young people's age, experience, and cultural background

Young people need to have information on all the following topics:

- Sexual development
- Reproduction

- Contraception
- Relationships

They need to have information about the physical and emotional changes associated with puberty and sexual reproduction, including fertilization and conception and about STDs, including HIV/AIDS. They also need to know about contraception, including what contraceptives there are, how they work, how people use them, how they decide what to use or not, and how they can be obtained. Some people are concerned that providing information about sex and sexuality arouses curiosity and can lead to sexual experimentation. There is no evidence that this happens. Sex education that works starts early, before young people reach puberty and before they have developed established patterns of behavior. The precise age depends on the physical, emotional, and intellectual development of the young people, as well as their level of understanding (Forrest & Kanabus, n.d.). Information is important as the basis on which young people can develop well-informed attitudes and views about sex and sexuality.

BIRTH CONTROL

Fertility control is an important aspect of life that has a tremendous impact on the growth of populations. Many individual factors may enhance or impair contraceptive behavior and impact the selection of birth control methods (Youngkin & Davis, 2004). Although recent trends have indicated that teenage pregnancy and birth rates are declining, the United States continues to have one of the highest teen pregnancy and birth rates among Western industrialized nations (Carter & Spear, 2002). Most adolescents and their parents believe that adolescents need information about abstinence and birth control. Both should have available family planning services or programs that offer a variety of safe, effective, acceptable, affordable contraceptive methods to help them prevent unwanted pregnancies and STDs. Today, when selecting a method, consideration must be given to whether the method offers any protection against STDs (Edelman & Mandle, 2002).

The health professional is responsible for providing the client with information regarding how each method works, the effectiveness, advantages, disadvantages, contraindications, and danger signs associated with each method. All presentation and educational materials should be compatible with the language, culture, and educational level of the client.

Natural methods are also termed rhythm method, menstrual cycle charting, natural family planning, or periodic abstinence because women abstain from sex on days that they are fertile. This method requires no drugs or internal devices but demands a well-motivated and knowledgeable woman. It involves making observation and charting of scientifically proven fertility signs that determine whether a woman is fertile. These signs include watching the basal body temperature, cervical mucus, and cervical position. The rhythm method is the original method based on periodic abstinence and is still widely used around the world, but it is not as reliable as newer contraceptive methods and is no longer recommended (Youngkin & Davis, 2004).

Barrier methods are some of the oldest methods of birth control. Women in ancient Egypt used vaginal suppositories to prevent pregnancy. Today's modern devices include the traditional diaphragm, as well as the smaller counterpart, the FemCap or cervical cap. The condom is used to provide a mechanical barrier to the entry of sperm and is also recommended as a protection from STDs. For protection against many STDs, the female condom is now a reality (Epigee Women's Health, 2008; Caufield, 2004).

Hormonal methods include all contraceptives that use synthetic female hormones as birth control. Most forms contain estrogen. The oldest of theses is the pill, which includes combined oral contraceptive pills with estrogen and progesterone, and the newer estrogen-free minipill. These hormones are used in the Ortho Evra patch and the Nuva vaginal ring. Depo-Provera is an estrogen-free 3-month birth control injection. These hormones prevent ovulation by chemically altering the usual endocrine cycle. High levels of estrogen prevent the release of follicle stimulating hormone by the pituitary gland; ovarian follicles are not stimulated to maturity, and ovulation is prevented. When progesterone is added, the endometrium of the uterus is stimulated to develop as during a normal cycle, and cessation of taking the pill causes a menstrual period to occur, which stimulates the normal ovulatory cycle. For women who are interested in birth control that lasts a year or more, the intrauterine device is often recommended or Implanon, which has recently been approved for use. This device is similar to the Norplant device that is placed subdermally in the medial area of the upper arm. It slowly releases levonorgestrel into the bloodstream. The low-dose progestin provides contraception by thickening cervical mucus, reducing peristalsis of the fallopian tube, and causing the endometrium to be inhospitable for implantation (Epigee Women's Health, 2008).

Chemical contraceptives without the need of a prescription are also available in drugstores. They come in the form of sponges, creams, jellies, and foams, and their use is relatively simple and inexpensive. These products contain nonoxynol-9, which kills and immobilizes sperm and may provide some protection against STDs. The drawback on their use is that they must be applied immediately before coitus, which may be considered messy and involves touching the genital area (Epigee Women's Health, 2008).

STD

One of the leading causes of infection and reproductive dysfunction in adults between the ages of 15 and 80 are STDs. STDs are infections that can be transferred from one person to another through sexual contact. Most STDs are treatable. Other STDs, such as herpes, AIDS, and genital warts, all of which are caused by viruses, have no cure. Many STDs can lead to long-term health consequences, such as STD-related neoplasia, reproductive health problems, adverse outcomes of pregnancy for both women and infants, and an increased risk of HIV transmission; therefore, education about these diseases and prevention is important. It is also important to recognize that sexual contact includes more than just intercourse. It includes kissing, oral–genital contact, and use of sex toys. When the HIV or STD status of a person is not certain, there is no such thing as "safe sex." The only true safe sex is abstinence. All forms of sexual contact carry some risk. Condoms may be useful in helping to prevent certain diseases such as HIV and gonorrhea. Unfortunately, they are less effective in protecting against herpes, trichomoniasis, and chlamydia. Furthermore, they provide little protection against human papillomavirus (HPV), the cause of genital warts (Epigee Women's Health, 2008; Schaffer, 2004).

One of the most common STDs in the United States is chlamydia. Chlamydia is caused by the bacterium Chlamydia trachomatis, which can damage women's reproductive organs. This asymptomatic infection is common among both men and women. Men primarily develop urethritis. In women, chlamydia is associated with cervicitis, acute urethral syndrome, salpingitis, pelvic inflammatory disease, and infertility (Schaffer, 2004).

One of the most prevalent forms of vaginitis among childbearing women is a clinical syndrome characterized by alterations in vaginal flora known as bacterial vaginosis (BV). Although research suggests a nonsexual mode of transmission for BV, almost all BV occurs exclusively in sexually active women. Consequently, the treatment of male partner does not reduce the risk of occurrence, but the use of the condom does. Clients may be asymptomatic or may have malodorous vaginal discharge. Treatment regimens for BV are only 80% effective, and up to 20% of women will have recurrences within 1 month of treatment. Oral metronidazole is recommended for treatment of BV.

Trichomoniasis vaginitis is the causative organism for trichomoniasis. The primary means of transmission is through sexual contact, although nonsexual transmission by fomites is theoretically possible. In this common form of vaginitis, the woman may be markedly symptomatic or asymptomatic. Men are asymptomatic carriers, and thus, counseling should include the need to treat male partners. Metronidazole is the drug of choice for both symptomatic and asymptomatic clients and partners. The need to avoid alcohol 24 hours before and 72 hours after treatment should be stressed. Routine treatment of the sexual partner is recommended.

Herpes simplex virus (HSV) has no known cure and is a recurring viral disease characterized with painful lesions. These lesions can occur in the mouth and genitalia of affected men and women. There is significant perinatal morbidity and mortality associated with neonates who contract the virus congenitally. After HSV enters the body, the virus never leaves. Clinical manifestations disappear as the virus becomes dormant in sensory ganglia, but recurrence can be triggered by local or systemic stimuli such as trauma, fever, menstruation, ultraviolet light, and emotional stress. HSV type 1 primarily produces oral lesions, and herpes simplex virus type 2 produces genital lesions. The procedures for diagnosis and treatment are the same. The use of antiviral drugs is helpful in reducing the frequency and severity of occurrences but do not cure the disease.

HPV infection is the most prevalent viral STD in the United States. HPV-mediated oncogenesis is responsible for up to 95% of cervical squamous cell carcinomas and nearly all preinvasive cervical neoplasm; nevertheless, prospective studies in young women screened for HPV DNA suggest that HPV is frequently a transient infection, with most initially positive DNA tests becoming negative within 1 year. Even though as many as 40% of women are positive for HPV by polymerase chain-reacting testing, genital warts are only present in 2% of women and men. HPV is a slow growing DNA virus of the papovavirus family with more than 100 strands. Twenty of these strains are associated with genital tract infections (Schaffer, 2004) (**Table 31-1**).

Table 31-1 Summary of Sexually Transmitted Diseases

Disease	Causative Agent	Risk or Complication	Focus of Teaching
Chlamydia	*Chlamydia trachomatis*	Infertility Urethral scarring Ectopic pregnancy Pelvic inflammatory disease (PID) Endocervicitis Epididymitis Urethritis Sterility Preterm labor Higher risk for HIV	Understand importance of completing medication Return for test of cure Refer partners for evaluation A latex condom can reduce but not eliminate the risk of contracting the disease Abstain from vaginal and anal sex with an infected person; 75% of women and 25% of men are asymptomatic
Bacterial vaginosis (BV)	*Gardnerella vaginalis*	Asymptomatic infection Nonspecific vaginosis Preterm labor PID	Understand medication Avoid alcohol 24 hours before and 72 hours after treatment Sexual abstinence or use condoms until partner treated
Trichomoniasis	*Trichomoniasis vaginalis*	Vaginitis Recurrence Excoriation of genital area Premature rupture of membranes and preterm delivery	Understand medication regime Use condoms to prevent new infection
Genital herpes	Herpes simplex virus	Urethra stricture Lymph node enlargement Higher risk for HIV Higher risk for preterm labor	Abstain from sex while symptomatic No known cure
Genital warts	Human papilloma virus	Cervical dysplasia Cervical cancer Neoplasia Carcinoma	Return for treatment Examine partner Biannual pap smears needed for 2 years after treatment and then annually No known cure

Table 31-1 Summary of Sexually Transmitted Diseases (*Continued*)

Disease	Causative Agent	Risk or Complication	Focus of Teaching
Hepatitis B	Hepatitis B virus		No known cure
			Disease can lead to cirrhosis, liver cancer
			Sharing contaminated drug needles
Gonorrhea	*Neisseria gonorrhoeae*	PID, infertility	Monitor antibiotic treatment
		Ectopic pregnancy	Examine partner
		Urethritis	Reculture
		Epididymitis	
		Premature delivery	
Syphilis	*Treponema pallidum*	Secondary or late syphilis	Monitor antibiotic treatment
			Test and monitor partners

MEN'S HEALTH ISSUES

Over the past decade, attention to the documented trends in greater mortality rates for men compared with women has increased. In general, the leading causes of death among men and women are the same; what differs are the age at the time of death, the number of deaths caused by each disease, and the ranking of the cause. Historically, limited attention and resources have been devoted to initiatives that emphasize men's constructive involvement in contraceptive practices and fertility issues. They are often marginalized by health services that do not have provisions for males. Men's health does not have the equivalent of a specialist (gynecologist) to provide care for the reproductive tract. Males should be empowered through the provision of information and services targeting boys, youth, and adults within the home, communities, and work settings. Young and old males must be educated about responsible sexual behavior, treat women as equals, and support the effort to respect women. The failure of families and schools to educate youth, including males, about sex is a primary cause of unplanned and unwanted pregnancies. The importance of male participation has become much greater with the emergence of the HIV/AIDS pandemic and the increasing prevalence of STDs (Alexander, 2007; Maja, 2007).

Among male-specific disorders, prostatic conditions are of most concern to men and have raised the most questions in the healthcare community about diagnosis, screening, and treatment. Sexual health issues, such as premature ejaculation and erectile dysfunction, are also of substantial concern to men. Beginning in the late 1990s, treatments for these conditions gained increased attention. The incidence of STDs is on the rise, especially among younger men, posing a significant public health problem. Infertility is an issue for many younger men, and interest in late onset hypogonadism has increased, primarily because of the debate about the use of testosterone replacement therapy (Alexander, 2007).

Case Study 31-1

Prostate Screening

The local community health center recently received a grant to offer a comprehensive free prostate screening for men aged 50 years and over in a diverse community. The overall goal was to bring in individuals from lower socioeconomic and diverse cultural groups who would be able to access screening. Statistics for the area reveal great disparity among the population in regards to prostate cancer. Black American men are at a higher risk for developing prostate cancer and dying from their illness because they often lack access to routine health care according to recent studies. Prostate cancer incidence rates in the area are approximately 50% higher in black men than in white men. The prostate cancer mortality rate among blacks is nearly 2.5 times the white rate.

Publicity, including press releases and screening event advertisements, occurred in all of the local papers, and screenings were conducted at different hours and different days of the weeks to accommodate the targeted group. Despite this, the results indicated that the targeted group did not use the service as hoped, and predominate individuals who participated in the services were white, middle-class, insured men.

Analysis afterward revealed several possible reasons for the problem with the service.

Primarily, no one from the community was involved in the planning for the events or given an opportunity to provide any input in the program. "It isn't about cultural beliefs, and it isn't that they're uneducated or uninformed. It is that many are poor, lack insurance, and have lousy access to health care" (Mozes, 2007).

Screening services often open Pandora's box because clients lack an ongoing relationship with a physician. Who will follow up when a problem is diagnosed? Will the community health center provide services for those who lack insurance? Community organization and key individual or groups should be included in the planning process to make the event a success for all involved in the community.

Resources

Mozes, A. (2007). Poorer health care ups black men's prostate cancer risk: too often, black males lack insurance or ongoing relationship with doctor, study finds. Health Day News Scout News, LLC. Retrieved March 1, 2008, from http://www.healthfinder.gov/news/printnewsstory.asp?docID==602666.

Truglio-Londrigan, M. & Macali, M. (2002). Screening. In C. L. Edelman & C. L. Mandle. *Health promotion throughout the lifespan* (5th ed.). St. Louis: Mosby.

Case Study 31–2

Sex Education

You have just started your new job as a health educator for the Sunshine School District, which is located in a rural area of Oregon and consists of a diverse group of conservative farm families. The school board is concerned about the rising pregnancy rate in the district and has asked you to implement a comprehensive sex education program that stresses abstinence and includes information about contraception. You develop a committee consisting of school counselor, a physical education teacher, and selected instructors with the goal of developing a curricula plan for implementing sex education classes in the fall. The decision is made to require all seventh- and ninth-grade students participate in sex education classes during their physical education classes during the first quarter of the semester.

The committee decides that the approach will include encouraging parent–child communication, promoting an appreciation of diversity, and teaching skills in making decisions based on individual values and accurate information. Surveys

(Continues)

Case Study 31–2 (*Continued*)

were sent to the parents to collect information on what parents want and what young people need in sex education. Parents were required to provide written consent for students to participate in the classes, and separate session were planned to orient the parent to the specific content that would be included in the student session. Parents were not allowed to attend any sessions along with the student. Complete clinical services were made available at the school through the school nurse and the school based clinic provided by a federal grant offering health care for rural communities.

As a result of the implementation of the program in the school system, pregnancy rates have begun to show a decline after 8 months. Before the establishment of the program, 30 of their 100 female students became pregnant. The latest figures now show that the number of pregnant students dropped to only 10 females out of 100. The success of the program was contributed to the input all of the participants had in planning the program, the time taken to plan the program, and the availability of services to make the possibility of obtaining contraceptives a reality. Surveys done after the classes revealed that not only did the rate of pregnancy decrease but that many teens also decided to delay having intercourse until later years.

Resources

Caufield, Kathryn. (2004). Controlling Fertility. In E. Q. Youngkin & M. S. Davis. *Women's health: A primary care clinical guide* (3rd ed.). Upper Saddle River, NJ: Pearson Prentice Hall, pp. 165–225.

Center for the Advancement of Health. (2007, December 23). Sex education linked to delayed teen intercourse, new study says. *ScienceDaily*. Retrieved March 1, 2008, from http://www.sciencedaily.com/releases/2007/12/071220231428.htm.

Haag, P. (1998). Single-sex education in grades K–12: what does the research tell us? Separated by sex: a critical look at single-sex education for girls. Washington, DC: U.S. Department of Education. Retrieved March 1, 2008, from http://www.education.com/reference/article/Ref_K_12_Single_Sex/.

WEB RESOURCES

Learn to be healthy.org: Health science educational activities for educators and students. www.learntobehealthy.org.

Coolnurse.com: Teen health and teen advice. www.coolnurse.com.

REFERENCES

Alexander, L. (2007). Men's health issue. *CME for Florida Nurses, 133,* 61–100.

American Conference on Population Development (ACPD). (1999). Sexual and reproductive health education and services for adolescents. In consultation with CEDPA, CFFC, CRLP, FCI, Ipas, IPPF, IWHC, Latin American & Caribbean Youth Network for Sexual and Reproductive Rights, NAPY and Youth Coalition for ICPD. Retrieved from http://www.reproductiverights.org/pdf/pub_fac_adoles_sexedservices.pdf.

Carter, K., & Spear, H. (2002). Knowledge, attitudes, and behavior related to pregnancy in a rural teenage population. *Journal of Community Health Nursing 19*(2), 65–75.

Coolnurse.com (n.d.). What is puberty. Retrieved February 27, 2008, from http://www.righthealth.com/Health/what%20is%20puberty-s?lid=goog-ads-sb-6800049797&gclid=CNDxi-G_5pECFQJvHgodxgcAaQ.

Delgado, H. M., & Austin, S. B. (2007). Can media promote responsible sexual behaviors among adolescents and young adults? *Current Opinion in Pediatrics 19*(4), 405–410.

Edelman, C. L., & Mandle, C. L. (2002). *Health promotion throughout the lifespan* (5th ed.). St. Louis: Mosby.

Epigee Women's Health. (2008). *STD overview.* Retrieved December 17, 2007, from http://www.epigee.org/health/stds.html.

Forrest, S., & Kanabus, A. (n.d). Sex education that works. Sex Education Consultant. Retrieved November 17, 2007, from http://www.avert.org/sexedu.htm.

Lindberg, L. D., Santelli, J. S., & Singh, S. (2006). Changes in formal sex education: 1995–2002. *Perspectives on Sexual and Reproductive Health, 38*(4), 182–189.

Maja, T. (2007). Involvement of males in promoting reproductive health. *Curationis, 30*(1), 71–76.

Schaffer, S. (2004). Vaginitis and Sexually Transmitted Diseases. In E. Q. Youngkin & M. S. Davis. *Women's health: A primary care clinical guide.* Upper Saddle River, NJ: Pearson Prentice Hall, pp. 261–287.

Sexuality and Reproductive Issues. (n.d.). The prevalence and types of sexual dysfunction in people with cancer. Retrieved February 2, 2007, from http://www.cancer.gov/cancertopics/pdq/supportivecare/sexuality/HealthProffesional/page1.

United Nations Population Fund (UNFPA) (2000.). Women's empowerment and reproductive health: links throughout the life cycle. Retrieved February 27, 2008, from www.unfpa.org/intercenter/cycle/index.htm

Youngkin, E. Q., & Davis, M. S. (2004). *Women's health: A primary care clinical guide.* Upper Saddle River, NJ: Pearson Prentice Hall.

Index

Sexually transmitted diseases
>birth control education, 612–614
>education about, 610, 612
>types and characteristics, 614–615, 616–617*t*
Shape Your Future pediatric weight loss program, 391–392
Shared decision-making tools, as teaching tools, 224–225
Shewhart, Walter, 126
Sight impairment
>assistive technology for people with, 80, 244–246, 250–251
>communication errors and, 64
>teaching about medications to patients with, 355
Sign-language interpreters, computer-based, 247
Simulation, as learning tool, 125
Singh, G., 576
Skiba, D. J., 230
Skinner, B. F., 8, 589
Slidecasting software, 235
>tutorials for creating, 253
Slides, as teaching tools, 219–220
SMART framework, for goal setting, 320
Smoking
>asthma and, 432–433, 447
>cancer and other diseases caused by, 539–540
>cessation program guidelines, 540–541
>5As intervention, 433
>nutrition in pregnancy and, 418, 419, 421
>oral cancer and, 369
>outpatient cessation program components, 541–543
>teaching cardiovascular disease risk due to, 493–494
Social bookmarking tools, 232*t*, 233
>tutorials for creating, 253
Social circumstances, life expectancies and, 280, 281*t*
Social class. *See also* Socioeconomic status
>communication errors and, 64
Social cognitive theory, 7, 311–312
Social dimension of wellness, 283*f*, 284
Social liberation, in behavior change, 308*t*
Social liberation, patient adherence and, 113
Social Marketing, community health promotion and, 331, 337, 338*t*, 339
Social networking tools, 230, 231–232
Social system (or norms). *See also* Support network
>behavior change and, 312
>Diffusion of Innovations Theory and, 333–334

relapses and, 313
>support from, 289, 478–479
Social-interpersonal theory, 588–589
Socioeconomic status
>asthma and, 426
>asthma education and, 435
>health disparities and, 276
>obesity and, 380, 494
>osteoarthritis and, 555
Source errors, 162
Source monitoring, in learning retention, 161–162
South Shore Medical Center, 391–392
Spaced repetition, working memory and, 160
Spanking children, 412–414
Speaking to patients, speed vs. loudness of, 165–166
Speech
>limitations, people with, assistive technology for, 82–83, 243–244
>mental health status and, 595–596
Speech recognition technology, 248
Spirit possession, 62
Spiritual dimension of wellness, 283*f*, 284
>information resources, 297
>relaxation response and, 318
Spirituality, stress management with, 289
Stage Theory, community health promotion and, 331, 334–337, 335*t*
Staged Self-Directed Learning Model, Grow's, 29, 29*t*
Stages of Change model
>characteristics, 106, 107*t*
>Diffusion of Innovations Theory and, 332–333
>oral health and education and, 372, 374
>smoking cessation teaching and, 493–494, 493*t*, 542
>in Transtheoretical Model of Behavior Change, 307, 308*t*, 309
>for understanding behavior change, 157–158
Sticky Keys (computer operating system), 81
Stimulus control, in behavior change, 308*t*
Stopping, in cognitive restructuring, 317
Story boards, as teaching tools, 217–219
Stress
>ability to learn and, 9
>caregivers and, 93–96
>considering alternative therapies, 97–99
>coping and, 90–93
>definition of, 315–316
>elevated, poverty and, 46
>health literacy and, 96–97

Teaching Strategies
Health Education
AND
Health Promotion

Working with Patients,
Families, and Communities

Edited by

Arlene J. Lowenstein, PhD, RN
Professor and Director, Health Professions Education Doctoral Program
School of Health Sciences
Simmons College
Boston, Massachusetts

Lynn Foord, MEd, PhD, PT
Assistant Professor of Physical Therapy
Director of Online Teaching and Learning
School of Health Sciences
Simmons College
Boston, Massachusetts

Jane C. Romano, MS, RN, CAGS
Education Specialist
Project Manager, Critical Care Medicine
Children's Hospital Boston
Boston, Massachusetts

JONES AND BARTLETT PUBLISHERS
Sudbury, Massachusetts
BOSTON   TORONTO   LONDON   SINGAPORE

World Headquarters

Jones and Bartlett Publishers
40 Tall Pine Drive
Sudbury, MA 01776
978-443-5000
info@jbpub.com
www.jbpub.com

Jones and Bartlett Publishers
Canada
6339 Ormindale Way
Mississauga, Ontario L5V 1J2
Canada

Jones and Bartlett Publishers
International
Barb House, Barb Mews
London W6 7PA
United Kingdom

Jones and Bartlett's books and products are available through most bookstores and online booksellers. To contact Jones and Bartlett Publishers directly, call 800-832-0034, fax 978-443-8000, or visit our website www.jbpub.com.

Substantial discounts on bulk quantities of Jones and Bartlett's publications are available to corporations, professional associations, and other qualified organizations. For details and specific discount information, contact the special sales department at Jones and Bartlett via the above contact information or send an email to specialsales@jbpub.com.

The authors, editor, and publisher have made every effort to provide accurate information. However, they are not responsible for errors, omissions, or for any outcomes related to the use of the contents of this book and take no responsibility for the use of the products and procedures described. Treatments and side effects described in this book may not be applicable to all people; likewise, some people may require a dose or experience a side effect that is not described herein. Drugs and medical devices are discussed that may have limited availability controlled by the Food and Drug Administration (FDA) for use only in a research study or clinical trial. Research, clinical practice, and government regulations often change the accepted standard in this field. When consideration is being given to use of any drug in the clinical setting, the healthcare provider or reader is responsible for determining FDA status of the drug, reading the package insert, and reviewing prescribing information for the most up-to-date recommendations on dose, precautions, and contraindications, and determining the appropriate usage for the product. This is especially important in the case of drugs that are new or seldom used.

Production Credits

Publisher: Kevin Sullivan
Acquisitions Editor: Emily Ekle
Acquisitions Editor: Amy Sibley
Associate Editor: Patricia Donnelly
Editorial Assistant: Rachel Shuster
Senior Production Editor: Susan Schultz
Associate Marketing Manager: Rebecca Wasley
Associate Marketing Manager: Ilana Goddess

Manufacturing and Inventory Control Supervisor:
  Amy Bacus
Composition: Appingo
Cover Design: Kristin E. Ohlin
Cover Image: © magicinfoto/ShutterStock, Inc.
Printing and Binding: Malloy Lithographing
Cover Printing: Malloy Lithographing

Library of Congress Cataloging-in-Publication Data

Teaching strategies for health education and health promotion : working with patients, families, and communities / [edited by] Arlene J. Lowenstein, Lynn Foord-May, Jane Romano.
     p. ; cm.
  Includes bibliographical references.
  ISBN 978-0-7637-5227-9 (pbk.)
  1. Health education—Study and teaching. 2. Health promotion—Study and teaching.
I. Lowenstein, Arlene J. II. Foord-May, Lynn. III. Romano, Jane, 1957-
  [DNLM: 1. Health Education—methods. 2. Teaching—methods. 3. Health Promotion—methods.
WA 590 T2537 2009]
  RA440.5.T43 2009
  613.071—dc22
                                    2008031558

6048

Printed in the United States of America
13 12 11 10 09   10 9 8 7 6 5 4 3 2